THE ENCYLOPEDIA OF

DIABETES

Second Edition

THE ENCYCLOPEDIA OF

DIABETES

Second Edition

William A. Petit, Jr., M.D., F.A.C.P., F.A.C.E.
Christine Adamec

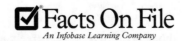

Facts On File
An Infobase Learning Company

The Encyclopedia of Diabetes, Second Edition

Copyright © 2011, 2002 by William A. Petit, Jr., M.D., F.A.C.P., F.A.C.E. and Christine Adamec

Facts On File, Inc.
An imprint of Infobase Learning
132 West 31st Street
New York NY 10001

Library of Congress Cataloging-in-Publication Data
Petit, William A.
The encyclopedia of diabetes / William A. Petit, Jr., Christine Adamec.—2nd ed.
p. cm.—(Library of health and living)
Includes bibliographical references and index.
ISBN-13: 978-0-8160-7948-3 (hardcover : alk. paper)
ISBN-10: 0-8160-7948-X (hardcover : alk. paper) 1. Diabetes—Encyclopedias. I. Adamec, Christine A., 1949– II. Title.
RC660.P424 2011
616.4'62003—dc22   2010025174

Facts On File books are available at special discounts when purchased in bulk quantities for businesses, associations, institutions, or sales promotions. Please call our Special Sales Department in New York at (212) 967-8800 or (800) 322-8755.

You can find Facts On File on the World Wide Web at http://www.infobaselearning.com

Text design by Cathy Rincon
Composition by Hermitage Publishing Services
Cover printed by Sheridan Books, Ann Arbor, Mich.
Book printed and bound by Sheridan Books, Ann Arbor, Mich.
Date printed: May 2011

Printed in the United States of America

10 9 8 7 6 5 4 3 2 1

This book is printed on acid-free paper.

CONTENTS

FOREWORD

Diabetes may well be the Black Plague of the 21st century, in terms of both its pervasiveness and pain. This plague upon us involves insulin resistance and Type 2 diabetes mellitus and is a growing threat to people all over the globe. In the United States, 23.6 million children and adults, which is 8 percent of the population, have diabetes. Although diabetes can be treated very effectively today and many complications can be prevented or slowed down, it is also a very insidious disease that people often suffer from for a long, long time. While they struggle with their diabetes, the disease costs them time, money, pain, aggravation and, sometimes, the price is also major sorrow and death.

Ignorance of the disease and how to manage it has caused too many thousands of people to lose their limbs as well as their eyesight. Yet, in most cases, this loss of sight and these amputations, as well as the other complications of diabetes, can be avoided by regular self-care and medical management.

Diabetes may well be the paradigm for all chronic diseases. It is a metabolic syndrome that affects every organ system in the body. Diabetes is also innately involved with the blood vessels and the heart. In fact, heart and blood vessel disease causes 80 percent of the deaths among patients with diabetes.

Yet if people with diabetes adhere to their medication plan and make the lifestyle changes that are recommended by their physicians and discussed in this book, they *will* live longer, happier, and healthier lives. This has been clearly proven by studies such as the Diabetes Control and Complications Trial (DCCT) and the United Kingdom Prospective Diabetes Study (UKPDS), and it is my mission to convey this information to as many people as possible.

Fortunately, recent years have seen a renaissance of the means to treat diabetes effectively, ranging from home blood glucose monitors to disposable syringes, effective new medications, and the increasingly used and very effective insulin pump. There are many medications available to help individuals with diabetes deal with their disease.

In this new edition of *The Encyclopedia of Diabetes,* my coauthor and I have completely revised many entries, such as the entries on children with diabetes, cardiovascular disease, and obesity, to name only a few. In addition, we have added important new topic overviews that provide information on insulin, medications for Type 2 diabetes, the issue of depression, and lifestyle adaptations to diabetes and also the topics of pregnancy and diabetes, carbohydrates and nutrition, diabetic eye diseases, alternative medicine, and many other subjects that we hope will intrigue and enlighten our readers. A great deal of important research on diabetes has been performed, and it is available in medical journals and sometimes is found in very obscure clinical publications. We have scoured these documents to identify the most useful items for readers with diabetes or who care about someone who has diabetes.

My goal as an endocrinologist and a physician is to educate people about diabetes. For those who do not have diabetes, I want to provide knowledge so that they can do everything in their power to try to prevent the development of the disease and to help others who are living with diabetes. For example, obesity is a major cause of Type 2 diabetes and about 25 percent of the population in the United States is obese, as of this writing in 2010. As a result, many of these individuals, often unknowingly, are at high risk for the development of diabetes. Weight loss, however, will plummet that risk, and even a modest weight loss significantly decreases the risk for diabetes.

Education for those who already *do* have diabetes consists of teaching them that they need to keep their blood glucose levels as close to normal as is safely possible, and this message has been brought home again and again in so many studies. I urge those of you with diabetes not to smoke and encourage you to exercise regularly and keep your cholesterol and blood pressure levels as low as possible to avoid developing diabetic complications. If people with diabetes follow this plan and avoid the irreversible complications, then when we finally do have a cure, these patients can partake of this cure and enjoy *wellness!*

Diabetes requires a lot of continuing education. This cannot be done by one person and necessarily involves a team centered around patients and their families, a team that includes physicians, nurses, dietitians, and many other folks. The education is also ongoing. You cannot learn it "all" and then "graduate." As physicians learn more about diabetes, the treatment paradigms and therapeutic focus change and evolve, and we share this knowledge with our patients.

Diabetes also requires advocacy. People with diabetes are often too quiet, perhaps afraid to offend or upset anyone; as a result, diabetes does not obtain nearly the level of federal funding that it deserves based on the destructive toll it takes upon our society. If you have diabetes, it is nothing to be ashamed of and you are one among many with diabetes.

The Encyclopedia of Diabetes is not meant to be read cover to cover, although, as I recall from medical school, there are some readers who are wired in a compulsive manner and will read through it, from A to Z. We welcome those who dip in for data on a specific topic as well as those who seek to extract every gem of information that we have included.

Maybe you have had diabetes for 20 years or perhaps you were diagnosed today. You may have a family member or friend with diabetes, and you are trying to educate yourself. We hope that this book will give you a good place to start in your quest for information about diabetes. We have tried to cover enough information to be useful as a first source and reference and a good overview of diabetes. In some areas, we cover a lot of what you need to know. In other areas, we can only scratch the surface, but we frequently provide leads to other written and computer based resources.

Keep learning and keep asking questions. Go back and take a class again, and call your local diabetes educators for a review of your health status. Call, fax, and e-mail your member of Congress whenever the issue of diabetes funding is in front of them—as well as when other issues affecting diabetes come up, such as drug laws, Medicare, insurance regulations, disability laws, and stem cell research. Join your local American Diabetes Association and help us move forward to improve your life and the lives of all those affected by diabetes!

—William A. Petit, Jr., M.D. Fellow of the American College of Physicians, Fellow of the American College of Endocrinology

ACKNOWLEDGMENTS

Many people have assisted us with their advice, recommending research or even readings and additions to entries. Special and grateful thanks to our editor, James Chambers, for his excellent editing of our manuscript.

William Petit, Jr., would like to acknowledge the examples and ideals of Jennifer, Hayley, and Michaela, Dr. Funmi Onobrakpeya, Karen McAvoy, R.N., C.D.E., Pat O'Connell, R.D., C.D.E., Dr. Neal Zimmerman, Dr. Marc Kawalick, Dr. Ann Rasmusson, Dr. Steven Hanks, Dr. Don Higgins, Dr. Robert Malkin, Dr. Joseph Dell'Orfano, and my mother and father and also thank the community for their support. In addition, special thanks to Jo Ann Ahern, A.P.R.N., M.S.N., C.D.E.; Kathleen M. Ahern, Insulin Pump Consultant; and Patricia O'Connell, R.D., M.S., C.D.E.

Christine Adamec would especially like to thank her husband, John Adamec, for his patience and support during this project.

A HISTORY OF DIABETES
FROM ANCIENT TIMES TO THE TWENTY-FIRST CENTURY

Most decidedly *not* just a modern problem, diabetes was known and feared as a killing disease and an illness without hope for thousands of years. Nothing that physicians tried, no medications, concoctions, treatments, or diets, could prevent an early and inevitable death. It was not until the 20th century that medical researchers developed miraculous lifesaving and life-prolonging treatments. The discovery of insulin in 1921 was the key to diabetes salvation for millions of patients worldwide, then and now.

As a result of further medical research performed in the early part of the 21st century, and that continues on even as we write, researchers are making astonishing medical breakthroughs that will eventually lead to cures for many people with diabetes. For example, in 2000, the successful transplantation of islets of Langerhans cells from the pancreases of recently deceased people by physician A. M. James Shapiro (transplant surgeon), Jonathan Lakey Ph.D., Dr. Edmond Ryan (endocrinologist), Gregory Korbutt Ph.D., Dr. Ellen Toth, Dr. Garth Warnock, Dr. Norman Kneteman, and Ray Rajotte Ph.D., at the University of Alberta Hospital and the Surgical-Medical Research Institute in Canada presented, for the first time, the possibility of a cure for diabetes. Thus far, this treatment has led to an apparent complete remission of the disease in a handful of patients. Since 2000, an estimated several hundred people have received islet transplants, and within a year from the transplant, up to 68 percent did not need to take additional insulin. However, within five years of the procedure, less than 10 percent were completely free of the need for daily insulin supplementation.

Other breakthroughs, such as complete pancreas transplants or joint pancreas-kidney transplants, although still rare, also offer hope for a cure. Genetic manipulation may bring new hope for future sufferers of diabetes.

Today, many people with diabetes and their families envision a bright future. They would probably feel even more optimistic and appreciative if they learned about how people with diabetes fared with the disease and were treated for it by physicians in the past.

Diabetes in Ancient Times

The first recorded mention of a medical condition that was distinguishable as diabetes was found in an ancient papyrus, discovered in 1862 by German Egyptologist George Ebers. The Ebers papyrus, which dates back to about 1500 B.C.E., revealed translations of several different prescriptive directions for concoctions that purportedly could "remove the urine, which runs too often."

In the early part of the first millennium, Celsus, a Roman writer who lived during the times of Hippocrates, translated Greek writings on medicine. He also wrote a summary of medicine and surgery. Wrote Celsus, for physicians whose patients apparently had diabetes, "The food should be astringent, the wine dry and undiluted . . . and in quantity the minimum required to allay thirst." Celsus also recommended exercise for these patients, advice still offered today for people with diabetes.

Although his contributions to the written medical knowledge of the time were major, Celsus made one serious mistake about diabetes. He claimed that people with diabetes urinated more than they drank. Strangely, this view was accepted for hundreds of years, until finally, in the 16th century, Girolamo Cardano measured the amount of fluid consumed by a diabetic patient and then compared it to the amount of urine produced. They were roughly equivalent; thus, Cardano refuted the long-accepted medical error.

In about the second century C.E., the ancient Ionian Greeks gave the illness its name of "diabetes," which translated to "pass through" or "siphon." They had observed that individuals afflicted with the disease drank copious quantities of fluid and that they also urinated a great deal. Generally, the name "diabetes" is specifically attributed to the Greek physician, Aretaeus of Cappadocia, who described the illness in this way in a translation of his medical treatise, "Of the Causes and Signs of Acute and Chronic Diseases,"

> Diabetes is a wasting of the flesh and limbs into urine from a cause similar to dropsy. The patient never ceasing to make water and the discharge is as incessant as a sluice let off. The patient does not survive long for the marasmus is rapid and death speedy. The thirst is ungovernable, the copious potations are more than equalled by the profuse urinary discharge, for more urine flows away . . . The epithet diabetes has been assigned from the disorder being something like passing of water by a siphon . . .

Aretaeus made one major mistake, however. He believed that diabetes was caused by a snakebite.

The great Greek physician Galen was also familiar with diabetes. Galen said diabetes was "a weakness of the kidneys which cannot hold back water." Some Greek physicians urged exercise as a therapy for diabetes, especially horseback riding, which was regarded as an especially good way to rid the body of excessive urination.

Japanese and Chinese physicians were also aware of the disease. Ghang-ke wrote about diabetes around 229 C.E., stating that diabetic urine was copious and sweet, and that it attracted dogs.

In the fifth and sixth century C.E., Susruta, a prestigious physician from India, wrote about his observations on diabetes. He noted that the urine of a person with diabetes had a honey-like taste, one that attracted ants and other insects. Dr. Susruta was also one of the first known physicians to recognize that there were actually two primary types of diabetes, including one that afflicted very thin people and another form that was more commonly seen among obese and more sedentary individuals.

Today we call one form of diabetes "Type 1" (generally seen in thin or average-sized children and adults) and we call the other form "Type 2" diabetes (the more commonly diagnosed form of diabetes in the West today among obese and sedentary middle-aged and older individuals.)

During this period, Dr. Susruta advised moderation in diet and recommended exercise for his overweight patients with diabetes, recommendations that are still offered today for people with Type 2 diabetes—albeit that they are also supplemented with oral medications.

Avicenna (980–1027 C.E.), an Arabian physician, attempted to codify all known medical knowledge. He was deemed a great medical writer of his time. Avicenna wrote of his knowledge of diabetes, "The kidneys attract humors from the liver in greater quantities than they are able to retain. The urine leaves a residue like honey." Avicenna also noted that his patients with diabetes had extreme thirst, were nervous and unable to work, and experienced sexual dysfunction.

Avicenna was also aware of diabetic gangrene, although he knew that it could not be treated at that time, and thus, the affected patients invariably worsened and died.

Diabetes from the Seventeenth through the Nineteenth Centuries

Thomas Willis, a 17th-century Oxford University physician, believed that diabetes was a disease of the blood. He said that the sugar found in the blood was later apparent in the urine of the person with diabetes. Willis also noted that the illness had been rare in ancient times but that diabetes was on the rise because of "good fellowship and gustling down chiefly of unallayed wine." Clearly, Willis was referring to what we now call Type 2 diabetes.

About 100 years later, Matthew Dobson first demonstrated the presence of "saccharine matter" in both the urine and the blood in experiments performed in 1772. Dobson let urine stand until it dried, after which he observed a substance that closely resembled brown sugar. Dobson also left blood standing and found that the remaining serum was sweet. He concluded that "the saccharine matter was not formed in the secretory organ (the kidneys), but previously existed in the serum of the blood." It was not until 1815, however, that French chemist M. E. Chevreul definitively identified the substance found in the urine of people with diabetes as glucose.

William Cullen, a professor of chemistry and medicine in Glasgow and Edinburgh, Scotland, in the late 18th century, stated his thesis that diabetes was essentially a disease of the nervous system. We now know that diabetes is actually an endocrine disorder, although it can also have profound effects on the nervous system as well, particularly after many years. However, Dr. Cullen is credited for adding the term "mellitus" to the word diabetes.

In 1853, Ernst Stadelmann discovered that the diabetic coma was a consequence of a greatly increased accumulation of acids, and was what we now call "diabetic ketoacidosis" or DKA.

However, it was Bernhard Naunyn, Stadelmann's teacher, who was the first to employ the term "acidosis." Naunyn was a very strong proponent of diet as a means to control diabetes. He wrote 10 principles of treatment, some of which are still applicable today. Here are his first seven principles:

1. The Alpha and Omega in the area of diabetes is dietetic treatment, and not drugs.
2. It must be known that diabetic glycosuria increases with time while the tolerance of the patient decreases.
3. When the diabetic is free from sugar, his tolerance usually increases. Therefore, aim to render the patient sugar free and keep him aglycosuric.
4. Limitation of the total diet with resulting disencumbrance of the entire metabolism brings about a favorable result.
5. Reduction of carbohydrates or proteins for the removal of glycosuria.
6. Sugar producing foods are the carbohydrates and proteins.
7. We should determine the exact qualitative and quantitative diet for every diabetic who comes under treatment.

In 1857, Claude Bernard isolated a substance he then called "glycogen" and illustrated the role that the liver played in the metabolism of glucose. He demonstrated through his experiments what some physicians had previously believed: that individuals with diabetes had excessive sugar in the blood, followed by excessive sugar in the urine. At this time, however, it was still unknown that the pancreas was the key organ involved in diabetes.

Then in 1869, German researcher Paul Langerhans wrote a dissertation about special clusters of cells that he identified within the pancreas. He was particularly intrigued by one type of cell in the pancreas. Wrote Langerhans: "This cell is a small irregularly polygonal structure with brilliant cytoplasm; free of any granule with distinct round nuclei of moderate size. The cells lie together in considerable numbers diffusely scattered in the parenchyma of the gland." Although the cells had been identified, the importance of the pancreas to the development of diabetes remained a mystery to researchers and physicians.

In 1889, Oskar Minkowski performed experiments on removing the pancreases of dogs, thus inducing diabetes in the animals and definitively proving the significance of the pancreas. As with many great discoveries, Minkowski did not start out to study diabetes, nor did he suspect that the pancreas was the key. Instead, his colleague, Joseph von Mering, wanted to know if and how the pancreas affected the digestion of fat, and what would happen if the pancreas was removed.

Minkowski removed the pancreas from a dog and the next day a laboratory technician complained that the dog, which had been completely house-trained, was now constantly urinating everywhere. Minkowski, who had been trained by Dr. Carl H. von Noorden to test for diabetes whenever he identified polyuria, found that the dog's urine was laden with glucose. Minkowski realized the significance of this study—that the pancreas was the primary organ involved in diabetes. However, he did not discover the secret of how to resolve diabetes.

Minkowski and many others sought to find what substance it was that made the difference between diabetes and no diabetes, but none of them succeeded. Years later, when another colleague complained to him that it was really *he* who first discovered insulin, not Doctors Frederick G. Banting and Charles H. Best, Minkowski said, "I, too, wish I had discovered insulin." Minkowski received one of the early batches of insulin from Banting and Best, and he told his students that if he could not be the father of insulin, he was happy to be the grandfather.

Author J. O. Liebowitz, in his article on the historical perspective of diabetes, wrote that the finding from Minkowski's experiment was

the "greatest single contribution to experimental research on diabetes" and further, "From here on a straight line can be drawn to the epoch-making work of Banting and Best."

In 1893, Edouard Laguesse noted the importance of the cells that had been identified by Langerhans, and, in honor of Langerhans, he dubbed them the "islands of Langerhans." (These cells are now called "islets of Langerhans.")

Medical Treatments for Diabetes before the Discovery of Insulin

There was little relief for people with diabetes before the 20th century, but there were plenty of ideas on how to treat it. Opium was a drug of treatment for people with diabetes from the 17th-century recommendation of Thomas Willis to use a "syrup of poppies" and onward through the late 19th century. Most doctors didn't believe that opium cured or even much helped the person with diabetes; however, they did believe that it made this distressing disease more tolerable. Doctors also relied on bloodlettings in the 19th century, believing that they would be of some medical value. (Getting rid of the "bad blood" was the plan.) As we now know, they were mistaken in this belief.

During this period, surgeons rarely performed amputations on patients diagnosed with gangrene, which was considered an inevitable death sentence. Many patients did develop ulcerations and infections that led to gangrene and thus, many died. In his article for a 1972 issue of *Medical History*, Frank Allan described his own childhood memories of people he knew who had diabetes prior to the discovery of insulin. He described a man in his fifties who began to have pain in his toe that was severe and constant and that prevented him from sleeping. Allan said,

> Then to his horror it began to turn black. His family doctor called it gangrene and confirmed the diagnosis of diabetes which he himself had feared, since a brother and several members of his family had been diabetic. A surgeon,

consulted in the hope that the gangrenous toe could be amputated, was unwilling to operate. He stated that, with diabetes, healing would fail to occur. The man was bedridden for months as the gangrene extended into his foot. Finally death came to end his suffering.

Dr. Banting, the discoverer of insulin, commented on the nontreatment of gangrene prior to the discovery of insulin, in a paper published in 1937 in *Science*. Banting said, "Another complication of diabetes that was met with in the older patients was gangrene. In the pre-insulin days operation was dangerous and the patients usually died following the operation. Now diabetics can be safely operated upon because insulin controls the blood sugar and acetone production."

Before Banting and Best's discovery of insulin, some unusual pancreatic experimentation occurred by doctors attempting to help their patients with diabetes. For example, in 1906, following on the work of Minkowski, Scottish scientists Rennie and Fraser reported on their experiments with extracts from the islets of fish they had purchased at the Aberdeen Fish Market. They selected a daily supply of fish for their experiments, seeking out species known to have unusually large islets. Their results were reported in *The Biochemical Journal*.

The doctors boiled part of the pancreas, specifically the islets of Langerhans from the fish, and subsequently administered this compound to patients who were very ill with diabetes; for example, one patient who was given the fish extract was nearly blind and he was also very weak.

According to the doctor's notes, this patient showed improvement after receiving the compound, producing much less urine and reporting to them that he felt better. Their own tests revealed that his urinary glucose levels were considerably decreased. When the substance was withheld, however, the patient's urine volume increased and he felt much worse.

Unfortunately, the doctors rapidly ran out of fish and they were unable to procure any more in the fish market. As a result, they could no longer provide the compounded substance that they had created to their patient, who rapidly deteriorated. Other patients had also received the extract and had shown improvement, but a prolonged trial was not possible at that time. Several patients died or became very sick and the doctors lost track of one patient who refused to participate in their study any longer. The doctors did not continue their research.

Most Cases of Diabetes Prior to the 1930s Were Type 1 Diabetes: Today Most Cases Are Type 2 Diabetes

Although physicians have been able to identify diabetes for thousands of years, their treatments were largely ineffectual and most individuals with diabetes sickened and died. It is safe to assume that most of these patients had Type 1 diabetes.

There are two key reasons for this assumption. First, most people prior to the mid-20th century were not obese nor were they sedentary. Hence, they were less likely to develop Type 2 diabetes. Secondly, several generations ago, the life span of most people was far shorter and few lived to be elderly or even middle-aged, when the onset of Type 2 diabetes is most commonly observed.

As a result, frustrated physicians concentrated on striving to help their very ill patients with Type 1 diabetes, despite the fact that few treatments were effective until the discovery of insulin.

Pre-Insulin Era Attempts to Treat Diabetes with Diet

Some well-intentioned physicians put their patients on starvation or semi-starvation diets, ordering them to subsist for days on foods such as oatmeal alone, or to follow a broad array of other rigorous and difficult dietetic recommendations.

Some recommendations were actually harmful; some physicians mistakenly assumed that the body needed much *more* sugar and they mistakenly urged their already hyperglycemic patients to eat large quantities of heavily sweet foods. One account was reported of a physician who had diabetes himself and who decided to follow the regimen of the heavy consumption of sweets. He quickly died.

Other physicians urged the consumption of alcohol to their patients as a means to stave off acidosis and to theoretically help with digestion. (In sharp contrast to today's medical recommendations, which are to avoid alcohol altogether or to drink very moderately.) Lacking the arsenal of medications available today, doctors had to rely on whatever methods they found that seemed to work, if only for a while.

In the latter part of the 18th century, British physician John Rollo was firm in his belief that diabetes should be treated by dietary changes and restrictions, and he was credited as one of the pioneers of this idea. Rollo recommended a diet that was high on protein and fat, with entrees such as blood pudding, and lime water with milk to wash it down. On this diet, vegetables were eliminated. Rollo, as with many other physicians of the time, also favored the use of opium with diabetic patients.

Another 18th-century physician, Apollinaire Bourchardat, took the idea of using diet to control diabetes even further. In addition to inventing diagnostic tests for diabetes, Bourchardat also came up with the recipe for gluten bread. Unlike Rollo, he encouraged his patients to eat green vegetables. Bourchardat also recommended days of fasting and undereating for his patients. He had noted that in times of severe scarcity of food, sugar in the urine of those afflicted with diabetes had virtually vanished and their conditions had improved. Bourchardat was also a strong proponent of exercise.

In the 19th century, Italian physician Arnaldo Cantani was noted for his dietary regimen, which was composed of days of fasting, followed by meat consumption. According to some experts, if Dr. Cantani didn't believe his patients were adhering to his regimen, he locked them up in his clinic and forced them to comply.

Dr. Frederick Allen was famous for writing about and recommending the "Allen Starvation Diet," which he began propounding in 1912, based on his research. He believed that the islets of Langerhans deteriorated because they were overworked and thus, he concluded that less food would not strain them so much and they would have the opportunity to rest. The diet was comprised of several days of fasting followed by a semistarvation diet.

Introduced in 1895 and alluded to earlier, another popular diet was the oatmeal diet, the brainchild of Dr. Carl H. von Noorden in Frankfort, Germany. Dr. von Noorden believed that oatmeal had special qualities that somehow alleviated the symptoms of diabetes.

In another diet that was popular during the early 20th century, Dr. Karl Petren, a Swedish physician, recommended very high fat diets for his patients who had diabetes.

Guelpa of Paris made regular fasting popular in Europe in 1896. He used periodic fasting to "disintoxicate" the patient with diabetes, along with saline laxatives. Other physicians, however, questioned this advice and stated their belief that fasting could lead to diabetic coma.

Although such diets may sound strange or wrongheaded to modern readers, it is important to keep in mind that prior to the discovery of insulin, physicians' attempts to control the diet of the person with diabetes were really the *only* treatment (other than the administration of opium) found to give any temporary relief to the majority of their patients with Type 1 diabetes.

The Discovery of Insulin

Everything changed with the discovery of insulin in 1921. It was a medical paradigm shift and ultimately a lifesaver for millions of people. For people interested in diabetes, it was the equivalent of the discovery of fire or the wheel.

It all began with Dr. Frederick Banting, who built on the knowledge of others but who also made a grand leap forward, and he was the one that made all the difference. Banting, a co-discoverer with Dr. Best of insulin therapy, was a Canadian physician who was fascinated by research on diabetes. Dr. Banting also had a more personal interest in finding a way to prolong life for people afflicted with diabetes. A little girl from his childhood in Alliston, Ontario, had died of diabetes many years ago, and this had continued to affect him deeply, as he sought to find a treatment or cure.

Dr. Best also had a personal drive to resolve the problem of diabetes. Best wrote in an article published in 1956 in *Diabetes*,

My own interest in diabetes began when my father's sister, who had gone from Nova Scotia to train as a nurse at the Massachusetts General Hospital, came to help my father in his small hospital on the Maine-New Brunswick border. She had developed diabetes some years previously and although her life was prolonged by the treatment administered by Dr. Joslin [a noted figure in the early 20th century], she died a few years before insulin became available.

In 1921, Dr. Banting, a recently returned wounded and decorated war veteran of the "Great War" (World War I), was planning to practice orthopedic surgery. He had received an appointment to the faculty of the University of Western Ontario in London, Canada. While preparing a lecture on physiology, Banting happened to read an article by Moses Barron in the November 1920 issue of *Surgery, Gynecology and Obstetrics*. The article discussed the physiology of the pancreas and also commented on the deterioration that occurred when the pancreatic ducts of an animal were cut. Banting read and reread the article, transfixed.

Inspired, Banting then and there developed the idea of using a hormone extracted from the pancreas of an animal to treat diabetes in humans. Consumed by his idea, Banting traveled to the University of Toronto to ask Dr. J. J. R. MacLeod, a prominent diabetes researcher, for permission to use his laboratory so that he could do pancreatic experiments on dogs. Dr.

Banting was not a medical researcher nor had he ever performed any research on diabetes. To his credit, MacLeod agreed to the request and asked Charles Best, a medical student at the time, to assist Dr. Banting in the laboratory. MacLeod went home for the summer to his native Scotland, with no idea of the drama that would follow the experiments of Banting and Best.

During an unseasonably sweltering summer and spending most of their time in the small laboratory, Banting and Best performed their experiments and successfully treated a diabetic dog with their insulin extract.

Best later wrote, "Every time one of our diabetic dogs responded to insulin we hoped that the effect on patients would be just as dramatic. When, in the autumn of 1921, we had demonstrated on 75 successive occasions in 10 completely depancreatized dogs, the invariably definitely and frequently very impressive lowering of blood sugar after the administration of our pancreatic extracts, we considered that the phase of the discovering was complete."

The first human trial on 14-year-old Leonard Thompson, who weighed 64 pounds at the time, was disappointing. Thompson developed abscesses at the sites of the injections and he became very sick, although his glucose levels dropped. Then biochemist James Collip, who had assisted Banting and Best, developed a refined extract, which he tested on Thompson. It worked amazingly well and Thompson's glucose levels plunged from 520 to 120 mg/dL within a day. Thompson lived another 15 years, dying of an unrelated ailment.

At first, however, Collip was unwilling to share the information about his refining process with Banting or Best. Through the course of the very stressful process of the experiments, relations between Collip with Banting and Best had become extremely strained. According to a later account by Best, when Collip announced that he was leaving to go patent the process himself, Best told him he was *not* leaving until Banting heard the news. Best then put a chair in front of the door, sat in it, and physically blocked Collip from leaving. When Banting came back and heard of Collip's plan, he was very upset. There are differing accounts of what happened next and whether or not a scuffle ensued between Banting and Collip. The men somehow resolved their differences and they subsequently worked together.

Banting and Best made their first report of their exciting discovery at a meeting of the American Physiological Society in December 1921 in New Haven, Connecticut. At first they met with considerable skepticism as Banting reportedly gave a halting and rambling presentation of his research and discovery. The physicians knew that Banting was a newcomer to diabetes research, and most of the attendees knew little or nothing about either him or his colleague.

The first impression of many people apparently was, who is this interloper that we've never heard of before? However, the mood changed, by some accounts, when Dr. MacLeod, who was also present and was well-known by the diabetes researchers, warmly embraced the discovery. The audience, mostly physicians, quickly realized that they were hearing about a remarkable and historic scientific breakthrough.

Joseph Barach wrote, in his 1928 article on the history of diabetes for *Annals of Medical History,* "It must have come as a great awakening to the savants in medicine, when the wished for remedy came so suddenly and so unexpectedly from such a quiet spot in the medical world. Today, millions of diabetics may eat and live because they have insulin to meet their metabolic requirement."

Also present at that momentous meeting in Connecticut was George Clowes, the director of research for Eli Lilly & Company, a pharmaceutical company. Perceiving the potential value of the discovery, Clowes offered Banting and Best the assistance of Lilly in developing a pure product that could be distributed on a large scale. They were interested; however, Banting did not patent his discovery but instead assigned the rights (for one dollar) to the University of Toronto.

Banting's course was not a smooth one and it was often only by sheer determination that he succeeded at all. For example, he visited the Lilly plant in Indianapolis, Indiana, in July 1922 to find out how they made drugs because he wanted to produce insulin in Canada. He learned that Lilly used a much more sophisticated process than he had available to him and that he would need vacuum stills to make insulin efficiently in Canada. This equipment was expensive and Banting would need $10,000 to buy it. In 1922, this was no small sum.

Undaunted, Banting went to see the chairman of the Board of Governors at the University of Toronto and asked him for the money to buy the vacuum stills. He was told he would have to wait until the entire Board was in session in September. Although September was only a few months away, that was still too long for Banting, who knew that every day that passed counted against the patients who were dying of diabetes, and for them, insulin meant the difference between life and death. The frustrated Banting asked the board chairman if the university would take the money if Banting could get it himself, somehow, and the startled chairman agreed.

Banting's next stop was New York, where he went to see Dr. H. Rowle Geyelin, a doctor treating children who were sick and dying from diabetes. On a previous visit, Geyelin had told Banting that he was going to keep his sickest patients in bed so they could stay alive until they could receive insulin. He had also told Banting that if he ever needed help, to let him know. Banting now asked Geyelin if he would help him obtain the money for the equipment he needed.

Geyelin called up a wealthy man whose daughter was dying of diabetes. The man's only question was who to make the check out to. Banting immediately wired ahead to Toronto to go ahead and buy the equipment and he also wired that Dr. Geyelin should be among the first to receive the insulin when it was ready. Geyelin received advance supplies of insulin in 1922. He used them on his patients, to dramatic effect. (Two of Geyelin's patients are depicted in the before and after photos in this section.)

In the summer of 1923, Eli Lilly & Company made an agreement with the University of Toronto to begin producing insulin in large quantities for North Americans and others with diabetes. At long last, there was true hope for the emaciated, ravaged, and dying victims of Type 1 diabetes.

Despite the lack of popular communications at the time—when very few people had a telephone—word rapidly spread throughout North America that there was a new "cure" for diabetes. Although insulin was not actually a cure of the disease but was instead a treatment (as it still is in modern times), in the eyes of the people who had diabetes and their families,

insulin meant continued life. Lack of insulin meant certain death. Thus, it is no wonder that they perceived insulin as curative rather than merely therapeutic.

The clamor for the new drug was very great and it astonished physicians. Dr. Joseph H. Barach wrote in 1928,

> After insulin was announced and given to a number of internists in America for clinical trial, the appeal to these clinics by diabetic patients was tremendous. In my service at the Presbyterian Hospital the demand for treatment was far greater than we could possibly meet. Hundreds of letters from patients and their families, coming from all over the country, reflected the actual plight of the diabetic. These patients wrote that they had had the disease for periods of from one to twenty years, that they had had all kind of treatment by numerous doctors, and that in spite of many efforts to regain health, they were growing progressively

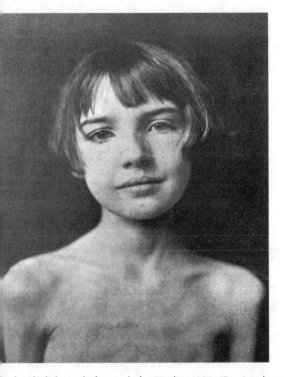 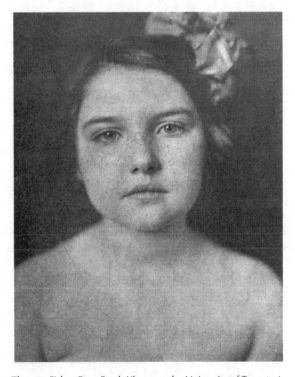

Girl with diabetes, before and after insulin, 1922 *(Reprinted courtesy the Thomas Fisher Rare Book Library at the University of Toronto.)*

worse. They invariably asked this one question, 'Was there really something that could be done to relieve them of their suffering?' Here were evidences of something very different from the complacent picture of the diabetic patient as described in books. The preceding medical treatment of these patients had been a failure, and they craved a return to health and to their occupations. These letters also made it clear that diabetes was not a disease of the rich, an idea which first appeared in the literature of the Hindus and writings of Avicenna, and apparently accepted by many writers even up to the 20th century.

Insulin transformed the lives of many people. For example, Robin Lawrence was a young British doctor who had developed diabetes and was dedicating what he thought were his remaining one or two years of life to treating patients in Florence, Italy. A biochemist friend sent him a telegram that said, "I have got insulin. It works. Come back immediately." Dr. Lawrence

returned to England and he received insulin treatment. He subsequently became an eminent diabetologist who treated thousands of patients, educated many doctors, and lived to the age of 76 years, reportedly suffering no complications of diabetes.

Physicians also quickly perceived the potential lifesaving capabilities of insulin for their child patients with diabetes. In 1922, in a paper for the *Journal for Metabolic Research*, Dr. Geyelin (the physician who helped Banting locate the money for his equipment) and his colleagues at the Presbyterian Hospital in New York described the impact of insulin on nine children with diabetes. This article included both "before" and "after" photos of the children, taken before the administration of insulin and afterwards.

Most of the children in the "before" photographs looked very emaciated, even skeletal. After the insulin therapy, the photographs clearly revealed children who looked thin but

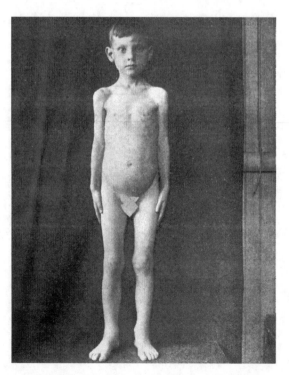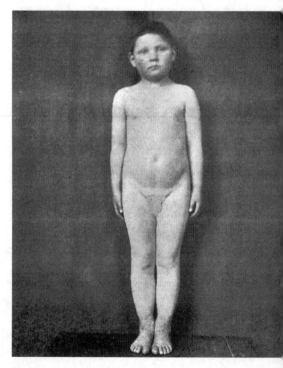

Boy with diabetes, before and after insulin, 1922 *(Reprinted courtesy the Thomas Fisher Rare Book Library at the University of Toronto.)*

normal. In fact, the children in the "after" pictures were barely recognizable as the same children in the "before" photographs.

The authors wrote,

One of the most striking and constantly observed effects of insulin in this group of diabetic children has been the rapid and complete disappearance of ketone bodies from the urine. When the initial ketosis was moderate in degree and accompanied by little or no evidence of an acidosis, the urine was occasionally found to be free from diabetic acid within 48 hours after the initiation of insulin therapy. In every case, the amount of diabetic acid in the urine was markedly diminished after the first week of insulin therapy, and in one case . . . did it persist for more than two weeks.

The doctors concluded, "In a series of nine children suffering from severe diabetes, treatment with insulin has been followed by certain definite results: (1) arrest of the downward course of the disease; (2) achievement of a total food intake approximating the normal age requirement in calories; (3) steady gain in weight and growth, with increase in mental and physical vigor; (4) absence of severe or permanent ill effects."

Noted physicians such as Dr. Elliott P. Joslin in Boston actively adopted and promoted the use of insulin. In one case, Joslin brought a five-year-old child before a spellbound audience of physicians, who listened to the child accurately describe a test for sugar in the urine and then expound about the meaning and importance of carbohydrates, proteins, and fats.

Doctors Banting and MacLeod were awarded the Nobel Prize for the discovery of insulin in 1923. Dr. Banting shared his prize with Dr. Best and Dr. MacLeod shared his prize with Dr. Collip. Banting was knighted in 1934 for his discovery, becoming Sir Frederick Banting, and he also received many other much-deserved honors.

There was considerable animosity for years between Banting and MacLeod because Banting made it clear that he felt that Best should have been the other recipient of the Nobel Prize and not Doctor MacLeod. MacLeod contended that he had provided the facilities for the work to be done and that he had also offered important advice and support and thus, his contributions were valuable. Banting's view has been largely vindicated in the judgment of history, which credits the discovery of insulin to Banting and Best.

Through the years, the ingredients and forms of insulin have been changed and improved upon. Insulin was made from beef and pork until the late 20th century, when synthetic forms of insulin were created. There are also different types of insulin in terms of their timeliness. For example, today there are long-acting, intermediate, and short-acting forms of insulin.

There are also various ways to introduce insulin into the body and the insulin pen or the implantable insulin pump are the most recent methods of insulin delivery, and inhaled insulin is another vehicle for introducing the drug into the body. It is easy to forget it but all these drugs and their different forms were predicated on the initial discovery of Doctors Banting and Best.

The American Diabetes Association

No book about diabetes or one that mentions the history of diabetes would be complete without a discussion of the American Diabetes Association (ADA), a powerful and important research and advocacy organization.

In 1940, the ADA was formed by physicians who had become concerned about the complications of diabetes and who wanted to learn more about treatment. The founder and first president was Cecil Striker, a clinician and medical professor at the University of Cincinnati.

In 1950, in concert with the American Dietetic Association and the U.S. Public Health Service, the ADA created the concept of meal exchanges. Foods were divided into six different groups with equivalent portions so that a diabetes patient could choose one food from one group one day and an equivalent food from that group (or another group) on another day.

Today the ADA publishes internationally acclaimed peer-reviewed journals on diabetes, including *Diabetes* and *Diabetes Care.* The ADA also publishes magazines and books for consumers with diabetes and their families.

The ADA has also been active in litigation, most notably in cases where children were barred from day-care centers because of their diabetes, as well as in cases where adults with diabetes have been unfairly denied employment.

The role of the ADA has evolved from an organization centering on treatment to one of research and advocacy as well as information-provider for doctors, patients, and their families. Today the ADA is one of the most powerful and effective nonprofit organizations in the United States.

Dr. Joslin and the Joslin Clinics

Elliott P. Joslin, a Boston physician, was a towering figure in diabetes until his death in 1962, leaving behind the Joslin Diabetes Center, which today is a large organization with affiliates at 23 locations in 12 states, serving more than 40,000 patients with diabetes.

Dr. Joslin's book *The Treatment of Diabetes Mellitus,* was published in 1916. He was globally regarded as one of the most influential and knowledgeable individuals in the field of diabetes. Joslin was one of the six doctors on the "Insulin Committee" that provided patients with the purified form of insulin that was first developed by Eli Lilly & Company in the early 1920s. Joslin also assisted with clinical trials.

Joslin's own mother, who was obese, had suffered from Type 2 diabetes. She died before the development of oral medications for people with diabetes. Perhaps in mind of his mother's weight problem, Joslin himself was said to be a man whose weight never varied more than a pound or so.

Joslin wrote about diabetes prior to the discovery of insulin by Banting and Best and after its introduction he was an immediate and very strong proponent of insulin. Dr. Joslin was also an ardent believer in the importance of careful diet as well as the need to educate patients on how they could best manage their diabetes.

Dr. Joslin's concern for his patients was evident in his work and writing. According to his biographer, Donald M. Barnett, MD, Dr. Joslin wrote in 1921,

> Although six of the seven persons, all head of families . . . living in [three] adjoining houses . . . on [a] peaceful, elm-lined . . . street . . . in a country town in New England . . . succumbed to diabetes . . . no one spoke of an epidemic. . . . Consider the measure which would have been adopted to discover the source of the outbreak to prevent a recurrence . . . [as it would] . . . if these deaths had occurred from scarlet fever, typhoid fever or tuberculosis. . . . Because the disease was diabetes, and because the deaths occurred over a considerable interval of time, the fatalities passed unnoticed.

Dr. Joslin founded the Joslin Diabetes Center in Boston in 1898 and the Joslin Clinics actively continue today throughout the United States, treating patients and performing pioneering research. Joslin pioneered the still-important concept of using a team of specialists to treat people with diabetes and he also favored the use of long and short-acting insulins. In addition, Joslin was a strong proponent of frequent testing of glucose levels.

Diabetes Treatment in Modern Times

A variety of important changes occurred in the second half of the 20th century. Insulins were improved upon and people with Type 1 diabetes could use long, intermediate, or short-acting insulins. Humalog and NovoLog, analogs, of a human-based insulin, replaced pork and beef insulin. Syringes were improved to be sharper and less painful. Special meters were developed, enabling people with diabetes to test their own blood from the comfort of their homes.

The Evolution of Insulin and Better Devices for People with Diabetes

If Drs. Banting and Best could see the changes to the original insulin that they developed, they would be very proud of how their brainchild has grown and matured. For example, Novo Nordisk Pharmaceuticals, Inc. developed the first slower-acting insulins, in 1936. In 1949, Becton Dickinson and Company produced a standardized syringe for insulin, approved by the American Diabetes Association. This standardization made life much easier for people with diabetes.

In the 1970s, portable glucose meters were introduced, enabling people with both Type 1 and Type 2 diabetes to easily test their blood glucose levels. Before this time, glucose monitoring was primarily managed only in the doctor's office, making daily monitoring difficult or impossible. The 1970s was also when the external insulin pump was first introduced, which was perfected further into the 21st century.

In 1986, the first insulin pen delivery system was developed, which ultimately led to the more convenient prefilled insulin pen. This device made injection easier and far less painful for people with diabetes.

Advances in DNA knowledge enabled researchers to create recombinant DNA insulin. The first human insulin analogue, Humalog (lispro) was developed by Eli Lilly & Company and approved by the Food and Drug Administration (FDA) in the United States in 1996. In 1998, studies began to show that inhaled insulin might work as effectively as insulin that was injected.

Development of Better Oral Medications

The 20th century, particularly the latter part of the century, was a time when many more cases of Type 2 diabetes were diagnosed. One disadvantage of an affluent lifestyle was that people had plenty/too much to eat and little need or incentive for physical labor. Rather than laboring in the fields, some people purchased memberships in health clubs.

Of course, not all people with Type 2 diabetes were or are affluent and many are individuals from lower socioeconomic strata. The middle to the end of the 20th century brought new and better oral medications for people with Type 2 diabetes. For example, in 1955, the first drugs in the sulfonylurea class were approved. These drugs induced the pancreas to produce more insulin. In 1961, Eli Lilly & Company developed glucagon for people with severe hypoglycemia.

In 1988, approval was given for angiotensin converting enzyme (ACE) inhibitor medications. These drugs decreased blood pressure and proteinuria (protein in the urine) and delayed the further development of kidney disease, which was and still is, a major problem faced by many people with diabetes.

In 1995, two major drugs were introduced for people with diabetes. The Bayer Corporation introduced acarbose (Precose). It was an alpha-glucosidase inhibitor that delayed the digestion of carbohydrates.

Bristol-Myers Squibb Company introduced metformin, or Glucophage, in 1995. This was a biguanide drug that prevented the liver from releasing excessive amounts of glucose. Subsequent studies have revealed that people with both Type 2 diabetes and coronary artery disease (CAD) who take metformin have a lower death rate than their peers who take other medications.

In 1997, troglitazone, or Rezulin, was introduced by Parke-Davis for patients with Type 2 diabetes. This drug was subsequently pulled from the market by the Food and Drug Administration (FDA) in 2000 after it appeared to cause serious medical problems in some users.

In 1997, Novo Nordisk Pharmaceuticals, Inc. introduced Prandin (repaglinide). This is an oral medication that is fast acting and is taken by people with Type 2 diabetes before meals.

Another major change came with the home-based management of diabetes. Although people with diabetes still needed to see their physicians in the latter part of the 20th century, blood glucose meters enabled patients to check their own blood levels rather than having to go to a clinic for a blood check. Blood checks were given on a periodic basis in the doctor's clinic. Medicare and most other health insurance companies now provide medical coverage for these devices, making them affordable to the average person.

A Global Look at Diabetes Today and into the Future

After millennia of suffering and death from diabetes, today we can at long last see ahead of us not only better and painless treatments for this disease but also that actual cures lie within our grasp. Experiments continue on identifying and implementing cures for the transplantation of islet cells from stem cells and other sources into individuals with diabetes. Replacement transplants of the entire pancreas also occur, either with the replacement of the pancreas alone or with multiple organ replacements, such as with kidney-pancreas transplants.

A study published in 2009 in the *New England Journal of Medicine* revealed that 87 newly diagnosed patients with Type 1 diabetes, ages eight to 40 years old, were treated with the arthritis medication rituximab for one year. The drug partially preserved the function of the beta cells of the pancreas, and as a result, the subjects in the group treated with rituximab required significantly less insulin than the subjects in the group treated with a placebo.

Researchers Mark D. Pescovitz, M.D., and colleagues said, "A single course of rituximab administered soon after diagnosis appears to preserve insulin secretion in part for at least one year." Continued immunotherapy research along this line should produce even further breakthroughs, with the hope that someday, individuals newly diagnosed with diabetes can be treated and cured.

There are also advances in the treatment of diabetes; for example, the insulin pump has made control of diabetes possible for many individuals who struggled greatly to get their blood sugar under control with insulin injections.

Researchers are also investigating the possibility of an inhaled form of insulin, which would replace the need for needles, syringes, and injections, if its promise is realized.

A cure is important because many experts predict a considerable increase in the number of diabetes cases over the next 25 years; for example, in a 2009 article in *Diabetes Care,* researchers Elbert S. Huang, M.D., and colleagues predicted that from 2009 to 2034, the number of people with both diagnosed and undiagnosed diabetes in America will nearly double from 23.7 million in 2009 to 44.1 million by 2034. The cost to treat individuals with diabetes is estimated to be staggeringly expensive; Huang and colleagues predicted spending on diabetes will nearly triple, from $113 billion in 2009 to $336 billion in 2034 (in 2007 dollars).

A large portion of this will be in Medicare dollars, and the projected increase in spending for Medicare recipients will escalate from $45 billion in 2009 to $171 billion in 2034. The projected increases are largely driven by an aging population, rather than by an obese population (although obesity plays a role because it often causes Type 2 diabetes; consequently, fewer obese people would translate into dollar savings).

Worldwide, the numbers are even more eye-popping with a World Health Organization prediction of 366 million people with diabetes by 2030, up from 171 million people worldwide in 2000. Clearly, diabetes is a problem that needs careful consideration and additional research.

Bibliography for the History of Diabetes

Allan, Frank N. "Diabetes Before and After Insulin." *Medical History* 16, no. 3 (July 1972): 66–73.

Allen, Frederick M., M.D. "Blueberry Leaf Extract: Physiologic and Clinical Properties in Relation to Carbohydrate Metabolism." *Journal of the American Medical Association* 89 (November 5, 1927): 1,577–1,580.

Allen, Frederick M., M.D. "Present Results and Outlook of Diabetic Treatment." *Annals of Internal Medicine* 2, no. 2 (August 1928): 203–215.

American Diabetes Association. "Milestones in Diabetes Treatment." *Diabetes Forecast* (November 1998): 76–82.

Banting, F. G., M.D. "Early Work on Insulin." *Science* 85, no. 2217 (June 25, 1937): 594–596.

———. "Insulin in the Treatment of Diabetes Mellitus." *The Journal of Metabolic Research* (November 1922): 547–604.

Banting, F. G., M.D., and Best, C. H. "The Internal Secretion of the Pancreas." *The Journal of Laboratory and Clinical Medicine* 8, no. 5 (February 1922): 251–266.

Barach, J., M.D. "Historical Facts in Diabetes." *Annals of Medical History* 10 (1928): 387–386.

Barnett, Donald M., M.D. *Elliott P. Joslin, M.D.: A Centennial Portrait.* Boston, Mass.: Joslin Diabetes Center, 1998.

Best, Charles H., M.D. "The First Clinical Use of Insulin." *Diabetes* 5, no. 1 (January–February 1956): 65–67.

Bliss, Michael. *Banting: A Biography.* Toronto, Canada: McClelland and Stewart, 1984.

———. *The Discovery of Insulin.* Chicago, Ill.: University of Chicago Press, 1982.

Foster, Nellis B., M.D. *Diabetes Mellitus: Designed for the Use of Practitioners of Medicine.* Philadelphia, Pa.: J. B. Lippincott Company, 1915.

Fulton, John F., M.D. "Reminiscences of the Discovery of Insulin." *Diabetes* 5, no. 1 (January–February 1956): 65–67.

Geyelin, H. Rawle, M.D., et al. "The Use of Insulin in Juvenile Diabetes." *Journal of Metabolic Research* 2, nos. 5 and 6 (1922): 767–791.

Huang, Elbert S., M.D. "Projecting the Future Diabetes Population Size and Related Costs for the U.S." *Diabetes Care* 32, no. 12 (2009): 2,225–2,229.

Joslin, Elliott, M.D. *The Treatment of Diabetes Mellitus with Observations upon the Disease Based upon Thirteen Hundred Cases.* Philadelphia, Pa.: Lea & Febiger, 1917.

Karlsen, Marie, Dorrine Khakpour, and Leslie Lobeda Thomson. "Efficacy of Medical Nutrition Therapy: Are Your Patients Getting What They Need?" *Clinical Diabetes* 14, no. 3 (May–June 1996): 54–61.

Leibowitz, J. O. "The Concept of Diabetes in Historical Perspective." *Israel Journal of Medical Sciences* 8, no. 3 (March 1972): 469–475.

MacCracken, Joan, M.D., guest editor with Donna Hotel. "From Ants to Analogues: Puzzles and Promises in Diabetes Management." *Postgraduate Medicine* 101, no. 4 (April 1997).

MacLeod, J. J. R. "History of the Researches Leading to the Discovery of Insulin." *Bulletin of the History of Medicine* 52, no. 3 (Fall 1978): 295–312.

Myers, Victor C., and Cameron V. Bailey. "The Lewis and Benedict Method for the Estimation of Blood Sugar, with Some Observations Obtained in Disease." *The Journal of Biological Chemistry* 2 (1916): 147–161.

Papaspryos, N. S., M.D. *The History of Diabetes Mellitus.* Stuttgart, Germany: Georg Thieme Verlag, 1964.

Pescovitz, Mark D., M.D., et al. "Rituximab, B-Lymphocyte Depletion, and Preservation of Beta-Cell Function." *New England Journal of Medicine* 361, no. 22 (2009): 2,143–2,152.

Pyke, D. A. "Preamble: the History of Diabetes." *The International Textbook of Diabetes.* London, England: John Wiley & Sons, 1997.

Rennie, John and Thomas Fraser. "The Islets of Langerhans in Relation to Diabetes." *The Biochemical Journal* 2, no. 1 (1907): 17–19.

Shapiro A. M. J., et al. "Islet Transplantation in Seven Patients with Type 1 Diabetes Mellitus Using a Glucocorticoid-free Immunosuppressive Regimen." *New England Journal of Medicine* 343 (2000): 230–238.

Striker, Cecil, M.D., comp. *Famous Faces in Diabetes.* Boston, Mass.: G. K. Hall & Co., 1961.

Wallace, George B., M.D. "Recent Advances in the Treatment of Diabetes Mellitus." *Journal of the American Medical Association* 55, no. 25 (December 17, 1910): 2,107–2,109.

ENTRIES A TO Z

abuse/neglect Causing harm or failing to provide needed help or medical care to a person who cannot provide that care to himself or herself, such as a child or a disabled person who is under the care of another. Individuals with diabetes need the ability/capability to check their glucose levels at least several times daily to be able to adjust their diet and activities accordingly. They also need to be able to take oral medication or insulin, or both, if necessary. In addition, individuals with diabetes (whether Type 1 or Type 2 diabetes) need to receive regular medical attention from a physician.

If a person is unable to check his or her own levels of blood glucose or administer medication appropriately, because he or she is a child or has a disabling condition that makes it impossible to do so, then it is generally up to family members or others to ensure that the person with diabetes receives such care. A failure to provide such assistance could be considered abuse or neglect under a state's law, particularly if the individual has Type 1 diabetes and must receive insulin in order to live. If the individual is a child under the age of 18 years and the parents or legal guardians fail to provide needed care, then they could be charged with child neglect or, more specifically, "medical neglect," under the state's child abuse laws. (Each state has its own statutes on what actions constitute child abuse.)

Sometimes religious beliefs collide directly with state laws on abuse or neglect, as when the parents of a child with Type 1 diabetes refuse to provide the child with medical care, preferring to rely on prayer alone, and the child then dies. In 2008, Madeline Kara Neumann, age 11, died in a coma from untreated DIABETIC KETOACIDOSIS (DKA). The child had allegedly not received any medical care since she was three years old. Prior to her death, the child was reportedly extremely ill with excessive thirst, nausea, and weakness for about a month. She had not been diagnosed with Type 1 diabetes but the autopsy ruled that her death was from DKA.

The child's parents were members of the Unleavened Bread Ministries, a Christian sect that eschews medical treatment. In 2009, and in two separate trials, Wisconsin juries found both parents guilty of second-degree reckless homicide. As of this writing in late 2010, the parents were sentenced to 10 years of probation, with six months of jail time that has been stayed pending an appeal. The Neumanns have three teenage children.

Local sentiment in Weston, Wisconsin, ran heavily against the Neumanns, and boycotts allegedly caused their coffee business to fail.

According to Scott St. Amand in his 2009 law article on spiritual healing exemptions to child protection laws for the *Richmond Journal of the Law and the Public Interest,* the Wisconsin exemption states that a "person is not guilty of an offense . . . solely because he or she provides a child with treatment by spiritual means through prayer alone for healing." St. Amand says that most states (45 of them) have legal accommodations for parents who wish to rely on spiritual healing.

St. Amand says that most of such exemptions occurred after the passage of the federal Child Abuse Prevention and Treatment Act (CAPTA) in 1974. He explains, "Such state spiritual exemption clauses, whose passage was monetarily rewarded through CAPTA funding, allow religious parents and faith-healers to escape criminal prosecution if their child was injured or died because the parents relied on spiritual healing in lieu of requisite conventional medical attention. In a twenty-year period following the passage of CAPTA, and the subsequent passage of state-by-state religious exemptions, an empirical study noted that an estimated 172 children have died as a result of the faith-based denial of medical care." St. Amand says that the U.S. Supreme Court has yet to rule on this issue. It is possible that the Supreme Court may be asked to rule in the case of the Neumanns, although it is unknown whether the Court will agree to hear the case.

See also RELIGION/SPIRITUALITY.

St. Amand, Scott. "Protecting Neglect: The Constitutionality of Spiritual Healing Exemptions to Child Protection Statutes." *Richmond Journal of the Law and the Public Interest* 12, no. 129 (2009): 139–161.

acanthosis nigricans   A skin condition that is characterized by many papillomas (benign skin tumors) and also by thickening of the skin (hyperkeratosis). The skin is often described as having a velvety texture and being hyperpigmented. Acanthosis nigricans is primarily found on the neck of the patient, although it may also appear in other areas such as the elbows, knees, groin, underarms, and knuckles. The acanthosis itself only causes cosmetic problems.

This condition is associated with Type 2 diabetes. It is also associated with severe INSULIN RESISTANCE. In addition, it is also found in many patients with lesser degrees of insulin resistance, polycystic ovary syndrome, hyperthyroidism and hypothyroidism, obesity, acromegaly, and Cushing's syndrome.

James Burke and his colleagues developed a scale to measure acanthosis nigricans, and this scale was published in a 1999 issue of *Diabetes Care*. The scale offers conditions to consider in

various parts of the body, as well as their severity, including the neck, axilla (underarm area), knuckles, elbows, and knees. For example, in considering "neck texture," the authors offer four levels, from 0 to 3. A "0" is defined as a neck texture that is "smooth to touch; no differentiation from normal skin to palpation." In contrast, a "3" level is "extremely coarse; 'hills and valleys' observable on visual examination."

As of this writing, there is no treatment for this disease.

Burke, James P., Ph.D., et al., "A Quantitative Scale of Acanthosis Nigricans." *Diabetes Care* 22, no. 10 (October 1999): 2,655–2,659.
Stuart, C. A., et al., "Acanthosis Nigricans As a Risk Factor for non-Insulin Dependent Diabetes." *Clinical Pediatrics* 37, no. 2 (1998): 73.

acarbose (Precose)   An alpha-glucosidase inhibitor that slows the absorption of carbohydrates from the small intestine and thus diminishes the increase in glucose after a meal. It is a medication that is occasionally used for people with Type 2 diabetes and occasionally for patients with Type 1 diabetes. It decreases hyperglycemia (high blood glucose levels) by affecting the absorption of carbohydrates within the intestines.

ACE inhibitors/ACE drugs   Angiotensin-converting enzyme (ACE) inhibitors are a class of medications used to reduce high blood pressure (HYPERTENSION), to reverse left ventricular hypertrophy (thickening of the main wall of the heart) and to improve quality of life and increase the survival rate among patients with congestive heart failure. They are also used to slow the progression of renal (kidney) disease, especially among patients who have DIABETIC NEPHROPATHY.

ACE medications were used in the HOPE STUDY among patients with a high risk of developing CARDIOVASCULAR DISEASE. Among the subjects, including patients with diabetes, the researchers found that the medication effectively decreased the risk of serious cardiovascular problems.

The effect of ACE inhibitors in slowing the progression of nephropathy is independent of their effect on blood pressure. This has been clearly demonstrated in patients with both Type 1 and Type 2 diabetes and patients with and without hypertension.

When patients with diabetes use ACE inhibitors, physicians order kidney tests such as BUN, CREATININE, urinary microalbumin/creatinine ratios and potassium to monitor patients, because in rare cases, this class of medication may cause changes that require adjustment of the dosage.

The use of nonsteroidal antiinflammatory (NSAID) medications, often used to reduce pain and inflammation in diseases such as arthritis, may slightly decrease the effectiveness of ACE drugs. Pregnant women should avoid ACE medications completely. The most common side effect found with an ACE medication is cough, and it is often mild and generally well tolerated.

Some examples of commonly prescribed ACE inhibitor medications as of this writing are: captopril (Capoten), enalapril (Vasotec), quinapril (Accupril), fosinopril (Monopril), and benazepril (Lotensin).

See also CORONARY HEART DISEASE; MYOCARDIAL INFARCTION; STROKE.

acquired immune deficiency syndrome (AIDS)
A chronic viral and severe degenerative illness, for which there is no cure as of this writing, although there are many medications that may help. AIDS results from the human immunodeficiency virus (HIV). Individuals who have both diabetes and AIDS need very careful monitoring.

In 2000, some researchers demonstrated that nondiabetic individuals with AIDS gained benefit from taking very small doses of INSULIN, improving their overall health status and enabling them to gain weight and strength. Further research is needed to determine the full implications of this finding.

Patients with AIDS can develop forms of lipodystrophy, which are abnormal deposits of fat that are usually seen in patients with Cushing's disease/syndrome. Cushing's disease is due to excess steroid effect (produced by the body or taken by the patient for medical reasons). Lipodystrophy is also found among patients with diabetes who inject insulin repetitively into one area of the body. Interestingly, researchers have been using diabetes drugs such as metformin, rosiglitazone, and pioglitazone to try to treat this problem.

acromegaly Very rare endocrine disorder of the pituitary gland that is usually caused by an excessive output of growth hormone. The disease is called *acromegaly* if it occurs after puberty and is denoted as *gigantism* if it occurs before puberty. In about 95 percent of the cases, the excess of growth hormone is caused by a noncancerous tumor in the pituitary gland. Rarely, it may also be caused by the secretion of growth hormone-releasing hormone (GHRH) that is made by a tumor located in another part of the body. Three to four people out of every million develop a new case of acromegaly each year, and an estimated 60 of every million people have acromegaly; however, these estimates may be somewhat low since the diagnosis is often missed. About 20 to 30 percent of those with acromegaly/gigantism have diabetes and about 30 to 45 percent have impaired glucose tolerance.

The prepubescent individual with gigantism will attain unusually tall heights because of accelerated bone growth, while the adult with acromegaly will not grow taller because the growth plates in the bones have already fused. Instead, when the disease has its onset in adulthood, the person will develop tissue deformities, such as swelling of the hands and feet, and eventually will also suffer from bony and cartilaginous facial changes that alter the individual's appearance.

The most serious health results of acromegaly are TYPE 2 DIABETES, hypertension, arthritis, and an increased risk for cardiovascular disease. Individuals with acromegaly are also at a greater risk for developing polyps in the colon and for the development of colorectal cancer. As a result, experts recommend that a colonoscopy be performed every two to four years, depending on the recommendation of the treating physician.

According to Shlomo Melmed in his article on acromegaly for the *New England Journal of Medicine* in 2006, an estimated 40 percent of patients with acromegaly are diagnosed by an internist and the remaining 60 percent are diagnosed by other doctors, such as their ophthalmologist because of visual disorders, their gynecologist for complaints of menstrual difficulties and infertility, their rheumatologist because of osteoarthritis, or their sleep specialist because of obstructive sleep apnea. Often by the time that the patient is diagnosed (in about 60 percent of the cases), patients have problems with HYPERTENSION and heart disease. Individuals with acromegaly also have a higher rate of death than others because of their elevated presence of diabetes, hypertension, cardiomyopathy, and sleep apnea.

Symptoms and Diagnostic Path

Swelling of the hands and feet is an early sign of acromegaly, and the individual may also notice that a wider size in shoes is needed. Some body organs, particularly the heart, may enlarge (although only a cardiac ultrasound or echocardiogram would reveal this change.

According to the National Endocrine and Metabolic Diseases Information Service, some other signs and symptoms of this disorder are as follows:

- oily skin
- achy joints
- impaired vision
- headaches
- hyperhidrosis (excessive sweating)

- skin tags
- in women, abnormal menstrual cycles and sometimes breast discharge
- in men, erectile dysfunction
- in both men and women, decreased libido
- hypertension
- excess enlargement of the mouth, nose, and tongue (acral growth)
- deepening voice due to enlarged vocal cords and sinuses
- deformities of teeth and facial bones
- carpal tunnel syndrome (compressed median nerve, accompanied by numbness, tingling, and weakness in the wrist, thumb, index, or middle finger)

The diagnosis of acromegaly is often delayed by 15 to 20 years because the onset is very slow and insidious. As a result, diagnosis may not occur until the individual is 35 to 50 years old, when the signs and symptoms have become much more prominent and obvious.

If the disease occurs during childhood, it is more apparent, although it still may go undiagnosed and untreated. The late actor Andre the Giant had gigantism. Some experts speculate that in the biblical story of David and Goliath, Goliath was a victim of this syndrome.

If the physician suspects that a patient may have acromegaly or gigantism, the doctor can order a fasting blood test of growth hormone; however, this test alone is not sufficient, because people with acromegaly may have instances of the normal production of growth hormone, interspersed with instances of abnormal production, and consequently, the blood test could occur when the body is producing a normal level. As a result, the blood test for growth hormone should be combined with an ORAL GLUCOSE TOLERANCE TEST, because when patients' bodies are overproducing growth hormone, the ingestion of the sugar glucose will not appropriately lower blood growth hormone levels.

Other blood tests, such as for IGF-1 levels, may be ordered. These levels are increased in people with acromegaly. Confirming tests such as a magnetic resonance imaging (MRI) scan or a computer tomography (CT) scan may also be used to detect the location and size of the tumor that is causing the excessive production of growth hormone. If the tumors cannot be located with these scans, sometimes they are identified elsewhere, such as in the chest, abdomen, or pelvis.

Treatment Options and Outlook

The goal of treatment is to decrease growth hormone levels to normal while preserving normal pituitary function and treating any hormone deficiencies that may be present. In addition, the physician also seeks to improve the symptoms of the disease.

Acromegaly is often treated with pituitary surgery (usually transsphenoidal through the sinuses), which is successful in about 80 to 90 percent of cases. Remission of many symptoms generally occurs within days after surgery. However, the patient will need to be monitored for the rest of his or her life for a possible return of the disease.

A risk with surgery is that the pituitary gland could be damaged, and thus the patient would need to take multiple hormones to replace the deficient pituitary hormones for the rest of his or her life. Another risk is that the posterior section of the pituitary, which stores antidiuretic hormone (ADH), a hormone that is vital in the balance of water in the body, could be temporarily or (rarely) permanently damaged, which would require further medical therapy.

Medications are also a common form of treatment. Somatostatin analogs (SSAs) are used to attempt to shut off the production of growth hormone, and these drugs are effective in the majority (50–70 percent) of patients. Long-acting SSAs are given by injection on a monthly basis. SSAs may have a side benefit of improving the blood glucose control in patients who have diabetes, and they also reduce the need for insulin. The primary risk with SSAs is the development of gallstones.

Drugs known as growth hormone receptor antagonists (GHRAs) such as pegvisomant (Somavert) are sometimes used to treat acromegaly. Pegvisomant has a 97 percent normalization rate of IGF-1 levels (which are used to monitor acromegalics, as it acts as a surrogate and more accurate marker than GH). Pegvisomant is injected subcutaneously daily. Common side effects include injection site reactions in 7.4 percent, elevated liver enzymes (3 times greater than normal) in 5.2 percent (3.1 percent spontaneously normalized during continued treatment), reported increase of pituitary tumor volume in 5.2 percent (which was verified in 3.1 percent), and headache in 1.7 percent.

In those with diabetes, there is an improvement in the glucose levels and hemoglobin HgbA1c levels that may be a bit better than with the improvement seen with SSAs. Thus after therapy is begun, medication doses for the treatment of the diabetes often need to be reduced gradually, or down-titrated.

Another category of drugs used to treat acromegaly is dopamine agonists such as bromocriptine, which are not as effective as SSAs or GHRAs. They may help patients with a mildly elevated level of acromegaly as well as those who have both acromegaly and hyperprolactinemia (excessive levels of the hormone prolactin, which can cause breast discharge). Sometimes dopamine agonists are used along with SSAs. Side effects of dopamine agonists are headache, nausea, and lightheadedness.

Radiation therapy may be used when other treatments have failed, although it is generally considered a last resort for treatment. Doctors may use radioisotope implantation with protein beam and alpha particles. Focused radiation may be performed with a gamma knife.

The outlook for the disease depends on when treatment is given and how successfully the body responds to treatment.

Risk Factors and Preventive Measures

This disease is very rare and only about 60 people per million have it. There are no known preventive measures.

Melmed, Shlomo. "Acromegaly," *New England Journal of Medicine* 355, no. 24 (December 14, 2006): 2,558–2,573.

Schreiber, I., et al. "Treatment of Acromegaly with the GH Receptor Antagonist Pegvisomant in Clinical Practice: Safety and Efficacy Evaluation from the German Pegvisomant Observational Study," *European Journal of Endocrinology* 156, no. 1 (2007): 75–82.

adolescents with diabetes Most adolescents with diabetes suffer from Type 1 diabetes but some adolescents have Type 2 diabetes, particularly if they are obese and sedentary. In fact, increasing numbers of children and teenagers in the United States are being diagnosed with Type 2 diabetes. Native American adolescents who have diabetes are more likely to have Type 2 diabetes than Type 1 diabetes, according to the Centers for Disease Control and Prevention (CDC). About 186,000 children and adolescents under age 20 in the United States have diabetes, according to the American Diabetes Association. About one person in every 400–600 children and adolescents has Type 1 diabetes.

There are also a very small number of primarily African-American adolescents who suffer from MATURITY ONSET DIABETES OF THE YOUNG (MODY). This is a rare genetic form (six known gene defects) of Type 2 diabetes that can develop in nonobese teenagers. It may account for 2 percent to 5 percent of all Type 2 diabetes cases in people under age 25, but it is often unrecognized and undiagnosed. MODY is rarely found in white adolescents.

Like adults, adolescents may also have secondary diabetes due to other ailments, such as cystic fibrosis.

Some adolescents have a hybrid form of diabetes, which is a mix between Type 1 and Type 2 diabetes. Measurements of insulin, GAD, and other antibodies as well as C-peptide are helpful in determining the appropriate therapy.

Adolescents with Type 1 Diabetes

Formerly called "juvenile diabetes," "juvenile-onset diabetes," or "insulin-dependent diabetes mellitus (IDDM)," the illness was renamed because it may be diagnosed in young adults or even older individuals. Type 1 diabetes is caused by the body's failed ability to make INSULIN. For this reason, people with Type 1 diabetes must take exogenous insulin to live. They may inject the insulin with syringes or an insulin pen or they may have an INSULIN PUMP that provides the needed insulin.

In general, WHITES/CAUCASIANS and HISPANICS are more likely to have Type 1 diabetes than are AFRICAN AMERICANS, ASIANS AND PACIFIC ISLANDERS, or AMERICAN INDIANS AND ALASKA NATIVES.

Some adolescents with Type 1 diabetes are at risk for developing EATING DISORDERS, particularly females in their early teens. Some girls or young women manipulate their insulin by taking a lower dose of insulin or not taking their insulin at all, in order to lose weight. One indicator of this behavior is weight loss in the face of an adolescent who is eating normally. The teenager may also have another form of eating disorder, called "bulimia," in which the person eats, sometimes to excess, and then induces vomiting.

In their 2005 article on "disordered eating behaviors" among youths with Type 1 diabetes, published in *Diabetes Educator,* Sarah Dion Kelly and colleagues discussed the underlying features of disordered eating (problematic eating that does not rise to the level of an eating disorder) as well as features of eating disorders, such as a poor body image and low self-esteem, combined with an extreme fear of gaining weight or a refusal to maintain the current body weight.

Some signs of disordered eating or eating disorders include unexplained hyperglycemia combined with a major body weight loss. The hemoglobin HgbA1c laboratory test can provide blood glucose data for the past three months, and it may also help to diagnose eating issues. Measures of serum electrolytes are also helpful; for example, the diagnosis of hypokalemia (below-normal potassium levels in the blood) may indicate the use or abuse of diuretics and self-induced vomiting. Individuals with anorexia nervosa may have hyponatremia, or below normal levels of sodium in the blood, due to excessive drinking of water to try to squelch the appetite. Recurrent cases of DIABETIC KETOACIDO-SIS (DKA) may also indicate an eating problem or failure to take insulin in an adolescent.

Once identified, the treatment of eating issues in youths with Type 1 diabetes involves a diabetes team as well as treatment by mental health professionals, and these physicians and other diabetes experts need to work together collaboratively. Kelly et al. say, "Treatment begins with emphasis on nutritional rehabilitation, weight restoration, and adequate diabetes control. Psychotherapy should begin immediately for the patient and family but is not effective for the patient when the patient is in a starvation mode."

In another study of adolescents and children with Type 1 diabetes and their weight-related concerns and behavior, Carol J. Howe and colleagues discussed these issues in the *Journal of the American Psychiatric Nurses Association* in 2008. They surveyed the subjects using a compilation of the Diabetes Eating Problem Survey and survey items from the Project EAT Survey. There were 295 respondents, including 158 males and 137 females, and the subjects ranged in age from students in grade five to college students. Most of the females (82.8 percent) had begun their menstrual cycles. The average BODY MASS INDEX (BMI) of the subjects was 23.3, which is in the normal range. (Underweight is a BMI of less than 18.5.) Most of the subjects (83.4 percent) were white, while 12.5 percent were black and 1 percent were Hispanic. Two-thirds of the subjects used insulin injections, using two to five injections daily, and the rest used an insulin pump.

The researchers found that nearly a third (30.8 percent) of the subjects reported trying to lose weight and 12.5 percent said that they were trying to gain weight. In general, the weight loss methods that the subjects endorsed were healthy choices, such as exercising, eating more fruits and vegetables and fewer sweets, and so on. However, some subjects also reported using unhealthy weight loss measures, such as fasting, eating little food, skipping meals, and smoking. Only a small percentage of the subjects reported using what the researchers classified as very unhealthy weight loss methods such as taking diet pills, vomiting, skipping insulin injections, or taking laxatives and diuretics.

There was a distinct difference in the percentages of specific behaviors exhibited by males and females as well as among subjects who were satisfied with their weight and those who were dissatisfied. For example, females wishing to lose weight were more likely to fast than males (6.7 percent of females vs. 2.6 percent of males); to eat very little food (20.7 percent of females vs. 3.9 percent of males); and to skip meals (16.3 percent of females vs. 5.2 percent of males). Females were also much more likely to use dangerous weight loss behaviors than males, such as using laxatives (2.9 percent of females versus 0 percent of males); to vomit (2.2 percent of females versus 0 percent of males); and to use less insulin than they needed (2.2 percent of females versus 0 percent of males).

In comparing those diabetics who were satisfied with their weight to those who were not, few of the satisfied subjects exhibited unhealthy or very unhealthy behaviors. For example, only 2.7 percent of the satisfied subjects fasted, compared to 10.4 percent of the dissatisfied subjects. In addition, 6.6 percent of the satisfied subjects reported eating very little, compared to the very high 59.8 percent of the dissatisfied subjects. It was also found that only 6.1 percent of the satisfied subjects skipped meals, compared to 22.1 percent of the dissatisfied youths.

None of the satisfied group used laxatives, compared to 5.2 percent of the dissatisfied group, and less than 1 percent reported vomiting or using less insulin, compared to 2.6 percent each of the dissatisfied group.

The researchers concluded, "All children and adolescents should be asked about weight satisfaction and weight perception. Older females with higher BMI and elevated A1C remain at increased risk. This population should receive routine education and counseling about healthy weight-control behaviors and review of the risks of unhealthy weight-control behaviors. Clinicians should discuss with parents the influence of media and parental attitudes on females' body satisfaction and subsequent weight-control behaviors. Formal classes for teens that allow group discussion of the pressure to be thin from family, peers, and socio-cultural messages, the dissonance between the super-model and the average person, and ways to negotiate all of this may prove to have impact. These classes should also include practical tips for incorporating healthy weight-control practices."

In another study which sought to identify adolescent characteristics linked to adverse outcomes of their Type 1 diabetes, Carla Johns and colleagues reported their findings in *Diabetes Educator* in 2008. The researchers obtained data from 108 adolescents and analyzed them based on the level of glycemic control, the number of hospitalizations the adolescents had had in the past year, and whether they injected their insulin or used an insulin pump. They also further analyzed the subjects by body mass index, insulin dose, calorie intake, annual family income, race, gender, and other factors.

The researchers found that the subjects who used an insulin pump were on lower insulin dosages and had better glucose control than the adolescents who injected their insulin. They also found that adolescents with inadequate glucose control were more likely to be members of an ethnic minority and to come from a single-parent lower-income family. However, poor adolescents who used insulin pumps had similar success with them as did wealthier adolescents using pumps.

One unique article discussed teacher victimizations of children and adolescents with Type 1 diabetes. For example, the authors cite one past shocking example of a teacher who ripped out a student's insulin pump, thinking it was a cell phone. In this study by Christine D. Peters and colleagues and reported in the *Journal of Child Health Care* in 2008, the subjects were 167 children and adolescents, ages eight to 17 years. Most (80.2 percent) were white, 13.8 percent were African American, 2.6 percent were Hispanic, and the rest were from other ethnic groups. None of the subjects used pump therapy or had serious psychopathology.

About 6 percent of the students reported that they avoided checking their blood sugar in school because the teacher could get angry, and 2 percent said that they often or always avoided giving themselves an insulin injection in school because the teacher might get angry. The researchers also found that youths who are visibly different from their peers (such as obese children) were more likely to report victimization by their teachers. They also found that youths and especially younger children victimized by teachers may avoid managing their diabetes in school.

The researchers said, "These avoidance behaviors may place youth at medical risk as their blood glucose levels may reach dangerously high or low levels without proper regulation."

Adolescents with Type 2 Diabetes

Formerly called "adult-onset diabetes" or "non-insulin-dependent diabetes mellitus" (NIDDM), Type 2 diabetes is a disease of insulin resistance and the inability to make enough insulin to normalize the blood glucose. This means that the body makes insulin, but for some reason, it is not used properly. Individuals with Type 2 diabetes must also test their blood glucose and follow appropriate nutrition and exercise plans. They may need to take oral medications or insulin to control the disease.

An increasing number of adolescents in the United States are developing classic Type 2 diabetes, particularly those who are obese. Some groups are at high risk for Type 2 diabetes; for example, American Indian teenagers have an elevated risk of developing Type 2 diabetes.

Teens with Type 2 diabetes are usually diagnosed between the ages of 12 and 14 years. Few of the oral medications for treating adult Type 2 diabetes have been tested on adolescents, but doctors must rely on these medications to treat children. Adolescents with Type 2 diabetes rarely need insulin, although insulin is an approved drug for children.

In a small study of 24 adolescents ages 12 to 21 years with Type 2 diabetes (mostly African American), researchers Shelagh A. Mulvaney and colleagues analyzed the self-management of diabetes from the adolescent perspective. They used small focus groups of three to six participants each. The researchers identified four primary domains that affected the self-management of the adolescents' diabetes, including adolescent psychosocial development, environmental influences, the roles of others with their diabetes, and the problem-solving and coping skills of the adolescent.

With regard to psychosocial development, the researchers further identified key issues affecting self-management, such as embarrassment/lack of normalcy, rebellion, and their peer relations. For example, with regard to embarrassment/ lack of normalcy, the researchers said, "Many participants stated they did not want friends to know [that they had diabetes] because friends would ask questions, express judgment, or have false beliefs about diabetes (e.g., that diabetes is contagious)."

With regard to rebellion, some adolescents reported an unwillingness to accept what adults told them and rejected the diabetes goals their parents promoted. Some of the adolescents said that they went so far as to purposely deceive their parents by taking the batteries out of their glucometer (the device that measures blood sugar) or by using another person's blood for a reading.

Many adolescents complained about school, which fit into the environmental context. The researchers said, "Negative behaviors on the part of teachers included stopping students from leaving class to check their blood and forcing a student to describe her diabetes in front of the class. One student could not check blood glucose at school because of a ban on needles. Participants generally agreed they did not want teachers to know they had diabetes."

With regard to problem-solving and coping behaviors, the adolescents reported many strategies, such as showing their friends how to check blood sugar, searching for information on the Internet, avoiding others when feeling down, playing with pets, and so forth.

Adolescents with diabetes may develop complications of diabetes, including DIABETIC RETINOPATHY, DIABETIC NEPHROPATHY, and DIABETIC NEUROPATHY, although typically these problems are not seen until after five to 10 years of diabetes and after puberty. Eye exams are recommended after the age of 10 in those with Type 1 diabetes and at the time of diagnosis with Type 2 diabetes. Blood pressure should be optimized (< 95 percent for age) and urine screened for microalbuminuria. LDL cholesterol should be less than 100 mg/dL and treated at first with diet and in some instances with medications if diet fails.

Treatment goals for glycemic control should be individualized in adolescents, but if the risk of hypoglycemia is under control then pre-meal glucose levels should be in the 90–130 mg/dL range and HbA1c less than 7.5 percent or should be as near normal as can be safely achieved.

Diagnosing Teenagers

Adolescents are diagnosed for diabetes in the same manner as adults are, based on their symptoms and the results of blood tests. Often it may not be clear at the start whether the child has Type 1 or Type 2 diabetes, and special blood tests are needed to measure diabetes indicators: islet cell antibodies, anti-GAD antibodies, and C-peptide levels. Some children and adolescents are diagnosed with diabetes for the first time when they are acutely ill, as with the case of diabetic ketoacidosis or severe HYPOGLYCEMIA.

Risk of Diabetic Ketoacidosis

Diabetic ketoacidosis is a dangerous result of diabetes that is out of control and can result in COMA and even death. In addition to occurring in undiagnosed adolescents, it may also occur in adolescents who know that they have diabetes but as mentioned earlier, they are purposely withholding insulin, possibly as a consequence of an eating disorder and/or an attempt to lose weight.

The other reason for DKA may be that the adolescent also has another illness. This is why it is so important to establish SICK DAY RULES. For example, many people including adolescents mistakenly believe that when people with diabetes are sick, then they do not have to be careful about their diet or take their medications. This is wrong. In fact, glycemic control is critical when one is ill because of the severe stress that the body is under. Patients usually need to check their blood glucose levels more frequently, monitor their urine for ketones, and may actually require more insulin even when they are eating poorly. If the teenager is so ill that he or she cannot eat or drink (and thus, is susceptible to DEHYDRATION), the risk for DKA increases further.

In several small studies of teenagers with diabetes who died, the majority of deaths were attributed to DKA (about 85 percent), and small percentages were attributed to hypoglycemia. Since hypoglycemia is another indicator of glucose levels that are out of control (at the low end of the scale), this further underlines the importance of monitoring glucose levels at home, especially when the person with diabetes is ill.

General Coping Difficulties and Possible Solutions

Because teenagers are often extremely self-conscious about their own bodies and their behaviors, it can be difficult for them to deal with their diabetes or even to admit that they have the illness at all. They may resent the questions of their parents or others about their diet and blood-testing regimens, even when those questions are reasonable.

Possible management solutions are alternative options to traditional medical emergency IDs, such as the option of shoe tags. Parents may also use the teen's own self-consciousness to encourage the adolescent to rotate the site of the injection; for example, by pointing out that rotating a site is less likely to make it noticeable.

Adolescents in the early years may be defiant and uncooperative, refusing to adhere to meal plans and becoming angry at reminders to test their blood. Experts say that it may be helpful to have the teenager see her diabetes team by herself. Counseling may also be helpful, because the counselor may be able to help the teenager cope with anger. Some experts say that some teenagers have a fatalistic view about their illness and mistakenly believe that they are doomed to die young. This may also be an excuse to avoid testing their blood and injecting insulin.

Teens who are 15 to 16 years old have other issues, such as an increased demand for independence and more instances of boundary testing. Teens of this age may experiment with tobacco, alcohol, or drugs. They may also become sexually active. To help teens of this age, experts recommend involving them more in decision making and using negotiation to affect behavior. Teens with diabetes should also be educated on substance abuse and how drugs, alcohol, and tobacco could affect them in relation to their disease. Teens also need to be educated about sexuality.

Older teens (ages 17 to 18) are often idealistic, and they may be interested in becoming involved at the local level with organizations such as the American Diabetes Association. Teens of this age are also beginning to think about their future and seek greater independence. Adolescents of this age may wish to see the doctor on their own. They also continue to need education about their diabetes. Adults may think teenagers already know what they need to know about diabetes but sometimes important issues that were discussed earlier may not have made an impression or were not understood at the time.

Attitude Is Key

Adolescents and children who believe that they can manage their diabetes have measurably better glucose levels than teenagers who believe that their disease controls them and that there is little they can do about it. There is an apparent self-fulfilling prophecy at work: those teenagers who think they can control their diabetes are successful at controlling it. Those who believe that there is little or nothing they can do about their illness often do not bother to take appropriate actions to manage their illness. As a result, they have poor control and they are at greater risk for consequences.

See also CHILDREN WITH DIABETES, SCHOOL-AGE; INSULIN; INSULIN PUMP; MEN WITH DIABETES; WOMEN WITH DIABETES.

American Diabetes Association. "Standards of Medical Care in Diabetes—2008." *Diabetes Care* 31, Suppl 1 (2008): S12–54.

Howe, Carol J., et al. "Weight-Related Concerns and Behaviors in Children and Adolescents with Type 1 Diabetes." *The Journal of the American Psychiatric Nurses Association* 13, no. 6 (2008): 376–385.

Johns, Carla, Melissa Spezia Faulkner, and Lauretta Quinn. "Characteristics of Adolescents with Type 1 Diabetes Who Exhibit Adverse Outcomes." *Diabetes Educator* 34 (2008): 874–885.

Kelly, Sarah Dion, et al. "Disordered Eating Behaviors in Youth with Type 1 Diabetes." *Diabetes Educator* 34, no. 4 (2005): 572–583.

Mulvaney, Shelagh A., et al. "Self-Management in Type 2 Diabetes: The Adolescent Perspective." *Diabetes Educator* 34 (2008): 674–682.

Peters, Christine D., et al. "Victimization of Youth with Type-1 Diabetes by Teachers: Relations with Adherence and Metabolic Control." *Journal of Child Health Care* 12 (2008): 209–220.

adult-onset diabetes   One of the former names for Type 2 diabetes, also formerly known as non-insulin diabetes mellitus or NIDDM. The name was changed because it is possible for the "onset" to occur in childhood or adolescence. In fact, increasing numbers of children in North America are being diagnosed with the disease, particularly if they are obese, sedentary, and have a family history of diabetes. Type 2 diabetes is as serious an illness as is Type 1 diabetes and should be treated as aggressively.

By definition, patients with this illness still make some insulin and may be treated with diet, exercise, and pills. In some cases, they may also require insulin. Patients with Type 2 diabetes both make insufficient insulin and are unable to properly use it.

If people with Type 2 diabetes are ill or stressed enough, they can develop DIABETIC KETOACIDOSIS (DKA), although this occurs much less commonly than among patients who have Type 1 diabetes. With very high glucose levels, these patients can also develop HYPEROSMOLAR COMA, a life-threatening condition.

See also TYPE 2 DIABETES.

African Americans with diabetes   Blacks in the United States who suffer from either Type 1 or Type 2 diabetes. According to the Centers for Disease Control and Prevention (CDC), 14.7 percent of all non-Hispanic blacks ages 20 years and older have diabetes, or 3.7 million people. Black women are at particular risk for the development of Type 2 diabetes, although black men also are at risk for diabetes.

African Americans with diabetes also have a higher prevalence of complications that are directly linked to diabetes than do individuals of other races and ethnicities (with the exception of American Indians, a group that also has a very high risk of complications) for several basic reasons. Some of the key factors that are involved in this elevated prevalence include:

- a genetic predisposition to diabetes
- a greater prevalence or predisposition to obesity
- high blood pressure that is more difficult to control
- high glucose levels and worse glycemic control compared to other groups
- a lower education level about diabetes (less knowledge about the risks and complications that are associated with the disease, which may affect medication and nutritional adherence and other factors)

Blacks in United States Have Higher Risk for Diabetes than Whites

Individuals who are of African-American descent have about twice the risk of developing Type 2 diabetes than do whites in North America. In addition, African-American children and adolescents, particularly when they are obese, are also at a high risk for developing Type 2 diabetes. However, African-American children in the United States are much less likely to have Type 1 diabetes than white or Hispanic children.

Age is another risk factor in the incidence of diabetes. Middle-aged and older African Americans are more likely to have been diagnosed with diabetes than are their younger same-race counterparts, just as the rates of diabetes increase with age in other racial and ethnic groups. However, black women are at greater risk for the disease than WOMEN WITH DIABETES of other races and ethnicities.

African-American Youths with Diabetes

In a study of diabetes among youths of different races and ethnicities, Elizabeth J. Mayer-Davis and colleagues reported on their findings of diabetes among African Americans in *Diabetes Care* in 2009. The prevalence of Type 1 diabetes was very low; for example, among black youths ages zero to nine years, the researchers found a prevalence of less than 1 percent, and among those ages 10 to 19 years, the prevalence of Type 1 diabetes was 2 percent. They also found that nearly half (44.7 percent) of African-American youths with Type 1 diabetes were overweight or obese.

In considering the prevalence of Type 2 diabetes among African youths, the researchers found that among youths ages 10 to 19 years, the prevalence was 1 percent. (Type 2 diabetes was not evaluated in youths under the age of 10 years.) Among the youths with Type 2 diabetes, more than 90 percent were either overweight or obese. The researchers also found that Type 2 diabetes among black youths older than 10 years was greater than twice as prominent among girls as among boys.

The researchers also found a high prevalence of elevated low density lipoproteins (LDL—the "bad" cholesterol) among the youths with either Type 1 or Type 2 diabetes; more than 90 percent had an LDL cholesterol of greater than 70 mg/dL and more than 60 percent had an LDL cholesterol of greater than 100 mg/dL. The researchers also found a low level of high density lipoprotein (HDL, the "good" cholesterol). These findings may be an indicator and a warning sign of risks for future cardiovascular disease.

The majority of the youths reported a low intake of fruits, vegetables, and dairy products, and many were physically inactive.

Socioeconomic Status May Be a Leveler for Everyone

Some researchers have noted that when only socioeconomic status and environmental factors are the factors that are considered, then blacks and whites have about the same prevalence of diabetes. For example, in their 2009 article in the *Journal of General Internal Medicine,* Thomas A. LaVeist and colleagues looked at poor blacks as well as poor whites from the same area. They found that the racial disparities in the prevalence of diabetes disappeared in this case. (It is unknown if wealthy blacks have about the same rate of diabetes as wealthy whites, but it seems probable.)

High Risk of Complications from Diabetes

African Americans with diabetes are twice as likely to suffer from BLINDNESS and three to five times as likely as whites to experience such severe kidney disease as END-STAGE RENAL DISEASE. According to the National Kidney Disease Education Program (NKDEP), among new patients whose kidney failure was caused by diabetes, nearly a third (31.3 percent) are African Americans.

The risk of suffering from AMPUTATION of a lower extremity such as a foot or leg is twice as high among African Americans as that for whites. In addition, blacks have a higher rate of DIABETIC RETINOPATHY than whites. In general, the medical care that diabetic blacks receive is inferior to the care that is received by whites, according to many studies, including a study by Loes C. Lanting in *Diabetes Care* in 2005. The reasons are unknown but may be less access, education, and financial resources.

African Americans with diabetes also have a higher rate of death from DIABETIC KETOACIDOSIS (DKA) than whites, according to the Centers for Disease Control and Prevention; for example, in 2001 (the latest data as of this writing in 2009), 56.5 black males per 100,000 males with diabetes died from DKA, as did 22.6 per 100,000 black females with diabetes. In contrast, however, the rate for white males with diabetes who died from DKA, was 21.7 per 100,000 males, and it was 15.3 per 100,000 females with diabetes. (Thus again illustrating that African Americans receive worse medical care or have less access to care than whites.)

As a result of the frequency and severity of complications that African Americans with diabetes can incur, particularly among females, African Americans need to be very vigilant about the prospect of diabetes and educated about associated risks and complications. Screening should begin in early adulthood if there is a family history of diabetes as well as other risk factors such as obesity.

Study after study has shown that EARLY DETECTION can prevent or diminish the impact of the severe complications that can result when diabetes has gone untreated for many years.

Interventions May Decrease ER Visits

A study published in a 2009 issue of *Archives of Internal Medicine* by Tiffany L. Gary and colleagues indicated that an intensive intervention that was culturally tailored and provided by a nurse care manager and a community health care worker reduced the use of the emergency room by 24 percent among 542 African Americans with diabetes in Baltimore, Maryland, who were followed up after 24 months. The "cultural tailoring" included the use of community health workers who were "part of participants' cultural group and spent time in participants' homes, received extensive training to enhance communication of shared experiences and personalization of interventions in their roles as educators and problem solvers, which may have contributed to the findings." They also noted that community health workers have been effective in other disease settings.

The "interventionists" (health care workers in the intervention group) triaged the diabetes patients based on their level of glycemic control and other issues; for example, a preprandial (before meal) blood glucose of 350 mg/dL was considered "very poor" and led the workers to call the subjects, counsel them to see their physician within seven days, plan a follow-up, and take other actions. The intervention group concentrated on such issues as nutrition, medication adherence, appointment adherence, foot care, and socioeconomic issues. If glucose control was rated as very poor, then the interventionist would seek to discover whether the patient understood the drug regimen, had any trouble obtaining the medication, or other issues. If the patient did not understand the regimen, then it would be discussed with the subject.

See also AMERICAN INDIANS/ALASKA NATIVES; ASIANS/PACIFIC ISLANDER AMERICANS; DEATH; HISPANICS/LATINOS; WHITE/CAUCASIANS.

Gary, Tiffany L., et al. "The Effects of a Nurse Care Manager and a Community Health Worker Team on Diabetic Control, Emergency Department Visits, and Hospitalizations among Urban Urban African Americans with Type 2 Diabetes Mellitus: A Randomized Controlled Trial." *Archives of Internal Medicine* 169, no. 19 (2009): 1,788–1,794.

Lanting, Loes C., et al. "Ethnic Differences in Mortality, End-Stage Complications, and Quality of Care Among Diabetic Patients." *Diabetes Care* 28, no. 9 (2005): 2,280–2,288.

LaVeist, Thomas A., et al. "Environmental and Socio-Economic Factors as Contributors to Racial Disparities in Diabetes Prevalence." *Journal of General Internal Medicine* 24, no. 10 (2009): 1,144–1,148.

Mayer-Davis, Elizabeth J., et al. "Diabetes in African American Youth: Prevalence, Incidence, and Clinical Characteristics: The SEARCH for Diabetes in Youth Study." *Diabetes Care* 32, Supplement 2 (2009): S112–S122.

age/aging and diabetes   The impact of growing older on the incidence of diabetes as well as how older people are affected by diabetes. In general, diabetes is an increasing risk with aging, rising with middle age and reaching its peak in individuals who are over age 60. However, people of any age, including children, may develop diabetes.

Aging also presents a risk factor for people with diabetes to develop COMPLICATIONS that can occur from diabetes. For example, the risks for CARDIOVASCULAR DISEASE, DIABETIC NEPHROPATHY, and DIABETIC RETINOPATHY all increase with age, as do risks for many other illnesses that are directly and indirectly associated with diabetes.

In the past, diabetes was primarily perceived as either a problem for children and adolescents, hence "juvenile-onset diabetes" or for middle-aged or older adults, hence "adult-onset diabetes." However, researchers have learned that adults may have the disease diagnosed primarily in children—and children may have the form of diabetes found in older adults.

As a result, rather than defining diabetes in terms of age alone, it is defined in terms of its primary symptoms. Type 1 diabetes is an illness in which the individual's body stops producing insulin and, as a result, he or she needs supplemental insulin in order to live. This condition is usually first diagnosed in children or adolescents but it may also be found in adults of any age.

Type 2 diabetes is a disease in which the person's body produces some insulin but the body fails to use it properly (INSULIN RESISTANCE) and the amount of insulin is inadequate to normalize the blood glucose (BETA CELL dysfunction). Both abnormalities worsen with age and are also modified by environmental factors, such as weight and activity levels, as well as medications and intercurrent illnesses. Type 2 diabetes is primarily diagnosed in middle-aged and older adults but is also on the rise among children and adolescents.

The incidence of Type 2 diabetes has increased and a study of nearly 150,000 individuals in the US, published in a 2000 issue of *Diabetes Care,* revealed an increase in the overall prevalence of 33 percent. The greatest increase was among people ages 30–39 years, where the prevalence increased dramatically by 76 percent. Researchers believe that most of this increase could be attributed to an increased incidence of obesity among the afflicted individuals.

See also ADOLESCENTS WITH DIABETES; CHILDREN WITH DIABETES, SCHOOL-AGE; ELDERLY.

See AMERICAN INDIANS/ALASKA NATIVES.

Mokdad, Ali H., et al. "Diabetes Trends in the U.S.: 1990–1998," *Diabetes Care* 23, no. 9 (September 2000): 1,278–1,283.

albuminuria   Albumin is a protein that is sometimes found in the urine and that may be noted in the urine of people who have had diabetes for many years. The presence of albumin in the urine can be a sign of HYPERTENSION (high blood pressure), and may also be an indicator or a possible precursor of kidney problems. It is very important to determine whether the person has hypertension, because when uncontrolled hypertension is combined with diabetes, it can lead to a rapid decline in kidney function. Yet if hypertension is identified, it is eminently treatable.

People with diabetes should have an examination for macroalbuminuria (large amounts of albumin in the urine) at least once a year. This can be done at the time of an office visit by dipping a REAGENT STRIP into a small amount of the patient's urine, to check for protein. If that examination is negative, then an examination for microalbuminuria (small amounts of albumin in the urine) should be performed. This can be done in the doctor's office with a different type of test or it can be sent to the laboratory for evaluation. Often the doctor may repeat this test on several occasions because there are several confounding variables such as fever, exercise, uncontrolled blood glucose, and other factors that may temporarily increase the amount of protein or albumin in the urine. Research published late in 2009 revealed that individuals who have Type 2 diabetes and albuminuria may be at risk for a silent subclinical cerebral infarction (STROKE). Further future research should provide more information and details.

See also PROTEINURIA.

alcohol   Wine, beer, or distilled spirits. According to the U.S. Department of Agriculture, the moderate use of alcohol is safe and without significant negative effect in patients with well-managed diabetes. Moderate consumption is defined as no more than one drink per day for women and no more than two drinks per day for men. A "drink" is defined as 12 ounces of beer or 5 ounces of wine or 1.5 ounces of 80 proof spirit.

An estimated 75 percent of the population in the United States drink alcohol and individuals in many other countries also imbibe alcoholic beverages. Alcohol affects people with diabetes beyond the intoxicating effects that alcohol can have on everyone. For example, alcohol has little or no nutritional value (although it does have calories), while at the same time, it decreases the liver's ability to produce glucose. It should also be noted that calories from alcohol increase the risk of OBESITY, yet another factor that is strongly linked to Type 2 diabetes.

As a result, if a person with diabetes who is drinking alcohol does not also consume food, then he or she risks developing HYPOGLYCEMIA. A further complication is the fact that often the effects of hypoglycemia are misinterpreted as intoxication, by the individual or by other people, and thus treatment does not ensue. This can be very dangerous for the person with diabetes. Note: if children with diabetes accidentally or purposely ingest alcohol, they may also suffer a severe bout of hypoglycemia.

Hypoglycemia and Chronic Alcoholism

Severe hypoglycemia is one consequence of chronic alcohol abuse by patients who have diabetes. A large study, reported in a 2000 issue of *Diabetes Care*, indicated that a regular high level of alcohol intake is associated with the later development of Type 2 diabetes in men. (A high

alcohol intake may also have the same effect on women, but such a study has not yet been reported, as of this writing.)

In this study, 8,663 nondiabetic men ages 30–79 were evaluated according to alcohol intake and other factors. The men were followed for six years and 149 of them developed Type 2 diabetes. The men were divided into five groups, including nondrinkers and four quartiles of drinkers.

The quartiles of drinkers were as follows: Quartile 1 drank between 1.0 to 61.8 grams per week. Those in Quartile 2 drank from 61.9 to 122.7 grams per week. Those in Quartile 3 drank 122.8 to 276.6 grams per week. Lastly, those in Quartile 4 drank any amount over 276.6 grams weekly.

The researchers found a statistical link between alcohol consumption at the higher quartiles and the subsequent development of Type 2 diabetes. The men in the third and fourth quartiles had a 2.2 to 2.4 greater risk of developing diabetes than the other groups, with the highest risk faced by heavy drinkers.

Interestingly, the nondrinkers had a 1.8 greater risk of developing diabetes, which the researchers could not explain, although they hypothesized that perhaps the nondrinkers were recovering alcoholics or were ill. The risk for the moderate drinkers of developing diabetes was actually lower than for the nondrinkers. Based on this study, it appears that excessive consumption of alcohol is a risk factor for the development of Type 2 diabetes among males.

In this study, heavy drinkers were more likely to also be heavy smokers. Smoking is yet another risk factor for the development of Type 2 diabetes.

Other studies have shown that moderate drinkers face an increased risk for developing Type 2 diabetes over nondrinkers. It is also known that excessive alcohol consumption can contribute to obesity.

Expert Advice

According to British authors Williams and Pickup, in their book, *Handbook of Diabetes*, alcohol should be "forbidden completely in those with hyperlipidaemia [hyperlipidemia], hypertension, pancreatic disease, or recurrent, severe hypoglycaemia [hypoglycemia]." They also note that alcohol consumption is associated with an increase in ERECTILE DYSFUNCTION (impotence).

If people with diabetes do choose to consume alcoholic beverages, experts offer the following basic tips:

- Do not drink more than one or two drinks per evening.
- Mix your own drinks so that you know exactly what is in them.
- Understand that some beers have a high alcohol content, as do liqueurs.
- Wear an emergency medical identification bracelet, necklace, or anklet, so that you are identified as a person with diabetes.
- Bring a fast-acting carbohydrate source such as juice or specially prepared items for people with diabetes, should you develop hypoglycemia.
- Consume food to avoid the risk of hypoglycemia as well as decrease the risk for intoxication.
- Check glucose levels every few hours.
- Learn what medications can have bad or even dangerous interactions when mixed with alcohol since many common medications for diabetes should not be mixed with alcohol.

See also ALCOHOL ABUSE/ALCOHOLISM.

Wei, Ming, M.D., et al. "Alcohol Intake and Incidence of Type 2 Diabetes in Men." *Diabetes Care* 23, no. 1 (January 2000): 18–22.

Williams, Gareth, and John C. Pickup. *Handbook of Diabetes*. London, England: Blackwell, 1999.

Zielke, J. "Alcohol: A Primer: How Does Alcohol Affect Diabetes?" *Diabetes Forecast* 52, no. 3 (1999): 64–66.

alcohol abuse/alcoholism   Excessive consumption of or addiction to alcohol. Alcoholism is also known as *alcohol dependence*. Alcohol abuse

and alcoholism together are known as *alcohol use disorders*. An abuser of alcohol may develop alcoholism if the abuse occurs on a regular basis and meets other criteria for alcohol dependence, such as *tolerance* (the need for consuming greater amounts of alcohol to achieve the same level of intoxication). Heavy drinking is very risky for a person with diabetes because he or she may fail to take needed diabetes medications appropriately as well as incur all the risks of those who drink to excess, such as suffering from accidents, injuries, and poor health consequences. In addition, alcohol interacts with some diabetes medications; for example, alcohol combined with some medications may lead to HYPOGLYCEMIA as well as other side effects. (See the table on page 17.)

According to the National Epidemiologic Survey on Alcohol and Related Conditions (NESARC) data for 2001–02, an estimated 4.7 percent of the U.S. population ages 18 years and older fit the criteria over 12 months for alcohol abuse and 3.8 percent meet the criteria for alcohol dependence. In addition, the lifetime rates (of ever having these disorders) were 17.8 percent for alcohol abuse and 12.5 percent for alcohol dependence. This means that an estimated 11.1 million people in the United States will have a 12-month alcohol abuse diagnosis in 2010, and an estimated 8.9 million will have a 12-month alcohol dependence—for a total of 20 million people with an alcohol use disorder. (An alcohol use disorder is either alcohol abuse or alcohol dependence.)

In one study of 89 patients with Type 2 diabetes published in the *Journal of the American Board of Family Practice* in 2004 and reported by researchers Michael Fleming, M.D., and Marlon Mundt, the researchers used an alcohol biomarker (carbohydrate-deficient transferrin or CDT) to detect alcohol abuse and alcoholism among their subjects. They found that the CDT test was useful in detecting or confirming heavy drinking in patients with both Type 2 diabetes and hypertension.

There were 209 patients with hypertension and diabetes, 299 with hypertension alone, and

TABLE 1: POSSIBLE ALCOHOL INTERACTIONS WITH DIABETES MEDICATIONS

Brand Name	Generic Name	Possible Reactions
Glucophage	Metformin	Abnormally low blood sugar levels, flushing reaction (nausea, vomiting, headache, rapid heartbeat, sudden changes in blood pressure)
Micronase	Glyburide	
Orinase	Tolbutamide	

Source: Adapted from National Institute on Alcohol Abuse and Alcoholism. *Harmful Interactions: Mixing Alcohol with Medicines.* Bethesda, Md.: National Institutes of Health, 2007. Available online. URL: http://pubs.niaaa.nih.gov/publications/Medicine/medicine.htm. Downloaded June 27, 2009.

202 subjects with neither hypertension nor diabetes. Interestingly, the researchers found a higher rate of alcohol abuse in these groups than identified in the NESARC research. According to the Fleming and Mundt research, of those subjects with diabetes only, 28 percent had a lifetime diagnosis of alcohol abuse and 11 percent had a lifetime diagnosis of alcoholism. In considering current alcohol issues, the researchers found that none of the subjects with diabetes were current alcohol abusers, while 1 percent were alcoholics.

Of those with both diabetes and hypertension, the rates of alcohol use disorders were high for alcohol abuse: 35 percent had a lifetime diagnosis of alcohol abuse, while 12 percent had a lifetime diagnosis of alcoholism.

Interestingly, the subjects with *neither* diabetes nor hypertension had higher rates of both alcohol abuse and alcoholism than those with only diabetes or with diabetes and hypertension; this group had a 42 percent rate of lifetime alcohol abuse and an 18 percent rate of alcoholism. The reasons for this finding are unknown.

The researchers also looked at the number of drinks that were consumed by their subjects and said, "Assuming there are 15 million patients with diabetes and 50 million patients with hypertension in the United States, the findings of our study suggest there are 1.35 million patients with diabetes and 7.5 million patients with hypertension who drink too much (28 or more drinks per month) who could benefit from brief physician advice."

Symptoms and Diagnostic Path

According to the National Institute on Alcohol Abuse and Alcoholism (NIAAA), in the United States, alcohol abuse is characterized by a drinking pattern that includes at least one of the following aspects over a 12-month period:

- failure to perform responsibilities at work, home, or school
- consumption of alcohol while driving a car or arrest for driving under the influence of alcohol or for assaulting someone while under the influence of alcohol
- consumption of alcohol despite relationship problems that are caused or made worse by alcohol

Alcohol abuse may escalate into alcoholism, a disease characterized by an urgent craving for and dependency on alcohol and a tolerance to alcohol, or a need for greater amounts of alcohol in order to achieve the same level of intoxication. Alcoholism is also characterized by symptoms of withdrawal when the person does not drink, for any reason (whether he or she chooses not to drink or for some reason the person cannot drink).

Alcoholism is a serious disease and one that is very dangerous for people with diabetes. It affects and can damage virtually every organ in the body, including the pancreas, the brain, the stomach, the heart, and all other vital organs. The person with diabetes is already at risk for many diseases and disorders, and excessive drinking further exacerbates these risks. Note that according to Michael S. Gold, M.D., author of *The Encyclopedia of Alcoholism and Alcohol Abuse,* up to 80 percent of drinkers also smoke, and smoking is very dangerous for individuals with diabetes, causing many health risks. Smoking has been proven to accentuate the complications caused by diabetes.

Treatment Options and Outlook

People with diabetes who have a problem with alcohol abuse or full-blown alcoholism should inform their physicians. Many people are embarrassed or afraid to report this behavior or to ask for help. The doctor may recommend a therapist who is an expert at treating people with alcohol-related problems. He or she may also advise that the individual attend support group meetings or self-help groups such as Alcoholics Anonymous. The doctor should also explain the health risks to the diabetic patient and recommend that drinking be cut back, with a follow-up date to discuss the subject. This is sometimes referred to as a "brief intervention."

In their article on "at-risk drinking" among diabetics, published in *Substance Abuse* in 2009, authors Susan E. Ramsey and Patricia A. Engler noted studies indicating that drinking is associated with inferior treatment adherence by individuals with diabetes as well as by poorer outcomes. They recommended that primary care physicians intervene to identify problem drinking among their patients and also use brief interventions to help patients change their behavior.

Ramsey and Engler said, "It is important to note that screening for at-risk drinking can be done very simply by asking patients how often they consume alcohol and how many drinks they typically have when they do consume alcohol." Studies have shown that brief interventions are effective when they involve feedback about how drinking affects health and include advice on how to reduce drinking and set goals to cut back on drinking. Even a five- to 10-minute session on advice on drinking that is delivered by primary care providers as part of a routine medical advice has had a positive effect on heavy drinkers.

Yet the authors also note that many physicians are reluctant to become involved in this issue, sometimes because of a fear of offending the patient and sometimes by the erroneous belief that if the patient is a young person, this behavior will inevitably be "outgrown."

Some people need intensive outpatient or inpatient care for their alcoholism. People with diabetes who enter such facilities should be sure that the facility is made aware of the diabetes diagnosis and the medications that the person takes, as well as the individual's complete medical history.

Some doctors believe that people with alcohol abuse problems are "self-medicating" because of an underlying problem with DEPRESSION. If so, the doctor may believe that a course of an antidepressant or another medication would be helpful. However, it should be noted that antidepressants may also interact with alcohol, causing drowsiness and dizziness and an increased risk for health risks or even death from an overdose.

There are also some medications that have shown success in decreasing the desire for drinking in some people who have problems with alcoholism, including such medications as naltrexone and acamprosate. One drawback is that these medications can be expensive and there is often poor compliance with taking them. Of course, it is essential that the person with diabetes verifies with the prescribing physician (as well as with the pharmacist) that such medications will not interfere with any medicine that is taken for diabetes.

Risk Factors and Preventive Measures

Individuals with a family history of alcohol abuse or dependence have an increased risk for developing an alcohol use disorder. There are no known preventive measures to the development of alcohol abuse or alcoholism, but if an alcohol use disorder develops, it is important to treat the problem. To avoid low blood sugar, diabetics should never drink alcohol on an empty stomach. They should also limit themselves to one drink if a woman and two drinks if a man. Even drinking as little as two ounces of alcohol (about two drinks) on an empty stomach can lead to very low blood sugar.

Chronic Risks of Alcohol Abuse/Alcoholism for People with Diabetes

One reason heavy drinking is particularly perilous for people with diabetes is that those who are heavy alcohol consumers may not consume any or enough food. As a result, in addition to the impaired judgment that all people who abuse alcohol experience, the person with diabetes also risks the development of hypoglycemia, which may be severe.

In addition, chronic alcohol abuse increases the risk of HYPOGLYCEMIC UNAWARENESS, when the intoxicated person does not recognize the classic signs of hypoglycemia, such as a racing heart, sweatiness, and other symptoms. Because he is unaware of these signs, he will not take appropriate actions such as drinking fruit juice or consuming special foods that are designed to combat hypoglycemia. As a result, the problem can escalate further and develop into a medical emergency.

It is also possible for a person with diabetes to become both severely intoxicated and also hypoglycemic, and yet not receive treatment from others in the environment who do not know about the person's diabetes or who may be unfamiliar with hypoglycemia. They may mistake hypoglycemic symptoms or even unconsciousness as a common result of excessive drinking. Thus, they fail to recognize a hypoglycemic crisis. (This could also be a mistake made by law enforcement people or even paramedics.) This is yet another reason why all persons with diabetes should wear a medical emergency identification in the form of a bracelet, necklace, anklet, or other easily visible item.

In some cases, the person with hypoglycemia may be asked to take a blood or a breath test for alcohol if he or she has some of the signs that may also indicate excessive drinking, such as slurred speech or confusion. The person should agree to the test because diabetes alone will not affect the results of a test for alcohol, even if the person is having a diabetic reaction or has a fruity smell to the breath because of high ketone levels. If asked to take a test for alcohol, the diabetic person who is not intoxicated and who has a choice should always choose a blood test because health care providers can also check the blood levels of glucose and ketones.

Among those who *do* eat normally, chronic alcohol consumption may result in HYPERGLYCEMIA, although researchers are not sure if one specific mechanism is to blame. The hyperglycemia may be the result of biochemical interactions in the liver or pancreas, or it could be attributed to the failure of heavy drinkers to take their prescribed medications. Probably the hyperglycemia results from a combination of causes.

Alcohol abuse causes disease Some studies have indicated that heavy alcohol consumption may lead to the development of Type 2 diabetes. Chronic and excessive alcohol consumption may also cause a variety of other diseases, most notably pancreatitis or cirrhosis of the liver. Pancreatitis may lead to the development of Type 1 diabetes because the islet cells in the pancreas are destroyed by excessive drinking. Thus, the person who formerly had Type 2 diabetes will then develop Type 1 diabetes, necessitating the use of insulin.

Alcoholism is also linked to the development of hypertension, heart disease, and many other illnesses. Excessive drinking is linked to the development of colorectal cancer. Female alcoholics are at risk for breast cancer. Women at risk for breast cancer because of a family history or a personal history should avoid all alcohol because even moderate drinking can cause breast cancer when there is a genetic risk for the disease.

Adolescents who drink When a teenager has diabetes and then complicates his or her illness with alcohol abuse, very severe complications, up to and including death, may be the end result. The most common complications of alcohol abuse among teenagers with diabetes are either DIABETIC KETOACIDOSIS (DKA) or hypoglycemia.

Peer pressure is a major problem for many teenagers, and it is also a driving force leading adolescents to drink alcohol, smoke, and use illegal drugs. Adolescents with diabetes may already feel out of the mainstream because of their disease, especially when they must frequently test their blood and inject themselves with insulin, and thus, it may be hard for them to resist social pressure to abuse alcohol and drugs. Parents who think that their children may be abusing alcohol need to consult with physicians and counselors immediately, particularly when that child also has diabetes. Even if parents are certain that their children do not drink, they should still educate them about the risks of alcohol abuse.

Medication interactions Many people who take medication on a regular basis do not realize that when they consume alcohol, the combination of the drug and the alcohol can sometimes cause very serious side effects. The medication and alcohol interact with each other even when they are not consumed at the same time, because many medications stay in the system for hours.

People with diabetes may take other medications for illnesses such as hypertension, arthritis, or other medical problems they may have. These medications may also interact negatively with alcohol. Even a medication as seemingly harmless as acetaminophen (Tylenol) can result in a harmful reaction when combined with excessive amounts of alcohol. Excessive alcohol intake with or without liver disease can lead to an increased risk of lactic acidosis in patients on METFORMIN (Glucophage).

Binge Drinking

Some individuals may engage in binge drinking, or drinking five or more drinks on at least one occasion in the past month. The individual may not fit the criteria for alcohol abuse or alcoholism, but binge drinking is still very dangerous for the person with diabetes.

In their article for the *Journal of the American Medical Association* in 2003, Timothy S. Naimi, M.D., and colleagues say, "Adverse health effects specifically associated with binge drinking include unintentional injuries (e.g., motor vehicle crashes, falls, drowning, hypothermia,

and burns), suicide, sudden infant death syndrome, alcohol poisoning, hypertension, acute myocardial infarction [heart attack], gastritis, pancreatitis, sexually transmitted disease, meningitis, and poor control of diabetes."

See also ALCOHOL.

Gold, Michael S., M.D., and Christine Adamec. *The Encyclopedia of Alcoholism and Alcohol Abuse.* New York: Facts On File, Inc., 2010.

Naimi, Timothy S., M.D., et al. "Binge Drinking Among U.S. Adults." *Journal of the American Medical Association* 289, no. 13 (2003): 70–75.

Ramsey, Susan E., and Patricia A. Engler. "At-Risk Drinking Among Diabetic Patients." *Substance Abuse: Research and Treatment* 3 (2009): 15–23.

alternative medicine/complementary medicine Nontraditional, nonprescribed medications, remedies, and treatments. Alternative medicine also includes treatments such as acupuncture, chiropractic, massage therapy, yoga, and other forms of therapies that need not generally be ordered by physicians (although occasionally such treatments are ordered by doctors). Alternative medicine is extremely popular among the general population, both with and without diabetes, as evidenced by the billions of dollars spent on alternative medications by consumers; for example, Americans spent $23.7 billion on dietary supplements in 2007 alone, according to the General Accounting Office (GAO).

A dietary supplement is defined by the federal government as a product that is intended for ingestion to supplement the diet, is labeled as a dietary supplement, and is not represented as a conventional food or an item of a meal. In 1994, there were about 4,000 dietary supplements available to consumers; by 2008, there were 76,000 dietary supplements available to consumers, according to the GAO.

The National Center for Health Statistics reports that Americans spent $33.9 billion on visits to alternative medicine practitioners as well as on purchases of products, classes, and materials in 2007.

Alternative remedies may be very helpful to many people; however, some drugs may also be dangerous, particularly if they purport to "cure" diabetes, cancer, and other serious ailments, and particularly if users are advised to avoid traditional therapies. Any person with or without diabetes who plans to take an herbal remedy or nutritional supplement should be sure to tell their physician beforehand, because some alternative remedies interact strongly with prescribed medications. For example, doctors know that individuals who are taking warfarin (Coumadin), a blood thinner, should avoid taking vitamin E or gingko biloba, because the patient's blood could become too thin and they could suffer from heavy bleeding as a result of the combination of the prescribed drug and the herbal remedy. Also, many alternative remedies may interact with psychiatric drugs or alcohol and should not be used unless the consumer checks first with a physician.

Alternative medications are offered in health food stores throughout the United States as well as in supermarkets and pharmacies. In addition, a proliferation of alternative medicines and remedies are offered to consumers worldwide over the Internet. These drugs are considered nutritional supplements, based on the Dietary Supplement Health and Education Act of 1994. As a result of this legislation, herbal remedies and vitamin supplements are regulated differently from both over-the-counter and prescribed medications.

The key difference: most pharmaceutical companies must offer considerable proof in the form of clinical studies to the Food and Drug Administration (FDA) before a new medication may be offered to the public. These studies must indicate not only that a new drug is safe but also that it is efficacious and that it improves the condition that it purports to treat. In contrast, the Dietary Supplement Health and Education Act of 1994 in the United States made the situation quite different for the sale of herbs and supplemental vitamins and minerals. In this case, it is the federal government, rather than the drug company, that must provide proof. Also, rather than prove

that the drug is safe and efficacious, the government must instead prove that the herbal remedy is actually harmful before it can be removed from the market.

This is a much more difficult burden of proof. Of course, the FDA can and does issue press releases when it believes an alternative remedy may be harmful to the public. In addition, some supplements have been removed from the market, such as ephedra, which was a weight-loss stimulant that caused some deaths.

Most medical experts believe that individuals with diabetes should not take any herbal remedies unless they are specifically advised to take them by their medical doctor. In addition, breastfeeding mothers, with or without diabetes, should avoid *all* supplemental herbs, minerals, and other alternative remedies, unless their physician specifically recommends them.

Studies of Individuals with Diabetes and Alternative Medicine

In a study by Donald Garrow, M.D., and Leonard E. Egede, M.D., of the use of alternative therapies by diabetics, the researchers analyzed data on 2,474 adults with diabetes, reporting their findings in *Diabetes Care* in 2006. They found that nearly half (48 percent) of the subjects used some form of alternative medicine. This is higher than the level of alternative medicine used by Americans in general, or 38 percent, according to the National Center for Health Statistics in their report in 2008.

Garrow and Egede also found that the use of alternative medicine was associated with receiving a pneumonia vaccination but not a flu shot. In addition, the researchers found that 67 percent of the adults with diabetes used vitamins, 22 percent used an herbal remedy, 21 percent used chiropractic therapy, and 17 percent received relaxation therapy. The users of alternative medicine were also more likely to be younger, more educated, with higher income, and employed compared to the non-users.

The researchers who looked at the use of alternative medicine by individuals with diabetes also found that the use of alternative medicine was not a barrier to the use of traditional medicine. For example, using alternative medicine was associated with visiting the emergency room of the hospital as well as with a greater number of visits with their primary care physicians compared to non-users. This last finding also tracks data from the National Center for Health Statistics, which reported in 2007 that the greater the number of visits to the doctor, the higher the percentage of patients who used alternative medicine; for example, among patients who visited their doctor four to nine times in the past year, nearly half (47.2 percent) used alternative medicine. Among those who saw their doctors 10 or more times in the past year, more than half (53.4 percent) used alternative medicine. One possible reason for the increased use of alternative medicine by sicker patients is that they are seeking relief that they believe they have not obtained through traditional medicine.

In another study of diabetic patients in India, researchers D. Kumar and colleagues analyzed 493 patients with diabetes, reporting on their results in *Public Health* in 2006. (Note that alternative remedies are even more popular in India and other countries than in the United States) They found that the use of alternative medicine was high (71 percent). However, less than half (42.2 percent) of the subjects said they had received any relief from their use of alternative therapies. When relief was perceived, the most common perceived relief was the lowering of blood sugar.

As found with other studies, younger individuals had the highest use of alternative remedies, and the researchers reported that awareness of alternative medicine was the highest among subjects ages 30–40 years, as well as among those of higher socioeconomic status and income. The researchers stated their opinion that "desire for quick and additional relief is the most common reason for using CAM [complementary alternative medicine] but most users are disappointed. Educating the community about CAM and self-care in diabetes is needed. A healthy clinical environment with improved doctor-patient relationships should be created to overcome reasons of dissatisfaction, if any, with the existing health care system. Clinicians should also explore CAM practices used by their patients in order to avoid misleading clinical decisions."

In another study reported by Jose A. Pagan and Jesus Tanguma in *Diabetes Care* in 2007, the researchers analyzed the use of CAM therapy by adults with diabetes based on federal data from 2002. They found that the majority (70.5 percent) of the subjects had used at least one form of alternative medicine in the past year. Herbal treatments were used by 15.1 percent, and some subjects used relaxation techniques (11.8 percent) and chiropractic care (6.6 percent). The researchers also found that, with the exception of megavitamins, CAM use was higher for diabetics whose treatment was delayed or who did not receive treatment because of cost.

For example, 77 percent of those who said their treatment was delayed or they did not receive treatment at all because of medical costs said that they used at least one CAM therapy, in contrast to 69.4 percent who said their treatment was not delayed or was not omitted because of cost. This finding seems to conflict with other study findings that those who are more well-off financially are more likely to use alternative medicine than those with less income. Interestingly, the researchers also found that more educated patients were more likely to use alternative medicine (as found in other studies).

The researchers also found that CAM users with diabetes were more likely to report their use of their CAM to their physicians (52 percent reported this use), compared to the minority statistic of only 39 percent of patients without diabetes who reported their CAM use to their doctors.

In a study by Thomas A. Arcury and colleagues, reported in the *Journal of Gerontology* in 2006, the researchers did a survey interview with 701 white, African-American, and Native American elderly people with diabetes living in rural environments on their use of alternative medicine. Most of the subjects were treated with oral agents only for their diabetes (60.3 percent), and 27.6 percent used insulin. Some of the participants (12.2 percent) took no diabetes medications.

The researchers found that most of the elderly used some form of alternative medicine but few used CAM as a therapy for diabetes. Instead, they used alternative remedies such as vitamins and minerals. They also used food home remedies, with the most popular being vinegar (used by 30.1 percent), lemon (27.2 percent), and honey (21.3 percent). Among those attempting to treat their diabetes symptoms, the most popular CAM therapies were salves (6.8 percent), vinegar (5.5 percent), and lemon (5.3 percent).

The researchers found that African Americans and Native Americans were more likely to use food remedies and home remedies than whites, both for diabetes and for other health problems. Many of the subjects took multivitamins (34.3 percent), while some took specific vitamins such as vitamin E (11.8 percent) or vitamin C (8.7 percent). About 17.3 percent of the subjects took minerals, with the most popular being calcium, used by 12.1 percent.

As with other research, the study showed that the use of alternative medicine was greater among those with poorer health.

A study by Colleen P. Gobert and Alison M. Duncan of the use of natural health products (NHPs) in Canada among adults with Type 2 diabetes with an average age of 59.2 years, published in the *Canadian Journal of Diabetes* in 2008, analyzed data from a questionnaire administered to 200 adults with Type 2 diabetes. They found that the majority (73 percent) used such products and the three products most commonly used were multivitamins/minerals, calcium, and vitamin C.

The most common reason for the use of NHPs was bone health (21.4 percent), followed by general health (15.9 percent), arthritis (15.3 percent), and diabetes (13.8 percent). As with other studies, the researchers found that the users were more likely to be educated and employed. The majority of users (60.7 percent) said that their diabetes was managed by medications, compared to 50.9 percent of the nonusers. The largest group of users said that they had received information about NHPs from their physicians (25.3 percent), followed by their pharmacists (23.2 percent) and registered dietitians (22.2 percent).

Among those who used NHPs, the majority agreed with the following statements: "NHPs allow me to have more control over my own health" (81.4 percent); "I am motivated to take NHPs because food cannot adequately support my nutritional needs" (75.2 percent); "I believe the labels on the NHPs I consume provide accurate information" (58.2 percent), and "I take NHPs because I believe that they are safer than medications" (41.4 percent). The researchers stated, "Overall, there appears to be confusion regarding the safety of NHP use, indicating a need for education."

The researchers found that both the fasting plasma glucose (FPG) and the HgbA1c for both users and nonusers were close to target ranges from the Canadian Diabetes Association, so the use of alternative medicine did not impede maintaining glycemic control. In addition, 91.0 percent of the NHP users and 96.4 percent of the nonusers said they owned a glucometer to test their blood.

More than half of the users also consumed alcohol, which is of concern since many alternative remedies interact with alcohol. As can be seen from the table, commonly used diabetes drugs do interact with alcohol, as do many other commonly used prescribed and over-the-counter (OTC) medications. (See Table 1.)

A Brief Overview of Alternative Medicine

In general, alternative medications encompass such categories as:

- herbal remedies
- supplemental vitamin or mineral therapy
- homeopathic remedies

**TABLE 1: COMMONLY USED MEDICATIONS (PRESCRIPTION AND OVER-THE-COUNTER)
THAT INTERACT WITH ALCOHOL**

Symptoms/Disorders	Medication Brand Name	Medication Generic Name	Some Possible Reactions with Alcohol
Allergies/Colds/Flu	Alavert	Loratadine	Drowsiness, dizziness; increased risk for overdose
	Allegra, Allegra-D	Fexofenadin	
	Benadryl	Diphenhydramine	
	Clarinex	Desloratadine	
	Claritin, Claritin-D	Loratadine	
	Dimetapp Cold & Allergy	Brompheniramine	
	Sudafed Sinus & Allergy	Chlorpheniramine	
	Triaminic Cold & Allergy	Chlorpheniramine	
	Tylenol Allergy Sinus	Chlorpheniramine	
	Tylenol Cold & Flu	Chlorpheniramine	
	Zyrtec	Cetirizine	
Angina (chest pain), coronary heart disease	Isordil	Isosorbide Nitroglycerin	Rapid heartbeat, sudden changes in blood pressure, dizziness, fainting
Anxiety and epilepsy	Ativan	Lorazepam	Drowsiness, dizziness; increased risk for overdose; slowed or difficulty breathing; impaired motor control; unusual behavior; and memory problems
	Klonopin	Clonazepam	
	Librium	Chlordiazepoxide	
	Paxil	Paroxetine	
	Valium	Diazepam	
	Xanax	Alprazolam	
	Herbal preparations (Kava Kava)		Liver damage, drowsiness
Arthritis	Celebrex	Celecoxib	Ulcers, stomach bleeding, liver problems
	Naprosyn	Naproxen	
	Voltaren	Dicloffenac	
Blood clots	Coumadin	Warfarin	Occasional drinking may lead to internal bleeding; heavier drinking also may cause bleeding or may have the opposite effect, resulting in possible blood clots, strokes, or heart attacks
Cough	Delsym, Robitussin Cough	Dextromethorphan	Drowsiness, dizziness; increased risk for overdose
	Robitussin A-C	Guaifenesin + codeine	
Depression	Anafranil	Clomipramine	Drowsiness, dizziness; increased risk for overdose; increased feelings of depression or hopelessness in adolescents (suicide)
	Celexa	Citalopram	
	Desyrel	Trazodone	
	Effexor	Venlafaxine	
	Elavil	Amitriptyline	
	Lexapro	Escitalopram	

Symptoms/Disorders	Medication Brand Name	Medication Generic Name	Some Possible Reactions with Alcohol
Depression (continued)	Luvox Norpramin Paxil Prozac Serzone Wellbutrin Zoloft	Fluvoxamine Desipramine Paroxetine Fluoxetine Nefazodone Bupropion Sertraline	Drowsiness, dizziness; increased risk for overdose; increased feelings of depression or hopelessness in adolescents (suicide)
	Herbal preparation (St. John's Wort)		
Diabetes	Glucophage Micronase Orinase	Metformin Glyburide Tolbutamide	Abnormally low blood sugar levels, flushing reaction (nausea, vomiting, headache, rapid heartbeat, sudden changes in blood pressure)
Enlarged prostate	Cardura Flomax Hytrin Minipress	Doxazosin Tamsulosin Terazosin Prazosin	Dizziness, light-headedness, fainting
Heartburn, indigestion, sour stomach	Axid Reglan Tagamet Zantac	Nizatidine Metoclopramide Cimetidine Ranitidine	Rapid heartbeat, sudden changes in blood pressure (metoclopramide); increased alcohol effect
High blood pressure	Accupril Capozide Cardura Catapres Xozaar Hytrin Lopressor HCT Lotensin Minipress Vaseretic	Quinapril Hydrochlorothiazide Doxazosin Clonidine Losartan Terazosin Hydrochlorothiazide Benazpril Prazosin Enalapril	Dizziness, fainting, drowsiness; heart problems, such as changes in the heart's regular heartbeat (arrhythmia)
High cholesterol	Advicor Altocor Crestor Lipitor Mevacor Niaspan Pravachol Pravigard Vytorin Zocor	Lovastatin + Niacin Lovastatin Rosuvastatin Atorvastatin Lovastatin Niacin Pravastatin Pravastatin + Aspirin Exetimibe +Simvastatin Simvastatin	Liver damage (all medications); increased flushing and itching (niacin); increased stomach bleeding (pravastatin + aspirin)

(table continues)

TABLE (continued)

Symptoms/Disorders	Medication Brand Name	Medication Generic Name	Some Possible Reactions with Alcohol
Infections	Acrodantin	Nitrofurantoin	Fast heartbeat, sudden changes in blood pressure; stomach pain, upset stomach, vomiting, headache, or flushing or redness of the face; liver damage (isoniazid, ketokonazole)
	Flagyl	Metronidazole	
	Grisactin	Griseofulvin	
	Nizoral	Ketokonazole	
	Nydrazid	Isoniazid	
	Seromycin	Cycloserine	
	Tindamax	Tiniadazole	
Muscle pain	Flexeril	Cyclobenzaprine	Drowsiness, dizziness; increased risk of seizures; increased risk for overdose; slowed or difficulty breathing; impaired motor control; unusual behavior; memory problems
	Soma	Carisoprodol	
Nausea, motion sickness	Chamomile	Various preparations	Alcohol may accentuate the drowsiness that is associated with these herbal preparations.
	Echinacea		
	Valerian		
Pain (such as headache, muscle ache, minor arthritis pain), fever, inflammation	Advil	Ibuprofen	Stomach upset, bleeding and ulcers; liver damage (acetaminophen); rapid heartbeat
	Aleve	Naproxen	
	Excedrin	Aspirin, Acetaminophen	
	Motrin	Ibuprofen	
	Tylenol	Acetaminophen	
Seizures	Dilantin	Phenytoin	Drowsiness, dizziness; increased risk of seizures
	Klonopin	Clonazepam	
		Phenobarbital	
Severe pain from injury, postsurgical care, oral surgery, migraines	Darvocet-N	Propoxyphene	Drowsiness, dizziness; increased risk for overdose; slowed or difficulty breathing; impaired motor control; unusual behavior; memory problems
	Demerol	Meperidine	
	Fiorinal with codeine	Butalbital + codeine	
	Percocet	Oxycodone	
	Vicodin	Hydrocodone	
Sleep problems	Ambien	Zolpidem	Drowsiness, sleepiness, dizziness; slowed or difficulty breathing; impaired motor control; unusual behavior; memory problems
	Lunesta	Eszopiclone	
	Prosom	Estazolam	
	Restoril	Temazepam	
	Sominex	Diphenhydramine	
	Unison	Doxylamine	
	Herbal preparations (chamomile, valerian, lavender)		Increased drowsiness

Source: National Institute on Alcohol Abuse and Alcoholism. *Harmful Interactions: Mixing Alcohol with Medicines.* Bethesda, Md: National Institutes of Health, 2007. Available at http://pubs.niaaa.nih.gov/publications/Medicine/medicine.htm. Downloaded June 27, 2008.

Herbal Remedies

There are a wide variety of roots, teas, berries, and other items that are sold as herbal remedies, some example of which are included in Table 2. These remedies are used to treat headaches, stomach pain, and many other health issues as well as to purportedly aid consumers in weight loss and increase their energy levels and muscle mass. According to The Herb Society of America's *New Encyclopedia of Herbs and Their Uses* by Deni Bown:

> The term "herb" also has more than one definition. Botanists describe an herb as a small, seed bearing plant with fleshy, rather than woody, parts (from which we get the term "herbaceous"). In this book, the term refers to a far wider range of plants. In addition to herbaceous perennials, herbs include trees, shrubs, annuals, vines, and more primitive plants, such as ferns, mosses, algae, lichens, and fungi. They [herbs] are valued for their flavor, fragrance, medicinal and healthful qualities, economic and industrial uses, pesticidal properties, and coloring materials (dyes).

Supplemental Vitamins and Minerals

Supplements are popular among individuals with diabetes. Among Americans in general, the most popular supplements are fish oil/omega 3/DHA, used by nearly 11 million Americans in 2007, followed by glucosamine, used by more than 6 million Americans.

In some cases, alternative remedies have proven very useful in helping those with diabetes; however, individuals should always check with their physicians first before instituting any new medication regimen, including vitamin or mineral therapy. Controlled studies have indicated that supplemental vitamin E may improve the health of individuals with diabetes; however, vitamin E in high doses may also result in bleeding disorders, as may some herbal remedies such as ginkgo biloba.

Some German studies of alpha-lipoic acid (ALA) have indicated that ALA can be effective in treating DIABETIC NEUROPATHY. Studies on ALA

TABLE 2: FREQUENCIES AND PERCENTAGES OF ADULTS 18 YEARS OF AGE AND OLDER WHO USED SELECTED TYPES OF NONVITAMIN, NONMINERAL NATURAL PRODUCTS FOR HEALTH REASONS IN THE PAST 30 DAYS, BY TYPE OF PRODUCT USED: UNITED STATES, 2007

Nonvitamin, Nonmineral, Natural Products	Number in Thousands	Percent
Fish oil or omega 3 or DHA	10,923	37.4
Glucosamine	6,132	19.9
Echinacea	4,848	19.8
Flaxseed oil or pills	4,416	15.9
Ginseng	3,345	14.1
Combination herb pill	3,446	13.0
Ginkgo biloba	2,977	11.3
Chondroitin	3,390	11.2
Garlic supplements	3,278	11.0
Coenzyme Q-10	2,691	8.7
Fiber or psyllium	1,791	6.6
Green tea pills	1,528	6.3
Cranberry (pills, gelcaps)	1,560	6.0
Saw palmetto	1,682	5.1
Soy supplements of isofavones	1,363	5.0
Melatonin	1,296	4.6
Grape seed extract	1,214	4.3
MSM (methylsufonylmethane)	1,312	4.1
Milk thistle	1,001	3.7
Lutein	1,047	3.4

Note that some respondents used more than one product.

Source: Adapted from Barnes, Patricia M., and Barbara Bloom. "Complementary and Alternative Medicine Use Among Adults and Children: United States, 2007." *National Health Statistics Reports* 18 (December 10, 2008): 12.

are currently under way in the United States. ALA is an accepted treatment in Germany. A July 2000 issue of *Alternative Medicine Alert Archives* included an article which provided an overview on studies of ALA in treating diabetic neuropathy. Most of the studies have concentrated on positive results from injected ALA, a treatment not available in the United States as of this writing. One 2006 study in Australia on oral alpha lipoic acid showed positive results, although most other studies using the oral formulation are poorly designed and inconclusive.

ALA is also found in red meat, although many people in the United States with and without diabetes have cut back on their consumption of red meat.

Scientists have also been studying the impact of minerals such as chromium and others on people with diabetes, but to date, they have not yet found any clear indications for recommending supplementation to patients with diabetes. Some experts believe that a magnesium deficiency can worsen the complications of diabetes, but further research is needed.

Impaired Glucose Tolerance and Type 2 Diabetes Mellitus

In 12 out of 15 controlled studies of people with impaired glucose tolerance, chromium supplementation was found to improve some measure of glucose utilization or to have beneficial effects on blood lipid profiles. Impaired glucose tolerance refers to a metabolic state between normal glucose regulation and overt diabetes. Commonly, blood glucose levels are higher than normal but lower than those accepted as diagnostic for diabetes. Impaired glucose tolerance is associated with increased risk for cardiovascular diseases but is not associated with the other classic complications of diabetes.

About 25–30 percent of individuals with impaired glucose tolerance eventually develop Type 2 diabetes. Generally, chromium supplementation in a variety of forms, at doses of about 200 mcg/day for two to three months, has been found to be beneficial. The reasons for the variation or lack of effect in some studies are not clear, but chromium depletion is not the only known cause of impaired glucose tolerance. Additionally, the lack of an accurate measure of chromium nutritional status prevents researchers from identifying those individuals who are most likely to benefit from chromium supplementation. A recent meta-analysis of 15 randomized clinical trials reported that chromium had no effect on glucose or insulin concentrations in nondiabetic individuals.

Homeopathic Remedies

Homeopathy is a system that was developed by German physician Samuel Hahnemann in the early 19th century. This physician had stopped practicing medicine but he continued experimenting on herbs. Hahnemann noted that large quantities of the drug quinine made healthy individuals feverish and shaky, with malaria-like symptoms. Much smaller doses, however, helped people who actually had malaria. Hahnemann devised his concept of the "law of similars," which was based on his belief that large quantities of substances may cause illness, but very tiny quantities of the same substance may provide relief. For example, belladonna, a deadly drug for most people, is used by homeopaths in tiny quantities to cure migraine headaches. Hahnemann's experiments are compiled in an 1811 reference guide called *Materia Medica*.

Many physicians in the United States discount the value of homeopathic remedies, although doctors in Germany and other European countries accept them.

Alternative Therapies

Alternative therapies such as chiropractic, massage therapy, acupuncture, and other options are popular among many Americans, and it is likely that adults with diabetes also avail themselves of such therapies; for example, as seen in Table 3, 38 million people used some form of alternative therapy in 2007, based on data from the National Center for Health Statistics. As can be seen from the table, chiropractic therapy was very popular, used by nearly half (49.2 percent) of those using CAM, followed in popularity by massage therapy (47.4 percent).

Acury, Thomas A., et al. "Complementary and Alternative Medicine Use as Health Self-Management: Rural Older Adults with Diabetes." *Journal of Gerontology: Social Sciences* 61B, no. 2 (2006): S62–S70.

Barnes, Patricia, M., and Barbara Bloom. "Complementary and Alternative Medicine Use Among Adults and Children: United States, 2007." *National Health Statistics Reports* 18 (December 10, 2008): 1–24.

TABLE 3: FREQUENCIES AND PERCENTAGES OF PERSONS AGES 18 AND OLDER WHO SAW ALTERNATIVE MEDICINE PRACTITIONERS DURING THE PAST 12 MONTHS, TOTAL PRACTITIONER VISITS AND TOTAL OUT-OF-POCKET COSTS PER YEAR, BY TYPE OF THERAPY, UNITED STATES, 2007

Therapy	Total persons		Total visits per year		Total out-of-pocket costs per year (dollars)	
	Number (thousands)	Percent	Number (thousands)	Percent	Number (thousands)	Percent
Total	38,146	100.0	354,203	100.0	11,938,611	100.0
Alternative medical systems	4,965	13.1	27,734	7.8	1,392,508	11.7
Acupuncture	3,141	8.2	17,629	5.0	827,336	6.9
Ayurveda	214	0.6	1,068	Not provided	18,793	0.2
Homeopathic treatment	862	2.3	3,411	1.0	167,416	1.4
Naturopathy	729	1.9	3,180	0.9	275,863	2.3
Biologically based therapies	1,828	4.8	9,600	2.7	630,439	5.3
Chelation therapy	111	0.3	426	0.1	31,913	0.3
Nonvitamin, nonmineral and natural products	1,488	3.9	8,273	2.3	566,650	4.7
Manipulative and body-based therapies	33,044	86.7	276,861	78.2	8,629,455	72.3
Chiropractic or osteopathic manipulation	18,740	49.2	151,220	42.7	3,901,894	32.7
Massage	18,068	47.4	95,296	26.9	4,175,124	35.0
Mind-body therapies	3,821	10.2	32,806	9.3	864,567	7.2
Biofeedback	362	1.0	1,991	0.6	83,542	Not provided
Relaxation techniques	3,131	8.3	28,882	8.2	707,175	5.9
Hypnosis	561	1.5	1,933	0.5	73,850	0.6
Energy healing therapy	1,216	3.2	7,203	2.0	421,602	3.5

Source: Adapted from Nahin, Richard L., et al. "Costs of Complementary and Alternative Medicine (CAM) and Frequency of Visits to CAM Practitioners: United States, 2007." *National Health Statistics Reports* 18 (July 30, 2009): 6.

Drake, Victoria. "Chromium." Linus Pauling Institute, Oregon State University. Available online. URL: http://lpi.oregonstate.edu/infocenter/minerals/chromium/. Updated September 2007. Downloaded September 30, 2009.

Garrow, Donald, M.D., and Leonard E. Edege, M.D. "Association between Complementary and Alternative Medicine Use, Preventive Care Practices, and Use of Conventional Medical Services among Adults with Diabetes." *Diabetes Care* 29, no. 1 (2006): 15–19.

General Accounting Office. *Dietary Supplements: FDA Should Take Further Actions to Improve Oversight and Consumer Understanding. Report to Congressional Requesters.* Washington, D.C.: General Accounting Office, January 2009.

Gobert, Colleen P., and Alison M. Duncan. "Use of Natural Health Products by Adults with Type 2 Diabetes." *Canadian Journal of Diabetes.* 32, no. 4 (2008): 260–272.

Kumar, D., S. Bajaj, and R. Mehrotra. "Knowledge, Attitude and Practice of Complementary and Alternative Medicines for Diabetes." *Public Health* 120 (2006): 705–711.

National Institute on Alcohol Abuse and Alcoholism. *Harmful Interactions: Mixing Alcohol with Medicines.* Bethesda, Md: National Institutes of Health, 2007. Available online. URL: http://pubs.niaaa.nih.gov/

publications/Medicine/medicine.htm. Downloaded June 27, 2008.

Pagan, Jose A., and Jesus Tanguma. "Health Care Affordability and Complementary and Alternative Medicine Utilization by Adults with Diabetes." *Diabetes Care* 30, no. 8 (2007): 2,030–2,031.

Yeh, Gloria Y., M.D., et al. "Systematic Review of Herbs and Dietary Supplements for Glycemic Control in Diabetes." *Diabetes Care* 26, no. 4 (2003): 1,277–1,294.

Ziegler, D., A. Ametov, A. Barinov, et al. "Oral Treatment with Alpha-lipoic Acid Improves Symptomatic Diabetic Polyneuropathy: The SYDNEY 2 Trial." *Diabetes Care* 29 (2006): 2,365–2,370.

Alzheimer's disease A brain disease and the most common form of dementia. Dementia is a disorder that causes a progressive and severe decline in memory and cognitive abilities. Alzheimer's disease represents from 60–80 percent of all cases of dementia and also accounts for 70 percent of all forms of dementia among individuals ages 71 years and older. The rate of deterioration in the person with Alzheimer's disease may be rapid or slow, depending on many factors, but it generally occurs over a period of from two to 20 years.

Some studies have indicated that people with diabetes are at much greater risk for developing Alzheimer's disease or other forms of dementia than are nondiabetics, although the cause for this is unknown. (Recent research indicates that there may be a genetic cause that triggers both diseases.) About 25 percent of all patients with Alzheimer's disease have diabetes.

Medical care for the person with Alzheimer's disease is more expensive than for older individuals without Alzheimer's. According to the Alzheimer's Association in Chicago, Illinois, the average total annual Medicare payment for the person with both diabetes and Alzheimer's in 2006 was $20,655. In contrast, the person with diabetes who did not have Alzheimer's used care that cost $12,979.

An estimated 5.3 million people in the United States had Alzheimer's disease in 2009 according to the Alzheimer's Association, including 200,000 individuals younger than age 65 who had early-onset Alzheimer's. In 2005, 71,599 people in the United States died of Alzheimer's disease. These numbers are anticipated to rise with an aging population.

The disease was first diagnosed by German physician Alois Alzheimer in 1906, after an autopsy on Auguste D., who had reportedly said poignantly at some point before her death, "I have lost myself." Auguste D. had experienced increasingly difficult and severe problems with her memory and behavior, and she died at age 51. (Auguste D. had an early onset of Alzheimer's disease; most people with Alzheimer's disease are 65 years or older.)

The autopsy on Auguste D. startled Dr. Alzheimer, who discovered brain cells that were shaped differently from the norm for the cerebral cortex of the brain. This is the area of the brain that is responsible for memory and reasoning. He also found tangles of a plaque substance, which are not seen in a normal brain. These lesions are still found in the brains of Alzheimer's victims after their deaths. Currently, they cannot be identified in brain tests on living individuals with techniques such as magnetic resonance imaging (MRI) or other radiologic tests.

Although Alzheimer's disease is more likely to be found among individuals who are over age 65, and the risk for the disease increases with age, it is still not "normal" for older people to have Alzheimer's disease. About 10 percent of North Americans over age 65 have Alzheimer's disease but the percentage of those afflicted increases to 30–50 percent of people who are older than age 85.

Symptoms and Diagnostic Path

Many middle-aged and older individuals may fear that they are showing signs of Alzheimer's disease merely because they misplace their car keys or forget someone's name. These are common memory errors and they are not indicative of Alzheimer's disease.

Some early symptoms and signs of mild Alzheimer's disease may include continued trouble with or an inability to remember recent events. Unlike with others who temporarily forget recent events and then remember them later, the person with Alzheimer's forgets these events and never remembers them, as if these events were erased from their memory. Apathy and depression are also common early symptoms of Alzheimer's disease.

Some possible indicators of progressing Alzheimer's disease (although other medical causes should be ruled out first) are:

- refusal to bathe
- failure to recognize people who have been known for a long time
- extreme suspiciousness of others or paranoia
- rages and combativeness
- disorientation and confusion
- difficulty with speaking
- poor judgment
- trouble with tying shoes or dressing that is unrelated to any physical disabilities
- wandering around the house (or outside) at night
- aphasia (difficulty in speaking or understanding the meaning of words used by others)

Doctors may use such tests as the Mini-Mental State Examination (MMSE) to determine both short- and long-term memory capabilities, as well as the patient's abilities in writing and speaking. They also question the individual and look at his or her medical history.

Physicians should be sure to perform a very careful evaluation of older individuals who seem confused, because Alzheimer's may be misdiagnosed in a person who suffers from undiagnosed diabetes or who may be more properly diagnosed with a variety of other ailments including DEPRESSION, vitamin B$_{12}$ deficiency, syphilis, Parkinson's disease, heart disease, and other medical problems. Alzheimer's disease may also be misdiagnosed in a person whose primary problem is that he or she is abusing drugs or alcohol.

Treatment Options and Outlook

Although Alzheimer's disease is not curable as of this writing, physicians work to delay the severity of the deterioration with medications. As of this writing, there are several medications used to slow the memory loss experienced by patients diagnosed with Alzheimer's disease, including donepezil (Aricept), rivastigime (Exelon), and galantamine (Razadyne), which are all medications used to treat mild to moderate Alzheimer's disease. Memantine (Namenda) is a medication used to treat moderate to severe Alzheimer's.

These medications can slow the deterioration caused by Alzheimer's for up to 12 months for about 50 percent of individuals who take them, but they are not a cure. Other medications are under development. Ultimately, the disease will progress and the individual will either die of it or die of another illness, such as CARDIOVASCULAR DISEASE, cancer, or the one of the many COMPLICATIONS OF DIABETES.

Experts report that the physician's goals for a diabetic patient with Alzheimer's disease may become less stringent. The reason for this is that tight control of glucose levels may lead to HYPOGLYCEMIA, and it may become very difficult or even impossible for a person with dementia to recognize the symptoms of hypoglycemia. It may also be very difficult for the caregiver assisting the person with Alzheimer's to maintain more than very basic levels of glucose control.

According to the Alzheimer's Association, "Some data indicate that management of cardiovascular risk factors, such as high cholesterol, Type 2 diabetes, high blood pressure and overweight, may help avoid or delay cognitive decline."

Risk Factors and Preventive Measures

Gender plays a role in Alzheimer's disease, and about 16 percent of women ages 71 years and older and 11 percent of men ages 71 and older have some form of dementia. An estimated two-thirds of elderly individuals with Alzheimer's are in fair to poor health.

Alzheimer's and Diabetes

Some research has indicated that people with either Type 1 or Type 2 diabetes may be at greater risk for developing Alzheimer's disease than are nondiabetics. New research in 2009 indicates that a gene linked to the development of Type 2 diabetes may also be a factor in the development of Alzheimer's disease. It is hoped that further research will lead to a treatment breakthrough or even preventive measures against the development of diabetes and/or Alzheimer's disease.

When a person who has diabetes also has Alzheimer's disease, there is definitely an increasing impact from both of these illnesses. For example, as the individual's cognitive abilities decline, others must take over the caregiving and make sure that the individual takes his or her medication and performs the necessary blood testing. Required insulin injections must eventually be performed for the person because he or she cannot manage them.

Some emerging research indicates that older individuals with stronger muscles have a reduced risk for developing Alzheimer's disease, although further research is needed. Other research has shown that muscular strength is inversely related to OBESITY in men; that is, the stronger the man, the less likely that he will be obese.

See also ELDERLY.

Alzheimer's Association. *2009 Alzheimer's Disease Facts and Figures.* Chicago: Alzheimer's Association, 2009.

American Indians/Alaska Natives Individuals who are descendants of tribal groups within the United States. According to the Indian Health Service (IHS), there were 3.3 million American Indians and Alaska Natives in the United States from 561 tribes in 2007. This group comprises less than 1 percent of the U.S. population. Many American Indians are at a very high risk for developing Type 2 diabetes. According to the IHS, the rate of diabetes among American Indian adults is about double that of the rate for WHITES/CAUCASIANS. An estimated16.3 percent of American Indians and Alaska Natives ages 20 years and older have been diagnosed with diabetes, compared to 11.8 percent of African Americans, 10.4 percent of Hispanics, 7.5 percent of Asian Americans, and only 6.6 percent of the same age group of non-Hispanic whites.

Nearly all of those with diabetes among American Indians and Alaska Natives have Type 2 diabetes. According to the Centers for Disease Control and Prevention (CDC), the rates of diabetes among American Indian tribes and Alaska Natives vary drastically; for example, the estimated rate of diabetes among Alaska Natives ages 20 years and older is only about 6 percent, while the rate is nearly a third (29.3 percent) among American Indians in southern Arizona, such as the PIMA INDIANS.

The Pima Indian tribe has been studied by the National Institutes of Health (NIH) since 1965. Over half of the members of this group over the age of 35 years have Type 2 diabetes. However, the high rate of Type 2 diabetes among the Pima Indians appears to be largely influenced by diet, OBESITY, and a sedentary lifestyle, because very few of the Pima Indians who live in Mexico have Type 2 diabetes.

The children of Pima Indians who develop DIABETIC NEPHROPATHY (kidney disease that is caused by diabetes and which may lead to kidney failure) also appear to inherit their parents' risk for this complication of diabetes. As a result, many Pima Indians will experience kidney failure, a very serious medical problem which is treatable only with either dialysis or kidney transplantation.

A Higher Rate of Problem Behaviors

According to data from the National Center for Health Statistics, American Indians and Alaska Natives are more likely to exhibit problematic health behaviors than many other groups, and many of these behaviors exacerbate the complications for diabetes. For example, an estimated 33.5 percent of American Indians and Alaska Natives are smokers, compared to the much lower rate of white adults (23.4 percent), African-American adults (22.4 percent), and the very low rate of Asian adults (12.7 percent). In considering moderate or heavy drinking of alcohol, American Indian males have a rate of 27.8 percent, compared to whites (29.3 percent), African Americans (20.5 percent), and Asian men (14.9 percent).

American Indians and Alaska Native adults in the United States are also much more likely (10.7 percent of this group) to fail to receive needed medical care due to the cost of care than are African Americans (7.9 percent), whites (5.7 percent) or Asian adults (3.5 percent). These factors taken together considerably increase the health problems that American Indian diabetics may experience.

More Complications from Diabetes than Other Groups

American Indians and Alaska Natives have an elevated risk of suffering from many complications that are associated with diabetes; for example, they have a 3.5 times greater risk of diabetes-related kidney failure when compared to the general population. Because of the high risk for diabetes among American Indians, the U.S. Congress established the Special Diabetes Program for Indians in 1997 to assist this group.

Navajo Youths with Diabetes

In a study of Navajo children and adolescents who were diagnosed with diabetes, Dana Dabelea, M.D., and colleagues found that diabetes infrequently occurred among children ages 10 years and younger. The majority of all the youths who had diabetes were diagnosed with Type 2 diabetes (80.4 percent). The researchers also found that of those Navajo youths who did have diabetes, it was common for them to have poor glycemic control and to exhibit unhealthy behaviors (such as SMOKING). The researchers also found that many youths with diabetes were severely depressed; for example, 14.3 percent

of the Navajo youths with Type 1 diabetes were depressed, as were 21.9 percent of those with Type 2 diabetes.

Among the Navajo youths with Type 2 diabetes, more than two-thirds (67.7 percent) were obese, and 17.7 percent of those diagnosed with Type 1 diabetes were obese. Most of those in both groups had a family history of diabetes, including 92.2 percent of those with Type 2 diabetes and 76.5 percent of those with Type 1 diabetes.

See also AFRICAN AMERICANS WITH DIABETES; ASIANS/PACIFIC ISLANDER AMERICANS; HISPANICS/ LATINOS; WHITES/CAUCASIANS.

Dabelea, Dana, M.D., et al. "Diabetes in Navajo Youth: Prevalence, Incidence, and Clinical Characteristics: The SEARCH for Diabetes in Youth Study." *Diabetes Care* 32, Supplement 2 (2009): S141–S147.
National Diabetes Information Clearinghouse. National Diabetes Statistics, 2007. Available online. URL: http://diabetes.niddk.nih.gov/DM/PUBS/statistics/ DM_Statistics.pdf. Downloaded October 23, 2009.

Americans with Disabilities Act (ADA) Signed into law in 1990, the Americans with Disabilities Act prohibits discrimination against disabled individuals in the workplace, schools, and in other areas used by disabled individuals.

Work and the ADA

In the workplace, the ADA applies when employers have 15 or more workers. There are many provisions in the ADA but several are key to keep in mind. For example, according to the Equal Employment Opportunity Commission, one provision is that employers who are interviewing job applicants may not question the prospective employee about his or her disability, even if it may be related to the job.

If the interviewer decides to make a conditional offer of employment at that point, he or she may inquire about disabilities and may also request medical examinations, if such inquiries would be made for others applying for the same type of job. After the person is hired, questions about a disability can be made only if they are related to the job. The same holds true about requiring a medical examination after the person has been hired: under the ADA, a medical examination can only be mandated if it is job-related. The specific wording is as follows:

> A covered entity shall not require a medical examination and shall not make inquiries of an employee as to whether such employee is an individual with a disability or as to the nature and severity of the disability, unless such examination or inquiry is shown to be job-related and consistent with business necessity.

Impact of the Americans with Disabilities Act

According to attorney Michael A. Greene, in his 1999 article for *Diabetes Spectrum,* the enactment of the ADA was "the sunrise of legal advocacy for diabetes." Greene also stated that the efforts of the American Diabetes Association that preceded its passage resulted in a "legislative history replete with medical and scientific references to diabetes."

Prior to the passage of the ADA, disabled individuals fell under a broad range of state statutes that varied greatly from state to state. The ADA, a federal law, provided one prevailing standard for all children and adults with disabilities, although many lawsuits have tested the law since its passage.

Lawsuits under the ADA

The American Diabetes Association has appeared as a plaintiff in some lawsuits filed under the provisions of the Americans with Disabilities Act. For example, in the case of *Stuthard and the American Diabetes Association v. KinderCare Learning Centers,* an Ohio day-care center refused to accept a child with Type 1 diabetes because he needed insulin injections. The day-care provider would not allow any staff members to give the injections even though the child was a toddler and was too young to perform self-glucose testing or to self-inject.

The case was resolved in favor of the family and the American Diabetes Association. Attor-

ney General Janet Reno said, "Children with diabetes shouldn't be left on the sidelines. We hope that other child care facilities will do the right thing and follow KinderCare's lead."

See also FAMILY AND MEDICAL LEAVE ACT; LAWSUITS.

Greene, Michael A. "The Age of Legal Advocacy for Diabetes." *Diabetes Spectrum* 12, no. 4 (1999).

amputation The surgical removal of a body part such as an arm, leg, finger, or toe; however, the overwhelming majority of amputations in individuals with diabetes are of the lower extremities, such as a toe, a foot, or all or part of a leg. Diabetes is the number one cause of nontraumatic amputations in the United States. According to the Centers for Disease Control and Prevention (CDC), 71,000 people in the United States with diabetes as their first diagnosis had a nontraumatic (non-accidental) lower extremity amputation in 2005, the most recent data as of this writing. Experts believe that as many as half of all the amputations that are experienced by people with diabetes could have been prevented had they received appropriate examinations and patient education.

According to the CDC in their 2009 analysis of risk factors for amputations among people with diabetes by their lower extremity disease status, diabetics with either peripheral arterial disease (PAD) or peripheral neuropathy have a three times greater risk of having an amputation compared to diabetic people without these conditions. The CDC also noted that fewer than 30 percent of individuals who experience a diabetes-related amputation survive for five years. (That is to say that the underlying problems that led to the amputation, such as peripheral arterial disease or DIABETIC NEUROPATHY, as well as other factors such as poor glycemic control, smoking, hypertension, dyslipidemia, and others, are all markers for significant vascular dysfunction.) In addition, they also noted that whites with diabetes have a lower risk of nontraumatic amputations than diabetic blacks. Amputations are more common among individuals with Type 1 diabetes, although those who have had Type 2 diabetes for many years may also be at risk for amputations.

Some studies have shown that the risk of an amputation is reduced by about 36 percent among patients taking fenofibrate to lower their blood cholesterol. Other studies have shown that patients with diabetes and dyslipidemia have a greater risk for lower extremity amputations than diabetics whose CHOLESTEROL levels are under good control. Other factors related to amputations are poor glycemic control, the presence of hypertension, microvascular complications, and stroke. Poor circulation in the legs and diabetic neuropathy have also been found to be relevant factors associated with an increased risk for a lower extremity amputation.

Reason for Amputation

If an injury progresses to the point of bacterial infestation and then GANGRENE or tissue death, then the gangrenous part must be amputated to avoid any further spreading of the gangrene and infection and subsequent certain death.

The main reason people with diabetes are at greater risk than nondiabetics for amputations is that they lose feeling in their feet and may not feel or notice an injury. This nerve damage is also called diabetic neuropathy. The injury becomes progressively worse and may deteriorate to the point of gangrene before it is even noticed by the individual or by his or her doctors.

Other risk factors It is also important to minimize or eliminate other risk factors that can contribute to future amputations, such as OBESITY, SMOKING, infections, and uncontrolled HYPERTENSION. Dyslipidemia is also a major risk factor.

In an analysis of 145 diabetic patients with necrotizing soft-tissue infections in their feet, Javier Aragon-Sanchez and colleagues sought to identify factors associated with limb loss and death. They found that specific medical conditions such as fasciitis and myonecrosis correlated with the loss of a limb. They also found that age

older than 75 years and high creatinine levels (signifying abnormal kidney function, DIABETIC NEPHROPATHY) were correlated with death from foot infections.

A study from Barbados reported by J. M. Anselm and colleagues in *Diabetes Care* in 2004 indicated that simply not wearing shoes tripled the risk of diabetes-related, lower-extremity amputation among Barbados residents. The risk of amputation was quadrupled for those wearing "fashion" footwear, as well as for female walkers who wore sneakers frequently. Thus appropriate footwear plays a critical role in preventing foot ulcerations that can lead eventually to amputation.

Preventive measures: The following patients with diabetes should see a podiatrist for prevention approximately every 12 weeks. Patients who:

- cannot see or assess their own feet for injuries, because of obesity or for another reason
- have DIABETIC RETINOPATHY or other causes of visual loss
- are on anticoagulants
- have known peripheral vascular disease (intermittent claudication)
- have had a prior amputation
- have insensate feet (diabetic neuropathy)

Medicare and many other health plans will cover an annual payment for therapeutic shoes for patients with diabetes. Patients need to obtain a prescription for the shoes from their medical doctor.

Foot Care Is Essential

To greatly reduce the risk of amputation, physicians emphasize the importance of good FOOT CARE, including the daily examination of the entire foot by the patient, particularly the bottoms of feet, but also including the heel and between the toes. Because it can be hard to study the soles of one's own feet, mirrors may help with this task, or family members may be taught to examine the individual's foot for injuries.

Experts say that when a person with diabetes visits the doctor, a yearly complete examination of the foot (inspection of skin, palpation of pulses, exam of toenails, testing of sensory function with a monofilament and or a tuning fork) should be as routine as is a blood pressure or weight check. Yet many physicians still do not perform regular foot examinations of their diabetic patients. To help their doctors, people with diabetes should remove their shoes and socks at doctor visits, before the physician even enters the room. Shorter exams can be done during follow-up visits.

Surgical procedures have improved greatly over the past 10 years, and referral to an experienced foot surgeon (orthopedist, podiatrist, and some general surgeons) can help minimize the amount of amputation required; often the lower extremity is re-vascularized via angioplasty, stenting, or bypass—usually the last—and then removal of gangrenous tissue. Today new types of rotational flaps are used during an amputation. This is where a blood vessel and muscular tissue are rotated down to cover the defect. The less of the lower extremity that is amputated, the less energy that is required for the patient to walk again on the stump or prosthesis.

Emotional Impact of Amputation

Clearly, the emotional impact of losing one or more limbs is a devastating one for patients as well as their families. The patient may develop problems with feelings of hopelessness and DEPRESSION and may require psychiatric intervention. Some patients are so depressed that they are suicidal.

Rajiv Singh and colleagues reported on their findings on depression and anxiety in amputees at three points: before the amputation, upon discharge after the procedure, and several years later, reporting on their findings in *Clinical Rehabilitation* in 2009. The researchers found that among 68 patients who were alive two to three years after a lower limb amputation, depression and anxiety were common problems immediately before the procedure; for example, 23.5

percent were both depressed and anxious at that point. However, the rates of depression and anxiety then fell dramatically to about 3 percent on discharge.

Interestingly, several years later, the rates of depression and anxiety had dramatically increased to 17.6 percent with depression and 19.1 percent with anxiety. Some depression that occurred several years later was linked to having depression or anxiety immediately after the surgery and anxiety was linked to a younger age of the amputees. The researchers hypothesized that older amputees may have had lower expectations and demands from their lives than did the younger amputees. They also found that depression correlated with the presence of other illnesses.

The researchers said, "Our finding that anxiety and depressive symptoms drop after amputation and then rise again after discharge is hitherto unreported. It is interesting to speculate that this may be due to initial adjustment reaction and learning of new skills followed by worsening of symptoms once discharged home and the reality of life sets in. Further work could look in more detail at the temporal relationships of symptoms after discharge especially in the first year after amputation as well [as] at possible treatment options."

A psychiatrist or therapist cannot bring back the missing limb to the patient, but may be able to provide assistance in developing ways to help the patient cope with the problem or help the patient connect with others who have dealt with their amputations. The patient may also benefit from taking antidepressant medication, although this option should be discussed between the patient and physician.

Anselm, J. M., et al. "Explanation for the High Risk of Diabetes Related to Amputation in a Caribbean Population of Black African Descent and Potential for Prevention." *Diabetes Care* 27, no. 11 (2004): 2,636–2,641.

Aragon-Sanchez, Javier, et al. "Necrotizing Soft-Tissue Infections in the Feet of Patients with Diabetes: Outcome of Surgical Treatment and Factors Associated with Limb Loss and Mortality." *International Journal of Lower Extremity Wounds* 8, no. 3 (2009): 141–146.

Dorsey, Rashida R., et al. "Control of Risk Factors among People with Diagnosed Diabetes, by Lower Extremity Disease Status." *Preventing Chronic Disease* 6, no. 4 (2009): 1–10.

Singh, Rajiv, et al. "Depression and Anxiety Symptoms after Lower Limb Amputation: The Rise and Fall." *Clinical Rehabilitation* 23 (2009): 282–286.

angiotensin receptor blockers (ARBs) A category of blood pressure medications that are given to people who suffer from HYPERTENSION. Many people who have diabetes also have hypertension. ARB drugs work to reduce protein in the urine (PROTEINURIA) as well as delay kidney damage. Some examples of ARBs are: losartan, valsartan, candesartan, and irbesartan. ARBS differ from the angiotensin converting enzyme (ACE) inhibitor drugs in that they block the effects of angiotensin by preventing it from binding to its receptor. The effect is to prevent the angiotensin in the system from increasing blood pressure.

ACE drugs work by blocking the conversion of angiotensinogen to angiotensin I, and thus, they cause lower levels of angiotensin II to be available. Angiotensin II is one of the most potent constrictors of blood vessels known. Therefore, if there are lower levels, there is also less constriction of the arteries, and thus the vessels are more relaxed and blood pressure decreases. In addition, if there is less angiotensin II, there is also less stimulation of the adrenal to make aldosterone, which would cause the retention of some salt and water and raise blood pressure. Aldosterone also causes loss of potassium by the kidney. If the formation of angiotensin I and II is blocked, then blood pressure will be lower and potassium levels will be increased.

Similar to ACE drugs, ARBs are very well tolerated, with as few side effects as a placebo. They do not cause cough, which is one of the most common side effects of ACE drugs, albeit a side effect that is often minor and tolerated by many people.

ACE drugs have been available for many years in the United States and are still considered first-line therapy for hypertension and for the prevention of development or progression of DIABETIC NEPHROPATHY; however an ARB medication is often used as a second choice if the patient is unable to tolerate the ACE drug. Multiple studies are underway to determine whether or not ARBs are as effective as ACE drugs in protecting the diabetic kidney.

animals and diabetes Nonhuman species, particularly dogs, cats, rats, and mice that have played a large role in the research and treatment of diabetes in humans as well as animals. Animals can also develop diabetes in their later years, and they are usually treated with insulin.

The first successful experiments on injected insulin, performed by Drs. Banting and Best in 1921 in Canada, were performed on a dog. Many subsequent experiments have been performed on other animals as well as mice and rats, some of which have been specially inbred so that they would develop diabetes. Experiments have been done on animals to determine the effects of diabetes, to find underlying genetic causes of OBESITY, and for many other purposes. Some people are opposed to experimentation on animals.

Animals may also develop diabetes, particularly as they age, and they may require oral medication or insulin injections in order to survive. According to *Diabetes Mellitus* by Porte and Sherwin, Type 1 diabetes occurs in about 1 in every 200 dogs and occurs in 1 of 800 cats. Other animals may also develop diabetes. The authors say,

> Diabetes has been reported in horses, ferrets, and ground squirrels. In zoological gardens, in which animals are liberally fed as compared to the nutrition available in their native habitat, diabetes has been reported in dolphins, foxes, and a hippopotamus.

Veterinarians are very familiar with diabetes among animals and have researched many ways to help animals. Some researchers seeking to help animals have made findings that could also benefit humans; for example, an article in a 2000 issue of *Veterinary Medicine* revealed that chromium and vanadium, trace elements needed by both humans and animals, may be useful as a supplemental treatment for both cats and people with Type 2 diabetes. Further research is needed on this topic.

Porte, Daniel, Jr., M.D., and Robert S. Sherwin, M.D. *Ellenberg & Rifkin's Diabetes Mellitus.* Stamford, Conn.: Appleton & Lange, 1997.

"Two Transition Metals Show Promise in Treating Diabetic Cats." *Veterinary Medicine* 95, no. 3 (March 1, 2000): 190–193.

antibodies to insulin Proteins made by B-lymphocytes that can bind to and neutralize insulin that it mistakenly considers as an intruder to the body.

Anyone who takes insulin will develop antibodies against insulin. These antibodies are generally in low levels that do not cause clinical effects.

In fact, patients who have Type 1 diabetes develop antibodies to insulin *before* the diagnosis of diabetes and before insulin therapy has begun. Part of their disease was the destruction of the beta cells that produced natural insulin.

Modern insulin is much purer than past formulations, and thus, antibody levels (titers) are less.

Stopping and starting insulin can increase a person's antibody levels to insulin, and consequently, is not recommended.

The Controversy over Insulin Antibodies

The effects of insulin antibodies are under debate. Theoretically, they can bind to insulin and worsen GLYCEMIC CONTROL, thus preventing insulin from working. They can also buffer large amounts of free insulin that is released from the body's subcutaneous (fat) stores and help with smoothing out insulin levels and improving glycemic control.

Insulin antibodies apparently may exacerbate complications of diabetes. They have been found in the eyes and kidneys of animals that experienced diabetic complications. But no one has yet proven a direct cause and effect link between insulin antibodies and complications of diabetes.

Appropriate Blood Pressure Control in Diabetes Trial (ABCD Trial) A clinical study of 470 patients who had both diabetes and HYPERTENSION. Patients were assigned to two groups, one treated with enalapril (an ACE drug) and the other group treated with nisoldipine (a calcium channel blocker not available in the United States but similar to amlodipine and felodipine). Patients averaged 57–58 years old and had had diabetes for eight and a half years.

The initial blood pressure for patients was 155/98 in both groups. After five years of follow up, there were 25 heart attacks in the nisoldipine group versus five in the enalapril group. There were also 43 strokes in the nisoldipine group and seven in the enalapril group. The blood pressure decline was the same in both groups. The use of the ACE drug enalapril clearly conferred an advantage to the patients who took it, and it had effects other than just lowering blood pressure. The nisoldipine did not make the patients worse: they just did not do as well as the ACE group.

Asians/Pacific Islander Americans (APIA) People of Chinese, Filipino, Japanese, Asian Indian, Korean, Hawaiian, Samoan, and Vietnamese origin as well as people from an additional 28 Asian and 19 Pacific Islander ethnic groups, although the groups that are studied vary by researcher.

Some researchers study Pacific Islanders alone. These are people who are ethnic descendants of individuals from Hawaii, Samoa, or the South Seas. The risk for the development of Type 2 diabetes is particularly high among Native Hawaiians, largely because of their high risk for obesity.

In general, Asians living in the United States have a greater risk of developing Type 2 diabetes than do Asians residing in Asian countries; for example, their risk for diabetes is two to four times greater than the risk for people of the same race but who live in China, the Philippines, and other Asian countries.

Asian and Pacific Islander Youths

In a study of the incidence (new cases in a year) and prevalence (all individuals) of both Type 1 and Type 2 diabetes among 245 Asian and Pacific Islander youths, researchers Lenna L. Liu, M.D., and colleagues reported their findings in *Diabetes Care* in 2009. Most of the youths with diabetes had Type 1 diabetes, but they found a very low prevalence of Type 1 diabetes; for example, the prevalence of Type 1 diabetes among Asian, Pacific Islander, and Asian-Pacific Islanders was 0.26 per 1,000 youths ages 0–9 years and 0.88 per 1,000 youths ages 10–19 years. Of those with diabetes, about 70 percent had Type 1 diabetes.

Among those with Type 1 diabetes, the prevalence was 0.52 per 1,000 youths ages 10–19 years. (The prevalence of Type 2 diabetes among children ages 0–9 years was not computed because it is likely extremely low.)

In looking at the percentages of youths with diabetes, there were some discrepancies between races and ethnicities; for example, 77 percent of those who were mixed Asian/Pacific Islanders had Type 1 diabetes, while the rate was 73.5 percent for Pacific Islanders and 70 percent for those who were Asians. This also means that 30 percent of the Asians with diabetes had Type 2 diabetes, compared to 26.5 percent of Pacific Islanders and 23.0 percent of the mixed Asian-Pacific Islanders.

Most of the youths with Type 2 diabetes were obese; for example 71 percent of the 22 Asians with Type 2 diabetes were obese, as were 72.7 percent of the eight Asian-Pacific Islanders. Among Pacific Islanders, 100 percent of the eight subjects were obese.

See also AFRICAN AMERICANS WITH DIABETES; AMERICAN INDIANS/ALASKA NATIVES; HISPANICS/LATINOS; WHITES/CAUCASIANS.

Liu, Lenna L., M.D., et al. "Type 1 and Type 2 Diabetes in Asian and Pacific Islander U.S. Youth: The SEARCH for Diabetes in Youth Study." *Diabetes Care* 32, Supplement 2 (2009): S133–S140.

aspirin therapy Aspirin taken on a daily basis as a preventive measure against heart disease or stroke. People who have diabetes face between double to quadruple the risk of death from cardiovascular disease (CVD) as nondiabetics. However, a regular dose use of aspirin, taken under the advice and care of a physician, has been found to be effective in decreasing deaths after heart attacks by about 23 percent. It has also been shown to cut the risk of a repeat heart attack by about 50 percent.

According to the American Diabetes Association, those who benefit the most from aspirin therapy are people with diabetes who are over age 65 and have HYPERTENSION or CARDIOVASCULAR DISEASE.

Patients with diabetes have very reactive or "sticky" platelets in their blood, and thus, these platelets are more likely to clot than the platelets of patients without diabetes. Thus, taking aspirin may particularly help patients with diabetes by blocking or decreasing this excessive clotting action.

According to a position statement from the American Diabetes Association in 2001, analyses of studies of cardiovascular diseases reveal that

> low dose aspirin therapy should be prescribed as a secondary prevention strategy, if no contraindications exist. Substantial evidence suggests that low-dose aspirin therapy should also be used as a primary prevention strategy in men and women with diabetes who are at high risk for cardiovascular events.

Aspirin is particularly recommended to reduce the risk of heart disease in patients who:

- have a family history of coronary heart disease
- continue to smoke cigarettes (although it is always best to cease all smoking)
- have hypertension
- have protein in their urine
- have an obesity problem
- have low density lipids (LDL) under 130 ("bad" cholesterol)

- have high density lipids (HDL) over 40 ("good" cholesterol)
- have triglycerides over 250

Aspirin has also been shown to be effective in decreasing risks for patients with the following medical problems:

- heart attack
- stroke
- transient ischemic attack ("mini-stroke")
- peripheral vascular disease
- angina (chest pains related to heart disease)

A clinical study that was comparing the results of low-dose aspirin therapy to Vitamin E in decreasing cardiovascular problems was actually halted prematurely when the researchers found clear evidence that aspirin had major benefits to patients. According to a 2001 article in *Lancet,* the researchers found that cardiovascular deaths were reduced from 1.4 percent to 0.8 percent and total cardiovascular events dropped from 8.2 percent to 6.3 percent in the aspirin group. In this study, vitamin E did *not* confer these benefits.

Since the researchers did not wish to deny these benefits to the non-aspirin group, they ended the study earlier than they had planned so they could advise the patients to begin aspirin therapy.

The authors said the results should give doctors "the confidence to recommend low doses of aspirin (80–100 mg daily) for primary prevention in individuals who have one or more risk factors but whose blood pressure is contained within the normal range."

Despite the advantages of aspirin therapy, many people with diabetes who have CVD are not taking aspirin. According to a 2001 study in *Diabetes Care,* about 27 percent of people with diabetes have CVD, but only about one third (37 percent) use aspirin on a regular basis.

African Americans and Mexican Americans are less likely to use aspirin than whites.

Side Effects

Side effects of aspirin therapy may be allergy as well as minor or major gastrointestinal bleeding. Coated and lower-dose aspirin may decrease this problem. For this reason, it's important for patients using aspirin therapy to report any problems to their physicians. Aspirin therapy is not recommended for those who are under age 21, or those receiving anticoagulant medication, or who have had recent problems with gastrointestinal bleeding, or have problems with easy bleeding.

American Diabetes Association. "Aspirin Therapy in Diabetes," *Diabetes Care* 24, Supp. 1 (2001): S62–S63.

Collaborative Group of the Primary Prevention Project. "Low Dose Aspirin and Vitamin E in People at Cardiovascular Risk: A Randomised Trial in General Practice." *Lancet* 357 (2001): 89–95.

Kajubi, Samuel K., M.D. "Aspirin in the Treatment of Type 2 Diabetes." *Archives of Internal Medicine* 160, no. 3 (2000): 394.

Rolka, D. B., et al. "Aspirin Use Among Adults with Diabetes: Estimates from the Third National Health Nutrition Examination Survey," *Diabetes Care* 24, no. 2 (2001): 197–201.

assisted living facilities (ALF) Refers to rooms or apartments for older and/or disabled individuals in a facility where the staff provides assistance to residents. These facilities usually don't provide as much care as a person would receive in a SKILLED NURSING FACILITY (nursing home), but they do offer more care than the individual would receive if he or she were living at a private home. For example, most assisted living facilities provide meals, social events, and a nurse available on the premises as well as a physician on call.

Many assisted living facilities also offer special care to residents with diabetes, cognitive impairments such as ALZHEIMER'S DISEASE, and who suffer from other medical problems. In addition, the staff in an ALF often assists residents in making sure that needed medication is taken. Most staff members also offer or arrange for transportation for residents to get to their doctor appointments and shopping facilities.

Demographics of Assisted Living Residents

According to a summary of a report in a 2000 issue of *Contemporary Longterm Care,* most residents (75 percent) of assisted living facilities are female. The average age of residents is about 84 years for women and 83 years for men. An estimated 41 percent of residents are wheelchair users. About 10 percent of ALF residents receive special assistance with managing their diabetes and about 29 percent of residents receive help with managing their medications.

Advantages of Assisted Living Facilities

Older individuals with diabetes may find it difficult to live completely independently and yet they may also be fairly self-sustaining. As a result, they don't need or want the high level of care and the more limited freedom of a skilled nursing environment. Instead, the mid-level care offered in an assisted living facility may be sufficient for their needs. Study after study has demonstrated that many people intensely dislike the idea of moving to a skilled nursing facility; consequently, the interim step of an assisted living facility may provide residents with the convenience and the care that they need.

Disadvantages of Assisted Living

Most assisted living facilities are "private pay," and thus Medicare or Medicaid will not cover the cost of residence fees. Residents must use their own income and savings or must liquidate assets or find some other means to afford fees.

It should not be assumed that assisted living facilities follow the same state and federal regulations as skilled nursing facilities. Instead, state laws vary greatly on requirements that ALFs must meet; however, in general, the requirements are not as strict as they are for skilled nursing facilities. Of course, new ALFs must meet state and local building code requirements.

In 2000, the average rate for a private studio apartment in an ALF was estimated at about $2,000 per month, although fees vary greatly from area to area. The cost also depends heavily on the type of facility that is chosen and the services provided; for example, some ALFs advertise that they offer gourmet meals to residents. As one might expect, fees at such facilities are higher than where facilities provide nutritious but nongourmet fare.

Medicaid Waivers May Cover ALF Fees

It should be noted that in many states, and in assisted living facilities that wish to participate and are approved, a limited number of units are set aside in a special program for Medicaid recipients. In this "Medicaid waiver" program, requested by the state to the federal government, individuals who are receiving Medicaid benefits may have all or part of their rent paid for out of Medicaid funds. This program may be expanded in the future; however, as of this writing, it represents only a tiny portion of all assisted living units.

"ALF Overview Preview" *Contemporary Longterm Care* 23, no. 6 (June 2000): 9.

atherosclerosis/arteriosclerosis A complex condition in which the surface of the blood vessel (endothelium) is remodeled as the result of various processes. Atherosclerosis is a medical problem faced by many people with diabetes. It is an active process involving lipids (fats), white blood cells, antibodies, platelets, and other hormones and proteins that are all participants.

If the process continues long enough, it may block a blood vessel. More frequently, the plaque that builds up in the vessel ruptures and exposes lipids and other proteins to the circulation, setting off an acute clot (thrombus). This results in the blocking of blood flow and oxygen to the affected organ. Depending on the severity of the blood flow blockage, atherosclerosis may lead to MYOCARDIAL INFARCTION (heart attack), STROKE, or other serious medical problems.

See also CARDIOVASCULAR DISEASE.

autonomic neuropathy Refers to nerve problems involving the automatic functions of the body, such as the emptying of the stomach, colon, and bladder, as well as nerve problems with sexual function (erectile dysfunction in men and vaginal dryness and arousal failure in women).

If the stomach does not empty well, the condition is called GASTROPARESIS DIABETICORUM. When the bladder is affected, it can cause neurogenic bladder. When the colon is affected, it can cause diabetic diarrhea. It may also cause colonic dysmotility, a malfunction of the colon that may result in severe constipation, sometimes to the point of requiring the surgical removal of part of the colon.

Autonomic neuropathy can also affect heart function and lead to cardiac arrhythmias and sudden death. The blood pressure can also be affected. ORTHOSTATIC HYPOTENSION is a condition in which the systolic blood pressure of the person falls by more than 20 mm Hg when the person moves from lying to standing and has symptoms of lightheadedness and faintness. The person may actually faint.

See also DIABETIC NEUROPATHY.

bariatric surgery Elective surgery that is used in obese individuals with Type 2 diabetes and with extremely obese individuals (with or without diabetes) to aid them in weight loss. Bariatric surgery is also sometimes referred to as *metabolic surgery*. This type of surgery has become an increasingly common therapy for individuals who are suffering from obesity and its associated issues, namely Type 2 diabetes as well as its complications, such as dyslipidemia, HYPERTENSION, and obstructive sleep apnea. The American Society for Metabolic & Bariatric Surgery in Gainesville, Florida, estimates that 220,000 severely obese adults in the United States underwent bariatric surgery in 2008. In addition, some severely obese adolescents also have had the procedure, and an estimated 349 adolescents had bariatric surgery in 2004, the latest data as of this writing.

The two most common bariatric surgeries as of this writing in 2010 are gastric bypass surgery and the laparoscopic adjustable gastric band or LAGB (often referred to as lap-band surgery). The gastric bypass was actually developed in the 1960s when several surgeons noticed that a partial removal of the stomach for ulcers caused a weight loss in these patients. It was later developed into a procedure to help obese patients lose weight.

According to the National Institute of Diabetes and Digestive and Kidney Diseases (NIDDK) in their 2009 report on bariatric surgery, about 10 percent of the patients who have bariatric surgery will not lose sufficient weight or they will regain the weight that they had lost initially subsequent to the surgery. However, conversely, 90 percent of patients *will* apparently achieve their goals. The NIDDK estimates that bariatric surgery costs about $20,000 to $25,000. Insurance may or may not cover the costs, and this determination must be made prior to the surgery.

Some research has shown that the majority of patients with Type 2 diabetes who had a gastric bypass experienced a remission of their diabetes. One study published in 2009 in the *American Journal of Medicine* by Henry Buchwald, M.D., and colleagues, based on an analysis of 621 studies of bariatric surgery that occurred from 1990–2006 found that diabetes was resolved in 80.3 percent of patients with gastric bypass and in 56.7 percent of those with laparoscopic adjustable banding surgery. The majority of patients remained diabetes-free when followed up for two years after the surgery. (They may have remained diabetes-free longer; the follow-up occurred two years subsequent to the procedure.) Other studies have found that the resolution of diabetes continues for up to 16 years. Some studies show that the earlier in the course of the diabetes the surgery occurs, the better the outcome, although other studies have found an improvement in long-term diabetes patients who have had bariatric surgery.

Complications from the gastric bypass or the LAGB are more likely to occur in patients with a past history of blood clots or sleep apnea; however, researchers have found that analyzing risk management ahead of time significantly reduces the risk of complications, as with using an instrument known as the Metabolic Acuity Score (MAS). This instrument shows patients that need more aggressive follow-up.

The death rate from bariatric surgery is very low (about 0.5 percent), based on a study by the Agency for Healthcare Research and Quality (a United States federal government agency) in 2007. The agency also noted that hospital readmissions subsequent to the surgery are about 7 percent, down from 10 percent in 2002. The study was based on 9,500 patients younger than 65 years who had surgery at 652 hospitals in the periods 2001–02 and 2005–06.

Procedure

The two primary bariatric procedures are the gastric bypass (nearly always the Roux-en-Y gastric bypass) or the LAGB. Both procedures can be performed laparoscopically but sometimes the gastric bypass is performed in an "open" procedure with a large incision in the abdomen.

The gastric bypass With the gastric bypass, the surgeon sews or staples the stomach into a very small size that holds only about four to 10 teaspoons in volume. As a result, the stomach volume shrinks from about the size of a football to the size of a golf ball. The absorption of food that is consumed by the individual is reduced by excluding not only most of the stomach but also most of the duodenum and the upper part of the small intestine. As a result, the food goes into the small pouch of the stomach that has been created and into the lower part of the small intestine. This procedure can be performed laparoscopically but an open incision may be required if patients are extremely obese and/or they have had prior abdominal surgery. The larger the pouch that is created during this surgery, the less the weight loss that is seen. Patients with diabetes lose a bit less weight than their non-diabetic counterparts, but typically lose enough that most come off nearly all their anti-hyperglycemic medications.

The gastric bypass is considered both a restrictive procedure (since it limits the capabilities of the stomach) and also a malabsorptive procedure because it limits food absorption as a result of excluding food from most of the stomach and the duodenum.

Prior to the gastric bypass, patients must be carefully screened with a comprehensive physical examination and a cardiology evaluation, including some form of stress testing, pulmonary (lung) function testing, and an array of blood work to check for liver dysfunction. In addition, a psychiatric evaluation is also important to be sure that patients will be able to handle this very new lifestyle and to rule out serious psychiatric disorders that need treatment before the procedure, such as depression, bipolar disorder, anxiety disorder, or adult attention deficit/hyperactivity disorder (ADHD). Very obese patients often lose on the order of 70 to 100 pounds with this procedure.

The laparoscopic adjustable gastric band With the other most popular form of bariatric surgery, the LAGB, the surgeon performs the procedure laparoscopically and inserts a silicone saline-filled band over the top of the stomach to limit the rate and amount of food that may enter the digestive tract. It does not bypass the duodenum as does the gastric bypass, and thus there are fewer beneficial metabolic changes than with gastric bypass surgeries. The weight loss with the lap band is often less than with the gastric bypass, or about 30 to 50 pounds. The band can be adjusted with saline solution to expand or contract it, allowing for more or less food to be consumed.

Risks and Complications

Both the gastric bypass and the LAGB have risks and potential complications, although the LAGB is often considered safer than the gastric bypass because the band can be adjusted or even removed. (Some authors believe the gastric bypass is safer because the rate of resurgery is lower.) The gastric bypass cannot be reversed. With both forms of surgery, infections are a risk, as with all surgeries. In most cases, any infections that may develop are easily resolved with antibiotics.

Gastric bypass The gastric bypass is partially a malabsorptive procedure and it is also a restrictive procedure. It is a malabsorptive procedure because the portion of the intestine that is bypassed is also the area where iron and calcium absorption occurs, and consequently, the gastric bypass presents risks for osteoporosis and anemia. As a result, supplementation with both calcium and iron is required. In addition, supplementation of vitamin B_1 and vitamin B_{12} is also essential. If patients fail to follow their doctors' recommendations for vitamin and mineral supplementation, they may develop diseases of malnutrition, which are diseases such as pellagra or beri beri, usually seen only in people from very poor countries.

In addition, there is a risk for the development of gallstones with a large weight loss, as often occurs with the gastric bypass, and individuals should be screened in advance to determine if there are any existing gallstones or issues with the gallbladder.

Some patients who have had bariatric surgery may develop hernias, such as incisional hernias or internal hernias. Hernias are more likely to occur with an open incision than with a laparoscopic incision.

With the incisional hernia, part of the digestive system extends out from the abdominal wall, and this form of hernia may cause a blockage in the intestine. With an internal hernia, the small bowel develops pockets within the lining of the abdomen, and these hernias are even more dangerous than are incisional hernias.

Dumping syndrome can occur with gastric bypass surgery, causing vomiting, light-headedness, diarrhea, cramps, heart palpitations, and other symptoms within 10 to 30 minutes after eating. This is most likely to occur after patients eat foods that are high in sugar content. According to the Agency for Healthcare Research and Quality, dumping syndrome occurs in about 19 percent of patients who have a gastric bypass.

Late dumping may also occur from one to three hours after eating and usually occurs in relation to low blood sugar (HYPOGLYCEMIA), and is characterized by shakiness, sweating, hunger, and even fainting. In this case, the situation can be resolved with a small amount of sugar (as in fruit juice), taken about an hour after eating.

Other risks include ulcers, deep vein thrombosis, and pulmonary embolisms, although the risks for these particular adverse results occur in, at most, 2 percent of gastric bypass patients.

The laparoscopic adjustable gastric band The LAGB is *not* a malabsorptive procedure, however, in many cases, patients are encouraged to take vitamin supplements because they can digest only a fraction of what they could digest earlier and there is a risk of deficiencies. Patients generally lose less weight with the LAGB procedure (30 to 50 pounds, versus up to 100 pounds or more with the gastric bypass).

Postoperative complications with the LAGB may include dumping syndrome, as with the gastric bypass procedure. This is particularly a problem when patients eat sweet foods and thus, they usually learn to avoid such foods, which also helps with weight loss. Some patients experience problems with diarrhea or constipation subsequent to the LAGB. As with the gastric bypass, hernias may develop with the adjustable gastric band procedure.

A complication that is specific to LAGB is acid reflux that is caused by a band that is overly tight. This can be corrected by loosening the band. In addition, the pouch itself can be stretched if patients overeat.

Rare complications are a slipping of the band or an erosion of the band, which requires surgical adjustment or replacement. This problem can be diagnosed with an X-ray.

Outlook and Lifestyle Modifications

In general, most people do well with bariatric surgery, although some patients regain the weight that they have lost by eating high-calorie foods and not exercising. However, if the recommendations of the physician are followed, many people maintain the weight loss, and some studies indicate that the majority of patients with diabetes lose a significant amount of weight and keep the weight off for many years.

Another factor that should be considered with bariatric surgery is that when obese people with diabetes lose a significant amount of weight, often their diabetes improves or even remits altogether. In contrast, if the same people did *not* have the surgery and they remained obese, then their diabetes would continue to affect them, as will the many complications that are associated with diabetes.

Another issue to consider is that the skin may have stretched out a great deal and not have retained sufficient elasticity to contract after a large weight loss. As a result, the individual may have large flaps of skin, especially in the abdominal area. Some individuals choose to have the extra skin flaps removed so that they have a flatter stomach. (This procedure may or may not be covered by insurance because it may be considered "cosmetic.")

Gastric bypass According to Stacy A. Brethauer, M.D., and colleagues in their 2009 article *Obesity Management,* more than two-thirds of excess weight is lost within two years after a gastric bypass and for most patients with diabetes, this weight loss is maintained for 14 years or longer. They also noted that longitudinal research has demonstrated that people with impaired glucose tolerance who have had bariatric surgery reduced their risk for progressing to Type 2 diabetes by an estimated 30 times.

The authors also noted that among those individuals who are severely obese (with a body mass index of greater than 40 kg/m2), the failure rate for diet therapy (going on a traditional diet) is nearly 100 percent at the five-year point. Thus, bariatric surgery is basically the only therapy with staying power for most individuals.

Patients who have had a gastric bypass need to make effective food choices; for example, it is important to consume foods that are high in protein, such as fish, meat, and beans. In addition, patients must learn to avoid consuming fluids during meals because this can decrease or eliminate satiety and cause the person to eat more.

Exercise is another important component, and patients need to incorporate exercise into their daily life.

LAGB The outlook with the LAGB is generally positive, although the weight loss is lower than with the gastric bypass. Individuals need to follow the recommendations of their physicians in order to keep the weight off. Patients who have had an LAGB are less likely than patients with gastric bypass to develop serious vitamin deficits.

Considering Bariatric Surgery

According to the NIDDK, individuals considering bariatric surgery should ask themselves the following questions:

- Am I likely to lose weight or keep it off over the long term with nonsurgical measures?
- Am I well informed about the surgical procedure and the effects of treatment?
- Am I determined to lose weight and improve my health?
- Am I aware of how my life may change after the operation, such as the need to adjust to the side effects of the surgery, including the need to chew food well and the inability to eat large meals?
- Am I committed to lifelong healthy eating, exercise, medical follow-up visits, and vitamin and mineral supplementation?

Further Research

In a study by Jeffrey A. Tice, M.D., and colleagues that was published in the *American Journal of Medicine* in 2009, the researchers analyzed 14 studies that compared the results for the gastric bypass (Roux-en-Y) with results from the laparoscopic adjustable gastric banding. They found that a greater weight loss occurred with the gastric bypass and that those with the laparoscopic banding had fewer short-term problems resulting from the procedure than those with the gastric bypass. They also found, however, that reoperation rates were higher among those receiving the LAGB.

In addition, the research also showed that about 80 percent of the patients who had gastric bypass said that they were very satisfied, and none said that they were unsatisfied or that they regretted having the procedure. However, among those who had the laparoscopic banding procedure, only 46 percent said that they were very satisfied and 19 percent said that they were either unsatisfied or regretted having the procedure. As a result, the authors concluded that the gastric bypass should be the main procedure used in bariatric surgery.

In another article about bariatric surgery in the *British Journal of Diabetes and Vascular Disease* in 2009, Peter Flatt, Caroline Day, and Clifford J. Bailey discussed the effect of gut hormones with gastric bypass as compared to the laparoscopic gastric banding procedure in relation to lowering the risk for diabetes associated with obesity or what they referred to as "diabesity."

They said, "While calorie reduction is common to both types of intervention and accounts for much of the glucose-lowering effect, the diversion of nutrients away from the proximal small intestine and into the ileum [with the gastric bypass] appears to alter the release of gut hormones. Increased GLP-1 [glucagon-like peptide-1] and reduced GIP [gastric inhibitory polypeptide/glucose-dependent insulinotropic polypeptide] provide an interesting concept that may contribute to the difference in glucose-lowering efficacy between the different bariatric procedures." These changes in intestinal hormones or incretins are likely part of the reason why patients with diabetes can often come off many and in some cases all of their diabetes medications immediately after surgery, even before they have had significant weight loss.

Bariatric Surgery: Now in the Mainstream

Weight loss procedures have become so accepted as a treatment therapy that the American Diabetes association provided recommendations for the surgery in its annual list of recommendations in 2009. These include but are not limited to the following:

- Bariatric surgery should be considered for interested adults with a BODY MASS INDEX (BMI) of greater than 35 kg/m2 and with Type 2 diabetes, especially if the individual has found that they cannot control their weight with lifestyle and weight loss medications.

- Patients with type 2 diabetes who receive bariatric surgery will need to receive lifestyle support and medical monitoring for the rest of their lives.

- Although some studies have shown glycemic benefit of bariatric surgery in patients with Type 2 diabetes and a lower BMI of 30–35 kg/m2, there is not enough evidence to recommend surgery in patients with a BMI that is lower than 35 kg/m2.

See also OBESITY.

Agency for Healthcare Research and Quality. *Complications and Costs for Obesity Surgery.* Press Release. April 29, 2009. Rockville, MD: Agency for Healthcare Research and Quality. April 29, 2009. Available online. URL: http://www.ahrq.gov/news/press/pr2009/barsurgpr.htm. Accessed December 9, 2009.

American Diabetes Association. "Executive Summary: Standards of Medical Care in Diabetes-2009." *Diabetes Care* 32, Supplement 1 (2009): S6–S12.

Buchwald, Henry, M.D., et al. "Weight and Type 2 Diabetes after Bariatric Surgery: Systematic Review and Meta-analysis." American Journal of Medicine 122, no.3 (2009): 248–256.

Campos, G. M., Mulligan, Rabl C. K., et al. "Factors Associated With Weight Loss After Gastric Bypass." *Archives of Surgery* 143, no. 9 (2008): 877–884.

Flatt, Peter R., Caroline Day, and Clifford J. Bailey. "Bariatric Surgery: To Treat Diabesity." British Journal of Diabetes and Vascular Disease 9 (2009): 103–107.

Longitudinal Assessment of Bariatric Surgery (LABS) Consortium. "Perioperative Safety in the Longitudinal Assessment of Bariatric Surgery." *New England Journal of Medicine* 361, no. 5 (2009): 445–454.

Minocha, Anil, M.D., and Christine Adamec. *The Encyclopedia of the Digestive System and Digestive Disorders.* 2nd ed. New York: Facts On File, 2011.

National Institute for Diabetes and Digestive and Kidney Diseases. *Bariatric Surgery for Severe Obesity.* Bethesda, Md.: National Institutes of Health, 2009.

Tice, Jeffrey A., M.D., et al. "Gastric Banding or Bypass? A Systematic Review Comparing the Two Most Popular Bariatric Procedures." *American Journal of Medicine* 121 (2008): 885–893.

behavioral modification A purposeful changing and shaping of behavior. For example, psychologists may use behavioral modification techniques to help patients with diabetes exhibit better medication adherence and improve their diet, lose weight, and quit smoking, among some of the available choices. In their 1998 article for *Clinical Diabetes,* authors Harris and Lustman note that the psychologist or social worker can help the patient improve his or her health. They also state that,

> The bulk of the psychological services in diabetes care are provided to patients who do not have diagnosable psychological problems. For example, nonadherence to the diabetes regimen is the most common reason for psychological referral, although in a statistical sense, it represents the norm and not the exception. Nonadherence to treatment is not itself evidence of a psychological problem.

Common psychological goals are:

- to improve adherence to diet and insulin/medication
- to promote exercise and a healthy lifestyle
- to aid the patient in eliminating harmful behavior such as smoking
- to evaluate psychological problems that may exist and make appropriate referral

Of course, sometimes patients with diabetes do have serious psychological problems, such as DEPRESSION, and it's estimated that at least one third of all patients with diabetes will experience depression or anxiety at some point in their lives. Sometimes antidepressants or other medications are prescribed. The psychiatrist or treating physician should carefully coordinate any medication that is prescribed for a patient with diabetes with the patient's primary physician. The patient should also be sure to tell his or her physician about the psychiatrist or any other medical doctor being seen, so that any risks of medication interactions are minimal.

See also MEDICATION ADHERENCE/COMPLIANCE.

beta cell Specialized cell found in the islets of Langerhans along with alpha cells (glucagon) and delta cells. It is this cell that produces insulin and that may become defective and stop producing insulin.

People with Type 1 diabetes have pancreases that produce no insulin because their immune system has destroyed the beta cells. In contrast, people with Type 2 diabetes usually have a pancreas with beta cells that produce some insulin; however, their bodies have developed a resistance to the effects of insulin.

Current research is focused on attempts to infuse/transplant beta cells to cure diabetes. The limiting issue, however, is the availability of pancreases from which to harvest the beta cells. Intense efforts are ongoing to grow beta cells in the laboratory in order to create a dependable and renewable supply.

biguanides A class of drugs used to treat people with Type 2 diabetes. As of this writing, the only drug in the class is Glucophage (METFORMIN). Drugs in this class work to boost or improve the use of glucose in the body and lower the amount of insulin in the body. Glucophage does not cause HYPOGLYCEMIA as do some other diabetes medications, nor does it cause weight gain. Since many people with Type 2 diabetes have a problem with OBESITY, this is an important asset.

Glucophage may cause nausea and can initially lead to changes in bowel habits, especially loose stools. Taking the pill with a meal and slowly titrating the dose up to 2,000 to 2,550 milligrams per day often diminishes these side effects. Glucophage should not be used in patients with renal insufficiency or moderate-to-severe liver dysfunction. Nor should it be used in patients with congestive heart failure.

See also CANCER.

birth control Devices used to prevent conception from occurring, such as birth control pills, intrauterine devices, condoms, diaphragms with spermicides, sponges, and "natural" methods, such as charting when conception is most likely to occur and avoiding intercourse at that time. (Also known as the "rhythm" method.) Women with diabetes can, in general, use most of the same methods and devices for birth control as women with normal glucose levels. Caution must be taken, however, in using oral birth control contraceptives.

Experts caution women with diabetes against using progesterone-containing intrauterine devices (IUDs) for contraception because of the risk of infection. However, it is felt that women with diabetes may safely use copper-containing IUDs.

Contraception Enables Preconception Care

Contraception is also important for the woman with diabetes because before conception, experts strongly advise that extra care should be taken to avoid later harm to both mother and baby. Preconception care has proven to provide significant health benefits to both mother and child.

See also PREGNANCY.

Birth Control Pills

If women with diabetes use birth control pills for contraception, they need to realize that the female hormone in the pills may affect their blood glucose levels. Birth control pills may increase insulin resistance. This is especially true for progesterone-only contraceptives. Women with diabetes who use birth control pills may require an adjustment in their therapy to continue to maintain their usual level of glycemic control. Monophasic pills (pills with a steady level of hormone on each day, with no variation) supply a steady level of hormone and thus

may cause fewer ups and downs in glucose levels. If a woman has diabetes, is over 30, is a smoker, or has high blood pressure, oral contraceptives may not be the safest option.

Women who are also at risk for diabetes, because of close family members with diabetes or whose doctors say they are at risk for another reason, should also be cautious in taking birth control pills. Women with normal glucose tolerance who have risk factors for diabetes and take birth control pills may develop IMPAIRED GLUCOSE TOLERANCE (IGT). In addition, women who already have IGT and who then take birth control pills may then progress to overt diabetes.

Birth Control for Women Who Had Gestational Diabetes

Birth control is also important for the mother who has had a previous experience with GESTATIONAL DIABETES MELLITUS (GDM) and who does not wish an active involvement in diabetes self-care. The rate for recurrent GDM is about 50 percent. To avoid unplanned pregnancies, contraception is important.

Tubal ligation, a form of surgical sterilization, is another option for women who do not wish to have any more children. It's important to realize, however, that it is usually difficult and may be impossible to reverse this procedure.

Male Contraception

There are fewer contraceptive options available for men, although condoms are about 90 percent effective when used correctly. Vasectomy is an excellent choice for couples who do not wish to have more children, and it is a much less invasive procedure than tubal ligation for women. As with tubal ligation, this decision needs to be taken very carefully, as reversal is very difficult and may prove to be impossible.

blindness The inability to see or the loss of vision. Diabetes mellitus is the main cause of blindness in individuals ages 20 to 74 years in the United States, and the disease accounts for up to 24,000 of new cases of blindness each year. People with diabetes have about 20 times the risk of nondiabetics for developing blindness. In the United States, there are about 65,000 new cases of proliferative retinopathy per year. The World Health Organization noted in a 2009 report that worldwide, 4.8 percent of blindness was caused by diabetic retinopathy. In many cases, an annual eye examination and subsequent diagnosis and treatment could have prevented, ameliorated, or at least delayed the subsequent loss of vision. (See DIABETIC EYE DISEASES.) Total blindness is a situation of no light perception (NLP).

In North America and most of Europe, legal blindness is defined as a best corrected visual acuity of 20/200 in the best eye. A white cane is the international sign for blindness and quite helpful for safe mobility of those with blindness. There are also definitions of blindness that include a loss of visual field. Many people with legal blindness have some light perception that helps them adjust to their daily circadian rhythm.

Although good medical treatment is available for many common eye diseases such as GLAUCOMA and CATARACTS when diagnosed early enough, many people with diabetes do not obtain such treatment, and as a result, they lose their eyesight; for example, the Centers for Disease Control and Prevention (CDC) estimates that 60 percent of individuals with diabetes fail to have their eyes checked annually with a dilated eye examination. This is an extremely crucial eye examination, which can reveal early signs of eye problems that may eventually lead to blindness.

Another reason for having an annual examination is that often serious eye diseases may have no noticeable symptoms until it is very difficult or too late to repair the damage, as in the case of DIABETIC RETINOPATHY. An ophthalmologist or an optometrist who is trained in diabetic eye diseases can detect such diseases in the early stages when treatment will often still be effective.

As a result of concern over this serious problem, individuals with diabetes who are over age

65 years and who are receiving Medicare may obtain free examinations and treatment and they should avail themselves of this opportunity. See also MACULAR EDEMA.

blood glucose meters Special hand-held devices that test the blood glucose levels, thus helping a person with diabetes determine if the glucose level is normal or not. Many devices require the person to prick a finger with a LANCET, so that a drop of blood may be tested. Some devices incorporate the blood extraction with the testing, enabling a person to extract the drop of blood from the forearm, where there are fewer nerve endings, and thus, less pain and to then obtain readout results in 8–30 seconds.

Many meters have memories, and an individual can make comparisons to previous readings. The patient may also be able to download the information to a computer for later use.

Many devices offer prompts to alert the patient to the presence of ketones or to advise the person to get a snack or adjust his or her insulin. Blood glucose meters may be small or very large and prices for them vary greatly. Insurance companies may provide payment for such devices. MEDICARE covers blood glucose meters for individuals with diabetes.

Most meters now automatically convert the whole blood glucose reading to a plasma level so that it would be comparable to a venous (vein) reading taken in a laboratory. *Diabetes Forecast,* a publication of the American Diabetes Association, includes a "Resource Guide" supplement at the end of each year that is devoted to reviewing blood glucose meters and other devices that are needed by or that are helpful to people with diabetes.

blood glucose monitoring Periodic testing of blood glucose levels, followed by possible action based on the results of the test. For example, if glucose levels are high, more medication may be needed. If they are very low or the person may be experiencing symptoms of HYPOGLYCEMIA, the individual will consume a glucose gel/tablet or a high carbohydrate food or drink.

One of the major developments in diabetes over the past 80 years is that patients can monitor their own glucose levels with a tiny drop of blood. Noninvasive options (bloodless testing) may be available to patients at some point in the early 21st century, thus alleviating the pain of the finger prick. Self-monitoring is really the cornerstone of care, and enables the person with diabetes to judge the effects of diet, exercise, medications, stress, insulin, and other factors.

See also GLYCEMIC CONTROL; HOME BLOOD GLUCOSE MONITORING.

blood pressure/hypertension See HYPERTENSION.

blood sugar Blood glucose levels, which are usually high (HYPERGLYCEMIA) in a person with untreated diabetes. If blood sugar drops to a low state, the person with diabetes is having an episode of HYPOGLYCEMIA, which can cause an array of serious problems and medical complications.

See also GLYCEMIC CONTROL.

blurred vision Clouded or distorted vision. For a person with diabetes, sudden blurred or clouded vision is a danger sign and means that he or she should see an ophthalmologist (doctor who specializes in eye diseases) immediately. The blurred vision could be a sign of the onset of DIABETIC RETINOPATHY with hemorrhage and impending BLINDNESS. If caught early, it may be possible to avert such severe complications. Blurred vision might also be a warning sign of CATARACTS. Untreated cataracts lead to blindness.

Blurred vision may also be caused by major shifts in glucose levels. Glucose gets into the lens of the eye, where it is converted to sorbitol. Water osmotically follows and the lens changes its shape. As a result, the person's eyes cannot refract properly. For these reasons, physicians recommend no change in eyeglass prescriptions until glucose levels have been stable for about four to six weeks.

body mass index (BMI) A specific formula that is based on height and weight, and which helps to determine whether a person is underweight, of optimal weight, or is overweight or obese. The United States and the World Health Organization rely primarily on the body mass index (BMI) to determine levels of OBESITY and to stratify a patient's risk for a variety of diseases and complications. It should also be noted that a BMI chart for an adult should not be used to determine whether a child is overweight or obese. Instead, physicians should refer to pediatric BMI charts for boys and girls. (See Appendix X.)

Research released in late 2009 revealed that body mass index is directly correlated to a risk for diabetes, and that the higher the BMI, the greater the risk. This research was based on more than 20,000 middle-aged and older men followed by a median of 23 years. The researchers also found that physical activity decreased the risk for developing diabetes among normal to obese men compared to men who failed to exercise.

In the past, physicians and other experts primarily relied on height/weight charts alone; however, the BMI measure is seen as a better measure of determining excessive weight. Because OBESITY is a strong predictor of Type 2 diabetes, BMI is an important concept in diabetes.

TABLE 1: BODY MASS INDEX CLASSIFICATION
Underweight: Less than 18.5
Normal weight: 18.5–24.9
Overweight: 25–29.9
Obesity (Class 1): 30–34.9
Obesity (Class 2): 35–39.9
Extreme Obesity: 40 or over

TABLE 2: BODY MASS INDEX (BMI) TABLE

BMI	19	20	21	22	23	24	25	26	27	28	29	30	31	32	33	34	35
Height									**Weight (in pounds)**								
4'10" (58")	91	96	100	105	110	115	119	124	129	134	138	143	148	153	158	162	167
4'11" (59")	94	99	104	109	114	119	124	128	133	138	143	148	153	158	163	168	173
5' (60")	97	102	107	112	118	123	128	133	138	143	148	153	158	163	168	174	179
5'1" (61")	100	106	111	116	122	127	132	137	143	148	153	158	164	169	174	180	185
5'2" (62")	104	109	115	120	126	131	136	142	147	153	158	164	169	175	180	186	191
5'3" (63")	107	113	118	124	130	135	141	146	152	158	163	169	175	180	186	191	197
5'4" (64")	110	116	122	128	134	140	145	151	157	163	169	174	180	186	192	197	204
5'5" (65")	114	120	126	132	138	144	150	156	162	168	174	180	186	192	198	204	210
5'6" (66")	118	124	130	136	142	148	155	161	167	173	179	186	192	198	204	210	216
5'7" (67")	121	127	134	140	146	153	159	166	172	178	185	191	198	204	211	217	223
5'8" (68")	125	131	138	144	151	158	164	171	177	184	190	197	203	210	216	223	230
5'9" (69")	128	135	142	149	155	162	169	176	182	189	196	203	209	216	223	230	236
5'10" (70")	132	139	146	153	160	167	174	181	188	195	202	209	216	222	229	236	243
5'11" (71")	136	143	150	157	165	172	179	186	193	200	208	215	222	229	236	243	250
6' (72")	140	147	154	162	169	177	184	191	199	206	213	221	228	235	242	250	258
6'1" (73")	144	151	159	166	174	182	189	197	204	212	219	227	235	242	250	257	265
6'2" (74")	148	155	163	171	179	186	194	202	210	218	225	233	241	249	256	264	272
6'3" (75")	152	160	168	176	184	192	200	208	216	224	232	240	248	256	264	272	279

Source: Evidence Report of Clinical Guidelines on the Identification, Evaluation, and Treatment of Overweight and Obesity in Adults, 1998. NIH/National Heart, Lung, and Blood Institute (NHLBI)

BMI is also usually a very effective measure to denote obesity. But it should also be noted that, in a few cases, such as the case of weightlifters or very athletic and heavily muscular people, they might appear to be overweight according to BMI charts, although they are not.

The converse is also true. Some studies indicate that in the case of some Asian individuals, because their bones and body build are smaller than the Western standard, Asians may be overweight or obese at lower weights than indicated by the BMI chart. As a result, some Asians may be at risk for diabetes or actually have diabetes, but because of the BMI chart, doctors think they do not have a weight problem and they do not realize when there is a risk for Type 2 diabetes.

According to a report on obesity in Asia, published in 2000, new criteria for overweight and obesity are needed. The authors say, "While in some Asian populations the prevalence of obesity is lower than that in Europe, the health risks associated with obesity occur at a lower body mass index (BMI) in Asian populations."

This source offered such criteria. For example, the normal range of BMI for an "adult Europid" (person from Europe) was 18.5–24.9. The authors proposed that a normal BMI for adult Asians should be 18.5–22.9. Thus, Asians would be considered overweight at lower levels than non-Asians.

See also DIABETES MELLITUS; OBESITY.

brain attack   See STROKE.

breast-feeding Directly providing breast milk to an infant, and a very highly regarded method of nutrition for babies. In past years, women with diabetes were discouraged from having children. If they did have babies, bottle-feeding rather than breast-feeding their infants was encouraged by doctors. Today, most doctors work with mothers who have diabetes to help them have an optimal pregnancy and a healthy child. Breast-feeding is now encouraged by physicians, who are aware of the strong bond that develops between the breast-feeding infant and the mother, as well as the nutritional and medical benefits that come with breast-feeding.

Some studies have shown that breast-feeding in infancy is protective against the development of Type 2 diabetes in childhood, adolescence, and adulthood. Note that most of these studies are performed on nondiabetic mothers, concentrating instead on whether breast-fed children have a lower probability of developing diabetes than non-breastfed children. In a study by Elizabeth J. Mayer-Davis and colleagues that was published in *Diabetes Care* in 2008, the researchers found that about a third (31.3 percent) of the youths had been breast-fed. Among the African Americans, Hispanics, and non-Hispanic white youths, ages 10 to 21 years, in each group, the prevalence of diabetes was lower among those who had been breast-fed. In addition, the children who were breast-fed had a significantly lower BODY MASS INDEX compared to those who were not breast-fed.

In an analysis of seven studies on breast-feeding that was published in 2006 by C. G. Owen and colleagues in the *American Journal of Clinical Nutrition,* the researchers found that breast-feeding in infancy was linked to a 39 percent reduced rate of Type 2 diabetes in childhood and adulthood.

More recently, in a study published in the September 2010 issue of the *American Journal of Medicine,* Eleanor Bimla Schwarz, M.D., and colleagues reported on their study of the relationship between breast-feeding and the later development of Type 2 diabetes. Of the 2,233

women studied ages 40 to 78 years old, 1,828 were mothers and 56 percent of the mothers had breast-fed an infant for at least a month. The researchers found that women who had breast-fed their infants had a decreased risk for the development of Type 2 diabetes. Said the researchers, "Mothers should be encouraged to exclusively breast-feed all of their infants for at least 1 month."

Breast-feeding may help decrease the risk for Type 2 diabetes by decreasing the risk for OBESITY, a primary cause of Type 2 diabetes. The Centers for Disease Control and Prevention (CDC) strongly supports breast-feeding, and in its 2009 report to prevent obesity in the United States, it has a strategy to encourage breast-feeding in communities. According to this report by Laura Kettel Khan and colleagues, "Breast-feeding is thought to promote an infant's ability to self regulate energy intake, thereby allowing him or her to eat in response to internal hunger and satiety cues. Some research suggests that the metabolic/hormonal cues provided by breast-milk contribute to the protective association between breast-feeding and childhood obesity."

Some researchers have looked at nondiabetic women who have breast-fed their infants to see if there was a relationship between breast-feeding and the subsequent development (or lack of development) of diabetes. In a study of the association between lactation history and the subsequent incidence of Type 2 diabetes among women by Alison M. Stuebe, M.D., and colleagues and published in the *Journal of the American Medical Association* in 2005, the researchers found that a longer period of lactation was associated with a reduced incidence of Type 2 diabetes, based on thousands of female subjects drawn from the Nurses' Health Study (121,700 women) and the Nurses' Health Study II (116,671 women). The women were all registered nurses.

Of the women in the first Nurses' Health Study, 83,585 reported having ever lactated and 64 percent of those who had lactated had ever breast-fed their children. In the Nurses' Health

Study II, 73,418 women reported ever having lactated and 85 percent of this group had breast-fed their infants.

The researchers said, "In both cohorts, higher parity [number of children they had] was associated with longer lifetime duration of breast-feeding. Women who breast-fed for longer periods were also less likely to have a family history of diabetes or to be smokers."

In another study in which the breast-feeding mothers were themselves diabetic at the time of breast-feeding their babies, the researchers studied the effect of the breast milk on the body weight of their children in the first year of life. This research by A. Kerssen and colleagues was reported in 2004 in the *European Journal of Clinical Nutrition*. The researchers studied 141 women with Type 1 diabetes in the Netherlands, and considered the duration of lactation, diseases in the child's first year of life, and other factors.

There were 39 mothers who breast-fed their infants, 43 who formula-fed them, and 59 mothers who did mixed feedings. The researchers found no significant difference between weight and body mass index of the infants at the age of one among those who were breast-fed, formula-fed, or mixed-fed (both formula- and breast-feeding). Although the researchers did not state this, this seems to indicate that the children breast-fed by diabetic mothers were as healthy as the children who were not breast-fed, indicating that breast-feeding is a viable option for diabetic mothers.

Some Difficulties to Overcome

WOMEN WITH DIABETES need to be aware that they must continue to be prudent in checking their glucose levels, a task that can become cumbersome among the many duties of a new mother. In addition, many new mothers are tired from lack of sleep, and sleep deprivation can upset glucose levels for the diabetic woman. A third risk for breast-feeding mothers who have diabetes is that they are more prone to infections than nondiabetic women and need to be sure to contact the physician if their breasts become painful or swollen. This may indicate a yeast or bacterial infection.

Women with diabetes who are breast-feeding will often need a small snack prior to breast-feeding a child, and they should also be sure to test their glucose levels about an hour after breast-feeding to make sure that there is no problem with excessively low levels of glucose (HYPOGLYCEMIA), which could lead to a dangerous situation for the mother and child.

Breast-feeding mothers should also be very careful about medications that they take. For example, oral hypoglycemic medications that can be secreted into breast milk should be avoided because they may cause the infant to suffer from hypoglycemia.

In very rare cases, breast-feeding should be avoided altogether. This is true in the case of women with diabetes who have proliferative retinopathy (an eye disease that can lead to blindness), because breast-feeding can further accelerate the retinopathy.

See also GESTATIONAL DIABETES MELLITUS; PREGNANCY.

Kerssen, A., et al. "Effect of Breast Milk of Diabetic Mothers on Bodyweight of the Offspring in the First Year of Life." *European Journal of Clinical Nutrition* 58 (2008): 1,429–1,431.

Khan, Laura Kettel, et al. "Recommended Community Strategies and Measurements to Prevent Obesity in the United States." *Morbidity and Mortality Weekly Report* 58, no. RR-7 (July 24, 2009): 1–30.

Mayer-Davis, Elizabeth J., et al. "Breast-Feeding and Type 2 Diabetes in the Youths of Three Ethnic Groups." *Diabetes Care* 31, no. 3 (2008): 470–475.

Owen, C. G., et al. "Does Breast-feeding Influence a Risk of Type 2 Diabetes in Later Life? A Quantitative Analysis of Published Evidence." *American Journal of Clinical Nutrition* 84, no. 5 (2006): 1,043–1,054.

Schwarz, Eleanor Bimla, M.D., et al. "Lactation and Maternal Risk of Type 2 Diabetes: A Population-Based Study." *American Journal of Medicine* 123, no. 9 (2010): 863e1–863e6.

Stuebe, Alison M., et al. "Duration of Lactation and Incidence of Type 2 Diabetes." *Journal of the American Medical Association* 294, no. 20 (2005): 2,601–2,610.

brittle diabetes A condition in which glucose levels are very variable and very difficult to control. When this type of problem occurs, it is nearly always diagnosed in patients with Type 1 diabetes and no immediate apparent or clear-cut cause is found. Further investigation is required to seek out the cause.

In their chapter on brittle diabetes in *Ellenberg and Rifkin's Diabetes Mellitus,* authors David S. Schade and Mark R. Burge define brittle diabetes as, "Specifically, a brittle diabetic patient is one who is either incapacitated or whose life-style is disrupted more than 3 times per week by repeated episodes of hyperglycemia or hypoglycemia *after the patient has been educated in the techniques of intensive insulin therapy.*" (Italic is per the original.)

Schade and Burge contend that until it is clear that the patient is fully educated and that the problem does not stem from misunderstanding about self-treatment, brittle diabetes should not be diagnosed.

They also state that in about half of the cases, once the underlying cause of the brittle diabetes is corrected, the patient then becomes "nonbrittle."

In his article on this topic in a 2000 issue of *Diabetes Forecast,* Dr. Michael Pfeiffer agrees that there are always reasons for wide swings in glucose levels. Some reasons that he suggested may be the causes are:

- insulin that has been improperly stored and as a result, has gone bad
- errors with insulin measurement or mixing
- digestive disorders such as GASTROPARESIS, or slow stomach emptying
- physical and/or psychological stress

Other causes noted by Schade and Burge include:

- narcotic drug addiction
- early morning hyperglycemia (dawn phenomenon)
- endocrine disorders
- insulin resistance
- psychological problems

Pfeiffer, Michael A., M.D. "Brittle Diabetes." *Diabetes Forecast* 53, no. 11 (November 2000): 13.

Schade, David S., and Mark R. Burge. "Brittle Diabetes: Pathogenesis and Therapy." In *Ellenberg and Rifkin's Diabetes Mellitus.* Oxford: Appleton & Lange, 1999.

calcium channel blockers (CCBs) A class of medications that is prescribed for people with HYPERTENSION (high blood pressure) in order to lower their blood pressure levels. Many people with diabetes also suffer from hypertension. The combination of diabetes and hypertension can cause severe complications including premature death. Some examples of calcium channel blocker medications are, as of this writing: nifedipine, amlodipine, isradipine, diltiazem, and verapamil.

CCBs are further broken down into the dihydropyridine (DHP) class and the non-DHP (NDHP) class. The DHP calcium channel blockers may cause mild headache and swollen ankles when given in large doses. The NDHP calcium channel blockers may cause constipation and may slow the heart rate, and they need to be used carefully with other drugs that could affect heart rate or any aspect of the heart's electrical conduction system. This has been an area of controversy as some studies have shown that although the DHP CCBs are very well tolerated and very effective, at the same time, they may be less effective than the NDHP CCBs at protecting kidney function in patients with diabetes.

Dr. George Bakris has done a number of studies showing that low-dose NDHP CCBs in combination with angiotensin-converting enzyme (ACE) inhibitor drugs or beta-blocker drugs may be the best choice. The exact combinations that are best will continue to be a source of controversy as newer drugs are developed. At this time, most experts feel that the most important issue is getting the blood pressure as low as the patient will tolerate, at a minimum under 135/85 or, ideally, as low as 120/70. If an optimal blood pressure can be achieved, then the exact choice of medications has less impact on the overall outcome.

See also CARDIOVASCULAR DISEASE; STROKE.

Bakris G., et al., "Effects of an ACE Inhibitor/Calcium Antagonist Combination on Proteinuria in Diabetic Nephropathy." *Kidney International* 54, no. 4 (1998): 1,283–1,289.

camps for children and adolescents with diabetes Summer camps for school-age children and adolescents who have diabetes. These camps are specifically oriented to their needs.

Summer camp can be a valuable experience, according to many experts, enabling children to meet new friends and providing an opportunity for children to learn that other children share the same struggles. It can help them feel less alone and more normal, as they discuss problems and solutions they have developed. Some children who have been resistant to self-injecting may overcome their fears when they see other children self-inject in a matter-of-fact manner. Camp counselors may also be adolescents and young adults who have diabetes and can be empathetic with the children about the disease and yet, at the same time, not overly fearful.

Camp can also be a break for parents or others who care for children with diabetes, and who must constantly consider issues such as blood checks, medication, and dealing with problems related to the disease.

According to Joanne D. Moore, R.N., C.D.E., in her article on sending a child to camp for the first time, in a 1996 issue of *Diabetes Self-Management*, parents should take the following steps to ease the way for both parent and child:

- talk to the child about the camp beforehand and emphasize its assets
- decide whether to send the child to a day camp or a residential camp. Day camps may be preferable for children under age nine
- make sure that the camp is accredited by the American Diabetes Association
- read camp brochures
- if the camp offers an open house opportunity to ask questions, attend it
- learn how the camp copes with medical problems and how they reach a physician if one is needed

The American Diabetes Association (ADA) has created a position statement on the management of diabetes at diabetes camps. According to the ADA, each camper should have a form that provides medical information on the child, as well as immunization information and the child's medication regimen.

While children are in camp, daily records of their blood glucose levels and insulin dosages should be recorded. Some modifications, such as reductions, may need to be made to insulin dosages because many children will be much more active at camp than at home. If the child uses an insulin pump, the camp director and medical staff should be familiar with the device and ensure that extra batteries are available.

American Diabetes Association, "Management of Diabetes at Diabetes Camps." *Diabetes Care* 24, Supp. 1 (January 2001): S113–S115.
Moore, Joanne D. "Sending Your Kid to Camp for the First Time." *Diabetes Self-Management* (March/April 1996): 23–26.

Canada and diabetes There are more than 2 million Canadians who have diabetes, according to the Canadian Diabetes Association. Of these, about 90 percent have Type 2 diabetes. Canadians also suffer from the complications of diabetes; for example, about 28 percent of the cases of severe kidney disease are experienced by Canadians with diabetes. ERECTILE DYSFUNCTION and many other illnesses are also problems.

Canada is comprised of diverse ethnic groups, and, as in the United States, minority groups are generally at a much greater risk for the development of Type 2 diabetes.

Interestingly, it has been Canadian scientists who have made great advances in helping people with diabetes. Most importantly, in 1922, Canadian scientists, Frederick Banting and Charles Best, proved that insulin could mitigate the impact of diabetes. Banting (with laboratory director Dr. MacLeod) later received the Nobel Prize for this work. It was truly an incredible lifesaving discovery, responsible for improving quality of life for millions of children and adults with diabetes.

In 2000, Dr. James Shapiro and his colleagues at the University of Alberta in Edmonton reported a breakthrough success with islets of Langerhans transplants, causing 11 patients to remain diabetes-free one year later. Dr. Shapiro attributed at least part of the success to the avoidance of steroid medications, which had apparently inhibited success in past trials. As of this writing, Shapiro's "Edmonton Protocol" is being tested and utilized on patients in the United States, Canada, and the United Kingdom.

Many other clinical studies on diabetes, too numerous to cite in this essay, have been performed by Canadian physicians and researchers.

See also ISLETS OF LANGERHANS.

cancer Some research indicates that people with diabetes have a greater risk for developing some forms of cancer, although the reasons for these elevated risks are unknown. In addition, diabetic patients who develop cancer have a greater risk for death over both the short term and the long term compared with those without diabetes, according to Andrew Renehan and colleagues in their 2010 article for the *Lancet*. They report that diabetic patients have an increased risk for developing the following cancers: postmenopausal breast cancer, colorectal cancer, endometrial cancer, liver cancer, non-Hodgkin's lymphoma, and pancreatic cancer. Note that these risks are not associated with OBESITY or BODY MASS INDEX.

The research indicates that the use of the biguanide drug METFORMIN (Glucophage, Glucophage XL) apparently decreases the risk for cancer, although the mechanism for this lowered risk is unknown.

Renehan et al. recommend that screening for cancer should be a standard part of diabetes care, and they contend that cancer-screening among diabetics is lower than among nondiabetics, despite the more frequent contacts that people with diabetes have with health professionals.

Renehan, Andrew, Ulf Smith, and M. Sue Kirkman. "Linking Diabetes and Cancer: A Consensus on Complexity." *Lancet* 35 (June 26, 2010): 2,201–2,202.

carbohydrates and meal planning   A carbohydrate is one of three energy-producing nutrients found in foods; the other two are fats and proteins. According to the American Diabetes Association, carbohydrates include sugars, starches and dietary fiber, and they contain 4 kilocalories per gram.

When the body cannot use glucose (sugar) for energy because of inadequate insulin (due to an absolute lack of insulin or an inadequate amount to overcome the body's resistance to insulin), then carbohydrates cannot be utilized properly. In such a situation, carbohydrates are stored as glycogen, mainly within the liver. During a fast, when the body has inadequate glucose to store as fuel, it then begins to break down stored glucose from glycogen. When those reserves are exhausted, the body begins to use its own fat, not a healthy situation. The breakdown of fats leads to the formation of ketoacids,

a substance that is seen in small quantities in nondiabetics; however, the formation of ketoacids can be deleterious to those with diabetes and to unborn fetuses. (See DIABETIC KETOACIDOSIS; GESTATIONAL DIABETES MELLITUS.)

The closer to normal that a person with diabetes keeps the blood glucose levels, the lower is the risk for many complications from diabetes, including such severe complications as AMPUTATION, BLINDNESS, kidney failure and an early DEATH. The person with diabetes who works toward tighter blood glucose control may be at a greater risk for developing HYPOGLYCEMIA, particularly when using certain MEDICATIONS FOR TREATMENT OF TYPE 2 DIABETES. Thus, prudence and regular blood glucose checking as recommended by the physician are important aspects of the lives of individuals with diabetes.

Note that in contrast to a popular misconception about diabetes, there is no evidence that the complete restriction of all sucrose (table sugar) is necessary for people with diabetes. However, at the same time, this does not mean that it is advisable for people with diabetes to eat large amounts of sugar-filled foods, which are usually high in calories and low in nutritional value. Instead, foods that are high in sugar should be consumed in moderation; for example, it is not necessary to forego special foods during the holidays or at other celebrations; however, one small piece of pumpkin pie or a slice of cake is sufficient for most people with or without diabetes.

There are various meal planning methods that people with diabetes can use to help them stay healthy and keep their glucose levels as close to normal as possible. These may include carbohydrate counting, following the diabetes food pyramid or plate method, and considering the glycemic index. It is also recommended that a person with diabetes meet with a registered dietitian to have a meal plan designed specifically for him or her.

Carbohydrate Counting: What Is It?

Carbohydrate counting is an important meal-planning tool for people with diabetes. It is a meal planning option that concentrates on the amount of carbohydrate that is consumed rather than on the individual food choices. Carbohydrates encompass many food items, and some examples are breads, pasta, starchy vegetables like corn or peas, fruits and fruit juices, milk and yogurt, and desserts. Many individuals with diabetes use carbohydrate counting to estimate the amount of foods containing carbohydrates that they will eat at each meal, working toward consistency and balancing their diet with their diabetes medications.

Patients with diabetes learn, for example, that one slice of bread is equivalent in carbohydrate grams to one small apple or 1 cup of milk or that 3 cups of popcorn is equal to 2 tablespoons of raisins or 1 tablespoon of sugar. Each of these choices will have about the same effect on blood glucose levels.

Karmeen D. Kulkarni explains carbohydrate counting this way in a 2005 issue of *Clinical Diabetes:* "Carbohydrate foods are identified as starches, fruit, milk, and desserts. Emphasis is placed on consistency in the timing, type, and amount of carbohydrate-containing foods consumed. Early on, discussion of portion sizes is also key to understanding the concept of what a serving of carbohydrate is. Carbohydrates are measured in grams and may be referred to in grams or servings. One carbohydrate serving is equal to 15 g of carbohydrate."

According to Kulkarni, a typical meal plan may include three carbohydrate servings for the breakfast (45 grams), three carbohydrate servings for lunch, and four carbohydrate servings for dinner (60 grams). It may also include a snack that is equivalent to one carbohydrate choice (15 grams).

Individuals who use carbohydrate counting as their meal-planning tool need to learn how to identify the serving size of a food, and also how to determine the grams of total carbohydrates in each serving. This is information that is available on the Nutrition Facts panel of ready-made products. Fresh fruits and vegetables do not have food labels. However, reference books provide the carbohydrate value for most foods. Using measuring cups or a special scale can help people with diabetes become familiar with portions and grams of carbohydrates.

Carbohydrate-insulin ratios People with diabetes who are treated with insulin can learn how much insulin they need to cover the carbohydrates that they eat. To establish a carbohydrate to insulin ratio, the person with diabetes needs to keep accurate records of the food eaten, the grams of carbohydrate and the blood glucose levels, both before and two hours after each meal. They may start with a generic carbohydrate to insulin ratio based on their total daily insulin dose (750 divided by total daily insulin). If a person's total daily dose of insulin is 50 units, their ratio would be 1 for every 15 grams of carbohydrate (750/50). If the postprandial (after meal) rise in blood glucose is under 40 points, the ratio is appropriate, if not, they would assess how a 1 to 12 or 1 to 10 ratio works.

Adolescents are poor at carbohydrate counting Teenagers are notoriously poor at medication adherence and they may need extra encouragement with understanding the concept of carbohydrate counting. In a study of 48 adolescents ages 12 to 18 years with Type 1 diabetes, reported in *Diabetes Spectrum* in 2009 by Franziska K. Bishop and colleagues, the teenage research subjects were asked to evaluate the amount of carbohydrates in 32 different foods that are often consumed by adolescents for breakfast, lunch, and dinner, such as pepperoni pizza, hash browns, peanut butter, spaghetti, chicken nuggets, and other common choices.

The researchers found that only 23 percent of the adolescents estimated the amount of carbohydrates within 10 grams of its true amount. In general, the adolescents overestimated the carbohydrate in 15 of 32 foods, such as spaghetti and hash browns, and underestimated the carbohydrate content in eight of 32 foods, such as cereal, French fries, and soda. The researchers concluded, "From a practical perspective, preliminary findings from this pilot project suggest that adolescents seen for diabetes care in a specialty clinic do not count carbohydrates of commonly consumed foods with acceptable accuracy."

Additional research is needed to determine if further training with adolescents could improve their ability to accurately count carbohydrates.

The Plate Method

Another method of food planning that is used by some individuals with diabetes is referred to simply as the Plate Method by the American Diabetes Association. With this method, the individual takes a dinner plate and draws an imaginary line in his or her mind that goes down the middle of the plate. Then on one side of the plate is drawn another imaginary line across the middle, so that there are three sections to the plate, including a large section that takes up half the plate and two sections of one-fourth the plate each.

In the largest section, a portion of non-starchy vegetables is placed, such as spinach, green beans, or broccoli. In one of the smaller sections, a starchy food is placed, such as rice, potatoes, or green peas. On the other small part of the place is placed the meat or meat substitute, such as skinless chicken or turkey, or fish (such as tuna, salmon or cod) or eggs. A beverage such as low fat or skim milk and a piece of fruit can be added to the meal. Note that a smaller plate should be used for breakfast.

The Diabetes Food Pyramid

The Diabetes Food Pyramid that is used by the American Diabetes Association (adapted from the food pyramid used by the U.S. Department of Agriculture's Nutrition Service) divides foods up into six groups. This pyramid can help people with diabetes make healthy food selections. Foods at the bottom and widest part of the pyramid can be consumed in greater quantities than foods at the top of the pyramid. For example, at the bottom of the diabetes pyramid are whole grain breads and other starches and on the next level of the diabetes pyramid are vegetables, alongside fruits and dairy products. The next level includes meat and meat substitutes. On

the top of the pyramid are fats, oils, and sweets which should be eaten in moderation.

Individuals with diabetes consider the appropriate amount of calories that they need when making their choices from the food pyramid. For example, non-starchy vegetables are low in carbohydrate and high in vitamins, minerals, and fiber. There are many different possible vegetable choices, such as peppers, carrots, broccoli, cauliflower, green beans, lettuce, cabbage, and peppers. In the diabetes meal plan, steamed or raw vegetables may be eaten freely, although they do contain a minimal amount of carbohydrate.

Fruits provide carbohydrate, vitamins, minerals, and fiber to the diet. There are many different fruits available. A few examples are apples, bananas, oranges, peaches, berries, and fruit juice. One serving of fruit is equal to one small apple or ½ cup of fruit juice or ½ grapefruit. Individuals who wish to eat two servings of fruit could eat one banana or a ½ cup of orange juice and 1¼ cups of whole strawberries.

Dairy products provide protein, calcium, carbohydrate, vitamins, and minerals to the diet. A cup of fat-free or low-fat yogurt is equivalent to 1 cup of fat-free or low-fat milk. Pregnant or breast-feeding women need to consume 4–5 servings of dairy products each day.

Individuals with diabetes need to eat small amounts of meat and meat substitutes each day. Meat and meat substitutes provide vitamins, minerals, and protein to the diet. Some examples of foods in this group include chicken, beef, turkey, lamb, pork, canned tuna or other fish, eggs, peanut butter, cottage cheese, and tofu.

An example of a one-ounce serving of meat or meat substitutes is one egg or two tablespoons of peanut butter. A two-ounce serving could include one slice of turkey (one ounce) and one slice (one ounce) of low-fat cheese. According to the National Institute of Diabetes and Digestive and Kidney Diseases (NIDDK), after cooking, 3 ounces of meat is about the size of a deck of cards.

Fats, oils, and sweets are on the top of the food pyramid, and should be eaten in moderation. They may lack nutritional value and be high in calories. Healthy fats, like olive oil, canola oil, avocado, nuts, and seeds are good sources of monounsaturated fats which may protect against cardiovascular disease; however, they are still high in calories. Other examples of fat include, butter, margarine, cream cheese, and bacon. One serving of fat may include a strip of bacon or a teaspoon of oil. An example of 2 servings is 1 tablespoon of regular salad dressing or 2 tablespoons of reduced-fat salad dressing or 1 tablespoon of reduced-fat mayonnaise. Sweets can be high in both carbohydrate and fat and may include saturated or trans fats as well as cholesterol, which may increase the risk of heart disease.

Some examples of sweets are cake, ice cream, pie, cookies, doughnuts, and syrup. One serving of sweets may include one 3-inch cookie or one plain doughnut or a tablespoon of maple syrup.

The Glycemic Index: Another Meal-planning Tool

Another way for people with diabetes to assess the impact of food and to plan their meals is to use the glycemic index. The glycemic index ranks how foods raise a person's blood glucose level. Foods are grouped into high, medium, or low, depending on their impact on the blood glucose level. The person with diabetes may find that choosing foods from the low or medium glycemic index categories help to improve their blood glucose control. Cooked and processed foods generally have a higher glycemic index than raw foods, and food that is cooked longer has a higher glycemic index than food cooked for a shorter period of time.

The glycemic index of one food can be balanced with the index of another food; for example, foods with a high glycemic index can be eaten with foods that have a low glycemic index, which may result in a meal within the moderate glycemic range.

According to Hope S. Warshaw in her book, *Making Diabetes Meal Planning Easy,*

Many of the foods that have a low glycemic index are healthy foods. Consider eating more whole-grain breads and cereals, legumes (beans), and some fruits and vegetables. Include these foods in your eating plan, but don't completely omit foods with a higher GI [glycemic index] if they are healthy foods and you enjoy them. You may find it helpful to create your own personal GI by recording the results of your after-meal blood glucose checks. Make notes about your experiences with certain foods and meals, and note what changes you might make when you eat that food or meal again. Perhaps you'll find that certain foods raise your blood glucose too much. You may want to eat smaller servings or just avoid them in the future.

For further information on using the glycemic index as a meal planning tool, contact a registered dietitian or a physician with expertise in treating diabetes.

Making Healthy Food Choices

When choosing starches to eat, the NIDDK recommends that individuals with diabetes eat whole-grain breads and cereals, as well as low-fat or fat-free dairy products. In addition, mustard is a better choice than mayonnaise on a sandwich.

Raw or cooked vegetables are best eaten with little or no fat, sauces, or dressings, although low-fat or fat-free salad dressing can be used. A small amount of vinegar or lime or lemon juice may also be used. If steaming the vegetables, water or low-fat broth can be used. Instead of adding fat to vegetables when they are cooking, a small piece of smoked turkey or lean ham can be added for flavor unless the individual has been advised to maintain a low sodium diet. Herbs and spices that are sprinkled on will enhance their flavor. If fat is used on the vegetables, it is best to use heart-healthy fats, such as canola oil, olive oil, or soft margarines instead of fat from shortening, or butter.

Fruits can be eaten raw or cooked. Experts recommend selecting small pieces of fruit rather than fruit juice, because whole fruit is more filling and has more fiber than fruit juice. High-fat and high-sugar desserts that contain fruits, such as cherry pie, should be eaten on special occasions and not as a regular daily choice.

Healthy choices for dairy products may include using low-fat plain yogurt in place of sour cream on a potato or other dishes. Fat-free or 1 percent milk is preferable to whole milk, as it is are lower in saturated fat and calories. In addition, there are other low-fat alternatives such as low-fat or fat-free yogurt and reduced fat cheeses which can be substituted for the high-fat versions.

Some healthy tips for eating meat and meat substitutes include the following:

- Cook eggs with cooking spray or a non-stick pan.

- Use vinegar, lemon juice, soy sauce, salsa, ketchup, barbecue sauce, herbs, and spices in place of fats, for more flavor.

- Cook meat and meat substitutes by broiling, grilling, stir-frying, roasting, steaming, or microwaving.

- Limit the amount of peanut butter, nuts, and fried foods that are eaten because these food choices are high in fat.

- Eat low-fat or fat-free cheese.

To satisfy a "sweet tooth," sugar-free popsicles, sugar-free gelatin desserts, low-fat ice cream, or sugar-free hot cocoa mix may be consumed. In restaurants, if a dessert is desired, individuals can try sharing the dessert with a dinner partner or consider boxing half up and eating the other half later.

Eating during holidays According to the National Diabetes Education Program (NDEP), individuals with diabetes can stay healthy during holidays by following these tips:

- Eat a healthy snack before leaving home. This can help prevent overeating at a party.

- Offer to bring a healthy dish to the party, like a salad or raw vegetables with a low-fat dip.

- Drink plenty of water/seltzer.

- Use a smaller plate to help with eating smaller portions of food.

- Trim off skin and fat from meat.

- Walk through the buffet table first, without a plate, checking out the party food before eating, making a mental note of what and how much to eat.

- Choose food from a buffet and then move away to avoid the temptation to eat finger foods while chatting with friends and family.

- Eat slowly and savor your food. This will help prevent overeating.

For those who are planning holiday parties, the following tips can help:

- Avoid frying. Instead, bake, broil, or grill meat.

- Increase fiber by serving whole-grain breads, beans, and peas as part of the meal.

- Use reduced-fat or margarine, reduced fat or fat-free mayonnaise, sour cream, and salad dressing. Try some of the spray fats.

- Serve fresh or canned fruits for dessert instead of pie, ice cream, or cake.

- Serve sparkling water and diet beverages to guests.

- Encourage family and friends to eat healthy foods.

See also ADOLESCENTS WITH DIABETES; CHILDREN WITH DIABETES, SCHOOL-AGE; INSULIN PUMP; LIFESTYLE ADAPTATIONS.

Bishop, Franziska K., et al. "The Carbohydrate Counting in Adolescents with Type 1 Diabetes (CCAT) Study." *Diabetes Spectrum* 22, no. 1 (2009): 56–62.

Kulkarni, Karmeen D. "Carbohydrate Counting: A Practical Meal-Planning Option for People with Diabetes." *Clinical Diabetes* 23, no. 3 (2005): 120–122.

National Institute of Diabetes and Digestive and Kidney Diseases. *What I Need to Know about Eating and Diabetes.* Bethesda, Md.: National Institutes of Health, 2007.

Povey, Rachel Claire, and David Clark-Carter. "Diabetes and Healthy Eating: A Systematic Review of the Literature." *Diabetes Educator* 33 (2007): 931–959.

Rovner, Alisha J. and Tonja R. Nansel. "Are Children with Type 1 Diabetes Consuming a Healthful Diet? A Review of the Current Evidence and Strategies for Dietary Change." *Diabetes Educator* 35, no. 1 (2009): 97–107.

Warshaw, Hope S. *Diabetes Meal Planning Made Easy: Making Smart Food Choices for a Healthier You.* 3d ed. Alexandria, Va.: American Diabetes Association, 2006.

cardiac dysfunctions See CARDIOVASCULAR DISEASE.

cardiovascular disease (CVD)   Diseases of the heart itself or of the blood vessels of the heart. Primarily includes CORONARY HEART DISEASE, HYPERTENSION, and STROKE. Cardiovascular diseases are the leading causes of death and disability in the United States, and coronary heart disease is the number one cause of death for both men and women. According to the Centers for Disease Control and Prevention (CDC), individuals who are middle-aged diabetics have at least twice the risk of nondiabetics of having heart disease or suffering from a stroke. It is also true that heart attacks among people with diabetes are much more serious than with nondiabetics and they are more likely to cause death, according to the CDC. Cardiovascular disease is particularly a problem for WOMEN WITH DIABETES, although it is also very problematic for MEN WITH DIABETES.

In 2010, researcher Michael A. Weber, M.D., and colleagues reported on the dramatically differing outcomes of patients with both diabetes and hypertension based on the medication therapies they received for their high blood pressure. This study included 6,946 diabetic patients, including a subgroup of 2,842 patients at very high risk for cardiovascular events because of a previous stroke or other cardiovascular event or a history of kidney disease. The subjects were compared with 4,559 hypertensive patients without diabetes. The researchers found that among the hypertensive and diabetic subjects, the type of drug therapy did matter significantly,

and a combination of benazepril (Lotensin), an angiotensin-converting enzyme (ACE) inhibitor medication together with amlodipine (Norvasc) was a superior therapy to the combination of benazepril with hydrochlorothiazide, a diuretic. This was also true among high-risk patients. The researchers said, "For the large proportion of diabetic patients whose blood pressure can be controlled with a two-drug combination, the use of amlodipine with a blocker of the RAS [renin-angiotensin system blocker or ACE inhibitor] should now be considered."

Intensive glucose control can reduce the risk of nonfatal heart attack, based on an analysis of studies performed from 1990 to 2009 and reviewed by Steven P. Marso and colleagues and published in *Diabetes & Vascular Disease Research* in 2010. The research included more than 27,000 subjects who were followed for more than five years. The researchers found that intensive glucose control did not prevent stroke, but there was a 14 percent reduction in heart attacks among the subjects with intensive glucose control, which is keeping blood sugar levels as close to normal as possible.

The Action to Control Cardiovascular Risk in Diabetes (ACCORD) study, whose results were reported in 2010 by the National Institutes of Health and other organizations, was a study to determine if intensive blood pressure control as well as the combination of lipid therapies would decrease the risk for cardiovascular events (such as heart attack) in adults with especially high-risk Type 2 diabetes. The researchers studied 4,733 adults with both elevated blood pressure and diabetes. They found that subjects in the intensive blood pressure control group, or those attempting to decrease their systolic blood pressure to less than a 120 mm Hg, did not significantly reduce the combined risk of fatal or nonfatal cardiovascular disease events compared to the standard control group that sought a decrease to 140 mm Hg.

There were, however, some significant improvements in some secondary outcome measures, noted the Endocrine Society in their statement to providers; for example, the total number of strokes were reduced by 41 percent in the intensively managed blood pressure group, or from 0.53 percent to 0.32 percent.

The ACCORD researchers also looked at individuals with dyslipidemia (bad CHOLESTEROL levels) concerning whether the combination of a fibrate drug with a statin medication would lower the risk of cardiovascular events compared with treatment with a statin alone. They studied 5,158 individuals in this part of the study and found no decrease in combined cardiovascular events with this combination.

The importance of this study is that although blood pressure needs to be monitored among those diabetics with hypertension, a goal of systolic pressure that is less than 140 mm HG appears to sufficiently decrease the risk for cardiovascular events and a more intensive reduction of blood pressure is not needed and may even be harmful because of the drugs that must be taken to achieve that lower level and their side effects. This information is being absorbed by professional groups as of this writing in late 2010. For example, the standard recommendation among many groups is to decrease systolic blood pressure to less than 130/80 mm Hg in patients with diabetes. Time will tell if groups will choose to raise their systolic blood pressure goals.

The researchers caution that these results might not apply to patients who are at lower risk of cardiovascular disease than those who participated in ACCORD or to people with more recently diagnosed Type 2 diabetes.

Risk Factors for CVD among Patients with Diabetes

Both Type 1 and Type 2 diabetes are risk factors for the development of CVD. Other risk factors for CVD that are common to many people with diabetes (in addition to the aforementioned risk of hypertension) are OBESITY (usually occurring among those with Type 2 diabetes) and a lack of exercise. Central obesity (or carrying extra weight around the waist rather than the hips, sometimes referred to as an "apple" shape) is a

risk factor for heart disease. Having abnormal CHOLESTEROL levels is another risk factor for cardiovascular disease. Cigarette SMOKING is also a known risk factor for the development of CVD.

INSULIN RESISTANCE, or the failure of the body to adequately use the insulin produced (a problem mainly for people with Type 2 diabetes), is also a risk factor for the development of CVD. Insulin resistance is also worsened in large part by obesity and lack of physical activity, as it is also improved by weight loss and increased levels of physical activity.

Heart Failure

Experts report that diabetes mellitus is a major risk factor for heart failure. This was first demonstrated in the 1980s with the Framingham Heart Study. Conversely, according to V. Baliga and R. Sapsford in their 2009 article for *Diabetes and Vascular Disease Research,* patients with heart failure are also at risk for developing diabetes. In one study of patients with heart failure who did not have diabetes, when they were followed up over three years, 29 percent had developed diabetes. The reasons for this are unknown.

Baliga and Sapsford report that heart failure occurs twice as often in men with diabetes compared to other men. It also occurs five times more frequently in women with diabetes when compared to women without diabetes. In addition, diabetes patients have twice the risk of hospitalization and death from heart failure as do nondiabetics.

Death from Cardiovascular Disease among Diabetics

According to Elizabeth L. M. Barr and colleagues in their article in *Circulation* in 2009 on the topics of cardiovascular and all-cause mortality among diabetics, there is a clear link between abnormal glucose levels and death, based on findings from the more than 10,000 subjects in the Australian Diabetes, Obesity, and Lifestyle Study (AusDiab). The researchers found a cardiovascular death rate among persons with known diabetes mellitus that was more than double the rate for nondiabetics. In addition, the rate was 50–60 percent higher for those with impaired glucose tolerance (IGT), or those with rates not sufficiently high to diagnose as diabetes.

Treatment for CVD

In addition to recommending that patients with diabetes attain good glycemic control and give up smoking, doctors also urge patients who are obese to lose weight and to become more physically active. However, these lifestyle changes alone may not be sufficient to control hypertension or dyslipidemia, and medications may also be needed.

Medications help considerably Studies such as the SCANDINAVIAN SIMVASTATIN SURVIVAL STUDY (4S) and other major studies have demonstrated that medications in the *statin* class such as simvastatin and pravastatin can lower lipid levels significantly and reduce the risk for heart attack.

Patients with diabetes benefited more than nondiabetics in the 4S study. The CVD risk decreased by 32 percent in patients who did *not* have diabetes but it decreased 55 percent in those who were diagnosed with diabetes.

Patients with cardiovascular disease may need medications such as beta-blockers or angiotensin-converting enzyme (ACE) inhibitors. The HOPE STUDY clearly demonstrated that ramipril, an ACE inhibitor, decreased the risk of myocardial infarction, stroke, and death. The findings were so positive that the study was ended early so that those patients on placebo could be given the drug too.

Drugs in the THIAZOLIDINEDIONES (TZDs) class can help patients who use insulin improve their glycemic control and may have direct effects on the endothelial layer of the blood vessels to help lower the risk of atherosclerosis. Some examples of drugs in this class are rosiglitazone and pioglitazone. However, the use of TZDs is also associated with some fluid retention and the development of congestive heart failure.

ASPIRIN THERAPY has also been proven to be a significant help in preventing cardiovascular disease, whether patients have diabetes or not, mainly in men over 50 years old.

As of this writing, the Look AHEAD (Action For Health Diabetes) Trial is attempting to show that an aggressive approach to increase activity, lower weight, and improve glycemic control and blood pressure will have an effect in lowering the risk of CVD in diabetic individuals. Four years worth of data are now available, and in the 5,145 people there are active treatment, and less active treatment groups. Those actively treated have lost 6.2 percent of their body weight and showed improved levels of high density lipoproteins (HDL), HgbA1c, and blood pressure.

The National Institutes of Health (NIH) is running the trial, and they intend to follow patients for an additional nine years and look at the primary outcomes of cardiovascular death, nonfatal heart attack, and stroke. Secondary end points include all-cause mortality, need for coronary artery bypass surgery, carotid endarterectomy, hospitalization for congestive heart failure leading to hospitalization, and peripheral arterial disease (intermittent claudication or discovered during evaluation for non-healing ulcers).

"If you look at the averages across the four years, we see that a lifestyle intervention produced significantly greater improvements across all four years for all of the cardiovascular-disease risk factors, except LDL cholesterol," lead investigator Dr. Rena Wing (Brown University, Providence, Rhode Island) told Heartwire. "The intensive lifestyle-intervention group spent considerably less cumulative time with lower cardiovascular disease risk, so we're hoping the intensive intervention will reduce cardiovascular morbidity and mortality. We're hoping people will live longer."

See also DEATH; DIABETES MELLITUS.

Baliga, V., and R. Sapsford. "Diabetes Mellitus and Heart Failure: An Overview of Epidemiology and Management." *Diabetes and Vascular Disease Research* 6 (2009): 164–171.

Barr, Elizabeth L. M., et al. "Risk of Cardiovascular and All-Cause Mortality in Individuals with Diabetes Mellitus, Impaired Fasting Glucose, and Impaired

Glucose Tolerance: The Australian Diabetes, Obesity, and Lifestyle Study (AusDiab)." *Circulation* 116 (2007): 151–157.

National Heart, Lung, and Blood Institute. "Questions and Answers: Action to Control Cardiovascular Risk in Diabetes." Available online. URL: //www.nhlbi.nih.gov/health/prof/heart/other/accord/q_htm. Accessed August 25, 2010.

National Institutes of Health. "Landmark ACCORD Trial Finds Intensive Blood Pressure and Combination Lipid Therapies Do Not Reduce Combined Cardiovascular Events in Adults with Diabetes." Available online. URL: http://public.nhlbi.nih.gov/newsroom/home/GetPressRelease.aspx?id=2696. Accessed August 30, 2010.

Weber, Michael A., M.D., et al. "Cardiovascular Events During Differing Hypertension Therapies in Patients with Diabetes." *Journal of the American College of Cardiology* 56, no. 1 (2010): 77–85.

CARE Trial (Cholesterol and Recurrent Events Trial)　A clinical study of heart disease, including subjects with and without diabetes. In this study, subjects were 4,159 patients, ages 21–75 years, who had suffered a MYOCARDIAL INFARCTION and were placed on either pravastatin or a placebo over five years. The study found that the drug lowered LDL cholesterol levels by 28 percent, and that fatal and nonfatal myocardial infarctions dropped by 24 percent. Patients with diabetes had an even more favorable result than did nondiabetics. Other studies, such as the SCANDINAVIAN SIMVASTATIN SURVIVAL STUDY (4-S), proved that simvastatin, another drug in the statin class, lowered fatality rates among patients at risk for heart attack.

See also CARDIOVASCULAR DISEASE; CORONARY HEART DISEASE.

Kris-Etherton, Penny, and T. A. Pearson. "For Your Information," *American Dietetic Association Journal* 100, no. 10 (October 1, 2000): 1,126–1,130.

cataract　An eye illness that causes an opaqueness of the lens of the eye. Cataracts are common among people with diabetes. A cataract is a clumping up of the protein in the lens of the eye and, once started, it continues to grow. As the disease progresses, it becomes more and more difficult for the individual to see through the cloudy film of the cataract.

People with diabetes have about twice the risk of developing cataracts than nondiabetics, according to the National Institutes of Health (NIH). Cataracts often appear in people with diabetes at a younger age and progress at a faster rate than among nondiabetics. Some studies have indicated that high blood glucose levels may be linked to the development of cataracts. Experts also believe that if glucose levels are kept at lower/near-normal levels, then the probability of cataracts developing will also be reduced.

Cataracts appear more commonly among people who smoke. However, people who neither smoke nor have diabetes may also develop cataracts, usually as an age-related disease among those over age 65. Ultraviolet light from sun exposure is also a risk factor for the development of cataracts.

Symptoms of Cataracts

When cataracts first develop, there may be no symptoms or may be only a slight clouding of a small area of what is seen. Some people experience a few early warning symptoms. For example, the person may find sunlight more glaring than in the past. Oncoming headlights of a car at night may seem far too bright. Colors may also seem duller than in the past. It is very easy to dismiss such symptoms as not important or as a normal part of aging. It is also easy for patients and even doctors not to realize that these can be signs of cataracts. It's better to be diagnosed and treated at an early stage of the disease. This is why experts recommend that people with diabetes have an annual eye examination.

As the cataract grows, it becomes harder to read and perform everyday tasks and the person eventually realizes that there is a serious problem.

Diagnosis and Treatment

An OPHTHALMOLOGIST or optometrist can diagnose the existence of cataracts. If surgery is required, the ophthalmologist can perform this procedure. The eye professional may decide on a "wait and see" approach if the cataract is small and does not significantly impair vision. If it begins to grow or is already large when it is diagnosed, the doctor may recommend surgery. The cataract will be removed and often a synthetic clear plastic lens will be implanted in the eye.

The National Eye Institute, a part of the National Institutes of Health, is researching whether some minerals or vitamins may be effective in delaying the growth of cataracts or in preventing them from forming altogether. Results should be available in several years.

See also BLINDNESS; DIABETIC RETINOPATHY; GLAUCOMA; GLYCEMIC CONTROL.

Charcot's arthropathy/Charcot's joint A condition that usually results from diabetes and which causes the joints and soft tissue, usually those of the feet, to become malformed and distorted. It can cause an acute painful destruction of the joint. It is also called "neuropathic arthropathy" or "Charcot's joint." It occurs when there is abnormal sensation in the feet although the circulation is usually normal.

Repeated minor traumas can lead to a widened foot that is shorter and with a flattened arch. It is most commonly found in the ankle and tarsal joints of the feet.

The patient is treated by an orthopedic or podiatric surgeon familiar with the disease. Treatment is nonweight bearing, which means that the patient can either remain in bed or the affected foot is placed in a special cast so that it is immobilized and has a chance to recover. The person may use crutches to walk. After the foot has recovered and the cast has been removed, the patient may still be considered at risk for future ulcerations. As a result, the physician may recommend a special leg brace and/or custom-molded shoes.

If Charcot's arthropathy is not treated, then ulceration may develop and progress to the point that gangrene develops and AMPUTATION of a limb is the only course of action to save the life of the patient.

Acutely ill patients may experience a warm to hot foot with an increased blood flow and pain. The bisphosphonate drugs, such as Fosamax (alendronate), Didronel (etidronate), and Actonel (risedronate) may be used to decrease the pain and inflammation, although they are not approved by the FDA for this specific indication. These drugs are used to treat OSTEOPOROSIS, Paget's disease, and other bone problems.

children of diabetic mothers The offspring of women who have Type 1 or Type 2 diabetes. Some studies indicate that children of mothers with diabetes are also affected by the illness, whether as a fetus, through genetic transmissions or by other means. The children may develop diabetes, whether they develop Type 1 diabetes as children or at an older age, or they develop Type 2 diabetes, usually later in life. In addition, they may not develop diabetes but may instead be more likely to suffer from other health problems than children of nondiabetic mothers.

In a study of the children of African mothers with Type 2 diabetes, published in a 2000 issue of *Diabetes Care*, researchers studied families in Cameroon and found that both diabetes and impaired glucose tolerance were much more common among the children of mothers with diabetes than among the African children who were born to nondiabetic mothers.

The researchers said, "The 4 percent prevalence of diabetes and 18 percent prevalence of IGT in the offspring of type 2 diabetic parents is four and nine times greater, respectively, than that found in the general population, which is estimated to be 1 and 2 percent in urban Cameroon." The researchers speculated that this problem may be driven by impairment of beta cells function.

See also GESTATIONAL DIABETES MELLITUS (GDM).

Dabelea, Dana, et al. "Effect of Diabetes in Pregnancy on Offspring: Follow-up Research in the Pima Indians." *Journal of Maternal-Fetal Medicine* 9, no. 1 (January–February, 2000): 83–88.

Mbanya, Jan-Claude N., M.D., et al. "Reduced Insulin Secretion in Offspring of African Type 2 Diabetic Parents." *Diabetes Care* 23, no. 12 (December 2000): 1,761–1,765.

Weiss, Peter A. M., M.D., et al. "Long-Term Follow-Up of Infants of Mothers with Type 1 Diabetes." *Diabetes Care* 23, no. 7 (July 2000): 905–911.

children with diabetes, school-age   Children from kindergarten age to about age 12 or 13 years who have diabetes (preadolescents). Children may have either Type 1 or Type 2 diabetes. Type 1 diabetes, formerly called juvenile-onset diabetes, is more common among children but researchers are finding an increasing incidence of Type 2 diabetes among children and adolescents. About 15,000 new cases of Type 1 diabetes are diagnosed each year among children and adolescents, according to the Centers for Disease Control and Prevention (CDC), and about 3,500 youths are diagnosed with Type 2 diabetes, although Type 2 diabetes is rarely diagnosed in children younger than age 10.

Children with Type 1 Diabetes

White children have a greater risk of developing Type 1 diabetes than children of other races, although the incidence of the disease varies greatly from country to country. (See the charts in this entry.) Children who are diagnosed with Type 1 diabetes must receive daily doses of insulin, either through injections or via an INSULIN PUMP. Most children who take injections can manage on two to three insulin shots per day, although some children need more frequent daily injections.

Because of the need for not only monitoring their blood glucose levels but also for administering injections (or having someone else test the child's blood and give the shots), school can become a much bigger problem for children with Type 1 diabetes than for those with Type 2 diabetes.

The primary risks for school-age children with Type 1 diabetes are the development of DIABETIC KETOACIDOSIS (DKA) among newly diagnosed children and the risk for HYPOGLYCEMIA, among children whose glucose levels are out of control because they are ill or for another reason.

Children with Type 2 Diabetes

Children who are AFRICAN AMERICAN have a higher risk of having or developing Type 2 diabetes than white children, although most people with Type 2 diabetes are adults or adolescents. AMERICAN INDIAN adolescents also have an elevated risk for the development of Type 2 diabetes.

In general, children and adolescents ages 10 to 19 years old who are diagnosed with Type 2 diabetes are obese, and they also lead sedentary lives. They also often have a parent or parents diagnosed with Type 2 diabetes. Many children with Type 2 diabetes have ACANTHOSIS NIGRICANS.

Girls older than 10 years appear to have a higher risk of developing Type 2 diabetes as children than do boys of that age.

Preventing Hypoglycemia

Hypoglycemia (low blood sugar) is a common problem among children with diabetes, particularly children with Type 1 diabetes. The following precautions can be made by parents or legal guardians to try to prevent the development of hypoglycemia in children diagnosed with diabetes:

- Ensure that the child does not miss meals or snacks. If the child must miss a meal or snack, then blood glucose checks need to be done more frequently.

- Monitor children's exercise. If a child has more exercise than usual, then extra snacks such as peanut butter and crackers should be given.

- Check the child's glucose levels at bedtime. If they are below 100 mg/dL, then they should be rechecked in the middle of the night. This is inconvenient but can also be life-saving.

- In the event of severely low blood glucose, and if the child is unable to eat or drink, GLUCAGON should be administered.

Preventing DKA

To prevent the development of DKA, regular blood glucose tests should be performed. Even if a child is using an insulin pump with continuous glucose monitoring, it is still important to be sure that the continuous sensor is providing accurate data by performing several finger-stick glucose checks daily. In addition, there is a time lag between the information provided by the sensor, which measures the glucose concentration of the interstitial fluid, compared to testing it directly from capillary blood from the finger.

Dental Issues

Children with diabetes have about a five-fold greater risk of developing periodontitis than do nondiabetic children. As a result, parents should ensure that their children have regular visits with their dentist, who should also be informed about the diabetes.

Children around the Globe

The rates of diabetes vary greatly depending on the country a child lives in. Type 1 diabetes is far more common among children than is Type 2 diabetes, and experts have analyzed the incidence of Type 1 diabetes in countries worldwide. (See Table 1.)

As can be seen from Table 1, the incidence (new development of diabetes in a year) of Type 1 diabetes in children ranges from a low of 0.1 per 100,000 children in some parts of China to a high of 36.8 per 100,000 children in Sardinia, Italy, and 36.5 in Finland.

Incidence also varies by gender. In some countries, the incidence among boys is higher and in other countries, the incidence among females predominates.

The age of the incidence of Type 1 diabetes in children also varies by country. (See Table 2.)

(text continues on page 76)

TABLE 1: WORLDWIDE AGE-STANDARDIZED INCIDENCE OF TYPE 1 DIABETES IN CHILDREN ≤ 14 YEARS OF AGE (PER 100,000 PER YEAR)

Region (country and area)	Incidence			Ratio of Boys:Girls	Cases		
	Boys	Girls	Total		Boys	Girls	Total
Africa							
Algeria							
Oran*	4.4	7.0	5.7	0.6	9	14	23
Tunisia							
Beja*	9.0	6.5	7.8	1.2	22	16	38
Gafsa*	10.0	7.5	8.8	1.3	31	22	53
Kairoan*	5.5	5.9	5.7	0.9	23	23	46
Monastir*	4.7	5.2	4.9	0.8	15	16	31
Sudan							
Gezira	5.6	4.4	5.0	1.3	17	12	29
Mauritius	1.3	1.5	1.4	0.9	10	11	21
Asia							
China							
Wuhan	5.2	3.8	4.6	1.4	13	9	22
Sichuan	1.8	2.7	2.3	0.7	9	13	22
Huhehot	1.1	0.7	0.9	1.6	10	6	16
Dalian	1.1	1.2	1.2	0.9	10	11	21

(table continues)

	Incidence				Cases		
Region (country and area)	**Boys**	**Girls**	**Total**	**Ratio of Boys:Girls**	**Boys**	**Girls**	**Total**
Guilin	0.6	1.0	0.8	0.6	2	3	5
Beijing*	0.7	1.1	0.9	0.6	38	52	90
Shanghai	0.7	0.7	0.7	1.0	24	23	47
Chang Chun	0.6	1.1	0.8	0.5	7	11	18
Nanjing	0.6	1.1	0.8	0.5	7	13	20
Jinan	0.4	0.4	0.4	1.0	12	11	23
Jilin	0.4	0.8	0.6	0.5	8	14	22
Shenyang	0.4	0.5	0.5	0.8	12	13	25
Lanzhou	0.5	0.3	0.4	1.7	5	3	8
Harbin	0.3	0.3	0.3	1.0	18	17	35
Nanning	0.3	0.7	0.5	0.4	4	10	14
Changsha	0.3	0.2	0.3	1.5	10	7	17
Zhengzhou	0.2	1.0	0.6	0.2	2	8	10
Hainan	0.1	0.2	0.2	0.5	6	11	17
Tie Ling	0.2	0.2	0.2	1.0	5	3	8
Zunyi	0.1	0.1	0.1	1.0	1	2	3
Wulumuqi	0.9	0.8	0.8	1.1	5	4	9
Hong Kong*	0.6	2.1	1.3	0.3	4	13	17
Kuwait	19.2	17.3	18.3	1.1	82	71	153
Israel†	5.5	6.6	6.0	0.8	167	194	361
Japan							
Chiba*	1.2	1.6	1.4	0.8	27	34	61
Hokkaido	2.2	2.1	2.2	1.0	45	44	89
Okinawa	1.0	1.8	1.4	0.6	6	11	17
Pakistan							
Karachi	0.5	0.9	0.7	0.6	9	16	25
Russia							
Novosibirsk	5.7	6.4	6.0	0.9	90	101	191
Europe							
Austria†	9.8	9.3	9.6	1.1	348	312	660
Belgium†							
Antwerpen	10.5	12.8	11.6	0.9	44	51	95
Bulgaria							
Varna	5.9	7.6	6.8	0.8	82	100	182
West Bulgaria	9.9	10.0	9.9	1.0	131	125	256
Denmark†							
4 counties	16.4	14.5	15.5	1.1	96	81	177
Estonia*	9.9	11.2	10.5	0.9	85	93	178
Finland*	37.0	36.0	36.5	1.0	915	853	1,768
France†							
4 regions	8.7	8.3	8.5	1.0	372	337	709
Germany†							
Baden-Württemberg	11.0	10.9	11.0	1.0	463	440	903

Region (country and area)	Incidence			Ratio of Boys:Girls	Cases		
	Boys	Girls	Total		Boys	Girls	Total
Greece†							
Attica	10.2	9.1	9.7	1.1	149	124	273
Hungary†							
18 counties	8.7	9.6	9.1	0.9	337	360	697
Italy							
Sardinia†	43.6	29.5	36.8	1.5‡	337	211	548
Eastern Sicily†	13.4	9.9	11.7	1.4	75	53	128
Pavia	11.6	11.9	11.7	1.0	17	17	34
Marche	10.5	8.9	9.7	1.2	55	44	99
Turin	11.9	10.1	11.0	1.2	86	69	155
Lazio*†	8.0	8.3	8.1	1.0	164	162	326
Lombardia†	7.6	6.8	7.2	1.1	239	204	443
Latvia	7.0	5.7	5.9	1.2	59	47	106
Lithuania	7.7	7.1	7.4	1.1	162	145	307
Luxemburg†	12.6	10.2	11.4	1.2	22	17	39
The Netherlands†							
5 regions	12.9	13.2	13.0	1.0	178	175	353
Norway†							
8 counties	22.4	19.9	21.2	1.1	222	187	409
Poland							
Krakow*	6.1	6.1	6.1	1.0	134	126	260
Wielkopolska	4.1	6.0	5.0	0.7	28	40	68
Portugal							
Algarve†	16.3	12.9	14.6	1.3	26	19	45
Coimbra	9.4	9.9	9.7	0.9	19	19	38
Madeira Island†	6.9	7.5	7.2	0.9	10	11	21
Portalegre†	15.9	26.7	21.1	0.6	9	14	23
Romania†							
Bucharest	4.2	5.9	5.0	0.7	52	65	117
Slovenia†	6.8	9.0	7.9	0.8	70	88	158
Slovakia	7.9	9.1	8.5	0.9	261	289	550
Spain							
Catalonia	12.5	12.6	12.5	1.0	358	338	696
Sweden*	28.1	26.9	27.5	1.0	1,135	1,031	2,166
U.K.							
Aberdeen	32.5	15.0	24.0	2.2	16	7	23
Leicestershire†	15.4	15.3	15.3	1.0	70	66	136
Northern Ireland†	20.1	19.3	19.7	1.0	202	185	387
Oxford*†	20.1	15.3	17.8	1.3‡	266	191	457
Plymouth	16.5	18.1	17.3	0.9	63	65	128
North America							
Canada							
Alberta	23.4	24.7	24.0	0.9	87	88	175
Prince Edward Island*	28.0	20.8	24.5	1.3	17	12	29

(table continues)

TABLE (continued)

Region (country and area)	Incidence			Ratio of Boys:Girls	Cases		
	Boys	Girls	Total		Boys	Girls	Total
U.S.							
Allegheny, PA	19.1	16.4	17.8	1.2	112	94	206
Jefferson, AL*	14.6	15.4	15.0	0.9	50	51	101
Chicago, IL§	10.2	13.3	11.7	0.8	131	169	300
South America							
Argentina							
Avellaneda	5.6	7.5	6.5	0.7	11	15	26
Córdoba	6.2	7.9	7.0	0.8	21	26	47
Corrientes	2.9	5.7	4.3	0.5	4	8	12
Tierra del Fuego	20.2	0	8.0		4	0	4
Brazil							
São Paulo	6.9	9.1	8.0	0.8	15	19	34
Chile							
Santiago	1.7	1.5	1.6	1.1	66	56	122
Colombia							
Santa Fe de Bogotá	4.7	2.9	3.8	1.6‡	35	21	56
Paraguay*	1.0	0.8	0.9	1.3	45	34	79
Peru							
Lima	0.2	0.6	0.4	0.3	4	12	16
Uruguay							
Montevideo	8.3	8.3	8.3	1.0	13	13	26
Venezuela							
Caracas							
(second center)*	0.1	0.2	0.1	0.7	18	25	43
Central America and West Indies							
Barbados*	2.4	1.6	2.0	1.5	3	2	5
Cuba	2.5	3.4	2.9	0.7	152	197	349
Dominica	6.6	4.9	5.7	1.5	3	2	5
Mexico							
Veracruz				0.5	3	6	9
Puerto Rico (U.S.)	16.2	18.7	17.4	0.9	398	445	843
Virgin Islands (U.S.)*	14.7	11.5	13.1	1.4	9	7	16
Oceania							
Australia							
New South Wales	13.1	15.9	14.5	0.8	335	387	722
New Zealand							
Auckland	12.3	13.6	12.9	0.9	65	70	135
Canterbury	23.9	19.8	21.9	1.2	43	35	78

*Primary source only; †EURODIAB ACE Study; §African-American and Hispanic, ‡Statistically significant

TABLE 2: WORLDWIDE AGE-SPECIFIC INCIDENCE OF TYPE 1 DIABETES IN CHILDREN ≤ 14 YEARS OF AGE (PER 100,000 PER YEAR)

Region (country and area)	Boys			Girls			Total		
	0–4 Years	5–9 Years	10–14 Years	0–4 Years	5–9 Years	10–14 Years	0–4 Years	5–9 Years	10–14 Years
Africa									
Algeria									
Oran*	2.8	4.3	6.1	5.8	5.8	9.4	4.3	5.0	7.8
Tunisia									
Beja*	11.0	6.1	10.0	1.4	6.4	11.6	6.3	6.2	10.8
Gafsa*	3.1	9.6	17.3	2.2	6.0	14.3	2.7	7.8	15.8
Kairoan*	6.4	4.7	10.9	1.0	9.1	13.5	3.8	6.8	12.1
Monastir*	1.9	3.6	8.5	2.9	1.8	11.0	2.3	2.7	9.7
Sudan									
Gezira	1.2	3.7	11.9	0.6	2.1	10.4	0.9	2.9	11.2
Mauritius	0.8	0.4	2.5	0.8	1.3	2.2	0.8	0.9	2.4
Asia									
China									
Wuhan	3.6	6.8	5.3	2.0	3.6	5.8	2.8	5.2	5.6
Sichuan	0.5	0.5	4.5	0.5	2.3	5.3	0.5	1.4	4.9
Huhehot	0.0	1.9	1.5	0.4	1.1	0.8	0.2	1.5	1.2
Dalian	0.5	0.9	2.1	1.0	0.9	1.8	0.7	0.9	1.9
Guilin	0.0	0.0	1.9	0.0	1.0	2.0	0.0	0.5	1.9
Beijing*	0.4	0.7	1.0	0.3	1.0	2.1	0.4	0.8	1.5
Shanghai	0.7	0.7	0.6	0.4	0.8	0.9	0.5	0.8	0.8
Chang Chun	1.1	0.3	0.6	0.3	1.1	1.8	0.7	0.7	1.1
Nanjing	0.2	0.5	1.0	1.3	1.0	1.1	0.7	0.7	1.0
Jinan	0.1	0.2	0.9	0.2	0.6	0.4	0.1	0.4	0.7
Jilin	0.5	0.5	0.3	0.2	0.5	1.7	0.3	0.5	1.0
Shenyang	0.2	0.4	0.7	0.2	0.6	0.6	0.2	0.5	0.6
Lanzhou	0.0	0.5	0.8	0.4	0.3	0.0	0.2	0.4	0.4
Harbin	0.2	0.3	0.3	0.0	0.3	0.5	0.1	0.3	0.4
Nanning	0.0	0.2	0.6	0.2	1.2	0.6	0.1	0.7	0.6
Changsha	0.2	0.2	0.5	0.1	0.0	0.6	0.2	0.1	0.6
Zhengzhou	0.3	0.4	0.0	0.3	0.8	2.0	0.3	0.6	1.0
Hainan	0.00	0.05	0.28	0.06	0.21	0.38	0.03	0.13	0.33
Tie Ling	0.13	0.30	0.25	0.00	0.32	0.13	0.07	0.31	0.19
Zunyi	0.00	0.17	0.00	0.00	0.00	0.28	0.00	0.09	0.13
Wulumuqi	0.0	0.6	2.1	0.5	0.6	1.1	0.3	0.6	1.6
Hong Kong*	0.5	0.5	0.9	0.0	3.0	3.4	0.3	1.7	2.1
Kuwait	16.2	17.0	24.4	10.0	18.6	23.3	13.2	17.8	23.8
Israel†	2.4	5.6	8.4	2.5	7.8	9.5	2.5	6.7	8.9
Japan									
Chiba*	0.8	0.7	2.0	1.2	1.6	2.0	1.0	1.2	2.0
Hokkaido	1.9	1.5	3.1	0.6	2.3	3.5	1.3	1.9	3.3
Okinawa	1.6	0.0	1.4	0.6	1.0	3.9	1.1	0.5	2.6

(table continues)

TABLE (continued)

Region (country and area)	Boys			Girls			Total		
	0–4 Years	5–9 Years	10–14 Years	0–4 Years	5–9 Years	10–14 Years	0–4 Years	5–9 Years	10–14 Years
Pakistan									
Karachi	0.2	0.9	0.3	0.5	0.3	2.0	0.3	0.6	1.1
Russia									
Novosibirsk	5.8	5.5	5.8	2.8	8.0	8.3	4.3	6.7	7.0
Europe									
Austria†	5.9	11.4	12.1	4.7	9.8	13.3	5.3	10. 6	12.7
Belgium†									
Antwerpen	6.3	10.2	15.3	6.6	12.9	19.1	6.4	11.5	17.2
Bulgaria									
Varna	3.3	5.5	9.0	4.4	7.7	10.8	3.8	6.6	9.9
West Bulgaria	5.9	10.6	13.0	7.3	9.0	13.5	6.6	9.8	13.3
Denmark†									
4 counties	8.6	16.5	24.2	6.4	14.9	22.2	7.5	15.7	23.3
Estonia*	8.1	8.1	13.5	7.4	9.7	16.4	7.8	8.9	14.9
Finland*	28.5	40.6	41.8	30.7	40.3	37.1	29.6	40.5	39.6
France†									
4 regions	4.6	9.9	11.6	4.8	8.7	11.4	4.7	9.3	11.5
Germany†									
Baden-Württemberg	6.7	10.5	15.8	7.6	11.6	13.5	7.1	11.1	14.7
Greece†									
Attica	6.6	8.3	15.7	7.0	9.6	10.8	6.8	8.9	13.3
Hungary†									
18 counties	5.7	9.2	11.1	5.8	10.1	12.8	5.8	9.6	11.9
Italy									
Sardinia†	32.6	48.3	49.9	25.7	34.1	28.6	29.2	41.4	39.6
Eastern Sicily†	10.5	18.1	11.6	7.7	11.1	11.1	9.1	14.7	11.3
Pavia	8.8	13.1	12.8	2.3	13.9	19.4	5.7	13.5	16.0
Marche	7.7	13.2	10.6	4.8	13.3	8.6	6.3	13.3	9.6
Turin	9.3	12.2	14.0	9.8	8.8	11.7	9.5	10.5	12.9
Lazio*†	6.5	9.0	8.4	6.7	9.8	8.4	6.6	9.4	8.4
Lombardia†	6.6	7.9	8.4	5.1	7.0	8.3	5.9	7.5	8.3
Latvia	3.3	5.6	12.0	3.1	4.8	9.3	3.2	5.2	10.7
Lithuania	4.7	8.0	10.3	3.1	8.7	9.4	3.9	8.3	9.9
Luxemburg†	9.5	10.4	18.0	8.3	11.0	11.3	8.9	10.7	14.7
The Netherlands†									
5 regions	9.3	12.3	17.1	9.7	15.0	14.8	9.5	13.6	15.9
Norway†									
8 counties	14.3	23.0	29.8	10.1	20.9	28.6	12.3	22.0	29.2
Poland									
Krakow*	3.0	5.7	9.6	3.5	7.3	7.5	3.2	6.5	8.6
Wielkopolska	2.9	4.2	5.2	2.0	6.9	9.0	2.5	5.5	7.1

Region (country and area)	Boys			Girls			Total		
	0–4 Years	5–9 Years	10–14 Years	0–4 Years	5–9 Years	10–14 Years	0–4 Years	5–9 Years	10–14 Years
Portugal									
Algarve†	12.8	8.1	28.0	11.1	15.0	12.6	12.0	11.4	20.5
Coimbra	3.8	11.4	13.1	2.0	15.5	12.2	2.9	13.4	12.7
Madeira Island†	9.1	6.1	5.5	7.1	2.2	13.2	8.1	4.2	9.3
Portalegre†	5.1	27.7	19.3	11.2	44.8	30.4	8.0	35.9	24.8
Romania†									
Bucharest	0.9	4.3	7.5	3.6	9.7	4.4	2.2	6.9	6.0
Slovenia	5.6	5.1	9.8	6.3	8.8	12.0	5.9	6.9	10.9
Slovakia	6.3	7.3	10.1	6.5	9.7	11.2	6.4	8.5	10.6
Spain									
Catalonia	5.6	12.8	18.9	5.0	13.5	19.2	5.3	13.1	19.0
Sweden*	19.6	28.9	35.7	17.4	31.8	31.5	18.5	30.3	33.7
U.K.									
Aberdeen	24.1	30.4	43.0	12.6	25.8	6.5	18.5	28.2	25.3
Leicestershire†	6.2	16.8	23.1	10.6	15.0	20.1	8. 4	15. 9	21.7
Northern Ireland†	11.4	22.4	26.6	10.4	22.4	25.1	10.9	22.4	25.9
Oxford*†	15.6	19.0	25.6	12.4	12.5	21.1	14.0	15.8	23.5
Plymouth	15.5	16.5	17.6	12.2	19.3	22.7	13.9	17.9	20.1
North America									
Canada									
Alberta	9.0	26.0	35.2	19.1	24.4	30.7	13.9	25.2	33.0
Prince Edward									
Island*	15.0	34.6	34.4	10.5	25.8	26.1	12.8	30.3	30.3
U.S.									
Allegheny, PA	7.4	19.4	30.4	10.1	19.2	20.0	8.7	19.3	25.3
Jefferson, AL*	9.7	13.8	20.3	6.5	15.1	24.6	8.1	14.4	22.4
Chicago, IL‡	4.4	9.1	16.9	5.0	12.4	22.6	4.7	10.7	19.8
South America									
Argentina									
Avellaneda	2.1	2.4	8.3	0.0	24.7	2.8	1.1	13.4	5.6
Córdoba	3.6	6.0	9.0	2.2	11.4	10.0	2.9	8.7	9.5
Corrientes	3.9	0.0	4.7	6.0	6.7	4.6	5.0	3.3	4.6
Tierra del Fuego	0	0	60.6	0	0	0	0	0	30.3
Brazil									
São Paulo	4.1	6.9	9.8	5.6	8.5	13.0	4.8	7.7	11.4
Chile									
Santiago	1.5	3.1	4.1	1.4	1.3	5.0	1.5	2.2	4.6
Colombia									
Santa Fe de Bogotá	3.0	3.9	7.3	2.0	2.8	3.9	2.5	3.3	5.6
Paraguay*	0.7	0.6	1.8	0.5	1.0	0.8	0.6	0.8	1.3
Peru									
Lima	0.1	0.0	0.4	0.4	0.7	0.6	0.3	0.4	0.5

(table continues)

TABLE (continued)

Region (country and area)	Boys			Girls			Total		
	0–4 Years	5–9 Years	10–14 Years	0–4 Years	5–9 Years	10–14 Years	0–4 Years	5–9 Years	10–14 Years
Uruguay									
Montevideo	0.0	3.6	21.2	2.0	14.8	7.9	1.0	9.1	14.7
Venezuela									
Caracas									
(second center)*	0.1	0.2	0.0	0.1	0.2	0.2	0.1	0.2	0.1
Central America and West Indies									
Barbados*	2.5	4.7	0.0	0.0	2.3	2.3	1.3	3.5	1.2
Cuba	1.1	2.9	3.5	1.9	3.8	4.5	1.5	3.3	4.0
Dominica	0.0	8.2	13.5	0.0	0.0	14.6	0.0	4.0	14.1
Mexico									
Veracruz							0.5	2.0	2.1
Puerto Rico (U.S.)	12.1	16.6	19.8	9.8	21.9	24.2	11.0	19.2	22.0
Virgin Islands (U.S.)*	15.9	14.3	13.9	10.8	9.7	14.1	13.4	12.0	14.0
Oceania									
Australia									
New South Wales	8.1	12.3	18.9	10.1	16.8	20.8	9.1	14.5	19.8
New Zealand									
Auckland	4.5	18.7	13.8	8.8	14.0	17.9	6.6	16.4	15.8
Canterbury	12.6	31.2	28.0	19.6	15.9	24.0	16.0	23.7	26.1

*Primary source only; †EURODIAB; ‡Statistically significant.

Permission granted to reprint tables by Marjatta Karvonen, Ph.D., senior researcher, Department of Epidemiology and Health Promotion, National Public Institute, Helsinki, Finland.

(text continued from page 69)

In some countries, there are few or no cases reported for ages 0–4, while in other countries, there are many cases. For example, in Finland, the rate of incidence for both boys and girls is 29.6 per 100,000 for ages 0–4, followed by Sardinia, with 29.2 per 100,000 cases in this age group. The incidence of diabetes rises for Finnish children ages 5–9 to 40.5 per 100,000. It also rises for children in Sardinia to 41.4 per 100,000 for children ages 5–9.

In some countries, the incidence of Type 1 diabetes is higher for younger children than older children; for example, in some parts of Portugal. As a rule, however, the incidence of Type 1 diabetes is greater among children ages five and older.

Schools and Diabetes

The federal Americans with Disabilities Act requires schools to let diabetic children test their blood and administer medications such as insulin as needed. Despite this law, some schools continue to fail to comply, insisting that nurses always administer medication, even to older children, and refusing to allow children to test their own blood, inject their insulin, or to have a snack if their glucose level is low or falling.

Astonishingly, some few teachers belittle or psychologically abuse children with diabetes; for example, demanding that they stand up in front of the class and give a lecture on diabetes. (See ADOLESCENTS WITH DIABETES.)

In other cases, the diabetic child may be treated as an invalid. For example, he or she is not allowed to participate in sports, despite the doctor's permission and opinion that the child should participate. Many children try to hide their diabetes from teachers because they fear (rightly or wrongly) that they will be mistreated or singled out. Parents of diabetic children report continuing to battle with schools over medical issues that are directly related to the child's diabetes. It is important for parents to act as advocates for their children, when needed. Banding together with other parents of diabetic children may also help parents feel (and become) more empowered.

Difficulties to anticipate and resolve Children with Type 1 diabetes require insulin to live. Yet many schools have been reluctant either to allow children to test their own blood and administer insulin themselves or to provide other individuals who will perform these functions if children cannot (or are not allowed to) perform these necessary tasks for their continued health and life.

The Americans with Disabilities Act requires accommodations for a disabled individual, including a disabled child, at school as well as in the workplace. The American Diabetes Association and other organizations have successfully prevailed in lawsuits where school boards attempted to block children with diabetes from receiving needed care. In some cases, parents have sued and prevailed because they wanted the school to be prepared to administer emergency glucagon in the event of an incident of hypoglycemia.

Another law that affects children with diabetes is Section 504 of the Rehabilitation Act of 1973, a law which is still in force in the United States. This law protects students from discrimination when they have a "physical or mental impairment that substantially limits one or more of major life activities." This law applies to all public schools and any private schools that receive federal dollars.

Parents can request that the accommodation that is needed by the child be placed in the child's school record. However, since many teachers do not ever review general student records, individual teachers should also be informed about the child's diabetes and what the child needs. Some teachers may need to be informed about the existence of both the Americans with Disabilities Act and Section 504 of the Rehabilitation Act of 1973 and their application to children as well as adults.

According to the American Diabetes Association, some types of accommodations that the school may be expected to make under Section 504 are:

- allowing a child to self-test glucose levels and act on the results
- permitting children to eat when they need to and to have enough time to eat
- allowing extra bathroom trips as well as trips to the water fountain
- planning for where the child's blood will be tested and insulin given

If the child is old enough and is allowed to test his or her blood and administer insulin, then the child needs a place and time to accomplish these tasks in the school, as well as the privacy to perform them.

Eating lunch in the cafeteria may present a problem for children with diabetes, if the fare that is offered is heavily laden with carbohydrates and is nutritionally suboptimal, making it difficult for them to have a balanced meal with appropriate carbohydrate content. In addition, if children in school are rewarded for good behavior with candy and sweets, this presents yet another problem for the child with diabetes. First, the child generally would like to eat the candy. Second, children may feel singled out if they refuse the candy in order to try to be compliant with their diabetes regimen. In addition, unaware adults often press candy on children, telling them that it is all right, one extra piece of cake will not hurt them. Conversely, adults may sometimes try to forbid diabetic children from eating any cake, which is usually unnecessary.

For these reasons, it is important for parents and children to inform teachers about the child's diabetes and his or her needs, and to repeat the information as often as needed.

Diabetic children and their parents and perceptions about the effect of missed medications In a study of the perception of both children with diabetes and their parents, as well as children with asthma and attention deficit hyperactivity disorder (ADHD) and their parents regarding the impact of missed medications at school, published in the *Journal of School Nursing* in 2008, researchers Daniel Clay and colleagues found that missing medicines in school has a major impact on children with diabetes; for example, 36.1 percent of the children and 69.8 percent of the parents said that missing medications at school caused high blood sugar. In addition, 29.2 percent of the diabetic children and 46.5 percent of their parents said that missing medications caused the children to have headaches or dizzy/blurred vision. With regard to missing their medication once a month to less than once a week, 4.2 percent of the diabetic children reported this was an issue. (There was no response from their parents.)

About 38 percent of the parents of the children with diabetes said that missing medicines at school affected their children's friendships a little, somewhat, or a lot, although their children had a much lower perception; about 7 percent of the diabetic children had the same perception regarding missed medications and friendships. About 28 percent of the parents of children with asthma felt that missing medications affected their children's friendships, as did about 7 percent of the children with asthma. Among children with ADHD, however, nearly 69 percent of their parents felt that missing medications affected their children's friendships, as did about 24 percent of the children. Clearly, children had a lesser concern for missing medications than did their parents, whether the children had diabetes, asthma, or ADHD. However, the most worried group of parents and children were parents of children with ADHD or children with ADHD.

As can also be seen from the table, most of the diabetic children (81.9 percent) never missed medication at school. However, in the case of children with diabetes (as also of children with asthma), missing a medication can result in a life-threatening situation, one which does not occur with ADHD. Thus, missing any medication at all is problematic for children with diabetes.

With regard to missed medication affecting their concentration, it is not surprising that 36.4 percent of the children with ADHD and 73.5 percent of the parents of the children with ADHD reported this problem. However, the inability to concentrate because of missed medication was also reported by 8.3 percent of the diabetic children and 30.2 percent of their parents, as well as by 15.9 percent of the asthmatic children and 26.8 percent of their parents. See Table 3 for further information.

Ethnic differences in children with diabetes receiving support in school In a disturbing report in a 2008 issue of *Diabetes Educator*, Farrah Jacquez and colleagues surveyed 309 parents of an ethnically mixed group of children with diabetes regarding issues surrounding their child's diabetes management in school. The majority of the children had Type 1 diabetes and most attended public schools.

Of the responses that were given, the parents of the white children had significantly higher percentages of "yes" responses with regard to needed issues related to their children than did the parents of Hispanic or black children, although the underlying reasons for these differences were unknown.

For example, 74 percent of the white parents said that their children had a written care plan, compared to 52 percent of the Hispanic parents and 46 percent of the black parents. In responding to whether the child's school had a nurse available, 78 percent of the white parents said "yes," compared to 54 percent of the black parents and less than half (48 percent) of the Hispanic parents. Whether insulin was allowed in class was about the same for whites (20 percent) and Hispanics (23 percent) but the response was only 10 percent for blacks. See Table 4 for further information.

TABLE 3: CHILD AND PARENT PERCEPTIONS OF THE IMPACT OF MISSING MEDICINES AT SCHOOL

	ADHD % (n=33)		Asthma % (n=44)		Diabetes % (n=72)	
	Child	Parent	Child	Parent	Child	Parent
Frequency of missing medicine at school						
Never	45.4	–	65.9	–	81.9	–
Once per year	12.1	–	6.8	–	12.5	–
Once per month to < once per week	27.2	–	25.0	–	4.2	–
Once per week	12.1	–	2.3	–	0	–
Affects schoolwork						
Not at all	27.3	0	59.1	30.0	44.4	6.5
A little	15.1	14.3	15.9	12.5	13.9	10.9
Some	12.1	28.6	4.5	10.0	5.6	19.6
A lot	15.1	51.4	6.8	35.0	11.1	45.7
Not sure	6.1	5.7	4.5	12.5	6.9	17.4
Affects friendships						
Not at all	54.5	11.4	84.1	48.8	72.2	37.8
A little	18.2	28.6	6.8	12.2	4.2	13.3
Some	6.1	34.3	0	4.9	1.4	20.0
A lot	0	5.7	0	9.8	1.4	4.4
Not sure	0	20.0	4.5	24.4	4.2	24.4
Effect on physical health						
Nausea/vomiting/stomach cramps	3.0	0	6.8	4.9	24.6	25.6
Breathing problems	0	0	36.4	68.3	2.8	0
High blood sugar	0	0	0	0	36.1	69.8
Headache/dizzy/blurred vision	12.1	5.9	20.5	22.0	29.2	46.5
Lack of energy	3.0	0	11.4	14.6	12.5	18.6
Feel anxious	12.1	8.8	2.3	17.1	6.9	9.3
Feel confused	15.2	8.8	2.3	2.4	4.2	16.3
Unable to concentrate	36.4	73.5	15.9	26.8	8.3	30.2
Other	30.0	0	15.9	7.3	2.8	23.3
Effect on schoolwork						
Have trouble paying attention	39.4	91.2	6.8	19.5	18.1	23.3
Misbehave in class	27.3	50.0	2.3	4.9	4.2	11.6
Do poorly on an exam	18.2	55.9	2.3	7.3	12.5	14.0
No effect	0	2.9	29.5	17.1	31.9	0

The researchers stated that, "In many instances, school personnel are not educated regarding diabetes care needs and therefore do not allow children access to the water, restrooms, glucose meters, and medications they need to care for themselves. Availability of school nurses is often limited, and many schools have a nurse only 1 or fewer days per week; however, in some schools, only nurses are authorized to provide diabetes care. Concerns about liability can prevent school personnel from participating in blood glucose monitoring, insulin injections,

TABLE 4: PARENT REPORT OF DIABETES SUPPORT IN SCHOOL BY ETHNICITY

Form of Diabetes Support in School	Percentage of "Yes" Responses Within Group			
	Hispanic	White	Black	Overall
Does child have written care plan?	52	74	46	55
Does school have a nurse?	48	78	54	55
Does child have glucagon kit at school?	45	70	43	49
Blood glucose checks in class allowed?	50	57	31	48
Blood glucose checks in special places allowed?	53	47	26	50
Insulin in class allowed?	23	20	10	21
Insulin in special places allowed?	57	55	46	54
Extra snacks allowed when needed?	86	90	70	84
Access to bathroom when needed?	80	93	69	81

Source: Jacquez, Farrah, et al. "Parent Perspectives of Diabetes Management in Schools." *Diabetes Educator* 34 (2008): 999.
Copyright 2009 by SAGE PUBLICATIONS INC. JOURNALS. Reproduced with permission of SAGE PUBLICATIONS INC. JOURNALS.

and glucagon administration, leaving children without any competent adult assistance in cases of emergency."

Emotional issues surrounding diabetes Jean Betschart Roemer discussed the emotional and psychological issues of diabetes in a 2009 article in *NASN School Nurse*. According to Betschart Roemer, children with diabetes may be anxious about their diabetes or depressed. Betschart Roemer says, "They might worry that they are not doing their diabetes tasks properly, thus displeasing their parents. They might worry about fitting their diabetes tasks into their school schedules without calling attention to themselves, worry that they have a low blood glucose [level], or worry about a host of other issues."

School nurses can help by reassuring the children and by testing them for hypoglycemia (or DKA) as needed. It is also a good idea for school nurses to ask children if they mind whether other people know about their diabetes and if they do, to minimize information given to others as much as is safely possible.

Betschart Roemer, Jean. "Emotional and Psychological Considerations of Children with Diabetes: Tips for School Nurses" *NASN School Nurse.* 24 (2009): 60–61.

Clay, Daniel, et al. "Family Perceptions of Medication Administration at School: Errors, Risk Factors, and Consequences." *Journal of School Nursing* 24 (2008): 95–102.

Jacquez, Farrah, et al. "Parent Perspectives of Diabetes Management in Schools." *Diabetes Educator* 34 (2008): 996–1,003.

cholesterol (good cholesterol/bad cholesterol)

One of several fats (lipids) that circulate in the body as lipoproteins, including low density lipoproteins (LDL) and high density lipoproteins (HDL). Although most people think of all cholesterol as "bad," it is LDL that is considered a "bad" form of cholesterol, while HDL is "good." Very simply put, HDL removes cholesterol from the blood vessels, while LDL clogs the vessels.

People with diabetes, even when they are adolescents or young adults (and the risk increases for middle-aged individuals and those who are older), are at risk for having abnormal LDL and low HDL. According to the National Cholesterol Education Program, people with diabetes have "diabetic dyslipidemia" when they have high triglycerides, low HDL, and small dense LDL.

Excessive levels of LDL can cause fatty deposits to collect within the arteries and can then result in medical problems such as strokes or heart attacks. People with diabetes are already at higher risk for cardiac ailments and strokes, even if their cholesterol levels are at optimal lev-

·ls. In one study done in Finland, patients with diabetes who had never had a heart attack had a higher risk of having a heart attack than did nondiabetic patients who had already had one or more previous heart attacks. Thus, patients with diabetes must keep their LDL levels as low as possible and their HDL levels as high as possible.

Testing Cholesterol Levels and Cholesterol Guidelines Created in 2001

To test for lipoproteins, physicians order a lipoprotein profile, which will provide data on levels of LDL, total cholesterol, HDL, and triglycerides (another fatty substance found in the blood).

In 2001, new guidelines were released by the National Cholesterol Education Program, coordinated by the National Heart, Lung, and Blood Institute (NHLBI). Earlier guidelines had been issued in 1993. These guidelines reinforced the concept that diabetes is a major risk factor for developing dyslipidemia as well as clinical heart disease. Other risk factors for the development of coronary heart disease are

- cigarette smoking
- high blood pressure
- low HDL cholesterol (under 40 mg/dL)
- family history of early heart disease
- age: men 45 or older and women 55 or older

According to the National Cholesterol Education Program guidelines, LDL should be less than 100 mg/dL in patients with diabetes (either type). Some research suggests that all patients with diabetes might benefit from an even lower level of less than 100, although this is a very controversial area. Conversely, high density lipoprotein levels (HDL) should be greater than 40 mg/dL.

In the Scandinavian Simvastatin Survival Study (the 4-S Study), patients with diabetes who reduced their cholesterol levels had a 54 percent risk reduction in major coronary events (fatal and near fatal myocardial infarctions) while the patients without diabetes had only a 32 percent risk reduction. This study yet again

proved the importance of cholesterol levels to the person with diabetes.

Treatment of High Cholesterol Levels

Dietary adjustments can lower LDL levels; for example, foods that are high in starch and fiber can help to lower the LDL level, as well as foods that are low in fat and cholesterol. It's also important to supplement changes in diet with an increase in exercise and weight loss for those who are overweight. Generally diet and exercise will lower total cholesterol levels by 5 to 20 percent, with 10 percent being a typical response. Given this fairly small effect, most patients with diabetes and dyslipidemia will require the use of cholesterol-lowering medications. For most patients with diabetes, the first class of medication that is usually considered is an HMG CoA reductase inhibitor drug, (or "statin"), such as pravastatin (Pravachol) or simvastatin (Zocor). These medications can lower LDL cholesterol levels by about 15–40 percent.

In 2001, the FDA removed Baycol (cerivastatin), a cholesterol-lowering drug, from the market after it was linked to deaths in 40 people worldwide. The drug resulted in rhabdomyolysis in a small number of people, which is muscle damage leading to pain and possible kidney failure. This problem has not been as severe in the five other HMG CoA reductase inhibitor medications that remain on the market. Mild myalgias (muscle aches) are not uncommon with this class of drugs, but usually are not severe enough to change muscle enzyme levels or to affect kidney function. Often a physician will change a patient from one drug to another if this occurs, as the effect is unpredictable; i.e., it may occur with one of the five and none of the other four medications.

Another treatment for high cholesterol levels is intermediate-release niacin, which can often be used, albeit with caution. Physicians and patients need to be aware that niacin can affect glucose levels and it can also increase uric acid levels, leading to the development of gout (a very painful acute inflammation of a joint, often in the foot). Prescribed niacin may also cause upset to the stomach, and it can affect liver function tests. In addition, it may cause an intense flushing syndrome; however, this reaction can be avoided with the use of aspirin 30 minutes prior to taking the niacin.

One study, reported in the *Journal of the American Medical Association* in 2000, found a positive effect with high doses of niacin on patients who had been diagnosed with peripheral arterial disease. Of the 468 patients who were studied, 125 of them had Type 2 diabetes and the other patients were nondiabetic. The study lasted for 60 weeks.

The researchers found that after 30 weeks, the niacin significantly increased the HDL levels of the patients with diabetes by 29 percent and decreased their triglycerides by 23 percent, both positive findings. They concluded,

> Our study suggests that lipid-modifying dosages of niacin can be safely used in patients with diabetes and that niacin therapy may be considered as an alternative to statin drugs or fibrates for patients with diabetes in whom these agents are not tolerated or fail to sufficiently correct hypertriglyceridemia or low HDL-C [cholesterol] levels.

TABLE 1: CLASSIFICATION OF LDL, TOTAL CHOLESTEROL, AND HDL CHOLESTEROL (mg/dL)

LDL Cholesterol	
100	Optimal
100–129*	Near optimal/above optimal
130–159	Borderline high
160–189	High
190 and higher	Very high

* Among people with diabetes, the recommended LDL is under 100.

Total Cholesterol	
200	Desirable
200–239	Borderline high
240 or higher	High

HDL Cholesterol	
40	Low
60 or higher	High

Source: National Cholesterol Education Program, 2001.

See also CARDIOVASCULAR DISEASE; DYSLIPIDEMIA; HDL; LDL; TRIGLYCERIDE.

Castelli, William P., M.D., and Glen C. Griffin, M.D. *Good Fat, Bad Fat: Reduce Your Heart-Attack Odds.* Tucson, Ariz.: Fisher Books, 1997.

Elam, Marshall B., M.D., et al. "Effect of Niacin or Lipid and Lipoprotein Levels and Glycemic Control in Patients with Diabetes and Peripheral Arterial Disease: The ADMIT Study: A Randomized Trial." *Journal of the American Medical Association* 284, no 13 (2000): 1,263–1,270.

National Cholesterol Education Program, National Heart, Lung, and Blood Institute. "Detection, Evaluation, and Treatment of High Blood Cholesterol in Adults (Adult Treatment Panel III): Executive Summary." NIH Publication No. 01-3670, May 2001.

chromium supplements Additional portions of chromium that are taken as dietary supplements. Some preliminary research has indicated that it is possible that diabetes may deplete the body or at least be associated with lower levels of important trace elements such as chromium and ZINC. As a result, supplements may be needed. However, individuals with diabetes should not take any dietary supplements without first consulting with their physicians.

In recent years, there has been a tremendous amount of interest in the trace mineral chromium. Much of this stems from basic research into the mechanism by which insulin is released from the beta cells in islets (ISLETS OF LANGERHANS) of the PANCREAS. When islet cells are cultured in a laboratory, if the media in which they are maintained is depleted of chromium, then the cells do not secrete insulin very well. If chromium is added back, the cells begin to secrete insulin robustly. Obviously, however, it is a large leap from animal islet cells grown in a laboratory to making assumptions about a human being.

There has also been interesting data from rural China, where subjects with diabetes received chromium supplements and their glucose levels subsequently improved. However, people in China eat a diet that is far different from what most people in America, Canada, and Europe consume, thus, these results are not easily generalized to Western cultures.

At the present time, there is no conclusive test for chromium deficiency in humans. In addition, it may be some time before the true impact of chromium on diabetes is answered definitively. It is also very difficult to measure chromium levels in humans. What we really need to know is the concentration of chromium in the tissues and specifically the concentration at the cellular levels, as opposed to the blood levels. At this time, such techniques are not readily available.

Studies have been done on genetically insulin-resistant rats whose insulin resistance decreased with supplementation with chromium picolinate. But there are no data on safe levels of chromium in the body and what medical problems that long-term exposure or build-up in tissues may lead to.

According to Richard Eastman, M.D., an endocrinologist at the National Institute of Diabetes and Digestive and Kidney Diseases (NIDDK), overweight people who have Type 2 diabetes can gain the same modest benefits as the Chinese subjects did with chromium supplements by losing some weight.

clinical studies/research Controlled experiments or studies that are usually peer-reviewed or evaluated by others who are expert in the field. Clinical studies are the basis for much of modern medical science, as well as the basis for the approval and introduction of new medications and treatments. Clinical studies may last as little as hours or days, or they may last as long as years.

Sometimes scientists return to the people in a previously studied clinical trial, as long as 10 years later, and follow-up on them or perform new studies on this group; however, such long-term follow-ups are not the norm because they are very costly. One example of such a follow-up/new research study group is the Epidemiology of Diabetes Interventions and Complications (EDIC) Research Group. In 1999, the EDIC Research Group reported that they had received permission from 96 percent of the Diabetes Control and Complications Trial (DCCT) subjects to study them further.

In general and in its simplest form, researchers study medications or treatments in an experimental group (the group that receives the medication or treatment) versus a control group which does not receive it, and the results are then compared to determine any significant differences.

Sometimes more than two groups are involved; for example, some researchers may compare a group of individuals with Type 1 diabetes to a group with Type 2 diabetes and sometimes to a third nondiabetic control group as well.

Some studies compare only people with Type 1 or Type 2 diabetes to a nondiabetic group. Or individuals with Type 1 or Type 2 diabetes may be separated into different groups and the results of the therapy or medication will be compared. Most studies are limited to using adult subjects, however, increasingly more studies are performed on children and adolescents who have diabetes. There are many possible combinations of groups that may be used to study a broad array of treatments and medications for diabetes.

Prior to publication in a professional medical journal, most clinical studies are "peer-reviewed," which means that individuals who are knowledgeable in the same field read the study to see if it seems feasible and logical and if enough information is provided so that others could duplicate the study. Scientists know they will be reviewed and this helps to ensure their carefulness (although not all clinical studies are rigorously performed).

For a new medication to obtain the approval of the FDA, in most cases, 2,000–10,000 patients must be studied to verify that the medication is not only safe but also efficacious. Researchers also look for possible side effects that the new medication may have.

Researchers seek to find statistical "significance." This means that statistical techniques are used to determine if the findings are more than what would occur with just random chance.

Individuals who do clinical studies also review what studies have gone on before them, not only so that they can learn from previous experience, but also because they may attempt to design their study in such a way as to avoid errors or problems that may have occurred in the past.

Clinical studies are vitally important to those interested in diabetes because researchers are constantly seeking to learn more about treatments and medications that directly impact people with diabetes. Researchers also study issues such as risk of developing diabetes or complications of diabetes, so that physicians can identify people who are most likely to develop specific medical problems. If they can act ahead of time, doctors may be able to advise their patients how to act to avoid the problem or at least limit its severity if it cannot be avoided.

There have been hundreds and probably thousands of studies on diabetes in recent years. Several prominent and often cited diabetes studies involved large numbers of individuals who were studied over extended periods of time; for example, the DIABETES CONTROL AND COMPLICATIONS TRIAL (DCCT) was a 10-year federally funded study of individuals with Type 1 diabetes in North America which ran from 1983 to 1993. The National Institute of Diabetes and Digestive and Kidney Diseases (NIDDK) conducted the study.

The DCCT was profoundly important because it conclusively proved that tight glucose control in patients with Type 1 diabetes could greatly reduce the risk of the development or slow progression of microvascular complications from diabetes, such as DIABETIC RETINOPATHY, kidney disease, and DIABETIC NEUROPATHY. As a direct result of this study, physicians now urge their patients to control their glucose levels as tightly as possible. If patients need proof for why they should take this action, doctors can justify their advice with the findings of this study.

The UNITED KINGDOM PROSPECTIVE DIABETES STUDY (UKPDS) was another major clinical study of diabetes. It was performed in the United King-dom and concentrated on the impact of tight glucose control on individuals who had Type 2 diabetes. The study also conclusively proved that tight glucose control greatly decreased the likelihood of later microvascular complications from diabetes.

coma An extended loss of consciousness that may last for days, weeks, or much longer. A coma may stem from glucose levels that are either too low (HYPOGLYCEMIA) or too high (HYPERGLYCEMIA). (See also HYPEROSMOLAR COMA.) Some individuals do not recover from a diabetic coma, and they die.

Coma may occur because the person did not adequately pay attention to diet or it could be due to other controllable or noncontrollable circumstances such as medication, illness, and excessive exercise.

The comatose individual needs emergency treatment and usually requires hospitalization.

See also COMPLICATIONS OF DIABETES AND ASSOCIATED DISORDERS; DIABETIC KETOACIDOSIS (DKA).

complications of diabetes and associated disorders Typically refers to chronic diseases or conditions that are caused or exacerbated by the underlying diabetes or that are commonly associated with diabetes. Some examples of the severe complications that are linked to diabetes are DIABETIC NEPHROPATHY, DIABETIC RETINOPATHY, and DIABETIC NEUROPATHY. Diabetic retinopathy, if not identified and treated, can lead to BLINDNESS. Other complications of diabetes include those that are acute such as DIABETIC KETOACIDOSIS (DKA) and HYPOGLYCEMIA, both of which can be life-threatening complications. There are also disorders that are directly linked to these complications; for example, the AMPUTATION of the limbs in diabetics is usually caused by a diabetic neuropathy which is related to a lack of appropriate FOOT CARE.

Other examples of complications that are associated with diabetes are CARDIOVASCULAR

DISEASE and also chronic kidney disease which, if undiagnosed and untreated, leads to kidney failure or END-STAGE RENAL DISEASE (ESRD). This complication stems from diabetic nephropathy. In fact, diabetes is the most common cause of kidney failure in the United States. In addition, many people with diabetes also have HYPERTENSION, which by itself is the second most common cause of kidney failure. The combination of *both* diabetes and hypertension further increases the risk for kidney failure. Individuals whose kidneys have failed will need to receive either kidney dialysis or kidney transplantation in order to survive.

Obesity is another condition that is commonly associated with Type 2 diabetes. In addition, many people with diabetes also have DYSLIPIDEMIA. The most typical type in those with Type 2 diabetes is a normal level of LDL, an elevated level of triglycerides, and a lower than normal level of HDL.

For a long time, it was believed that large-scale studies, such as the DIABETES CONTROL AND COMPLICATIONS TRIAL (DCCT) and the UNITED KINGDOM PROSPECTIVE DIABETES STUDY (UKPDS), had definitively proven that for patients both with Type 1 diabetes and the far more common Type 2 diabetes, tight glucose control greatly decreased the risk for the microvascular complications of diabetes. In addition, it was also assumed that if complications had already occurred, then an effort at attaining tight glycemic control could often delay a worsening of the problem. However, more recent studies have revealed that very tight control of diabetes may also lead to risks, such as an increased risk for hypoglycemia. Despite this, it is still important for individuals with diabetes/hypertension and/or kidney disease to maintain as tight a glycemic control as is possible, to avoid an increased risk for kidney failure.

Complications of Diabetes

Diabetic complications are common and require a careful overview, not only by the physician but also by patients themselves.

Diabetic ketoacidosis Diabetic ketoacidosis (DKA) is an acute diabetic complication that is caused when there is no or insufficient insulin in the body, which prevents cells from using glucose (helping to lead to hyperglycemia) as a fuel, and then they begin to breakdown fats, leading to a build-up of ketoacids in the blood. These ketoacids (acetoacetate and beta-hydroxybutyrate) lead to a build-up of acid in the blood. Most individuals with DKA have Type 1 diabetes but the disorder can also occur with individuals with Type 2 diabetes, especially after a severe illness or if the individuals are AFRICAN AMERICAN or HISPANIC.

Symptoms of DKA may include

- flushed face
- fruity breath
- nausea and vomiting
- deep and rapid breathing
- fatigue
- frequent urination and extreme thirst

According to the Centers for Disease Control and Prevention (CDC), in 2003 (the latest data as of this writing), DKA represented 8.3 percent of all hospital admissions.

Diabetic nephropathy According to the National Institute of Diabetes and Digestive and Kidney Diseases (NIDDK), about 180,000 people with diabetes in the United States have kidney failure that was caused by diabetes. End-stage renal disease is the last stage of chronic kidney disease and is the final no-turning-back stage at which the kidney fails and cannot recover, and the individual must have either dialysis or a kidney transplant to survive. Kidney damage usually does not begin until the individual has had diabetes for at least 10 years; however, many people with Type 2 diabetes are not diagnosed for years after their actual onset of the disease. According to the NIDDK, if there are no signs of kidney failure after more than 25 years of living with diabetes, then the probability of its later development is decreased.

Most people with chronic kidney disease (CKD) have no symptoms in the early years of their disease, and only vigilant testing by physicians can detect potential markers so that the individual can be treated before it is too late. For example, the presence of microalbuminuria (albumin in the urine) is an indicator of kidney disease, and individuals with diabetes should receive annual testing for microalbuminuria. If protein is present in the urine (PROTEINURIA), this indicates that the kidney disease has advanced further.

According to the NIDDK, kidney disease is present when there are more than 30 milligrams of albumin per gram of creatinine in the urine. The American Diabetes Association and the National Institutes of Health both recommend that all people with Type 2 diabetes receive an annual assessment of their urinary albumin excretion. For individuals with Type 1 diabetes, individuals should be assessed when they have had the disease for five or more years.

If kidney disease is found to be present, medications that are often used to treat hypertension may be effective at treating kidney disease, such as angiotensin-converting enzyme (ACE) inhibitors and ANGIOTENSIN RECEPTOR BLOCKERS (ARBs). Other medications such as diuretics, beta blockers or calcium channel blockers may also be used to treat kidney disease, mainly by helping lower blood pressure.

According to the NIDDK, one effective ACE inhibitor is lisinopril (Prinivil, Zestril). In addition to lowering blood pressure, this medication may also protect the glomeruli of the kidneys. (The kidneys are comprised of about a million tiny filters comprised of blood vessels, and these filters are called glomeruli. One vessel alone is a glomerulus.) An example of an ARB is losartan (Cozaar), a medication that is used to treat hypertension, and which also protects kidney function and lowers the risk for cardiovascular events.

According to the NIDDK, people with diabetes should take the following actions to protect their kidneys:

- have their health care provider measure their HgbA1c level at least twice a year. This is a blood level that provides blood sugar data for the past three months. It is best to keep the HgbA1c level at less than 7 percent.

- cooperate with the health care provider with regard to insulin injections, medications, meal planning, physical activity, and blood-glucose monitoring

- have their blood pressure checked at least several times per year. If the blood pressure is high, follow the health care provider's plan for keeping it as close to normal as possible. Aim for a blood pressure of less than 130/80 mmHg

- ask their health care provider if they might benefit from taking an ACE inhibitor or an ARB

- ask their health care provider to measure their estimated glomerular filtration rate (eGFR) at least once per year to learn how well their kidneys are functioning. The eGFR determines how much blood the glomeruli filter in a minute, based on the amount of creatinine, a waste product that is found in the blood sample.

- ask their health care provider to measure the amount of protein in their urine at least once per year to check for kidney damage

- ask their health care provider if they should reduce the amount of protein in their diet, and ask for a referral to a registered dietitian to help with meal planning

Diabetic neuropathy According to the NIDDK, 60–70 percent of individuals with diabetes have some form of nerve damage (neuropathy), and the risk for its development increases with age and the duration of time that they have had diabetes. Neuropathies also appear more common among people who are not controlling their blood sugar as well as among those who have a high volume of body fat and who are hypertensive and overweight.

The NIDDK says that the following factors can lead to nerve damage among diabetics:

- metabolic factors, such as high blood sugar, a long duration of diabetes, abnormal blood fat levels, and possibly also low levels of insulin
- neurovascular factors that lead to damage to the blood vessels which carry nutrients and oxygen to the nerve
- autoimmune factors that cause inflammation in the nerves
- inherited traits that increase the susceptibility to nerve disease and damage
- mechanical injuries to the nerves, as with carpal tunnel syndrome
- lifestyle factors, such as SMOKING or alcohol use

There are different forms of neuropathies that diabetics suffer from, including peripheral neuropathy (the nerves in the toes, feet, legs, hands, and arms are affected); autonomic neuropathy (the nerves in the heart, stomach, intestines, bladder, sex organs, sweat glands, eyes, and lungs may be affected); proximal neuropathy (the motor nerves in the thighs, hips, buttocks, or legs are affected, usually on one side only); and focal neuropathy or mononeuropathy (the nerves in the head, torso, or leg are affected).

Diabetic neuropathies often cause pain which may be severe, and individuals in pain may need prescribed analgesics as well as other medications, such as antidepressants and anticonvulsants. Pregabalin (Lyrica) has been approved by the FDA to treat diabetic neuropathy. Duloxetine (Cymbalta) is also FDA-approved for the treatment of diabetic neuropathy.

Diabetic retinopathy According to the CDC, about 5.3 million Americans ages 18 years and older, have diabetic retinopathy. In the early stages of this disease, it is nearly always readily treatable. However, if the disorder is not diagnosed and treated, there is a risk for blindness. (See DIABETIC EYE DISEASES.) It is best for individuals with diabetes to have regular eye examinations, to rule out the possibility of diabetic retinopathy as well as other serious eye diseases, such as CATARACT, GLAUCOMA, and macular degeneration.

Hypoglycemia Hypoglycemia is abnormally low blood sugar, also known as low blood glucose, and often incorrectly referred to as "insulin shock."

Individuals with diabetes can experience hypoglycemia as a result of their diet, medications, or for other reasons, such as an increased level of strenuous exercise or the consumption of alcoholic beverages. Hypoglycemia can occur suddenly, which is why it is important for individuals with diabetes to check their blood on a regular basis, as recommended by their physician. Some symptoms of hypoglycemia including the following:

- difficulty speaking
- sweating
- anxiety
- weakness
- hunger
- confusion
- sleepiness

Nocturnal hypoglycemia refers to a low blood glucose that is experienced only at night, especially while an individual with diabetes is asleep. Nearly 50 percent of severe hypoglycemia occurs when patients are asleep and thus, their response to it is much slower. Testing blood glucose levels at bedtime is critically important.

If a person experiences a sudden and severe drop in blood sugar during sleep, they may experience the following symptoms:

- nightmares or crying out
- sweating so much that their pajamas and the sheets are damp
- anxiety, irritation, or confusion that is present upon awakening

People with Type 1 diabetes need to be vigilant about their food intake and blood glucose levels and to be especially watchful that they work to avoid a lapse into hypoglycemia while asleep. To avert such a problem, most people with Type 1 diabetes are advised to eat a small snack before bedtime, especially if the glucose level is less than 140 mg/dL. Milk and graham crackers is one commonly recommended snack.

Working with their physicians and registered dietitians, people with nocturnal hypoglycemia may adjust the timing and dosage of their insulin to avoid hypoglycemia altogether. If nocturnal hypoglycemia is recurrent, the use of the continuous glucose monitor with the INSULIN PUMP may be helpful.

Some questions that people with diabetes should ask their doctors with regard to hypoglycemia include the following:

- Can my diabetes medications cause hypoglycemia?
- When should I take my diabetes medications?
- Should I keep taking my diabetes medications when I am sick? (Generally, the answer is a resounding "yes.")
- Should I adjust my diabetes medications before physical activity?
- If I skip a meal, should I adjust my diabetes medications? (It is best to avoid skipping meals, whenever possible.)

Individuals with a blood sugar of less than 70 mg/dL can raise their blood glucose by taking one of the following items to raise their blood sugar quickly (the amounts may need to be smaller for young children):

- 3 or 4 glucose tablets
- 1 serving of glucose gel
- ½ cup or 4 ounces of any fruit juice
- ½ cup or 4 ounces of regular (not diet) soft drink
- 1 cup or 8 ounces of milk
- 5 or 6 pieces of hard candy
- 1 tablespoon of sugar or honey

In the case of severe hypoglycemia, as when an individual with diabetes has fainted, an intra-muscular injection of glucagon administered by others can help the person regain consciousness. Family, friends, and coworkers of a person with diabetes should learn how to give a glucagon injection from an emergency glucagon kit, and to learn when it is necessary to call 911 for emergency treatment.

Amputation of limbs When neuropathy proceeds in the body of the diabetic, particularly in the feet, often wounds and injuries cause little or no pain until foot or leg ulcers become gangrenous and the limb must be amputated. Many experts report that in the wide majority of cases, these injuries could have been prevented.

Disorders Associated with Diabetes

Some disorders are associated with diabetes, such as cardiovascular disease, hypertension, obesity, and dyslipidemia (abnormal blood levels of lipids). These disorders increase the risk for further problems, such as kidney disease and kidney failure. In addition, people with diabetes may suffer from sexual or urologic problems.

Cardiovascular disease Individuals with diabetes mellitus face an increased risk for cardiovascular disease, including myocardial infarction (heart attack), heart failure, and stroke. According to the NIDDK, individuals with diabetes have at least twice the risk of experiencing a stroke or heart attack compared to nondiabetics. In addition, individuals with diabetes also have an elevated risk for the development of peripheral arterial disease (PAD). This is a condition in the blood vessels of the legs and feet in which there is a decreased blow flow. This poor circulation increases the risk of a heart attack or stroke, and it also increases the risk of amputation.

According to the CDC, in 2007, 20.2 percent of diabetics ages 35 and older had coronary heart disease. In addition, 7.9 percent of this population suffered from a stroke and 17.1 percent had other heart conditions than coronary heart disease. In their 2009 article on the macrovascular (large vessels) complications of diabetes mellitus in the *Journal of Pharmacy Practice*, Donald

S. Nuzum and Tonja Merz said that diabetes is associated with a two to four times greater risk of coronary heart disease. They also noted that LIFESTYLE ADAPTATIONS are the most cost-effective means to decrease cardiovascular risks, such as losing weight among those who are overweight or obese, ending smoking among smokers, and controlling hypertension.

Individuals with diabetes should eat a healthy diet, and they often need to take prescribed medications to lower both their blood glucose and their high blood pressure, as well as to reduce cholesterol levels in the blood. The NIDDK says that controlling the ABCs of diabetes can help considerably, referring to the "A" of HgbA1c (glucose level), the "B" of blood pressure, and the "C" of cholesterol.

Anyone with diabetes who smokes should immediately stop smoking. Individuals who are overweight or obese should lose weight. With any signs of a heart attack or a stroke, early treatment can often preserve heart and brain function.

Signs of a heart attack are

- chest pain or discomfort
- shortness of breath
- pain or discomfort in the arms, back, jaw, neck, or stomach
- sweating
- nausea
- light-headedness

Signs of a stroke are

- sudden dizziness, loss of balance, or trouble walking
- sudden weakness or numbness of the face, arm, or leg on one side of the body
- sudden confusion, trouble talking, or trouble understanding
- sudden trouble seeing out of one or both eyes or sudden double vision
- sudden severe headache

TABLE 1: AGE-ADJUSTED PERCENTAGE OF HYPERTENSION FOR ADULTS WITH DIABETES, UNITED STATES, 1996–2007

Year	Percent
1995	46.2
1997	45.9
1999	47.8
2001	52.9
2003	52.4
2005	54.2
2007	56.0

Source: Adapted from the Centers for Disease Control and Prevention. "Age-Adjusted Percentage of Hypertension for Adults with Diabetes, United States, 1995–2007." July 21, 2009. Accessed November 9, 2009.

Hypertension   According to the CDC, 56.0 percent of individuals with diabetes were hypertensive in 2007, up from 54.2 percent in 2005. (See Table 1 above.) Hypertension is the second leading cause of kidney failure, after diabetes, the first leading cause. Unfortunately, many people with diabetes are also hypertensive. Hypertension can be treated with medications, weight loss, exercise, and a healthy diet.

Hypercholesterolemia   At least half the adult population in the United States has high cholesterol blood levels, and the use of medications to control hypercholesterolemia substantially increased from the period 1988–94 to 2001–06, according to Dana E. King, M.D., and colleagues in their article for the *Southern Medical Journal* in 2009. They noted that the diagnosis of hypercholesterolemia has increased from 30.2 percent of individuals in the United States ages 40–74 years in the period 1988–2004 to 37.7 percent in the period 2001–06.

According to Nuzum and Merz in their article, levels of triglyceride and cholesterol in the lipoproteins of the blood are markers for the development of coronary heart disease. The authors say, "Patients with dyslipidemia typically have made poor lifestyle choices related to diet and exercise, have a predisposing genetic condition, and/or face a metabolic condition such as diabetes that promotes alteration of lipoproteins. The most common pattern of dyslipidemia seen in patients with diabetes is elevated triglyceride concentrations, with decreased high-density lipoprotein cholesterol (HDL-C) concentrations. Low-density lipoprotein cholesterol (LDL-C) concentrations may be elevated as well, but this finding is not as consistent across all patients with diabetes."

In other words, people with diabetes often have a low level of the "good" form of cholesterol (HDL-C), and they may or may not have a high level of the "bad" cholesterol (LDL-C.)

Obesity   About 25 percent of all American adults are obese, and obesity is an even greater problem among people with diabetes; according to the CDC, in 2007, 53.0 percent of adults with diabetes were obese. The rates of obesity were much lower in the 1990s. (See Table 2.) Obesity is linked to an increased risk for cardiovascular disease, hypertension, cancer, and many other disorders. Diabetic individuals who are obese should seek to lose weight on a plan recommended by their physician and also a dietitian. Some diabetes medications can cause weight gain, and most physicians try to avoid

TABLE 2: AGE-ADJUSTED PERCENTAGE OF OBESITY FOR ADULTS WITH DIABETES, UNITED STATES, 1994–2007	
1994	34.9
1995	37.1
1996	35.7
1997	40.0
1998	41.8
1999	43.4
2000	45.4
2001	48.3
2002	48.3
2003	49.9
2004	52.2
2005	52.9
2006	55.8
2007	53.07

Source: Adapted from Centers for Disease Control and Prevention. "Age-Adjusted Percentage of Obesity for Adults with Diabetes, United States, 1994–2007. July 21, 2009. Available online. URL: http://www.cdc.gov/diabetes/statistics/comp/fig7_obesity.htm. Accessed November 9, 2009.

prescribing such medications to already-obese individuals.

Sexual and urologic problems   Because of damage caused by diabetes to the nerves and small blood vessels, diabetics may suffer from both sexual and urologic problems. Urologic problems are often linked to autonomic neuropathy, especially as concerns control of the bladder.

Among men, diabetes may cause erectile dysfunction (ED), and diabetics are two to three times more likely than nondiabetics to have ED. They may also suffer from ED as young as age 45 or younger because of their diabetes. There are other disorders that cause or contribute to the development of ED, such as hypertension, alcohol abuse, and kidney disease. In addition, ED may be caused by the side effects of some medications or by hormonal deficiencies. Smoking may also contribute to the risk for ED.

Among women, diabetes can decrease sexual desire and also affect vaginal lubrication.

Other Complications of Diabetes

Diabetes is also associated with some less common but also very troublesome disorders, such as diabetic cheirarthropathy, a rheumatologic (arthritic) disorder; pancreatitis and gallbladder diseases; and malignant otitis externa and POLYCYSTIC OVARIAN SYNDROME. Some individuals with diabetes suffer from serious skin problems, while others suffer from restless legs syndrome, a sleep disorder.

Diabetic cheirarthropathy   Diabetic cheirarthropathy is a joint immobility, causing an inability to fully extend the fingers. A classic sign of this disorder is the inability to flatten out or to touch the palms together with fingers spread in the diagnostic "prayer sign." This disorder is found primarily among children and adults with Type 1 diabetes but it is also seen in those with Type 2 diabetes. From 10-50 percent of patients with diabetes experience some level of diabetic cheirarthropathy.

Diabetic cheirarthropathy is characterized by a limited mobility of the extension of the small joints of the hands and also by a thickening and stiffness of the overlying skin. This condition may be related to changes in collagen that have been induced by higher glucose levels. As a result, diabetic cheirarthropathy may improve with better glycemic control. No treatment is known or required.

Cancer Some studies show diabetic individuals have an increased risk for some forms of CANCER.

Malignant otitis externa Malignant otitis externa is a noncancerous outer ear infection (in the external auditory canal) that is found in some individuals with diabetes, often in those who are over age 65. It is usually caused by bacteria in the *Pseudomonas* genus. This potential problem needs to be considered in all external ear infections diagnosed among patients who have diabetes so that appropriate antibiotics may be started. Malignant otitis externa can affect the facial nerves and cause a facial droop.

The standard antibiotics that are usually used for ear infections typically will not kill *Pseudomonas*. In the worst case, surgery may be needed.

Acute pancreatitis and biliary disease Some studies have shown that individuals with Type 2 diabetes have an elevated risk for the development of acute pancreatitis (a serious and sudden inflammation of the pancreas) as well as for disease of the gallbladder (biliary disease). In a retrospective study of health care claims for the period 1999–2005, Rebecca A. Noel and colleagues reported on their findings in *Diabetes Care* in 2009.

The researchers found that 337,067 patients in the sample had Type 2 diabetes. They then compared their risk for acute pancreatitis and biliary disease to the risk for nondiabetics. The individuals with Type 2 diabetes had nearly a three-fold greater risk for the development of acute pancreatitis and a nearly two-fold greater risk for the development of biliary disease. They also found that diabetic patients younger than age 45 years had the greatest risk for pancreatitis; for example, diabetics ages 18–44 years had more than a five times greater risk of pancreatitis than nondiabetics of the same age.

With regard to biliary disease among diabetics, the researchers found that the incidence rate was highest at two age points; those who were 18–30 years old and those who were 65 years and older. More than half of the cases of biliary disease were individuals with cholelithiasis (gallbladder stones). The incidence of cholelithiasis was 1,229 cases per 100,000 diabetic subjects, compared to 647 cases per 100,000 subjects without diabetes.

The reasons for these findings were unknown and require further study.

Polycystic ovarian syndrome (PCOS) Polycystic ovarian syndrome is a condition that, if untreated, may cause enlarged cystic ovaries, though a woman may have the metabolic signs of the condition and ovaries that appear normal on ultrasound. In the modern era, it is typically identified by history (irregular menses, infertility), examination (hirsutism, which is hairiness), and presence of ACANTHOSIS NIGRICANS. If found at a later time, the ovaries may be abnormally sized and shaped when palpated on examination or seen on ultrasound. Polycystic ovarian syndrome (PCOS) is frequently accompanied by irregular menstruation and problems with infertility. Women who have INSULIN RESISTANCE syndrome or Type 2 diabetes are at greater risk for this medical problem than others.

Previously known as Stein-Leventhal syndrome, PCOS is more common among women who are obese. Other co-occurring syndromes are acanthosis nigricans and hypertension. Many individuals with this disorder also have hyperlipidemia. The women with this condition also have a problem with excessive body hair (hirsutism).

Treatment is aimed at lowering insulin resistance with medications such as metformin, rosiglitazone, or pioglitazone, although these drugs are not FDA-approved for this indication. An overweight woman who has not menstruated or who menstruates erratically and who is then placed on one of these drugs is advised to use birth control unless pregnancy is her intention. The drugs may alleviate years of infertility.

Treatment will decrease the levels of male hormones, and thus the hirsutism will decrease.

Dermatologic problems   Skin problems are common in individuals with diabetes. Some individuals with diabetes have a serious problem with dry and itchy skin and, consequently, they need to use skin moisturizers on a regular basis. It is also important for people with diabetes to perform regular checks of their feet because they are more prone to developing problems, which can become very serious, particularly if the person suffers from diabetic neuropathy and/or PERIPHERAL VASCULAR DISEASE.

Some examples of skin problems that may occur in people with diabetes are

- acanthosis nigricans
- acquired perforating dermatosis. This is a condition of small dome-shaped papules (flat lesions) or nodules (small bumps with a crust-filled center.
- diabetic bullae (blisters)
- granuloma annulare (fleshy red papules or plaques that are arranged like pearls on strings in a semicircle. The center is unaffected and the borders are raised. This is most commonly seen on the backs of hands or on the feet or legs)
- xerosis (very dry skin)
- fungal infections, such as Tinea pedis (feet), Tinea cruris (groin), and Tinea capitis (scalp)

One uncommon form of skin disorder in some people with diabetes is *necrobiosis lipoidica diabeticorum*. This disease was first described in 1929, and it is strongly associated with Type 1 diabetes. The disease is four times more common in women than men. Sixty percent of those with the disorder have diabetes, and most of the remaining patients have impaired glucose tolerance or impaired fasting glucose levels. In 10–20 percent of the cases, the problem resolves on its own. No therapies are effective.

Scleroderma diabeticorum is another skin condition that is sometimes associated with diabetes.

It slowly evolves without any preceding infection or trauma. It typically starts as a nonpitting thickening in the neck area, and it can involve the neck, back, trunk, and even the legs. It is four times more common in men than women, usually those with long-term diabetes. Scleroderma diabeticorum is usually not painful and there is no known treatment. The cause is unknown.

Restless legs syndrome (RLS)   Restless legs syndrome is a sleep disorder. Research has indicated that 21 percent of individuals with diabetes have this problem. This prevalence is about three times higher than among individuals in the general population, according to Norma G. Cuellar and Sarah J. Ratcliffe in their article on restless legs syndrome among patients with Type 2 diabetes, published in *Diabetes Educator* in 2008. RLS is a disorder that causes uncomfortable feelings in the legs that are relieved only by movement, hence the "restless legs" nomenclature. RLS is also usually much worse at night, preventing people with the disorder from sleeping, which is why it is considered a sleep disorder.

These researchers studied 121 patients with Type 2 diabetes and found that 54 subjects (45 percent) met the criteria for RLS. They also found that many subjects had other health problems, such as hypertension, neuropathy, irritable bowel syndrome, kidney failure, and rheumatoid arthritis, yet only 18 participants of the 54 with RLS were being treated for their RLS.

Of those subjects who were treated, the researchers noted that their diagnosis of RLS occurred about a year and a half after their diagnosis of Type 2 diabetes. The researchers also noted that nearly half (44.4 percent) of the subjects with RLS needed insulin to control their diabetes, which the researchers said indicated poor control of diabetes. In addition, the subjects were obese, with an average body mass index (BMI) of 32.3. They also noted that exercise worsens the symptoms of RLS, and this may complicate the treatment of patients with Type 2 diabetes, who are usually encouraged to exercise. They concluded that all patients with Type 2 diabetes be evaluated for sleep disorders, including RLS as well as other sleep disorders that may be present.

See also EMERGENCY ISSUES IN DIABETES; MEN WITH DIABETES; WOMEN WITH DIABETES.

Cuellar, Norma G., and Sarah J. Ratcliffe. "Restless Legs Syndrome in Type 2 Diabetes: Implications to Diabetes Educators." *Diabetes Educator* 34 (2008): 218–234.

King, Dana E., M.D., et al. "Medication Use for Diabetes, Hypertension, and Hypercholesterolemia from 1988–1994 to 2001–2006." *Southern Medical Journal* 102, no. 11 (2009): 1,127–1,132.

National Institute of Diabetes and Digestive and Kidney Diseases. *Diabetic Neuropathies: The Nerve Damage of Diabetes.* Bethesda, Md.: National Institutes of Health, 2009.

Noel, Rebecca A., et al. "Increased Risk of Acute Pancreatitis and Biliary Disease Observed in Patients with Type 2 Diabetes: A Retrospective Cohort Study." *Diabetes Care* 32, no. 5 (2009): 834–838.

Nuzum, Donald S., and Tonja Merz. "Macrovascular Complications of Diabetes Mellitus." *Journal of Pharmacy Practice* 22, no. 2 (2009): 135–148.

coronary heart disease (CHD)   Diseases of the heart, such as MYOCARDIAL INFARCTION (heart attack) and/or angina pectoris (chest pains from heart disease) that are due to blockages in the coronary arteries. Also known as coronary artery disease. People with diabetes have a much higher risk for CHD than nondiabetics, and thus, a diagnosis of diabetes is considered a major risk factor for developing CHD. Other risk factors for heart disease are high levels of LDL cholesterol, HYPERTENSION, SMOKING, and OBESITY.

Diabetes and Heart Disease

Based on an analysis of ten studies by Warren Lee and his colleagues and also reported in *Diabetes Care* in 2000, women who have diabetes experience more than a two and a half times greater risk of coronary death than nondiabetic women. Men with diabetes have about twice the risk of death as nondiabetic men.

Coronary artery disease (CAD) may result in a sudden heart attack (myocardial infarction) or a sudden cardiac death. According to experts, CAD is the cause of death in more than half of all patients who have diabetes. CAD also causes disability in many others.

In the UNITED KINGDOM PROSPECTIVE DIABETES STUDY (UKPDS), researchers studied the effect of the drug METFORMIN on patients with diabetes and made the dramatic finding that the drug resulted in significantly lower death rates from heart disease among all treatment groups.

This was very valuable data because, according to the report "Conquering Diabetes: A Strategic Plan for the 21st Century," released in 1999 by the Diabetes Research Working Group, a Congressionally established group, individuals with diabetes are two to four times more likely to suffer from a variety of cardiac problems than are those who are nondiabetic. In addition, people with diabetes have a higher DEATH rate from heart problems than do their nondiabetic peers.

Studies have also shown that African American WOMEN WITH DIABETES are at particular risk for suffering from coronary disease and death. Clearly, cardiac conditions are an area of concern for the person with diabetes as well as his or her family members.

See also CARDIOVASCULAR DISEASE; DIGAMI STUDY; DIURETICS.

American Heart Association. *2001 Heart and Stroke Statistical Update.* American Heart Association, 2000.

Bell, David, and Fernando Ovalle, M.D. "Diabetes as a Risk Factor for Ischemic Heart Disease." *Clinical Reviews* (Spring 2000): 88–92.

Bloomgarden, Zachary, M.D. "Cardiovascular Disease in Type 2 Diabetes." *Diabetes Care* 22, no. 10 (1999): 1,739–1,744.

Centers for Disease Control and Prevention. "American Heart Month—February 2001." *Morbidity and Mortality Weekly Report* 50, no. 6 (February 16, 2001): 89–93.

Cooper, Stephanie, M.D., and James H. Caldwell, M.D. "Coronary Artery Disease in People with Diabetes: Diagnostic and Risk Factor Evaluation." *Clinical Diabetes* 17, no. 2 (1999).

Lee, Warren L., M.D., et al. "Impact of Diabetes on Coronary Artery Disease in Women and Men." *Diabetes Care* 23, no. 7 (July 2000): 962–968.

counterregulatory hormones Reactive hormones such as cortisol (the body's natural cortisone), GLUCAGON, epinephrine, and GROWTH HORMONE. HYPOGLYCEMIA leads to a release of these hormones. For example, if a person develops hypoglycemia, then glucagon should be released to counteract the low blood sugar by helping stimulate the breakdown of glycogen from the liver. Unfortunately, within five years of the diagnosis of diabetes, most patients lose the ability to secrete glucagon in response to hypoglycemia.

If the body no longer releases glucagon in response to hypoglycemia, then epinephrine may be released to protect the body. If the hypoglycemia continues, then cortisol and growth hormone may be released, although they take a much longer time to become effective.

Some people with diabetes have reduced rates of responses from their counter-regulatory hormones. This can be due to tight glycemic control or autonomic neuropathy. This will cause HYPOGLYCEMIC UNAWARENESS, a state when the person does not have identifiable symptoms of hypoglycemia. Most of the typical symptoms of hypoglycemia, such as shakiness, sweating, nausea, and nervousness, are caused by epinephrine.

C-peptide The "connecting peptide" that is derived from pro-insulin after it is cleaved to form insulin. A peptide is a protein or part of a protein that is made from amino acids. The body releases C-peptide in equal proportions to the amount of insulin that is also released.

A laboratory test for C-peptides can determine how much insulin the body is releasing; however, it is only rarely used by physicians to make clinical decisions. C-peptide may be measured to determine if a patient still makes insulin. It is also measured in cases of severe HYPOGLYCEMIA, to determine if patients are making too much insulin (high C-peptide) or if they have been surreptitiously taking insulin by injection (causing low C-peptide levels). Some individuals who are weight lifters, but who do not have diabetes, use insulin illegally, as do others for a variety of reasons.

As of this writing, MEDICARE requires a C-peptide test with a specific result before it will approve the payment for an insulin pump.

creatinine A body chemical that is found in the blood and that is excreted through the urine. It is a measure of kidney function and the higher the creatinine level, the worse the kidney function. Creatinine as measured in the blood stream is also proportional to muscle mass, and more muscle mass means a higher creatinine level. As a result, because men generally have larger muscle masses than women, they also have higher creatinine levels, although men do not necessarily have lesser kidney function than women do.

Typically, creatinine levels in a healthy person range from approximately 0.5 to 1.5 mg/dL. Physicians caring for patients with diabetes should measure this blood level at least one time per year to monitor their patients' renal (kidney) function. When the creatinine measure is greater than or equal to 1.8 to 2.0 mg/dL, then it is appropriate to refer the patient to a NEPHROLOGIST (another member of the diabetes care team), because of his or her expertise in kidney diseases.

It is important to understand that because a referral to a nephrologist (physician expert in kidney disease) is made does not automatically mean that the patient is in dire straits. Instead, the specialist's insights into kidney function are sought, to ensure that both the referring M.D. and the patient are doing all they can to stabilize and protect the remaining kidney function. Some examples of actions that may be taken are to adjust medications (especially antihypertensive drugs), suggest dietary changes, and look for other possible risk factors that can be adjusted/corrected, such as avoidance of nonsteroidal antiinflammatory medications.

A 24-hour urine collection may also be ordered. This test will provide a better estimate of kidney function (creatinine clearance) as well s measure if excess amounts of protein are being lost in the urine. Test results will show exactly at what level the kidneys are functioning. Since many people with diabetes also suffer from kidney disease, but often they have no symptoms, this is an important test.

critically ill nondiabetic patients who become hyperglycemic Severe life-threatening illness may induce diabetes in some patients and can contribute to their deaths, if not treated. According to a study reported in the *New England Journal of Medicine* in 2001 by physicians in a Belgium hospital, this HYPERGLYCEMIA may lead to complications and even death. Patients were assigned to either the intensive therapy group or the conventional therapy group.

Researchers instituted intensive insulin therapy in 765 critically ill patients, and found that deaths (mortality) were reduced to 4.6 percent from 8.0 percent for patients with conventional care. In terms of numbers, 35 patients died in the intensive treatment group, versus 63 patients in the conventional treatment group. The patients suffered from a variety of medical problems including cardiac surgery, neurologic disease, cancer and other illnesses.

The authors concluded,

> The use of intensive insulin therapy to maintain blood glucose at a level that did not exceed 110 mg per deciliter substantially reduced mortality in the intensive care unit, in-hospital mortality, and morbidity [sickness] among critically ill patients admitted to our intensive care unit.

Greet Van Der Berge, M.D., et al. "Intensive Insulin Therapy in Critically Ill Patients." *New England Journal of Medicine* 335, no. 19 (November 8, 2001): 1,359–1,367.

Cushing's syndrome/Cushing's disease Any syndrome, regardless of the source, that leads to excess cortisol levels. Cushing's disease results from the pituitary gland making excessive levels of ACTH. It is also known as hypercortisolism.

Hyperglycemia (a high glucose level) is one sign that is found in adults with Cushing's syndrome, along with other symptoms that may accompany the illness.

Cushing's syndrome is a rare endocrine disease caused by the excessive secretion of cortisol, a hormone that is released by the adrenal glands. It has a prevalence of about 10–15 cases per million people each year. In 90 percent of the cases, the patient is an adult and in 10 percent of the cases, the patient is a child or an adolescent.

The disease may result from a variety of causes, including

- long-term use of steroids such as prednisone
- cancerous tumors in other parts of the body which cause the adrenal glands to overproduce cortisol
- benign or cancerous tumors of the adrenal glands

Symptoms and Diagnostic Path

Symptoms of Cushing's syndrome in a child or adolescent include

- delayed growth
- excessive weight gain, particularly in the face, neck, and abdomen (also called central obesity)
- hypertension
- either delayed or very early onset of puberty in a child or adolescent
- amenorrhea (missed periods in females)
- extreme fatigue

Symptoms of Cushing's syndrome in an adult include

- sleep disorders
- hyperglycemia
- menstrual disturbances
- osteoporosis
- muscle weakness (more prominent in the shoulder and hip girdle muscles)

- depression
- thin skin that is easily bruised
- hirsutism (excess hair growth and in atypical areas) in women, especially on the face, neck, chest, and abdominal area
- decreased fertility among men and/or lack of interest in sex and diminished libido

The illness is diagnosed through laboratory tests such as measurement of urinary free cortisol and the dexamethasone suppression test. Other radiologic tests may be ordered, such as computerized tomography (CT) scans of the adrenal glands and magnetic resonance imaging (MRI) scans of the pituitary.

Treatment Options and Outlook

Once diagnosed, the treatment depends on the underlying cause. Cushing's can be treated with medication, chemotherapy, radiation treatments, surgery, or a variety of other treatments. Sometimes surgery is indicated, especially when the patient has a cancerous tumor. If the primary cause is steroid use, often the medication level is steadily reduced to the lowest dose the physician considers efficacious for the other illness the patient may have (rheumatoid arthritis, lupus, etc.).

Risk Factors and Preventive Measures

The excessive and chronic use of steroids can lead to Cushing's syndrome. Thus, when steroids are needed, they should be used for the shortest possible time. It is also important to note the family history, because some rare syndromes are associated with an increased incidence of Cushing's syndrome, including familial primary pigmented micronodular adrenal disease and the multiple endocrine neoplasia syndrome Type I (MEN I).

For Cushing's disease, a family history may indicate that the symptoms are caused by MEN I.

cystitis   An inflammation of the bladder and a medical problem that is commonly caused by a urinary tract infection (UTI). Cystitis is a frequent complication of individuals with diabetes, particularly females. (Women in general are more likely to suffer from cystitis than men.)

The key symptoms of cystitis are: frequency of urination, urgency, burning (dysuria), and incontinence. Afflicted individuals also often strain when they are urinating. However, there may be no symptoms and asymptomatic bacteriuria (bacteria found in the urine) is actually more common among people with diabetes than in non-diabetics.

The physician may choose to culture the urine or may decide to treat the patient immediately, based on the cloudy appearance of the urine, microscopically visible bacteria, and the patient's symptoms. There may also be visible or microscopic blood found in the urine.

Treatment of a urinary tract infection is best done with an antibiotic with a narrow spectrum of efficiency or one that is picked based on urine culture results. Treatment of UTIs in patients with diabetes is not only done to alleviate infection but also to protect the kidneys from damage.

Once diagnosed, treatment usually involves prescribing an antibiotic that may be taken for as few as one to three days. Longer courses of treatment may be used for patients who have frequent infections or who have structural abnormalities or resistant bacteria.

Some individuals with undiagnosed diabetes, as well as patients with poorly controlled diabetes, may suffer from recurrent bouts of cystitis.

See also INFECTIONS; URINARY TRACT INFECTION (UTI).

dawn phenomenon A sudden rise in the blood glucose level of patients with diabetes, usually between 2 A.M. and 8 A.M., and prior to eating. Individuals with Type 1 diabetes may experience this early morning hyperglycemia, but it is less common in those who have Type 2 diabetes. Individuals with BRITTLE DIABETES are prone to suffering from this condition, although all patients experience the dawn phenomenon to some extent.

The dawn phenomenon is caused by the effects of counterregulatory hormone levels, such as adrenaline/epinephrine, noradrenaline/norepinephrine, and so forth. These hormone levels rise in the early morning and enable the individual to awake and "face the day." However, at the same time, they also lead to increased levels of glucose and blood pressure. These hormones do this by counteracting the effects of insulin and causing a rise in glucose as the person sleeps. Many people mistakenly believe that early morning hyperglycemia is mainly caused by what the individual ate the night before. Much of the excess morning hyperglycemia is due to the overproduction of glucose from the liver partly due to this dawn phenomenon.

The increases in counterregulatory hormones, which lead to increased glucose levels, increased blood pressure, elevated heart rate, and changes in lipids and in blood clotting, are why more heart attacks and strokes occur in the early morning than at other times.

For people with Type 1 diabetes who experience a problem with dawn phenomenon, physicians may suggest taking a long-lasting insulin before bedtime. They may also be good candidates for an INSULIN PUMP.

death Cessation of life. Diabetes was the sixth leading cause of death in the United States in 2006, according to 2009 data from the Centers for Disease Control and Prevention (CDC), and 72,449 people died of diabetes in 2006, or 3 percent of all deaths. The CDC says that diabetes is likely to be underreported as a cause of death. The largest percentages of deaths by population occurred among black females with diabetes, or a rate of 34.1 per 100,000 people, followed by the rate among black males with diabetes, or a rate of 30.6 per 100,000 males. In the category of black females, 7,041 females of all ages died from diabetes, out of a total black female population of 20,668,780. (See Table 1.)

Of those who died, the largest number of individuals were ages 75–84 years old (21,763 deaths) followed by 15,483 deaths among those ages 65–74 years.

The risk of death from diabetes is about double the death risk for people without diabetes who are the same age, according to the CDC. This is at least in part due to the fact that people with diabetes are more likely to have kidney failure and CARDIOVASCULAR DISEASE, as well as other related diseases and ailments.

The World Health Organization (WHO) reports that an estimated 1.1 million people worldwide died of diabetes in 2005, and about 80 percent of these deaths occurred among people living in low- to middle-income countries. The WHO also reported that about half of the deaths worldwide from diabetes occur to people younger than age 70. In addition, an estimated 55 percent of the worldwide deaths from diabetes are women. WHO predicted that diabetes deaths would increase by 80 percent

TABLE 1: DEATHS FROM DIABETES BY GENDER AND RACE, ACTUAL COUNT COMPARED TO POPULATION AND RATE PER 100,000

Gender	Race	Deaths from Diabetes	Total Population	Rate Per 100,000
Female	American Indian or Alaska Native	449	1,602,260	28.0
	Asian or Pacific Islander	809	7,467,989	10.8
	Black or African American	7,041	20,668,780	34.1
	White	28,144	122,147,303	23.0
	Total	**36,443**	**151,886,332**	**24.0**
Male	American Indian or Alaska Native	362	1,599,082	22.6
	Asian or Pacific Islander	812	7,073,288	11.5
	Black or African American	5,772	18,889,595	30.6
	White	29,060	119,950,187	24.2
	Total	**36,006**	**147,512,152**	**24.4**
	Total	72,449	299,398,484	24.2

Source: Adapted from Centers for Disease Control and Prevention, National Center for Health Statistics. Compressed Mortality File 1990–2006. CDC WONDER On-line Database, compiled from Compressed Mortality File 1999–2006 Series 20, No. 2L, 2009. Accessed at http://wonder.cdc.gov/cmf-icd10.html on October 26, 2009.

in upper-middle income countries between the years 2006 and 2015.

Among children and adolescents with diabetes, of the few numbers of deaths that occur, most are caused by either DIABETIC KETOACIDOSIS or HYPOGLYCEMIA, both conditions in which blood glucose levels are out of control.

See also COMPLICATIONS OF DIABETES AND ASSOCIATED DISORDERS; DIABETES MELLITUS; DIABETIC NEUROPATHY; MEN WITH DIABETES.

Heron, Melonie, et al. "Deaths: Final Data for 2006." *National Vital Statistics Reports* 57, no. 14 (April 17, 2009): 1–136.
World Health Organization. "Diabetes: What Is Diabetes?" Available online. URL: http://www.who.int/mediacentre/factsheets/fs312/en/print.html. November 2008. Accessed October 26, 2009.

dehydration   Severe and harmful lack of fluid, with the primary symptoms of thirst, dry skin and mucous membranes, lightheadedness, and nausea. HYPERGLYCEMIA is one cause of dehydration because excessive levels of glucose filtered through the kidneys pulls water out in a process that is called an "osmotic diuresis."

The primary causes of dehydration are as follows:

• inadequate fluid intake
• vomiting
• diarrhea
• diuretic medications
• high glucose levels (hyperglycemia)
• bleeding

Dehydration is treated by determining the cause of the problem and by replacing fluids to an adequate level. The dehydrated person may need to be hospitalized, depending on the severity of the dehydration.

Dehydration can become a serious problem if untreated, and dehydration may lead to or definitely contribute to and exacerbate DIABETIC KETOACIDOSIS (DKA) or HYPEROSMOLAR COMA.

See also HYPOGLYCEMIA.

dementia   A process that leads to very diminished cognitive ability, behavioral changes, and the inability to perform activities of daily living

The person may have ALZHEIMER'S DISEASE or he or she may have another form of dementia. Often the person may have emotional outbursts or rages. Some studies indicate that people with diabetes are at greater risk for developing dementia than are nondiabetics. In a study reported by Ott et al., in a 1999 issue of *Neurology*, the researchers described their findings on dementia drawn from the Rotterdam study, a study of 6,370 older people and chronic disorders. Of the total, there were 692 patients who had diabetes.

The subjects were followed for about two years and 126 of the patients with diabetes developed dementia. Of these, 89 developed Alzheimer's disease. Researchers found that subjects with diabetes had nearly double the risk of developing dementia over those who did not have diabetes, although they could not identify the underlying cause for this occurrence. Patients with newly diagnosed diabetes had a lower probability of developing dementia, while those who were receiving insulin were most likely to be diagnosed with dementia. This does not indicate that insulin was the cause of dementia. Instead, it was likely that these patients had diabetes for a longer period and required more therapy.

Signs of Dementia

The person with dementia and diabetes often cannot recognize the signs and symptoms of low and high glucose levels and often cannot respond appropriately because the person's brain is not functioning well. Wide swings in glucose levels may also exacerbate acute changes in cognitive skills and behavior.

The ill person with severe dementia may not recognize her own children, may not know the purpose of a wristwatch, and may experience paranoia, hallucinations, and other psychotic behaviors. These individuals are extremely difficult to care for in a home environment and may require care in an ASSISTED LIVING FACILITY or a SKILLED NURSING FACILITY.

Often medical doctors allow patients with dementia to have slightly higher levels of glucose (in the 120 to 250 range) to try to avoid HYPOGLYCEMIA, a problem that is more frequent with tight control.

See also ELDERLY.

Ott, A., et al. "Diabetes Mellitus and the Risk of Dementia: The Rotterdam Study." *Neurology* 53 (1999): 1,937–1,942.

denial (of diabetes) Refusal to accept that one has diabetes and/or refusal to accept that actions must be taken as a result of the disease. When a child, adolescent, or adult is first diagnosed with diabetes, it may be very difficult for the individual and other family members to accept the illness and the steps that must be taken to control it. The person and his or her loved ones may also fear immediate death, although such a consequence is rare. They may also worry about or resent the idea of taking lifelong medications, having to periodically check their blood glucose levels and, in some cases, needing to self-inject with INSULIN.

It's important for newly diagnosed individuals with diabetes to receive a complete EDUCATION about their illness, including a general overview of either Type 1 or Type 2 diabetes (whichever they are diagnosed with), as well as an explanation of what medications will be needed and what lifestyle changes are recommended.

The individual needs to be shown how to test his or her own blood and to understand what the meanings are of the findings. If the person must self-inject insulin, then he or she must be taught how to prepare the tools they need and where they can be obtained, and how to self-inject and they also must be taught how to identify and react to immediate symptoms or problems that may sometimes occur subsequent to injections.

If the denial persists, the physician may refer the patient to a social worker, psychologist, psychiatrist, or other mental health professional.

depression and diabetes Depression is a continued feeling of severe and profound sadness and hopelessness, which, in its most extreme state, can lead an individual to contemplate or even to seek to carry out a plan for suicide. Depression is also known as *depressive disorder* or *major depressive disorder.* Depression is far more than a temporary sad or a "down" mood, which itself is a common occurrence among most people with the common strains of daily life. Instead, depression is characterized by a persistent and very negative and/or apathetic mood which is also accompanied by changes in appetite (increased or decreased eating), changes in sleep patterns (increased or decreased sleeping), and a lack of interest in the activities that formerly appealed to the individual (hobbies, sexual drive).

Depression makes it difficult to impossible for an individual to attend to work requirements or even to the pressing needs of family members. Depression also seriously impedes the diabetic patient's ability and interest in managing diabetes and its complications. Yet depression is common among patients with diabetes and should be screened for by physicians. In fact, depression screening should occur at periodic intervals rather than only at the time of the initial diagnosis or the first visit with an endocrinologist or other physician treating the patient for diabetes, because research indicates that long-term diabetes patients are at increased risk for developing depression.

An Increased Risk for Death with Depression

Some researchers have pointed out that the presence of both diabetes and depression increases the risk for death. In a study by Elizabeth H. B. Lin and colleagues reported in a 2009 issue of *Annals of Family Medicine,* the researchers studied the link between depression and diabetes as well as mortality. The researchers studied 4,184 subjects with Type 2 diabetes, and they found that major depression was significantly related to death by all causes. They concluded that patients with both diabetes and clinical depression had substantially elevated risks for death. Minor depression, however, was not a factor in death among the diabetic subjects.

Some experts believe (and studies have supported) that identifying depression early on in the course of diabetes will improve glycemic control (control of blood glucose, sometimes referred to as "blood sugar"), and they also say that treating depression is cost-effective.

In a study by G. E. Simon and colleagues reported in *Archives of General Psychiatry* in 2007, the researchers identified 329 patients with diabetes (nearly all with Type 2 diabetes) and depression. The study subjects were placed in either the usual care group or in the intervention group. The intervention group received in-person nurse visits and telephone follow-ups over a one-year period. The researchers found that the intervention patients had outpatient health care costs that were $314 lower than the costs associated with usual care for diabetes.

Others say that their research shows that the true link between depression and diabetes lies among patients with Type 2 diabetes who use insulin (as opposed to oral medications). For example, in a study by J. E. Aikens and colleagues and published in *Diabetic Medicine* in 2008, the researchers found a significant link between patients taking insulin and who also suffered from depression. The researchers studied 103 patients with Type 2 diabetes who used insulin and compared them to 155 patients with Type 2 diabetes controlled with oral medications alone. The researchers recommended that clinicians be especially vigilant in checking for depression among patients with Type 2 diabetes who used insulin.

People with Type 1 and Type 2 diabetes are at least three times more likely to suffer from depression than are people without diabetes, and depression is also a common problem among those individuals who are diagnosed with prediabetes, which is usually an insulin resistant state manifested by the inability of the body to synthesize adequate amounts of insulin to normalize the blood glucose levels under all conditions. This causes elevated glucose levels but which are not high enough to reach the diagnostic level of diabetes.

Most studies show that women with diabetes are more likely to be diagnosed with depression than men with diabetes. The same is true in the general population, as women are more frequently diagnosed with depression than men are. However, a study that was published in *Morbidity and Mortality Weekly* in 2004 indicated that males with diabetes had a greater risk for serious psychological stress, which includes symptoms of both depression and anxiety.

According to the *Diagnostic and Statistical Manual of Mental Disorders, DSM-IV-TR* (American Psychiatric Association, 2000), a reference source which is used by many psychiatrists as well as other mental health professionals, "Up to 20–25 percent of individuals with certain general medical conditions (e.g., diabetes, myocardial infarction, carcinomas, stroke) will develop Major Depressive Disorder during the course of their general medical conditions." Some researchers such as Saba Moussavi and colleagues in their 2007 article for *Lancet* have reported that the physical health of diabetics with depression is significantly worse than among diabetics without depression, based on worldwide studies of depression and medical problems.

Many patients with diabetes who are treated routinely as outpatients may have depressive symptoms, based on a study by Bijal M. Shah and colleagues and reported in the *Journal of the American Pharmacists Association* in 2008. Shah et al. studied 217 primary care patients who were 18 years and older with Type 2 diabetes. The majority of the subjects were Hispanic (60.7 percent) and female (62.2 percent). The researchers used the Zung Self-Rating Depression Scale (Zung SDS) to ascertain the presence of depressive symptoms and found that 72.1 percent of the diabetic patients had depressive symptoms. They also found that 13 percent of diabetic patients previously diagnosed with depression were currently not receiving any treatment for depression. The researchers found that a past history of depression, the receipt of Medicaid health insurance, and the use of insulin were all factors that were significantly associated with patients with diabetes having depressive symptoms.

Said the researchers, "Only 62 of the 112 patients with possible depression had a documented diagnosis of the disease; this represents considerable unrecognized disease in those with type 2 diabetes. Disparities in detecting and treating depression in Hispanic patients with type 2 diabetes have been documented, potentially as a result of health literacy issues, somatic presentation of the disease, and use of cultural idioms of distress."

The Bidirectional Nature of Diabetes and Depression

Some experts have written about the "bidirectional" nature of diabetes and depression; i.e., some research indicates that depressed adults have an increased risk for developing diabetes and also that diabetic adults have an increased risk for developing depression. Thus, diabetes may trigger or tip a susceptible patient over into a clinical depression *or* depression itself may trigger diabetes (because of inadequate care of self, poor eating habits, less activity, and increased stress, in a susceptible individual, especially one with prediabetes).

Others have written about the coexistence (also known as comorbidity) of the presence of both diabetes and depression in relation to the many features that are common to both conditions, such as obesity, insufficient exercise, and a sedentary lifestyle, as well as overall poor health and a poor diet. Diabetes together with depression often worsens blood glucose levels and increases the risk for diabetic complications.

Said Wayne J. Katon, M.D., in his article on the comorbidity of diabetes and depression for the *American Journal of Medicine* in 2008, "Depressive symptoms are associated with decreased glycemic control and increased diabetic complications; conversely, poor metabolic control and functional impairment due to increasing complications may cause or worsen depression and lessen response to antidepressant medication."

Katon says that even low levels of depressive symptoms may worsen the self-management of diabetes. It is also true that diabetic complications themselves may trigger depression, and Katon says, "The burden of caring for diabetes, which includes managing complications, adhering to dietary restrictions, and monitoring glucose levels, can significantly diminish quality of life and contribute to affective [mood] disturbance."

Depression in Diabetic Individuals Often Goes Undiagnosed and Untreated

Physicians may fail to screen diabetic patients for depression because they may not recognize depressive symptoms or because they may believe that diabetes treatment is much more urgent; however, it is important to understand that depressed individuals often have difficulty in complying (or they fail to comply) with medical recommendations for treatment, such as at least once-daily blood testing (depending on what the doctor's recommendations are), and also taking action based on the results of blood tests (such as eating more or fewer carbohydrates or taking emergency actions as needed).

Serious Psychological Distress and Diabetes

In a study reported in 2004 by K. H. McVeigh, F. Mostashari, M.D., and L. E. Thorpe in *Morbidity & Mortality Weekly* on the effects of "serious psychological distress," a category that encompasses depression, anxiety, and other major psychological disorders, the researchers used data drawn from the New York City Department of Health and Mental Hygiene (DOHMH) on nearly 10,000 adults in New York City. The researchers found that adults with diabetes had twice the risk for serious psychological distress as did the subjects without diabetes.

Serious psychological distress was measured with the K6 Screening Scale, a scale developed by Dr. Ronald Kessler at Harvard Medical School. It is comprised of six items to which individuals respond with "all of the time," "most of the time," "some of the time," "none of the

time," "don't know," or that the patient refused to answer. For example, the self-rating scale asks a patient about how often in the last four weeks he or she felt "so sad that nothing could cheer you up," responding with one of the time items discussed. Each response to an item is coded with points ranging from 0 to 4, and patients who respond "all of the time" receive 4 points, while those who respond "most of the time" receive 3 points and so on. Those individuals who score 13 points or greater are considered to have serious psychological distress, and it is recommended that they should be referred to a mental health professional for a further evaluation.

The researchers analyzed data on 857 total individuals, including those with diabetes alone (777 subjects) as well as those with both diabetes and serious psychological distress (80 subjects), 10.4 percent of all the diabetics. They found that adults with both diabetes and serious psychological distress (SPD) had a much higher rate of reporting themselves with fair or poor health (78.2 percent) compared to those with diabetes only (39.8 percent). In addition, individuals with SPD were about three times more likely (64.2 percent) than diabetics without SPD (22.2 percent) to report experiencing three or more days in the past 30 days in which their poor physical health limited their usual activities. They were also much more likely to report that their poor mental health impeded their activities.

The researchers found that adults with diabetes and SPD had less access to health care, and more often lived in poverty compared to the adults with diabetes only. For example, 42.0 percent of the adults with both diabetes and serious psychological distress said that they did not fill a prescription that was written for them, compared to only 16.5 percent of adults with diabetes who did not have psychological distress. In addition, 47.1 percent of the adults with both SPD and diabetes said that they did not go to a doctor when they had a medical problem, about twice as high as the 23.1 percent of patients with diabetes only who said that they did not go to the doctor when they had a medical problem.

Many diabetics are overweight or obese, and the researchers found that more than two-thirds (68.9 percent) of the New York City subjects with diabetes but without SPD were overweight (with a BODY MASS INDEX between 25 and 29.9) or obese (with a body mass index of 30 or greater. However, the situation was even worse among those with *both* diabetes and SPD: 81.6 percent of these subjects were overweight or obese.

The subjects with both diabetes and serious psychological distress were also more likely than those with diabetes only to be divorced, separated, or widowed (48.7 percent) than the adults with diabetes only (25.3 percent). In considering other demographic features, the researchers found that Hispanic adults with diabetes had the highest rate for diabetes and SPD (45.2 percent), followed by blacks (23.0 percent).

In addition, in contrast to most categories of people with depression, men rather than women represented a greater proportion of those with both diabetes and SPD, or 55.5 percent. See Table 1 for further information.

TABLE 1: DEMOGRAPHIC, HEALTH CARE UTILIZATION AND HEALTH STATUS CHARACTERISTICS OF ADULTS WITH DIABETES, BY SERIOUS PSYCHOLOGICAL DISTRESS STATUS, NEW YORK CITY COMMUNITY HEALTH SURVEY, 2003. PERCENTAGE.

Characteristic	With SPD (n=80)	Without SPD (n=777)
Age group (years)		
18–44	21.9	16.5
45–64	55.9	46.7
≥65	22.3	36.8
Gender		
Men	55.5	55.1
Women	44.5	44.9
Race/Ethnicity		
White, non-Hispanic	18.3	23.9
Black, non-Hispanic	23.0	25.1
Hispanic	45.2	33.5
Asian/Pacific Islander	12.7	14.3
Other	0.8	3.2
Marital Status		
Married/partnered	33.4	51.7
Divorced/separated/widowed	48.7	25.3
Never married	18.0	23.0
Household income		
Less than $25,000	70.2	42.8
$25,000–$49,999	9.6	28.7
≥$50,000	3.5	16.7
Unknown	16.7	11.8
Health-care insurance		
Private insurance	11.0	41.6
Medicaid/Medicare insurance	67.7	45.8
Uninsured	21.3	12.6
Because of cost		
Did not fill a prescription	42.0	16.5
Did not go to a doctor when had a medical problem	47.1	23.1
Usual source of medical care		
Primary care physician	45.4	62.9
Emergency department	25.6	9.8
Had a primary care physician	82.3	77.9
Health status		
Good or excellent health	21.8	60.2
Fair or poor health	78.2	39.8
Days of limited activity caused by poor physical health		
Less than or equal to 3 days	35.8	77.8
More than 3 days	64.2	22.2
Days of limited activity caused by poor mental health		
Less than or equal to 3 days	36.7	90.9
Greater than 3 days	63.3	9.1
Smoking status		
Never smoker	53.0	57.1
Current smoker	23.2	19.6
Overweight or obese (body mass index equal to or greater than 25)	81.6	68.9
No physical activity	50.7	39.0

Source: Adapted from McVeigh, K. H., F. Mostashari, M.D., and L. E. Thorpe. "Serious Psychological Distress among Persons with Diabetes—New York City, 2003." *Morbidity and Mortality Weekly* 53, no. 46 (2004): 1,089.

Poor Quality of Life and Diabetes

Particularly when the depression is untreated, individuals with both diabetes and depression have a generally poor quality of life. In an analysis of 20 studies of diabetes and depression by Miranda T. Schram, Caroline A. Baan, and François Pouwer, published in 2009 in *Current Diabetes Reviews,* the authors found that all of the studies they analyzed reported a negative association between at least one aspect of quality of life among those subjects with both diabetes and depressive symptoms.

Depression and Diagnosed Prediabetes

It is distressing for individuals to learn that they are at a high risk for developing diabetes and that if they fail to control their risk factors (such as obesity, hypertension, and related issues that are within their control), then their prediabetes is likely to accelerate to a diagnosis of Type 2 diabetes.

In a study of 185 Australian adults (116 women and 69 men) with prediabetes by Michael Kyrios and colleagues and published in the *Medical Journal of Australia* in 2009, the researchers measured the subjects' depression and anxiety scores at baseline (the start of the study) as well as their measures of oral glucose tolerance, body mass index, and other factors. They then performed an intervention, providing a diabetes prevention program.

Said the researchers, "While depression is associated with poorer outcomes in diabetes, our study indicates that, rather than depression necessarily having a direct effect on physical outcomes, there is a complex set of interrelationships between mood, psychosocial, lifestyle, anthromometric, and health-related variables in prediabetes." The researchers said that they did not find high levels of anxiety or depression in their subjects; however, of those who were depressed there were significant improvements in their depression after the completion of a diabetes prevention program.

Risk Factors for Depression among People with Diabetes

Research has indicated that people with diabetes are more prone to depression when they are not at least high school graduates and/or they suffer

from two or more medical complications that are associated with diabetes. There are many possible medical complications of diabetes, ranging from severe eye problems such as DIABETIC RETINOPATHY or other eye complications up to and including BLINDNESS, as well as serious kidney disease (DIABETIC NEPHROPATHY) and loss of sensation or pain (manifestations of peripheral sensory neuropathy). In fact, diabetes is the number one cause of kidney failure in the United States, leading to the need for either kidney dialysis or kidney transplantation in order for the patient to survive, as well as the leading cause of adult blindness and non-accidental AMPUTATION.

Type 2 patients who suffer from depression are more likely than others to have a problem with OBESITY, and they may also be treated with INSULIN rather than oral medications.

The divorce or death of a patient's spouse are other factors that have been found to be associated with depression among those with diabetes. (These issues and the related depression are also a problem for people who do not have diabetes as well.) Some studies have found that retirement from work may be significantly related to the presence of depression among individuals with diabetes.

Racial and Ethnic Groups and Depression

Individuals with diabetes who are members of some specific racial and ethnic groups are more likely to suffer from depression than others; for example, AFRICAN AMERICANS WITH DIABETES are highly prone to problems with depression. In one study of 183 African Americans with diabetes, reported by Tiffany L. Gary and colleagues in a 2000 issue of *Diabetes Care,* the researchers found that 30 percent of the subjects had symptoms of depression. Because African Americans are at risk for serious complications from diabetes, such as suffering from limb amputations, this factor may account for at least part of the reason for this high rate of depression among African Americans.

More recent research has found increasing rates of problems with diabetes and depression among Hispanics, particularly Latinas (Hispanic women). According to Anna E. Pineda Olvera and colleagues in their 2007 article in *Cultural Diversity and Ethnic Minority Psychology,* up to 10 percent of Latinas have diabetes and many are depressed. In their study, the subjects were Latinas with Type 2 diabetes, between ages 18 and 65 years, and free of severe diabetic complications, such as blindness or amputations. Of the 96 subjects, the researchers found that age was negatively correlated with glycemic control; i.e., the longer that the individual had had diabetes, the less likely she was to have good metabolic control.

The researchers also found that Latinas who did not have good control over their diabetes were more likely to be depressed than those Latina diabetics who did have good control. Depression was also related to social support; those subjects with lower social support measures were more likely to be depressed. Concluded the authors, "More attention should be focused on Latinas with diabetes because this sector of the population is rapidly increasing. In addition, depression could be prevented in these women if caught in the early stages by a screening instrument. The link between metabolic control and depression emphasizes the importance of early cost-effective interventions that may prevent the vicious bidirectional cycle of depression and diabetes complications."

Native Americans also have a high rate of diabetes as well as an elevated rate for depression. According to researchers Darren Calhoun and colleagues in their 2009 article in the *Journal of Diabetes and Its Complications,* the researchers reported on the linkage between diabetes, depression, and glycemic control among 2,832 American Indians. They found that depression was significantly higher in AMERICAN INDIANS with diabetes than in those without diabetes. They also found that worse glycemic levels were linked to severe depressive symptoms and individuals with moderate or no depression had better levels. The researchers found that individuals who had diabetes with depression were most likely to be female and with higher body mass index scores than nondepressed individuals.

Elderly and Diabetes and Depression

Elderly people in general have an elevated risk for depression, and some research indicates that older depressed people have a higher likelihood of developing diabetes than their nondepressed peers. Yet treatment of either depression or diabetes improves the outcome of both diseases. Many researchers have found a link between diabetes and depression among older people; for example, Mercedes R. Carnethon and colleagues reported in their 2007 article for *Archives of Internal Medicine* that older adults (ages 65 and older) with depressive symptoms were more likely to develop Type 2 diabetes than nondepressed older adults. The research was based on 4,681 participants from the Cardiovascular Health Study who were followed up annually from 1989 to 1999 and who did not have diabetes at the beginning of the study in 1989. Thus, depression appeared to act as a trigger to the development of diabetes.

The researchers noted that the association could not be explained away by the subjects' risk factors for developing diabetes, such as weight gain or poor health habits. The researchers also noted that more than a third (39 percent) of the diabetes in older adults in general is diagnosed after the age of 65, and they noted further that about 2 million older adults may have depression; thus, if depression is a risk factor for diabetes, this is an important finding for researchers as well as for the affected subjects.

Further Research on Diabetes and Depression

In a study by Paul S. Ciechanowski, M.D., Wayne J. Katon, M.D., and Joan E. Russo on the impact of depressive symptoms on medication adherence, function, and costs, published in *Archives of Internal Medicine* in 2000, the researchers studied 367 patients in their late 50s and early 60s with Type 1 and Type 2 diabetes. They found that there was a direct impact of moderate to severe depression and that the subjects with medium to highly severe depressive symptoms were much *less* compliant with the dietary and medication recommendations of their doctors; for example, subjects with a high severity of depression had a rate of 15 percent noncompliance with their oral regimens, compared to 7 percent of other subjects.

The severely depressed subjects also had 86 percent higher total health care costs than the other subjects. In addition, 67 percent of the severely depressed patients had one or more complications from their diabetes, compared to 37 percent with low depressive symptoms and 59 percent with a medium level of depressive symptoms.

A study by Gretchen A. Brenes on symptoms of anxiety and depression in 919 primary care patients was published in 2007 in *Primary Care Companion to Journal of Clinical Psychiatry.* Brenes reported that nearly 40 percent of the subjects reported symptoms of anxiety and 30 percent reported symptoms of depression. Patients with anxiety or depression had worse outcomes than patients with diabetes only. Brenes also looked at the diseases with the most significantly negative effect on the subjects' quality of life and found that they were osteoarthritis, diabetes, osteoporosis, and chronic obstructive pulmonary disease (COPD). It seems logical to assume that patients with both anxiety and/or depression and diabetes (as well as osteoarthritis, etc.) have a high risk of a poor quality of life.

Depression Is a Treatable Illness

Depression is highly treatable in most cases, according to psychiatrists. Studies on depressed individuals who have diabetes have revealed that a class of antidepressant medications called serotonin selective reuptake inhibitors (SSRIs) are often highly effective in treating depression. This class includes medications such as Prozac (fluoxetine) and Zoloft (sertraline). Other medications known as serotonin norepineprine reuptake inhibitors (SNRIs) are also effective in treating depression, including such medications as duloxetine (Cymbalta) and venlafaxine (Effexor, Effexor XR).

Psychiatrists are medical doctors who treat emotional disorders such as depression and anxiety. Although any physician may treat these disorders, and many primary care physicians treat depression, psychiatrists are generally the most knowledgeable experts on the best medications and treatments for depression. Of course, it is very important for the psychiatrist to coordinate any prescribed medication with the diabetic person's primary care physician and to ensure that any likely or possible problems with medication interactions are prevented or minimized.

Many people have an unfairly negative and fearful view of psychiatrists, assuming, for example, that psychiatrists treat only individuals who are severely mentally ill. The reality is that most patients of psychiatrists experience common and treatable ailments such as depression and anxiety, and few patients are psychotic. However, it should be noted that when depressed patients are psychotic, antipsychotic medications should be used with care, because some antipsychotics can trigger or worsen diabetes. For example, a study by R. A. Baker and colleagues reported in *Psychopharmacology Bulletin* in 2009 found that there were elevated risks for triggering diabetes among some drugs, such as olanzapine (Zyprexa), risperidone (Risperdal), clozapine (Clozaril), and quetiapine (Seroquel). Lower risks were seen with other antipsychotics. As a result, patients taking antipsychotics for depression (or any other reason) should be monitored for a possible onset of diabetes.

Some people with diabetes may also benefit considerably from seeing a psychologist or social worker in order to gain insight to their feelings and learn better coping skills. Some individuals also benefit from joining support groups where they can not only empathize with other people in a similar situation but also learn practical and useful information from other members.

See also DENIAL OF DIABETES.

Aikens, J. E., et al. "Association between Depression and Concurrent Type 2 Diabetes Outcomes Varies by Diabetes Regimen." *Diabetic Medicine* 25, no. 11 (2008): 1,324–1,329.

Baker, R. A., et al. "Atypical Antipsychotic Drugs and Diabetes Mellitus in the U.S. Food and Drug Administration Adverse Event Database: A Systematic Bayesian Signal Detection Analysis." *Psychopharmacology Bulletin* 42, no. 1 (2009): 11–31.

Brenes, Gretchen A. "Anxiety, Depression, and Quality of Life in Primary Care Patients." *Primary Care Companion to Journal of Clinical Psychiatry* 9, no. 6 (2007): 437–433.

Calhoun, Darren, et al. "Relationship between Glycemic Control and Depression among American Indians in the Strong Heart Study." *Journal of Diabetes and Its Complications* 23, no. 4 (2010): 217–222.

Carnethon, Mercedes R., et al. "Longitudinal Association between Depressive Symptoms and Incident Type 2 Diabetes Mellitus in Older Adults: The Cardiovascular Health Study." *Archives of Internal Medicine* 167 (April 23, 2007): 802–807.

Ciechanowski, Paul S., M.D., Wayne J. Katon, M.D., and Joan E. Russo. "Depression and Diabetes: Impact of Depressive Symptoms on Adherence, Function, and Costs." *Archives of Internal Medicine* 160 (November 27, 2000): 3,278–3,285.

Gary, Tiffany L., et al. "Depressive Symptoms and Metabolic Control in African-Americans with Type 2 Diabetes." *Diabetes Care* 23, no. 1 (January 2000): 23–29.

Katon, Wayne J., M.D. "The Comorbidity of Diabetes Mellitus and Depression." *American Journal of Medicine* 121 (2008): S8–S15.

Kyrios, Michael, et al. "The Influence of Depression and Anxiety on Outcomes after an Intervention for Prediabetes." *Medical Journal of Australia* 190 (2009): S81–S85.

Lin, Elizabeth H. B., M.D., et al. "Depression and Increased Mortality in Diabetes: Unexpected Cause of Death." *Annals of Family Medicine* 7, no. 5 (2009): 414–421.

McVeigh, K. H., F. Mostashari, M.D., and L. E. Thorpe. "Serious Psychological Distress among Persons with Diabetes—New York City, 2003." *Morbidity and Mortality Weekly* 53, no. 46 (2004): 1,089–1,091.

Moussavi, Saba, et al. "Depression, Chronic Diseases, and Decrements in Health: Results from the World Health Surveys." *Lancet* 370 (2007): 851–858.

Pineda Olvera, Anna E., et al. "Diabetes, Depression, and Metabolic Control in Latinas." *Cultural Diversity and Ethnic Minority Psychology* 13, no. 3 (2007): 223–231.

Schram, Miranda, Caroline A. Baan, and François Pouwer. "Depression and Quality of Life in Patients with Diabetes: A Systematic Review from the European Depression in Diabetes (EDID) Research Consortium." *Current Diabetes Reviews* 5, no. 2 (2009): 112–119.

Shah, Bijal M., et al. "Depressive Symptoms in Patients with Type 2 Diabetes in the Ambulatory Care Setting: Opportunities to Improve Outcomes in the Course of Routine Care." *Journal of the American Pharmacists Association* 48, no. 6 (2008): 737–743.

Simon, G. E., et al. "Cost-effectiveness of Systematic Depression Treatment among People with Diabetes Mellitus." *Archives of General Psychiatry* 64 (2007): 65–72.

Diabetes Control and Complications Trial (DCCT) An extremely important federally funded study of individuals with Type 1 diabetes which studied 1,441 subjects and followed them from 1983 to 1993, amassing enormous amounts of data and analyzing the many ramifications and effects of the illness among adults. The Diabetes Control and Complications Trial Research Group in Bethesda, Maryland conducted the study, under the auspices of the National Institute of Diabetes and Digestive and Kidney Diseases (NIDDK).

The study information has been used by many different medical experts and some subgroups have also been contacted for further studies. In addition, an outgrowth of this study, the Epidemiology of Diabetes Interventions and Complications (EDIC) Research Group, continues to study the DCCT group. In 1999, the EDIC Research Group reported that they had received permission from 96 percent of the DCCT subjects to study them further.

This clinical study was the largest diabetes study that has ever been performed. It was carried out in 29 medical centers in the United States and Canada. Although the design changed somewhat from the onset, it ultimately involved patients who were divided into two groups.

One group was given traditional diabetes therapy, which generally involved one insulin injection per day. The glucose was initially monitored with urine glucose testing and later, with once per day blood glucose monitoring. The other group received intensive control, involving multiple daily blood glucose measurements (four or more times per day) and insulin that was delivered either four times daily through injections or administered continuously through an insulin pump.

The intensively managed group also received a diet and exercise plan. In addition, members of this group received weekly phone calls from educators, monthly visits with a team comprised of a doctor, a nurse, a dietitian and also a therapist, all assets that were not provided to the group receiving the standard therapy. The intensively treated group had an average HgbA1c that was 2 percent lower than the other group. (Seven percent versus nine percent.)

The Results

The DCCT study clearly established that tight control of blood glucose decreased the probability of complications related to diabetes. For example, the risk of eye disease was reduced by 76 percent with tight control. In addition, the group that successfully tightly controlled their diabetes had a 50 percent reduced risk for kidney disease and a 60 percent reduced risk for nerve disease. These are very dramatic results and people in the medical community took notice.

Problem with Tight Control

One problem with very tight control is that it is very difficult for most patients to achieve. Most people with diabetes find it hard to test their blood four times a day and self-inject four times. Also, few patients have monthly access not only to a doctor but also to a team of interested and highly motivated specialists.

Another problem with attempting very tight control is that it also involves a greater risk of the development of severe HYPOGLYCEMIA. The intensively treated group had three times the rate of severe hypoglycemia as that experienced by the standard-treatment group. As a result

of this risk, physicians as of this writing do not recommend such tight control for the following groups of people:

- those with severe diabetic complications
- those with hypoglycemic unawareness
- those with an inability to monitor glucose levels
- those with autonomic neuropathy

A related study, the UNITED KINGDOM PROSPECTIVE DIABETES STUDY (UKPDS), studied tight glucose control in individuals with Type 2 diabetes.

Importance of Team Approach to Treatment

The DCCT illustrated to physicians the important role of the diabetes team approach in assisting people with diabetes to maintain good glycemic control. It also became clear that dietitians should be a part of the team.

Relatives of DCCT Subjects

In a subsequent study based on the relatives of DCCT subjects, published in a 1997 issue of *Diabetes*, the researchers located biological relatives of the subjects and found a high degree of illness among them. Of 448 relatives with diabetes who were identified, about half (45 percent) had Type 1 diabetes and about half (45 percent) had Type 2 diabetes. (It was unknown what type of diabetes the remaining 10 percent had.)

The researchers contacted 241 relatives who provided further information. They learned that when the DCCT subjects had DIABETIC RETINOPATHY, about 40 percent of their relatives with diabetes also had retinopathy.

When the DCCT subjects had MICROALBUMINURIA, about 62 percent of the relatives with diabetes also had microalbuminuria. It seems clear that there are familial risks, not only to diabetes but also to the complications of diabetes. It is also likely that there may be other commonalities that will be discovered in the future.

The DCCT also showed that there did not appear to be a numerical threshold for glycemic complications below which level one is "safe" and above which one is at risk. Instead, there appears to be a continuous and graded relationship between the HgbA1c level and the risk of development or progression of a complication.

The economic analysis of the DCCT showed that although the initial cost of therapy is higher than standard therapy costs, the benefits that accrue with tight glycemic control mean that the individual is less likely to require kidney dialysis because he is less likely to experience END-STAGE RENAL DISEASE (ESRD). The person is also less likely to face an amputation of a limb due to neuropathy. Thus, the long-term savings in both dollars, human lives, and suffering make tight control worth the expenses involved.

American Diabetes Association. "Implications of the Diabetes Control and Complications Trial." *Diabetes Care* 24, Supp. 1 (2001): S25–27.

Diabetes Control and Complications Research Group. "Baseline Analysis of Renal Function in the Diabetes Control and Complications Research Trial." *Kidney International* 43 (1993): 668–674.

Diabetes Control and Complications Research Group. "Clustering of Long-Term Complications in Families with Diabetes in the Diabetes Control and Complications Trial." *Diabetes* 46 (November 1997): 1,829–1,839.

Diabetes Control and Complications Research Group. "Effect of Intensive Diabetes Management on Macrovascular Events and Risk Factors in the Diabetes Control and Complications Trial." *The American Journal of Cardiology* 75 (May 1, 1995): 894–903.

Diabetes Control and Complications Research Group. "Effect of Intensive Diabetes Therapy on the Development and Progression of Neuropathy." *Annals of Internal Medicine* 122, no. 8 (April 15, 1995): 561–568.

Diabetes Control and Complications Research Group. "Effect of Intensive Diabetes Treatment on the Development and Progression of Long-Term Complications in Adolescents with Insulin-Dependent Diabetes Mellitus: Diabetes Control and Complications Trial." *The Journal of Pediatrics* 125, no. 2 (August 1994): 177–188.

Diabetes Control and Complications Research Group. "Effect of Intensive Therapy on the Development and Progression of Diabetic Nephropathy in the Diabetes Control and Complications Trial." *Kidney International* 47 (1995): 1,703–1,720.

Diabetes Control and Complications Research Group. "Effect of Intensive Treatment of Diabetes on the Development and Progression of Long-Term Complications in Insulin-Dependent Diabetes Mellitus." *The New England Journal of Medicine* 329 (September 30, 1993): 977–986.

Diabetes Control and Complications Research Group. "Epidemiology of Severe Hypoglycemia in the Diabetes Control and Complications Research Trial." *The American Journal of Medicine* 90 (April 1991): 450–459.

Diabetes Control and Complications Research Group. "Expanded Role of the Dietitian in the Diabetes Control and Complications Trial: Implications for Clinical Practice." *Journal of the American Dietetic Association* 93 (July 1993): 758–764.

Diabetes Control and Complications Research Group. "Factors in Development of Diabetic Neuropathy: Baseline Analysis of Neuropathy in Feasibility Phase of Diabetes Control and Complications Trial (DCCT)." *Diabetes* 37 (April 1998): 476–481.

Diabetes Control and Complications Research Group. "Hypoglycemia in the Diabetes Control and Complications Trial." *Diabetes* 46 (February 1997): 271–286.

Diabetes Control and Complications Research Group. "Progression of Retinopathy with Intensive versus Conventional Treatment in the Diabetes Control and Complications Trial." *Ophthalmology* 102, no. 4 (April 1995): 647–661.

Epidemiology of Diabetes Control and Complications (ERIC) Research Group. "Epidemiology of Diabetes Interventions and Complications." *Diabetes Care* 22 (January 1999): 99–111.

Epidemiology of Diabetes Control and Complications (ERIC) Research Group. "Progression of Retinopathy in the DCCT Cohorts After 4 Years. Followup in the Epidemiology of Diabetes Interventions and Complications (ERIC) Study." *Diabetologia* 41, Supp. 1 (1998): A281.

diabetes insipidus A rare metabolic disease stemming from the kidneys or pituitary gland rather than the pancreas, and completely unique from Type 1 or Type 2 diabetes mellitus. Some forms of this disease are hereditary while other forms occur subsequent to brain surgery or an injury. The symptoms of the person with diabetes insipidus may be similar to those of the person with Type 1 or Type 2 diabetes, such as frequent urination, fatigue, and excessive thirst. However, the person with diabetes insipidus does not have HYPERGLYCEMIA, the hallmark feature of diabetes mellitus. Unless the person drinks copious quantities of fluid, he or she will become severely dehydrated and constipated.

The disease may occur abruptly in individuals of any age. If infants with the disease are not treated quickly, they may suffer from brain damage or developmental delays such as mental retardation. Symptoms of diabetes insipidus in a baby are fever, vomiting, and convulsions with high levels of sodium found in the blood upon laboratory examination.

Diabetes insipidus is usually treated with desmopressin acetate (DDAVP), a hormone that is available as a nasal spray, liquid, or tablets. Drugs are also prescribed to limit excessive urination. Paradoxically, diuretic drugs, usually effective in increasing urination, will reduce urine volume in the person with diabetes insipidus, in whom the cause is a kidney problem.

diabetes mellitus Diabetes mellitus is an increasingly dominant problem in the world today, particularly in the case of Type 2 diabetes, which represents about 95 percent of all cases of diabetes. According to the American Diabetes Association, one in every five health-care dollars in the United States is spent on diabetes, and this figure is anticipated to rise considerably as increasing numbers of obese "Baby Boomer" Americans (born 1946–64) grow older and many of them develop Type 2 diabetes. The National Institute of Diabetes and Digestive and Kidney Diseases (NIDDK) reports that in 2007, an estimated 23.6 million people, or 7.8 percent of the entire population in the United States, had some form of diabetes. Of this number, 17.9 million people had been diagnosed with diabetes, but 5.7 million people were yet to be diagnosed, and thus, they were not receiving any treatment. In

addition, according to the International Diabetes Federation, there are 314 million people worldwide with prediabetes and by 2025 there will be 418 million people with prediabetes.

Some experts predict a virtual explosion of the numbers of people with diabetes in future years. For example, researchers Elbert S. Huang, M.D., and colleagues predicted in a 2009 article in *Diabetes Care* that from 2009 to 2034, the number of people in the United States with both diagnosed and undiagnosed diabetes will nearly double, increasing from 23.7 million people in 2009 to 44.1 million individuals by 2034. Huang and colleagues also predicted that spending on diabetes will nearly triple, from $113 billion in 2009 to an estimated $336 billion in 2034 (in 2007 dollars).

The longer that a person has Type 2 diabetes, the greater is the risk for the development of serious COMPLICATIONS OF DIABETES (whether the individual knows he or she has diabetes or not). In addition, often these complications initially have few or no symptoms, such as DIABETIC EYE DISEASES or DIABETIC NEPHROPATHY (kidney disease that is caused by diabetes). This is why the diagnosis of diabetes is so important: individuals who are diagnosed can then receive treatment and take needed actions to prevent or at least delay the many serious complications that are associated with diabetes.

Considering Prediabetes

Prediabetes, which is a condition that is indicated by a blood test for diabetes, is a risk factor for the subsequent development of diabetes, and it is also a major issue in the United States today. According to the National Diabetes Education Program (NDEP), an estimated 57 million adults in the United States have prediabetes. Not all of these individuals with prediabetes will develop diabetes, but it is best for people with prediabetes to know that they *could* develop diabetes so that they can make the needed lifestyle changes to decrease their risks, such as ending a smoking habit, limiting or ending their consumption of alcohol, managing existing hypertension, and losing weight if they are overweight or obese. The importance of prediabetes is that with aging and obesity, the person with prediabetes has an elevated risk for developing Type 2 diabetes. Aging is not a modifiable risk factor but overweight and obesity can be managed, at least, theoretically. (About 20 percent of people with diabetes are severely obese and clearly have considerable difficulty with their weight.)

Prediabetes refers to a prediabetic glucose level that is lower than the diagnostic level for diabetes—but it is close to it. Specifically, prediabetes is diagnosed when the fasting plasma glucose (FPG) is within the range of 100–125 mg/dL after an overnight fast, according to the NDEP. Alternatively, prediabetes can also be measured with a two-hour post 75g glucose challenge when the resulting range is 140–199 mg/dL, or so-called impaired glucose tolerance (IGT).

Note that some authors and even some doctors confuse the diagnosis of METABOLIC SYNDROME with prediabetes. Metabolic syndrome is a condition that includes abdominal obesity, dyslipidemia, and other factors. Even more confusingly, people with prediabetes may also have metabolic syndrome. But prediabetes itself refers solely to the laboratory test result of a glucose level that is close to—but not as high as—the level for diabetes.

Types of Diabetes Mellitus

There are two primary types of diabetes, including Type 1 and Type 2 mellitus. There is also a third form of diabetes that is known as GESTATIONAL DIABETES, a diabetes that occurs during pregnancy. Type 1 diabetes, formerly known as *insulin-dependent diabetes* or *juvenile diabetes,* is an autoimmune disease that occurs when the body's own immune system destroys the beta cells of the pancreas. These are the cells that create insulin, which is a substance that is necessary in order to survive. Individuals with Type 1 diabetes need to inject insulin or to use an INSULIN PUMP that delivers insulin directly to the body.

Some people with Type 1 diabetes receive a pancreas implant, thus essentially curing their Type 1 diabetes, but this procedure is expensive and rare as of this writing. Sometimes diabetics whose kidneys have failed will receive a joint kidney-pancreas transplant.

In contrast to Type 1 diabetes, Type 2 diabetes is characterized by INSULIN RESISTANCE, which means that the pancreas does make at least some insulin, at least until the later stages of the disease, but the body is unable to use all of this insulin sufficiently. Thus there is both insulin resistance and an inability of the body to make adequate insulin to normalize the blood glucose levels. Obese individuals are at an elevated risk for developing Type 2 diabetes, as are those with a family history of diabetes. Individuals with Type 2 diabetes may need to take oral medications, and sometimes they need insulin as well, particularly after many years of having diabetes.

The third form of diabetes, gestational diabetes, occurs to some women during pregnancy, and remits soon after the delivery of the child. Some women, however, are diagnosed with gestational diabetes when they actually have had a previously undiagnosed Type 2 diabetes prior to their pregnancy. Others have a true form of gestational diabetes, which resolves after their child is born. Women with gestational diabetes have a high risk of developing Type 2 diabetes within five to 10 years after the birth of their child. In addition, they are also at risk of having gestational diabetes with each successive pregnancy that occurs.

Considering the Demographics of Diabetes

There are distinctive age, racial, and other differences between those who are at risk for diabetes and those with a lower risk. For example, individuals ages 65 years and older have an increased risk for Type 2 diabetes, and individuals who are AFRICAN AMERICANS, AMERICAN INDIANS/ALASKA NATIVES, and HISPANICS all have a higher risk for the development of Type 2 diabetes than do WHITES/CAUCASIANS.

Age Most people with diabetes are older than age 20. According to the NIDDK, in 2007, an estimated 186,300 people under age 20 had diabetes (either Type 1 or Type 2). This is less than 1 percent of all people in this age group. The risk for the development of diabetes increases with age, and the highest risk occurs among middle-aged and elderly individuals.

Gender   Women and men are about equally likely to develop Type 2 diabetes, although the complications of diabetes do not always impact them equally; for example, men are more likely to develop kidney disease and kidney failure than women.

Racial and ethnic risks   Whites and Hispanics have a higher rate of Type 1 diabetes than other races; however, African Americans and American Indians have significantly higher rates of Type 2 diabetes. Data from the Indian Health Service (IHS) indicates that about 16.5 percent of all American Indian adults in the United States have been diagnosed with Type 2 diabetes, although the rates of diabetes vary considerably between tribes; for example, the rate of diabetes is only 6 percent among Alaska Natives and is as high as 29.3 percent among American Indians living in southern Arizona.

Diagnosis of Diabetes

The decision to test for diabetes may be made as a result of symptoms that a person is experiencing that indicate the possibility of diabetes (such as extreme thirst and/or hunger, repeated minor infections, and frequent urination). The diabetes or prediabetes may also be detected from a panel of tests that a doctor routinely orders each year. If the panel shows high glucose levels, then the physician will usually order a blood test that is specifically oriented to test for diabetes, such as the oral glucose tolerance test or the fasting plasma glucose test. A preliminary diagnosis of diabetes is also considered by physicians based on underlying risk factors that the patient has (OBESITY, a sedentary lifestyle, ethnicity, a family history of diabetes, history of gestational diabetes, or current steroid use).

These risk factors may be discovered as a part of a routine checkup or during an employment physical examination. Sometimes, however, the diagnosis of diabetes is not discovered until an individual is hospitalized with emergency symptoms and is subsequently diagnosed with DIABETIC KETOACIDOSIS or HYPEROSMOLAR COMA.

Important elements of a diagnosis   The diagnosis of diabetes should result from the following elements:

- a careful medical history, including questions about the patient's biological relatives (particularly parents and siblings), the presence of gestational diabetes, the past delivery of large babies (greater than 9 pounds), or information on whether the patient was a large or small baby

- a physical examination

- a review of any symptoms that the patient that may exhibit, such as extreme thirst, frequent urination, slow healing cuts/wounds, blurred vision, unexplained weight loss, and other symptoms that are typically found among people who have diabetes

- blood glucose testing, such as the fasting plasma glucose (FPG) or the oral glucose tolerance test (OGTT). The doctor may also choose to order other tests.

Predicting the risk for diabetes   In a 2009 issue of *Diabetes Care,* the American Diabetes Association offered criteria for ordering diabetes testing in asymptomatic adults who may have prediabetes or diabetes or asymptomatic children who may have Type 2 diabetes. As can be seen from Table 1, the criteria include individuals who are overweight or obese, as well as those who are age 45 or older. Among children, overweight is also a factor as are family history and a maternal history of diabetes. (See Table 2.)

Considering the possibility of Type 2 diabetes in oneself   Sometimes individuals suspect that they may have diabetes and would like to know if they could do a preliminary self-analysis before checking with the doctor. Researchers Heejung Bang and colleagues developed a simple but proven effective self-test for individuals who

TABLE 1: CRITERIA FOR TESTING FOR DIABETES IN ASYMPTOMATIC ADULT INDIVIDUALS

1. Testing should be considered in all adults who are overweight (BMI ≥ 25 kg/m^{2*}) and have additional risk factors:

   - physical inactivity
   - first-degree relative with diabetes
   - members of a high-risk ethnic population (e.g., African American, Latino, Native American, Asian American, Pacific Islander)
   - women who delivered a baby weighing >9 lb or were diagnosed with GDM [gestational diabetes mellitus]
   - hypertension (≥140/90 mmHg or on therapy for hypertension)
   - HDL cholesterol level (<35 mg/dL (0.90 mmol/l) and/or a triglyceride level >250 mg/dL (2.82 mmol/l))
   - women with polycystic ovary syndrome
   - A1c ≥5.7%, IGT, or IFG on previous testing
   - other clinical conditions associated with insulin resistance (e.g., severe obesity, acanthosis nigricans)
   - history of CVD [cardiovascular disease]

In the absence of the above criteria, testing for diabetes should begin at age 45. If results are normal, testing should be repeated at least at three-year intervals, with consideration of more frequent testing depending on initial results and risk status.

*At-risk BMI may be lower in some ethnic groups

Source: American Diabetes Association. "Clinical Practice Recommendations." *Diabetes Care* 3, supplement 1 (2010): S14.

© 2010 American Diabetes Association. From *Diabetes Care*. Vol. 33 (2010): pp. S11–S61 Reprinted with permission from the American Diabetes Association.

TABLE 2: TESTING FOR TYPE 2 DIABETES IN ASYMPTOMATIC CHILDREN

Criteria: Overweight (BMI>85th percentile for age and sex, weight for height >85th percentile, or weight >120% of ideal for height)

Plus any two of the following risk factors:

- Family history of Type 2 diabetes in first- or second-degree relative
- Race/ethnicity (Native American, African American, Latino, Asian American, Pacific Islander)
- Signs of insulin resistance or conditions associated with insulin resistance (acanthosis nigricans, hypertension, dyslipidemia, polycystic ovary syndrome, or small for gestational age birthweight)
- Maternal history of diabetes or GDM during the child's gestation

Age of initiation: Age 10 years or at onset of puberty, if puberty occurs at a younger age

Frequency: Every three years

Source: American Diabetes Association. "Clinical Practice Recommendations." *Diabetes Care* 3, Supplement 1 (2010): S15.

© 2010 American Diabetes Association. From *Diabetes Care*. Vol. 33 (2010) pp. S11–S61. Reprinted with permission from the American Diabetes Association.

want to know if they may be at risk for diabetes, publishing their test in *Clinical Diabetes* in 2009. (See Table 3 on page 114.)

This test takes into account such factors as age, family history, gender, the presence or absence of hypertension, and the presence or absence of overweight or obesity and then helps the person predict whether he or she should receive a test for diabetes.

All the questions are easily answered with a yes or no, with the exception of the individual determining whether he or she is overweight or obese, based on the body mass index. This number can be determined with the BODY MASS INDEX (BMI) offered in Table 4 on page 116, which includes height in inches and pounds, and individuals simply find their height and weight to determine their BMI. For example,

a woman or man (BMI is a unisex measure) who is 66 inches (5 feet and 6 inches) and who weighs 200 pounds has a BMI of about 32.4. If an individual's BMI is less than the lowest BMI on this chart (25), then that person is not overweight.

Individuals can also find their exact BMI by using the Internet and going to http://www.nhlbisupport.com/bmi. The person simply types in his or her height and weight, and within seconds, the BMI is provided.

Note that if you answer no to question 6, "Are you physically active," you receive no points, but if you answer "yes," then you get -1 point, which means you can deduct a point from your total score. So if questions 1–5 added up to 4 but then you said that you are physically active, your final score is a 3, and you probably do not have diabetes or prediabetes. (Although this decision is still best left to your doctor and this is a screening tool only.)

For individuals who find that their self-assessment score indicates that they may have diabetes, it is important to follow up with a

TABLE 3: SELF-ASSESSMENT SCREENING SCORE FOR UNDIAGNOSED DIABETES OR PREDIABETES

Question	Answer (Score)	Enter Your Score (Enter 0 If You Don't Know)
1. How old are you?	<40 years (0 point)	
	40–49 y (1 point)	
	50–59 y (2 points)	
	60 y or more (3 points)	
2. Are you a woman or man?	Woman (0 point)	
	Man (1point)	
3. Do your family members (parent or sibling) have diabetes?	No (0 point)	
	Yes (1 point)	
4. Do you have high blood pressure or are you on medication for high blood pressure?	No (0 point)	
	Yes (1 point)	
5. Are you overweight or obese? (See chart on page 116 to answer this question more accurately)	Not overweight or obese (0 point)	
	Overweight (1 point)	
	Obese (2 points)	
	Extremely obese (3 points)	
6. Are you physically active?	No (0 point)	
	Yes (-1 point)	
TOTAL SCORE (add points from questions 1–6)		

If your TOTAL SCORE is 4 or greater, you are at high risk for undiagnosed diabetes or prediabetes
If your TOTAL SCORE is 5 or greater, you are at high risk for undiagnosed diabetes.
See your doctor for a blood test to look for diabetes if your score is high.

Source: Bang, Heejung, et al. "Development and Validation of a Patient Self-assessment Score for Diabetes Risk." *Annals of Internal Medicine* 151 (2009): 780. Annals of Internal Medicine Online by Heejung Bang et al. © 2009 by American College of Physicians—Journals. Reproduced with permission of American College of Physicians—Journals in the format tradebook via Copyright Clearance Center.

physician. He or she will take a complete medical history and order a test for diabetes, which will confirm or refute the self-assessment. If the individual does have diabetes, then he or she can begin receiving treatment, which is very important.

Diagnostic Tests

To diagnose Type 2 diabetes for the first time, doctors generally use the fasting plasma glucose (FPG) test or the oral glucose tolerance test (OGTT). There are also other available tests, such as the capillary glucose test or the urinary glucose test. A random plasma glucose (RPG) test can also be performed. It should also be noted that some physicians order a panel of tests, of which glucose screening is one. Some doctors or insurance companies feel that these panels are too expensive, however, and refuse to pay for them. In 2010, the American Association of

Clinical Endocrinologists (AACE) approved the A1c blood test as an additional diagnostic tool to diagnose Type 2 diabetes. The A1c provides a measurement based on an individual's blood glucose levels for the previous three months and requires only one blood draw. In addition, the results are available within a day. The advantage of the A1c is that it provides long-term as well as current data. With the A1c, if the level is 6.5 or greater, then the individual has Type 2 diabetes.

Once an individual has been diagnosed with diabetes and has been treated for at least three months, doctors may also order an HgbA1c test to help doctors (and patients) know if patients are complying with their medication and nutritional regimens. Once diagnosed, the goal with the A1c is 6.5 or less. See Table 4 and 5 on page 116 and 118. For further information on the various diagnostic tests that are currently available for nonpregnant adults and their pros and cons, recommendations for use, and whether they are generally recommended for screening for diabetes.

Diagnosing Type 1 diabetes Individuals who have Type 1 diabetes are usually easier to diagnose because their bodies produce *no* insulin and thus they are typically in a more acute state of distress, with more symptoms, and they are also often sicker than individuals with the early stages of Type 2 diabetes. Their symptoms of excessive thirst, extreme urination, poor appetite, low body weight, and other typical symptoms of Type 1 diabetes cannot be ignored by any competent physician. Most people with Type 1 diabetes are diagnosed by age 20.

Diagnosing Type 2 Diabetes The diagnosis of Type 2 diabetes is often made much later after its onset than with Type 1 diabetes because the person with Type 2 diabetes may be exhibiting no symptoms or, if symptoms are present, they are often very mild and easily ignored by the patient. As a result, many people in the United States with Type 2 diabetes are not diagnosed for years after the onset of their illness. Unfortunately, if the disease progresses for years without diagnosis or treatment, then serious complications of the disease may occur as well.

Knowing the risk factors for diabetes helps doctors determine if a person is a likely candidate to develop the illness, and as a result, they can periodically test to check if blood glucose levels have worsened. Obesity and a family history for the disease are the two major risk factors, and if a patient is obese and also has parents or siblings with diabetes, then physicians should check for the illness. In addition, as people age, they are more at risk for developing the disease.

People from certain ethnic groups are at particular risk for developing Type 2 diabetes, such as African Americans, Hispanics, and some Native American tribes. However, a person who is white, of medium or even small build, and who is not obese can still have Type 2 diabetes— it is less likely to occur, although it still happens.

When screening can occur Diabetes can be screened for at any time of the day, although some tests for diabetes require fasting, such as the fasting plasma glucose test. The first abnormality that is seen prior to the development of overt diabetes is an abnormal increase in the glucose levels after a meal. Thus, many physicians favor an oral glucose tolerance test in an attempt to diagnose and ascertain the risk for diabetes as early as possible.

The test will reveal whether the person has euglycemia (a normal glucose level), impaired glucose tolerance (IGT), impaired fasting glucose (IFG), or overt diabetes mellitus. As a practical matter, many patients are screened at the time of an office visit via a fingerstick glucose test, and thus many are being checked after a meal.

Many experts suggest that if the fasting glucose level is 100–110, then the person should be tested with an oral glucose tolerance test (OGTT) because there is a progressive risk for people with impaired glucose tolerance to develop overt diabetes. The OGTT can better screen for those people who fall into this category. Also, more people have impaired glucose tolerance than have impaired fasting glucose.

The DECODE trial from Europe showed that patients with impaired glucose tolerance appear to have a higher risk of developing

TABLE 4: BODY MASS INDEX

BMI	Normal						Overweight					Obese					
	19	20	21	22	23	24	25	26	27	28	29	30	31	32	33	34	35
Height (Inches)							Body Weight (pounds)										
58	91	96	100	105	110	115	119	124	129	134	138	143	148	153	158	162	167
59	94	99	104	109	114	119	124	128	133	138	143	148	153	158	163	168	173
60	97	102	107	112	118	123	128	133	138	143	148	153	158	163	168	174	179
61	100	106	111	116	122	127	132	137	143	148	153	158	164	169	174	180	185
62	104	109	115	120	126	131	136	142	147	153	158	164	169	175	180	186	191
63	107	113	118	124	130	135	141	146	152	158	163	169	175	180	186	191	197
64	110	116	122	128	134	140	145	151	157	163	169	174	180	186	192	197	204
65	114	120	126	132	138	144	150	156	162	168	174	180	186	192	198	204	210
66	118	124	130	136	142	148	155	161	167	173	179	186	192	198	204	210	216
67	121	127	134	140	146	153	159	166	172	178	185	191	198	204	211	217	223
68	125	131	138	144	151	158	164	171	177	184	190	197	203	210	216	223	230
69	128	135	142	149	155	162	169	176	182	189	196	203	209	216	223	230	236
70	132	139	146	153	160	167	174	181	188	195	202	209	216	222	229	236	243
71	136	143	150	157	165	172	179	186	193	200	208	215	222	229	236	243	250
72	140	147	154	162	169	177	184	191	199	206	213	221	228	235	242	250	258
73	144	151	159	166	174	182	189	197	204	212	219	227	235	242	250	257	265
74	148	155	163	171	179	186	194	202	210	218	225	233	241	249	256	264	272
75	152	160	168	176	184	192	200	208	216	224	232	240	248	256	264	272	279
76	156	164	172	180	189	197	205	213	221	230	238	246	254	263	271	279	287

cardiovascular disease. This may confirm earlier observations that seem to suggest that elevated postprandial glucose levels (levels taken after a meal) are a better predictor of the development of coronary heart disease than the level of the fasting glucose.

The Diabetes Prevention Program of over 3,000 patients with impaired glucose tolerance (68 percent female) showed that 150 minutes of exercise per week and 5–7 percent weight loss led to a 58 percent decrease in the numbers of subjects who progressed to overt Type 2 diabetes. The group treated with METFORMIN (Glucophage) had a 33 percent decrease in the risk of progression.

Medical Issues That Increase the Risk for Diabetes

Some medical issues increase the risk of the development (or current presence) of diabetes, such as obesity (for Type 2 diabetes), a family medical history and thus a genetic risk for diabetes, and the presence of high blood pressure (HYPERTENSION). In addition, smokers have an increased risk for developing diabetes.

Obesity Obesity is a major cause of Type 2 diabetes, and in the early stages of the disease, weight loss can bring remission. Unfortunately, many people who are overweight or obese have a significant problem with either losing weight or maintaining a weight loss. For this reason,

Obese				Extreme Obesity														
36	37	38	39	40	41	42	43	44	45	46	47	48	49	50	51	52	53	54
172	177	181	186	191	196	201	205	210	215	220	224	229	234	239	244	248	253	258
178	183	188	193	198	203	208	212	217	222	227	232	237	242	247	252	257	262	267
184	189	194	199	204	209	215	220	225	230	235	240	245	250	255	261	266	271	276
190	195	201	206	211	217	222	227	232	238	243	248	254	259	264	269	275	280	285
196	202	207	213	218	224	229	235	240	246	251	256	262	267	273	278	284	289	295
203	208	214	220	225	231	237	242	248	254	259	265	270	278	282	287	293	299	304
209	215	221	227	232	238	244	250	256	262	267	273	279	285	291	296	302	308	314
216	222	228	234	240	246	252	258	264	270	276	282	288	294	300	306	312	318	324
223	229	235	241	247	253	260	266	272	278	284	291	297	303	309	315	322	328	334
230	236	242	249	255	261	268	274	280	287	293	299	306	312	319	325	331	338	344
236	243	249	256	262	269	276	282	289	295	302	308	315	322	328	335	341	348	354
243	250	257	263	270	277	284	291	297	304	311	318	324	331	338	345	351	358	365
250	257	264	271	278	285	292	299	306	313	320	327	334	341	348	355	362	369	376
257	265	272	279	286	293	301	308	315	322	329	338	343	351	358	365	372	379	386
265	272	279	287	294	302	309	316	324	331	338	346	353	361	368	375	383	390	397
272	280	288	295	302	310	318	325	333	340	348	355	363	371	378	386	393	401	408
280	287	295	303	311	319	326	334	342	350	358	365	373	381	389	396	404	412	420
287	295	303	311	319	327	335	343	351	359	367	375	383	391	399	407	415	423	431
295	304	312	320	328	336	344	353	361	369	377	385	394	402	410	418	426	435	443

increasing numbers of experts are recommending that BARIATRIC SURGERY (weight loss surgery, also known as metabolic surgery) be considered for some obese individuals. Prior to the surgery, individuals should be thoroughly screened for health and psychiatric issues that could present complications.

Family medical history and genetic risks A family medical history is a strong risk factor for the development of diabetes. In addition, if an individual is obese and hypertensive and also has a family history of Type 2 diabetes, this person is at risk for the development of diabetes too, particularly if he or she is older than age 40.

Hypertension High blood pressure is frequently associated with diabetes, and it increases the risk for cardiovascular disease and kidney disease and kidney failure. Hypertension should be kept as close to normal as possible with medications and with lifestyle changes, such as weight loss, a minimal (or no) consumption of alcohol, and no smoking.

Treatment of Diabetes: Type 1

Type 1 diabetes is treated with INSULIN, LIFESTYLE ADAPTATIONS, and careful meal planning, as with carbohydrate counting and with careful attention to nutrition. (*See* CARBOHYDRATES AND MEAL PLANNING.) It is also important for the individual

TABLE 5: SUMMARY OF DIAGNOSTIC TEST CHARACTERISTICS FOR NONPREGNANT ADULTS

Test	Pros	Cons	Recommendations for Use	Use in Screening
Urinary glucose	Does not require blood sample; rapid Processing time; inexpensive	Unable to measure glucose above the renal threshold; not fully quantitative	Not recommended	Not recommended
FPG	Single plasma glucose level; highly correlated with presence of complications; inexpensive	Patient must be fasting; potential for processing error; point measurement can be affected by short-term term lifestyle changes	Diabetes diagnosis with FPG ≥ 126 mg/dL; prediabetes diagnosis with FPG 100–126 mg/dL	Informal recommendation for follow-up testing with FPG≥100 mg/dL
RPG	Single glucose level; component of routine lab testing; inexpensive	Potential for processing error; point measurement can be affected by multiple factors (time since prior meal, short-term lifestyle changes, etc.)	Diabetes diagnosis with RPG ≥ 200 mg/dL and symptoms of polyuria, polydipsia, and unin-tentional weight loss	Informal recommendation for follow-up test with RPG ≥ 130
OGTT	Most sensitive test for impaired glucose tolerance (IGT)	Impractical in clinical setting, lower reproducibility than other diagnostic tests	Diagnosis of IGT with 2-hour hour plasma glucose ≥ 200 mg/dL	Diagnostic criteria apply
Capillary glucose	Rapid test; does not require phlebotomy	Not standardized	Not recommended for diagnostic testing	Confirm any hyperglycemia with central laboratory glucose level of A1C
A1C	Gold standard for measuring glucose control; easy to obtain; does not require fasting; point-of-care testing available	Potential for nonglycemic causes of error; insensitive for IGT	A1C ≥ 6.5% diagnostic for diabetes; should be confirmed with a second A1C	High-risk group with A1C ≥ 6.0% and <6% and other risk factors are still eligible for preventive measures

Source: Cox, Mary E., M.D., and David Edelman, M.D. "Tests for Screening and Diagnosis of Type 2 Diabetes." *Clinical Diabetes* 27, no. 4 (2009): 134. © 2009 American Diabetes Association. From *Clinical Diabetes*. Vol. 27 (2009) pp. 132–138. Reprinted with permission from the American Diabetes Association.

to test his or her blood sugar level at least once each day, depending on the schedule provided by the physician, and to act on the information that the blood test provides; for example, if the blood sugar is high, then the individual needs to adjust carbohydrate intake for the rest of the day as well as adjusting his or her insulin dosing appropriately. If the blood sugar is low, then the individual needs to consume carbohydrates to bring glucose levels up to normal.

Individuals with Type 1 diabetes require careful monitoring to try to reduce the risk of complications.

Treatment of Diabetes: Type 2

Type 2 diabetes is treated with oral medications and sometimes with insulin as well, particularly in older individuals with long-term diabetes. In general, metformin (Glucophage, Glucophage XL) is the first-line oral medication that is used to treat Type 2 diabetes. Other medications may also need to be added to boost the effect of metformin.

A study reported in 2009 confirmed earlier research in the United States on metformin as the best initial treatment for Type 2 diabetes. In this study, reported in the *British Medical Journal,* the researchers analyzed results among more than 91,000 patients for the period 1990–2005. They found that oral sulfonylurea medications were not as effective at controlling diabetes as was metformin. In addition, they analyzed whether rosiglitazone (Avandia) had a worse outcome than metformin in terms of cardiovascular outcomes, but did not find it to be worse. The researchers said, however, that "pioglitazone [Actos] was associated with reduced all cause mortality compared with metformin and it had a favourable risk profile compared with rosiglitazone, which requires replication in other studies."

Meal planning and nutrition is also very important in the treatment of Type 2 diabetes. Many people with Type 2 diabetes are overweight or obese, and weight loss is an important component of improved health. Good meal planning will help keep the blood glucose level close to normal, and the person with diabetes should keep their blood glucose level as close to normal as possible to significantly decrease the risk of complications.

Daily testing of the blood on a schedule recommended by the physician is an important part of managing Type 2 diabetes.

General Treatment Goals

Whether the person has Type 1 or Type 2 diabetes, there are some basic treatment goals. For example, according to the NIDDK, the goal for the blood glucose before meals (the preprandial plasma glucose) is to stay within the range of 90–130 mg/dL. The goal for one to two hours after the start of eating a meal (the peak postprandial) is less than 180 mg/dL.

The HgbA1c is another important test, formerly known as the hemoglobin HgbA1c test. This blood test is taken by a laboratory and measures the average blood glucose over the course of 3 months. The goal for most people is an HgbA1c of less than 7 percent. An HgbA1c of 7 is equivalent to an average blood glucose level of 150 mg/dL.

Some factors can make the blood glucose levels go up or down; for example, exercising

TABLE 6: COMMON FACTORS THAT CAN MAKE GLUCOSE LEVELS RISE OR FALL

Reasons Blood Glucose Levels Rise	• Eating a meal or snack
	• Eating more food or more carbohydrates than usual
	• Being physically inactive
	• Having an infection, surgery, injury, or being ill
	• Being under stress
	• Having changes in hormonal levels, such as during times before a women's menstrual cycle
	• Taking too little diabetes medications or not taking the medicine
Reasons Blood Glucose Levels Fall	• Missing or delaying a meal or snack
	• Eating less food or fewer carbohydrates than usual
	• Being physically active
	• Drinking alcoholic beverages, especially on an empty stomach
	• Having changes in hormone levels, such as during menstruation
	• Taking some medications (side effects)
	• Taking too much diabetes medication

Adapted from Office on Women's Health. *The Healthy Woman: A Complete Guide for All Ages*, p. 76. Washington, D.C.: U.S. Department of Health and Human Services.

generally drives the glucose levels down, and as a result, the individual may need to eat a snack to compensate for lower glucose levels. Severe stress, on the other hand, may make the glucose levels go up. See Table 6 for some key factors which may make blood glucose levels go up or down.

Complications of Diabetes

There are many possible complications of diabetes, some acute and many chronic, including kidney disease (diabetic nephropathy) and kidney failure; diabetic ketoacidosis, or an extreme and dangerously high level of blood sugar (hyperosmolar state); diabetic neuropathy (nerve damage), which can lead to the need for the AMPUTATION of limbs; hypoglycemia, which is a severely low level of blood sugar; diabetic eye diseases, particularly DIABETIC RETINOPATHY, which can lead to BLINDNESS if it is not diagnosed and treated. Diabetic retinopathy causes from 12,000 to 24,000 new cases of blindness each year, according to the NIDDK. Diabetes is also the leading cause of blindness among all individuals age 20 to 74 years old.

Diabetic nephropathy Kidney disease that is caused by diabetes is very common, and in fact, diabetes is the number one cause of END-STAGE RENAL DISEASE (ESRD), or kidney failure that results over the long-term from chronic kidney disease. According to the National Center for Health Statistics, in 2005, there were 152.8 people per million people in the United States with diabetes and ESRD. The next highest rate was for those with hypertension, or 95.4 individuals per million population.

If the individual has both diabetes and hypertension (as many people do), then the risk for kidney disease is accelerated even further. Diabetes is a major problem in the United States, and according to the United States Renal Data System (USRDS), in comparison to many other countries, the United States has the third highest rate of kidney failure that is caused by diabetes. (See Appendix VIII for country-by-country information.)

The presence of kidney disease is also a predictor for a poor outcome with diabetic foot ulcers, according to Edouard Ghanassia, M.D., and colleagues in their 2008 article for *Diabetes Care.* The researchers analyzed 80 subjects who were hospitalized for diabetic foot ulcers, and they found that although the ulcers for which the patients with kidney disease were hospitalized did heal, the long-term outcome over six and a half years was poor, and about 60 percent reexperienced foot ulcers. Nearly half of the subjects (43.8 percent) had to have a limb amputated at a subsequent date.

According to Erika B. Rangel and colleagues in their 2009 article on kidney transplants in diabetic patients in *Diabetology & Metabolic Syndrome,* diabetics who receive kidney transplants have a higher survival rate than diabetics continuing dialysis therapy for kidney failure; however, individuals with diabetes have a higher rate of infectious complications and cardiovascular events than nondiabetic transplant patients.

One reason for the lower survival rate among diabetic transplant patients is that these patients are generally older than are the nondiabetic transplant patients; they also usually have a higher body mass index (BMI) and are more likely to be obese than the other transplant patients.

Diabetic ketoacidosis Diabetic ketoacidosis (DKA) is a serious complication of diabetes that occurs when the body has inadequate insulin activity and as a result, draws its energy from fat stores instead. The breakdown of these fats causes an accumulation of acids that are very deleterious to all organs and furthers the dehydration being caused by the high glucose levels. These dangerously high glucose levels and acids can quickly lead to a state of medical emergency. Up to 40 percent of individuals who are diagnosed with Type 1 diabetes were first admitted to the hospital and subsequently diagnosed with DKA. DKA can also develop in individuals with Type 2 diabetes.

Diabetic neuropathy Nerve damage caused by diabetes is common among individuals with diabetes, and the outcomes can be very serious; for example, if the diabetic person loses feeling in the feet and then steps on a sharp object, then he or she feels nothing, and this injury can cause serious damage to the foot over time. For this reason, doctors recommend that people with diabetes check their feet every day for injuries or lacerations, even if they still retain some feeling in their feet. Physicians should also check the feet of diabetic patients at every patient encounter.

Hypoglycemia Hypoglycemia is an unusually low level of blood glucose, and it can become a life-threatening emergency situation. Some individuals suffer from HYPOGLYCEMIC UNAWARENESS, which means that they have no warning signs that their blood sugar is dropping, such as feeling fatigued or ill. People with this problem should be sure to wear emergency medical identification with information on the hypoglycemia, the doctor's name, and the person to contact in an emergency.

Sometimes hypoglycemia is misconstrued as drunkenness by others because the person may stagger and behave in a confused manner, even though their blood alcohol level would register as zero. This is yet another reason for individuals with diabetes to wear an emergency identification bracelet.

Diabetic eye diseases   Diabetic retinopathy is a very common diabetic eye disease, but individuals with diabetes also have an elevated risk for CATARACTS, GLAUCOMA, and MACULAR EDEMA. The best defense against diabetic eye disease is an annual eye examination. Experts disagree on whether it is best to see an ophthalmologist or an optometrist, but what is most important is that the eye examination occurs once every year.

Other complications   Diabetes can affect every system of the body, so it is not surprising that the disease can be harmful to disparate areas. For example, diabetes can cause a slowing of digestion which is known as GASTROPARESIS DIA-BETICORUM. It can also lead to disorders of the skin and to an increased risk for some infections, such as thrush (a yeast infection), VAGINITIS, and dental infections of the gum.

People with diabetes are also at risk for some anatomic abnormalities; for example, CHARCOT'S ARTHROPATHY is a malformation of the foot that is caused by diabetes. Many people with diabetes need to wear special shoes that are prescribed by a podiatrist (and which may be covered by Medi-care or Medicaid, depending on many different variables). Individuals with diabetes also have an increased risk for developing carpal tunnel syndrome, a compression of the median nerve.

It is also true that many individuals with diabetes may suffer from DEPRESSION. Whether the depression develops from their concerns and fears related to diabetes and its treatment or is an independent issue is often difficult to determine, and often it is a combined issue. It is important for individuals with diabetes and depression to have the depression treated. Untreated diabetics with depression are less likely to take their diabetes medications and perform needed actions to manage their disease, thus increasing the risk for developing complications. There are many different antidepressants used to treat depression, and many primary care doctors treat this disorder, although a psychiatrist is an expert who is the most knowledgeable about treating depression.

Note that most psychiatrists do not treat severely mentally ill people, such as those with schizophrenia, but instead treat average individuals who have problems with depression and other disorders. Thus, there should be no shame or embarrassment related to seeing a psychiatrist; it does not mean that the person is "crazy."

Imaging to detect diabetic complications   According to Elizabeth Church in her article in *Radiologic Technology* in 2009, there are many important complications that are related to diabetes and which imaging tests may reveal, such as problems that the diabetic person has with the bones and eyes. For example, ultrasound studies have revealed that middle-aged pre-menopausal women with Type 1 diabetes have a lower bone mineral density than nondiabetic women. In addition, a study in Taiwan showed that both males and females with diabetes have an elevated risk for hip fracture.

Individuals with diabetes also have a greater risk for complications associated with hip- and knee-replacement surgery, although patients with Type 2 diabetes generally fare better than do patients with Type 1 diabetes, according to Church. Research has also shown that bone infections (osteomyelitis) are more common among people with diabetes.

Ultrasound is a safe technique to image the kidneys and the remainder of the urogenital tract in assessing possible diabetic nephropathy. Doppler ultrasound is often the first test used to assess the vascular system for adequacy of the circulation, especially the carotid, and femoral arteries as well as the aorta. Cardiac echo (ultrasound) is used to determine if the heart and its valves are structurally sound and can determine if the muscle itself is pumping effectively.

With regard to eye damage caused by diabetes, some experts believe that the imaging of the eyes of diabetic patients (fluorescein angiogram) to detect early retinal changes can provide important information for risks of other microvascular diabetic complications.

Risk factors for and preventive measures against complications of diabetes Some lifestyle choices as well as some health factors increase the risk for the development of complications from diabetes, including such health factors as current smoking, overweight or obesity, physical inactivity, hypertension, and a high blood cholesterol. According to the Centers for Disease Control and Prevention (CDC), an estimated 15.5 percent of adults with diabetes in the United States in 2007 were smokers, and 38.2 percent of this group were also physically inactive.

A broad majority of these individuals were overweight (83.5 percent) and more than half of adult diabetics in the United States were obese (51.1 percent). Nearly two-thirds (62.6 percent) had high levels of blood cholesterol (See Table 7). All of these factors, either alone or taken together, increase the risk for diabetic complications.

Preventing complications There are basic measures that every person with diabetes should take to decrease the risk of suffering

TABLE 7: PERCENTAGE OF RISK FACTORS FOR COMPLICATIONS AMONG ADULTS WITH DIABETES, UNITED STATES, 2007

Risk Factor	Percent
Current smoking	15.5
Physical inactivity	38.2
Overweight	83.5
Obesity	51.1
Hypertension	67.0
High blood cholesterol	62.6

Adapted from Centers for Disease Control and Prevention. "Percentage of Risk Factors for Complications Among Adults with Diabetes, United States." Available online. URL: http://www.cc.gov/diabetes/statistics/comp/fig10.htm. Accessed November 9, 2009.

from the distressing and often painful complications of diabetes, such as having an annual dilated eye examination; seeing the doctor at least once each year (preferably two to four times per year); monitoring their blood glucose each day and acting on its findings; having at least an annual foot examination by the physician as well as examining the feet oneself each day; having two or more HgbA1c blood tests each year (blood tests that show blood levels for a three-month period); having an annual influenza shot and having ever had a pneumonia vaccine; and attending a diabetes self-management class.

The majority of adults with diabetes in 2007 performed these tasks, although the rates were a low majority for the completion of some tasks, such as having had a pneumonia vaccine (51.7 percent) or having attended a diabetes self-management class (55.4 percent). Higher rates of performance of these tasks would translate into lower rates of diabetic complications. See Table 8 on page 123 for the percentage of adults with diabetes in 2007 who performed these important preventive tasks.

Diabetes and Women and Men

Both men and women with diabetes face an increased risk for complications from diabetes, but some risks are gender-specific. For example, WOMEN WITH DIABETES may suffer from frequent URINARY TRACT INFECTIONS (cystitis) and from vaginal yeast infections. They may also experience sexual dysfunctions, such as a diminished sexual desire and difficulty achieving orgasm, and they may experience pain during intercourse. Pregnancy can be especially challenging for the woman with diabetes, as discussed in the next section.

MEN WITH DIABETES may experience problems with erectile dysfunction, and some may experience problems with fertility as well because of a lower level of testosterone. Men also have a higher risk than women of developing diabetic retinopathy and of suffering from lower extremity amputations.

TABLE 8: PERCENTAGE OF PREVENTIVE CARE PRACTICES FOR ADULTS AGES 18 AND OLDER WITH DIABETES, UNITED STATES, 2007

Preventive Care Practice	Percent
Annual dilated eye examination	71.7
Daily self-monitoring of blood glucose	63.2
Annual foot examination	70.2
Annual doctor visit	87.6
Daily self-examination of feet	67.9
Had two or more HgbA1c tests in last year	73.7
Attended diabetes self-management class	55.4
Annual influenza vaccine	60.9
Ever had pneumococcal vaccine	51.7

Adapted from Centers for Disease Control and Prevention. "Percentage of Preventive Care Practices for Adults Ages 18 and Older with Diabetes, United States, 2007." Available online. URL: http://www.cdc.gov/diabetes/statistics/preventive/fAllPractices.htm. Accessed November 9, 2009.

Special Populations

Diabetes is not easy for anyone with this disease, but some groups have a particularly difficult time with diabetes, such as ADOLESCENTS WITH DIABETES, CHILDREN WITH DIABETES, the ELDERLY, and pregnant women with diabetes or gestational diabetes.

Children and adolescents with diabetes   Most adolescents with diabetes have Type 1 diabetes but whether they have Type 1 or Type 2 diabetes, they may be embarrassed by their illness and try to hide it from others, including fellow students and teachers. Unfortunately, diabetes is a disease that, if not managed, crops its head up with symptoms and problems, and as a result, teenagers who fail to manage their diabetes may develop serious complications from failing to test their blood and failing to watch their diet. The NDEP also notes that overweight children and teens may develop a hybrid form of diabetes, including the features of the insulin resistance that is associated with obesity and Type 2 diabetes as well as the autoimmunity and antibodies against their own pancreatic islet cells that is associated with Type 1 diabetes. As a result, treatment may include both insulin and glucose-lowering medications.

Another important factor to consider in children and adolescents is that they are growing and changing, and their glucose needs may vary with life stages as well; for example, in mid to late puberty, some experts say that adolescents may experience a decreased insulin sensitivity, which basically means that the hormones that are involved in growth and development (growth hormone, estrogen, testosterone, cortisol, and so forth) actually act against insulin, that is, they increase the body's resistance to the effects of insulin and push glucose levels higher.

The elderly   Older individuals are more likely to develop Type 2 diabetes than younger individuals or to face increasing problems with already-existing diabetes. It is estimated that at least 20 percent of all older adults have diabetes, and with this disease comes an elevated risk for cardiovascular disease, hypertension, coronary heart disease, and stroke, as well as kidney disease and kidney failure. However, some research shows that, even among older individuals, lifestyle factors affect the development of new-onset diabetes. Note that older people need not be obese to have Type 2 diabetes.

For example, in a study reported by Dariush Mozaffarian, M.D., and colleagues in a 2009 issue of the *Archives of Internal Medicine,* the researchers found that lifestyle factors directly corresponded with the development or the lack of development of diabetes among 4,883 men and women ages 65 years and older. The subjects who were in the "low-risk group" because of their active physical activity level, good nutritional diet, lack of smoking, and lack of or limited drinking had an 82 percent lower incidence of diabetes. The researchers said, "Even later in life, combined lifestyle factors are associated with a markedly lower incidence of new-onset diabetes mellitus."

They also added, "In this large, prospective cohort study of older US adults, lifestyle factors including physical activity level, dietary habits, smoking habits, alcohol use, and adiposity measures, assessed late in life, were each independently associated with risk of new-onset diabetes. In combination, these basic lifestyle risk factors strongly predicted diabetes incidence, with an approximately 50% lower risk with only physical activity level and dietary habits in the low-risk group and an approximately 80% lower risk with physical activity level, dietary habits, smoking habits, and alcohol use in the low-risk group. In sum, 8 in 10 cases of diabetes in this population of older adults appeared attributable to these 4 lifestyle factors, suggesting that, if these associations are causal, 8 in 10 new cases of diabetes might have been prevented if all older adults were in the low-risk group for these lifestyle factors."

Pregnant women and women of childbearing Age Women with diabetes who wish to bear children need special monitoring, preferably monitoring that occurs well before the conception of their children, because maximally good health prior to the conception also improves the odds of having a healthy infant. Women with diabetes who have unplanned pregnancies are at an increased risk for having problem pregnancies and for fetal abnormalities.

GESTATIONAL DIABETES MELLITUS, or diabetes that occurs only during pregnancy, also needs to be carefully monitored. Each subsequent pregnancy should also be carefully planned and monitored by physicians. Even if the woman never has another pregnancy, she is still at an elevated risk for developing Type 2 diabetes in the future. See Table 9

TABLE 9: RECOMMENDATIONS FOR WOMEN WITH A HISTORY OF GESTATIONAL DIABETES

Time	Test
Post-delivery (1–3 days)	Fasting or random plasma glucose (PG)
6 to 12 weeks postpartum	2-hour PG post 75g glucose challenge
1 year postpartum	2-hour PG post 75g glucose challenge
Annually	Fasting PG
Every 3 years and before another pregnancy	2-hour PG post 75g glucose challenge

Source: National Diabetes Education Program. *Guiding Principles for Diabetes Care: For Health Care Professionals*, p. 4. Bethesda, Md.: National Institutes of Health.

for the testing recommendations for women who have a history of gestational diabetes.

Most physicians strongly recommend that diabetic mothers use BREAST-FEEDING to provide nutrition to their infants. In fact, in a 2008 issue of *Diabetes Care*, researchers Elizabeth J. Mayer-Davis and colleagues found that breast-feeding provides an apparent protective factor against the development of Type 2 diabetes in youths born to women with diabetes, based on a study of mothers and youths who were African Americans, Hispanics, and non-Hispanic whites.

See also PREGNANCY.

Bang, Heejung, et al. "Development and Validation of a Patient Self-assessment Score for Diabetes Risk." *Annals of Internal Medicine* 151 (2009): 775–783.

Church, Elizabeth. "Imaging Diabetes." *Radiologic Technology* 80, no. 4 (2009): 340–360.

Ghanassia, Edouard, M.D., et al. "Long-Term Outcome and Disability of Diabetic Patients Hospitalized for Diabetic Foot Ulcers." *Diabetes Care* 31, no. 7 (2008): 1,288–1,292.

Huang, Elbert S., M.D., et al. "Projecting the Future Diabetes Population Size and Related Costs for the U.S." *Diabetes Care* 32, no. 12 (2009): 2,225–2,229.

Mayer-Davis, Elizabeth J., et al. "Breast-Feeding and Type 2 Diabetes in the Youth of Three Ethnic Groups." *Diabetes Care* 31, no. 3 (2008): 470–475.

Mozaffarian, Dariush, M.D., et al. "Lifestyle Risk Factors and New-Onset Diabetes Mellitus in Older Adults: The Cardiovascular Health Study." *Archives of Internal Medicine* 169, no. 8 (2009): 798–807.

National Diabetes Education Program. *Guiding Principles for Diabetes Care: For Health Care Professionals.* Bethesda, Md.: National Institutes of Health, 2009.

Rangel, Erika B., et al. "Kidney Transplant in Diabetic Patients: Modalities, Indications and Results." *Diabetology & Metabolic Syndrome* 1 (2009). Available online. URL: http://www.dmsjournal.com/content/pdf/1758-5996-1-2.pdf. Accessed August 28, 2010.

Tzoulaki, Ioanna, et al. "Risk of Cardiovascular Disease and All Cause Mortality among Patients with Type 2 Diabetes Prescribed Oral Antidiabetes Drugs: Retrospective Cohort Study Using UK General Practice Research Database." *British Medical Journal* 2009. Available online. URL: http://www.bmj.com/content/339/bmj.b4731.full.pdf. Accessed August 28, 2010.

Diabetes Prevention Trials   Refers to two large clinical trials launched by the National Institutes of Health in the 1990s including the Diabetes Prevention Trial for Type 1 Diabetes (DPT-1) and the Diabetes Prevention Program (DPP) for people with Type 2 diabetes. The DPT-1 is an ongoing study and the DPP ended in 2001. The purpose of these studies was to screen people who are at high risk for developing either Type 1 or Type 2 diabetes, to provide treatments, and to determine which approach is most effective at preventing the development of diabetes.

The DPT-1 Study

The purpose of this study is to screen for autoimmune abnormalities that predispose people to developing Type 1 diabetes. In the North American and Puerto Rican sites of the DPT-1 study, nondiabetic relatives of patients with Type 1 diabetes were recruited from nine centers. Eligible subjects were required to have impaired first phase insulin response (which means that they did not secrete insulin appropriately), a pre-diabetic condition, and also to have islet cell antibodies with a normal or impaired glucose tolerance test. These individuals are anticipated to have a 50 percent chance of developing Type 1 diabetes within five years.

In this phase, 89,827 relatives were screened. About 4 percent tested positive for islet cell antibodies. Of these, 338 were enrolled in the study, including 169 to the therapy group and 169 to the control group, which will be observed only.

Subjects in the treatment group receive insulin intravenously for four days each year and also receive ultralente insulin twice each day. They receive oral glucose tolerance tests every six months.

Preliminary results for this study have shown that there are risk factors for the rapid development of Type 1 diabetes, including

- younger age
- positive blood tests for more than one islet cell antibody
- a history of impaired glucose tolerance (IGT)

The subjects are closely followed. Individuals whose laboratory tests show that they have antibodies to insulin but their insulin levels are still in the normal range are treated with oral medications. Preliminary results have shown that small doses of insulin do not appear to prevent the development of Type 1 diabetes in susceptible individuals.

The DPP

Individuals who were at risk for developing Type 2 diabetes were the volunteers for the DPP, including women who have had GESTATIONAL DIABETES, members of ethnic groups with high rates of diabetes, people with a family member who has Type 2 diabetes, and others. Individuals are tested to determine if they have abnormal glucose levels but have not yet developed diabetes. Those who don't have diabetes are placed into one of three groups and followed up.

One group provided members with lifestyle recommendations and a placebo (sugar pill). The second group was given an even more intensive lifestyle management program that emphasized exercise and a personal trainer. The third group received an oral antidiabetic medication, either a sulfonylurea drug or metformin. The goal was to determine which of these three approaches is most effective at prevention.

The DPP ended in 2001 and Allan Spiegel, director of the National Institute of Diabetes and Digestive and Kidney Diseases (NIDDK) said that its results offered hope to an estimated 10 million Americans who were not diabetic but were "perilously close to the brink."

The study found that a relatively small weight loss of 10 to 15 pounds, accompanied by exercise for 30 minutes each day, enabled the subjects to reduce their risk for developing diabetes by a dramatic 58 percent. The study also found that metformin taken twice a day reduced the risk of developing diabetes by nearly one-third (31 percent). The drug worked best in obese and younger individuals ages 25–44.

diabetic eye diseases Illnesses that occur to one or both eyes of individuals with either Type 1 or Type 2 diabetes. Diabetics are more likely than others to develop eye diseases such as CATARACTS, DIABETIC RETINOPATHY, GLAUCOMA, and MACULAR EDEMA. If undiagnosed and untreated, eye diseases that stem from diabetes can eventually lead to BLINDNESS, although annual checkups can usually detect problems in the early stages of disease, when still treatable. In those cases, effective treatment can often be initiated well before the complete loss of eyesight.

The number of individuals with diabetic eye diseases is expected to increase, largely because of greater numbers of obese baby boomers (born 1946–64) with Type 2 diabetes. However, if these individuals receive annual eye examinations, then their risk for worsening eye disease or for blindness will be significantly averted.

When to Start Annual Eye Examinations

People recently diagnosed with Type 1 diabetes are advised to have their first annual eye examination within three to five years of diagnosis; however, people with Type 2 diabetes should have an eye examination concurrent with or soon after their diagnosis. The reasons behind these recommendations are that most people with Type 1 diabetes are diagnosed early on in their disease because of severe symptoms that are difficult to miss; however, people with Type 2 diabetes may not be diagnosed for years after the onset of their disease. As a result, individuals with Type 2 diabetes may have serious eye disease that has gone undiagnosed.

Cataracts

A cataract is a clouding of the lens of the eye, and it is often related to aging. An estimated half of all individuals in the United States ages 80 years and older (with or without diabetes) will develop cataracts or have already had cataract surgery; however, individuals with diabetes have an increased risk for developing cataracts. Other risk factors for the development of cataracts, according to the National Eye Institute, include SMOKING and alcohol use, as well as prolonged exposure to sunlight and steroid exposure.

Unlike some other serious eye diseases, cataracts often do have symptoms, such as having blurred or cloudy vision or viewing faded colors. In addition, it may appear that a halo surrounds headlights or lamps that a person with cataracts views. The person with cataracts also has poor night vision and may experience double vision. Frequent changes in the prescriptions for glasses or contact lenses are also common.

Cataracts are diagnosed with a visual acuity examination as well as a dilated eye examination. In addition, the pressure inside the eye is measured with tonometry.

Antiglare sunglasses may improve the symptoms that are associated with cataracts, as may the use of bright lights or magnifying glasses; however, eventually, many people with cataracts will need surgery. The surgeon will replace the clouded lens with a clear artificial lens. One benefit is that the individual may no longer need glasses or contact lenses because the cataract replacement will provide normal vision.

Cataract surgery The two types of cataract surgery are *phacoemulsification* and *extracapsular surgery.* With phacoemulsification, the doctor makes a tiny cut on the side of the cornea, and inserts a probe into the eye which breaks up the lens, which can then be removed with suction. Most surgery for cataracts in the United States is performed with phacoemulsification, also known as *small incision cataract surgery.*

With extracapsular surgery, the doctor makes a longer cut on the side of the cornea and removes the cloudy part of the lens as one piece. The remainder of the lens is then removed with suction.

The new lens is inserted into the eye with both types of surgery. The new lens is referred to as an *intraocular lens* (IOL).

According to Jinan B. Saaddine, M.D., and colleagues in their 2008 article for *Archives of Ophthalmology,* about 3 million people with diabetes had cataracts in 2005, and this number was projected to more than double to 6.2 million individuals by 2020 and to further increase to nearly 9 million people by 2030. In terms of numbers alone, white women ages 75 years and older had the greatest number of cases of cataracts in 2005, followed by white men, black women, and then black men.

Diabetic Macular Edema

Diabetic macular edema is considered by some to be a subset of diabetic retinopathy, while others regard it as a separate disease. It results from the leaking of blood from the retina and it is a leading cause of blindness among individuals with diabetes. This condition leads to swelling and blurred vision, and it also often leads to blindness, if untreated. About half of those individuals with the proliferative retinopathy (Stage 4) of diabetic retinopathy will also have diabetic macular edema.

Diabetic macular edema is diagnosed with a visual acuity test and a dilated eye examination. If present, this disorder is treated with laser surgery. If the individual has a great deal of blood in the eye, the physician may perform a vitrectomy to remove the fluid that is clouded by blood. This condition may also occur with diabetic retinopathy.

Treatment of diabetic macular edema Diabetic macular edema is treated with laser surgery. Some patients in whom laser surgery has failed have been treated with injections of an anti-cancer drug known as bevacizumab (Avastin). The results were promising, although large-scale clinical trials are needed before such a treatment can become accepted as standard.

An increased risk with some diabetes drugs Some research has indicated that the use of medications in the glitazone category of diabetes drugs can lead to an increased risk for the development of diabetic macular edema. Researchers D. S. Fong and R. Contreras analyzed the results of about 170,000 subjects with diabetes and compared their use of glitazone drugs, particularly rosiglitazone (Avandia), and looked at their subsequent diagnosis of diabetic macular edema. They reported in a 2009 issue of the *American Journal of Ophthalmology* that they found an elevated risk for macular edema in this population.

According to a report by Claire Kendall in the *Canadian Medical Association Journal* in 2006, those patients taking rosiglitazone who seem to be most at risk for macular edema are those using insulin or who have kidney insufficiency or heart disease. These patients also often have fluid retention, weight gain, or peripheral edema.

Medications that may improve diabetic macular edema In one very small (four subjects) study of patients with diabetic macular edema, Hibba Soomro, Lesley Burnett, and Nigel Davies reported in the *British Journal of Diabetes and Vascular Disease* in 2007 that patients who began taking or who increased their dosage of statin medications for dyslipidemia showed an improved reduction in their retinal thickness as well as their vision. Said the authors, "Ultimately the control of diabetic dyslipidaemia could become a powerful addition to the management options available to prevent this sight-threatening disease."

Diabetic Retinopathy

Diabetic retinopathy causes an estimated 12,000 to 14,000 people with diabetes to develop blindness every year. It is the number one cause of blindness among people of working age. According to the National Eye Institute, up to 45 percent of individuals who are diagnosed with diabetes in the United States have developed one of the four stages of diabetic retinopathy. Over time, high blood sugar levels cause the blood vessels within the eye to leak, become blocked or to break down. New abnormal vessels may develop, and these vessels are very fragile and easily broken.

According to the National Diabetes Education Program (NDEP), one in 12 diabetics age 40 years and older in the United States is at risk for the development of diabetic retinopathy. Diabetic retinopathy is often highly treatable, once identified; yet disturbingly, the NDEP says that only about half of individuals with diabetes have their eyes examined or have an examination in time for treatment to work. This is particularly disturbing since the NDEP also says that early detection and treatment can prevent or delay blindness in 90 percent of those with diabetes.

Diabetic retinopathy is on the increase According to Jinan B. Saaddine, M.D., and colleagues in their 2008 article for *Archives of Ophthalmology,* in 2005, 5.5 million Americans age 40 years and older had diabetic retinopathy, and 1.2 million people had vision-threatening diabetic retinopathy, or diabetic retinopathy that is likely to lead to blindness if not treated. The disease is more prominent among adults age 65 years and older; for example, 2.5 million adults, or about half of all adults with diabetic retinopathy in 2005, were older Americans, and 0.5 million with vision-threatening diabetic retinopathy were elderly.

Stages of diabetic retinopathy There are four stages of diabetic retinopathy, including Stage 1, which is mild nonproliferative retinopathy; Stage 2, which is moderate nonproliferative retinopathy; stage 3, which is severe nonproliferative retinopathy; and Stage 4, which is proliferative retinopathy. With Stage 1, tiny microaneurysms develop within the retina of the eye, although symptoms noticeable to the patient rarely occur until Stage 4.

With Stage 2, some of the blood vessels that normally provide nourishment to the retina are blocked and thus prevented from functioning. With Stage 3, many blood vessels are blocked and the retina is stimulated to grow new blood vessels to provide needed nourishment to the retina. With Stage 4, the new blood vessels are actually grown and they are very fragile. When they leak blood, they cause vision loss or blindness. If bleeding occurs in Stage 4, individuals may see spots or "floaters" going across the eyes. This is an indication for seeing an eye professional immediately.

Diabetic retinopathy is an indicator of coronary heart disease It should also be noted that research has indicated that the presence of diabetic retinopathy in an individual also correlates with an increased risk for the diagnosis of coronary heart disease. Research by Ning Cheung and colleagues, which was reported in *Diabetes Care* in 2007, followed 214 patients with diabetic retinopathy for nearly eight years. They found that the subjects had twice the risk of having coronary heart disease events and three times the risk of death from coronary heart disease compared to diabetics without diabetic retinopathy. Clearly, an annual eye examination is extremely important, not only to protect against blindness but also to identify individuals at risk for heart disease.

Diagnosis of diabetic retinopathy Diabetic retinopathy is diagnosed with a visual acuity test (the test in which one reads the letters or numbers off an eye chart), as well as with a dilated eye examination in which the pupils of the eyes are dilated.

Managing diabetic retinopathy According to Paul M. Dodson in his 2007 article on the treatment and prevention of diabetic retinopathy in *Diabetes and Vascular Disease Research,* the management of hyperglycemia as well as of dyslipidemia and hypertension are also priority issues with diabetic retinopathy. Dodson said that diabetic retinopathy affects an estimated 40 percent of those with diabetes in the United Kingdom, and about 10 percent of diabetics have advanced retinopathy that threatens their sight.

Although laser treatment is used with diabetic retinopathy, Dodson says that actions to prevent the development of the disorder are important. Medications can also help; for example, Dodson reported that the use of fenofibrate (Tricor) in the Fenofibrate Intervention and Event Lower in Diabetes (FIELD) study showed that after five years, fenofibrate decreased the risk of needing laser therapy to 3.6 percent, compared to a higher rate of 5.2 percent among the subjects who were given a placebo (sugar pill) drug.

Individuals at high risk Some groups have an increased risk for the development of diabetic retinopathy; for example, in addition to the high risk seen among the elderly, according to the Indian Health Service, the risk for diabetic retinopathy is 2.2 times greater among American Indians and Alaska Natives compared to the U.S.

population as a whole. In addition, some tribes have very high rates of diabetic retinopathy; for example, nearly half of the Sioux with diabetes in South Dakota have diabetic retinopathy.

Glaucoma

Glaucoma is an eye disease that damages the optic nerve of the eye. According to the NDEP, about 2.2 million people in the United States age 40 and older have been diagnosed with glaucoma. An additional 1.1 million people have glaucoma but they have not yet been diagnosed with this serious eye disease. Glaucoma is about twice as common among older AFRICAN AMERICANS as among WHITES/CAUCASIANS. Diabetes increases the risk for the development of glaucoma.

According to Jinan B. Saaddine, M.D., and colleagues in their 2008 article for *Archives of Ophthalmology*, there were 233,000 adults with diabetes age 40 and older with glaucoma in 2005. That number was projected to increase to 650,000 people by 2020 and further to 1,087,000 individuals with diabetes who have glaucoma by 2030.

Blindness

People with diabetes are an estimated 25 times more likely to become blind compared to individuals without diabetes, according to the NDEP. Diabetic retinopathy that is untreated is a major cause of blindness among adults with diabetes; however, untreated cataracts, glaucoma, and macular edema may also lead to blindness. In many cases, annual eye examinations could prevent blindness from ever occurring, which is why every person who is diagnosed with either Type 1 or Type 2 diabetes should have their eyes tested each year by an ophthalmologist (medical doctor who specializes in eye diseases) or an optometrist (health professional who is not a medical doctor but who does specialize in eye diseases).

Other Eye Complications among Diabetics

Individuals with diabetes may suffer from other eye complications in addition to blindness, dia-betic retinopathy, cataracts, glaucoma, and macular edema; for example, double vision may be caused by diabetes, and if such a problem occurs, the individual should consult with an ophthalmologist or optometrist right away. This ocular complication may sometimes be misinterpreted as a stroke or other neurological problem by physicians.

Some people with diabetes also suffer from fluctuations in their vision, and this is often due to poor control of their blood sugar. Elevated glucose levels can cause a thickening of the lens of the eye, leading to changes that can increase either nearsightedness or farsightedness. Then when the blood glucose level drops back to normal, the vision again returns to normal. Among individuals who need glasses to correct their vision, frequent fluctuations in their vision can become problematic.

A Lack of Knowledge of Serious Eye Diseases among Diabetics

In a study of 90 diabetics who received a comprehensive eye examination, reported by Heidi Wagner and colleagues in *Diabetes Educator* in 2008, the researchers found significant knowledge gaps in the subjects. Some of the patients received the eye examination alone while others received patient education. There were significant misconceptions among both groups, including the group who subsequently received education.

For example, the majority (75.6 percent) of all subjects believed that diabetic eye disease usually has early warning signs. (It does not.) Another area where subjects were misinformed was in whether people with diabetes are at a low risk for developing glaucoma; about half responded correctly that this is a false statement. (Diabetics have an elevated risk for glaucoma.) Only about a third realized that laser surgery could halt the worsening of diabetic retinopathy, and about half knew that cataracts were common among individuals with diabetes. It seems likely that many people with diabetes share the mistaken beliefs of this group.

The subjects who received education on eye disease became significantly more aware of the realities of diabetic eye disease.

See also CARDIOVASCULAR DISEASE; HYPERTENSION.

Cheung, Ning, et al. "Diabetic Retinopathy and the Risk of Coronary Heart Disease: The Atherosclerosis Risk in Communities Study." *Diabetes Care* 30, no. 7 (2007): 1,742–1,746.

Dodson, Paul M. "Diabetic Retinopathy: Treatment and Prevention." *Diabetes and Vascular Disease Research* 4 (2007): S9–S11.

Fong, D. S., and R. Contreras. "Glitazone Use Associated with Diabetic Macular Edema." *American Journal of Ophthalmology* 147, no. 4 (2009): 583–586.

Kendall, Claire. "Rosiglitazone (Avandia) and Macular Edema." *Canadian Medical Association Journal* 174, no. 5 (2006): 623.

Saaddine, Jinan B., M.D., et al. "Projection of Diabetic Retinopathy and Other Major Eye Diseases among People with Diabetes Mellitus.: United States, 2005–2050." *Archives of Ophthalmology* 126, no. 12 (2008): 1,740–1,747.

Soomro, Hibba, Lesley Burnett, and Nigel Davies. "Quantifying Changes in Retinal Anatomy after Interventions for Diabetic Maculopathy." *British Journal of Diabetes and Vascular Disease* 7 (2007): 181–185.

Wagner, Heidi, et al. "Eye on Diabetes: A Multidisciplinary Patient Education Intervention." *Diabetes Educator* 34, no. 1 (2008): 84–89.

diabetic ketoacidosis (DKA)   An acute metabolic complication of diabetes that involves a combination of hyperglycemia, excess acid in the bloodstream, and dehydration. Diabetic ketoacidosis (DKA) is a very serious emergency condition that is seen primarily in people with Type 1 diabetes rather than Type 2 diabetes. It is one of the two leading causes of death among children and adolescents who have Type 1 diabetes. (HYPOGLYCEMIA is the other leading cause.) Sometimes the diagnosis of diabetes is made at the same time as the diagnosis of DKA.

Patients with Type 2 diabetes who experience DKA will need to take some INSULIN to treat the DKA. If they had previously been maintained on oral medication, they may be able to return to taking oral medications at a later date if their glycemic control improves and stabilizes.

The blood glucose level of the person afflicted with DKA is very high, and chemicals that are known as ketones can also be identified in the urine and in the blood. In most cases, the patient will need to be hospitalized, often in the intensive care unit, in order to stabilize and carefully monitor the person.

Symptoms and Diagnostic Path

Some common symptoms of DKA are blurred vision, nausea, abdominal pains, and a lack of appetite. The individual may also experience increased urination and extreme thirst.

Treatment Options and Outlook

In the 1970s and earlier, physicians favored very high doses of insulin (20–100 U/h) to treat this condition; however, the current medical thinking is to provide lower doses of insulin, such as 5–10 U/h. This is done in order to alleviate the risk of an immediate drop in the blood glucose levels, which may also be dangerous to the patient. A recent study suggested that a priming dose of insulin is not necessary in the treatment of DKA if the treatment dosing is adequately calculated, typically about 10 units of regular insulin in a 155-pound patient. In addition to the administration of insulin, an aggressive program of "rehydration" or providing adequate fluids and also replenishing the depleted potassium levels of the patient are instituted as standard parts of the treatment for DKA. Potassium therapy is usually never started until it is determined that the patient is making urine.

Patients who have been hospitalized for DKA should be very carefully followed by their doctors, initially with hourly clinical and blood monitoring, and should also be extremely vigilant with regard to monitoring their blood glucose levels. Fluid and electrolyte levels should be closely monitored as well.

A person who has had DKA once is at risk for experiencing it again unless the reasons for its onset have been resolved.

Risk Factors and Preventive Measures

Ethnicity appears to be a factor in the incidence of DKA: blacks are more than twice as likely to be admitted to the hospital for DKA as whites. DKA is also a more common problem among older people of all races, and people over the age of 75 years have the highest death rates of this complication.

Poor glycemic control may also lead to DKA.

Studies indicate that patients with DKA who are seen by endocrinologists have a briefer and less costly stay than do patients who are treated by general practitioners. Endocrinologists order fewer tests, and they are apparently more confident about their treatment plan than are general practitioners.

See also COMPLICATIONS OF DIABETES AND ASSOCIATED DISORDERS; EMERGENCY ISSUES IN DIABETES.

Kitabchi, A. E., M. B. Murphy, J. Spencer, R. Matteri, and J. Karas. "Is a Priming Dose of Insulin Necessary in a Low-Dose Insulin Protocol for the Treatment of Diabetic Ketoacidosis?" *Diabetes Care* 31, no. 11 (2008): 2,081–2,085.

diabetic nephropathy Kidney damage that is directly or indirectly linked to diabetes mellitus and that may cause chronic kidney disease and may ultimately lead to kidney failure. Diabetic nephropathy is also known as *diabetic kidney disease.* (Past names included diabetic glomerulosclerosis and Kimmelstiel-Wilson disease.) Diabetes is the leading cause of kidney failure in the United States, followed by HYPERTENSION. Many individuals with diabetes also have hypertension, thus greatly escalating their risk for kidney disease and kidney failure. For patients who have both high blood pressure and diabetes and develop kidney disease, the risk for death is escalated.

The person with kidney failure must have either kidney dialysis or kidney transplantation in order to survive. Unfortunately, kidney disease usually has no symptoms until less than 25 percent of kidney function remains. However, there are excellent laboratory markers of early kidney disease. As a result, all patients with diabetes mellitus should be carefully monitored for the possible development of kidney disease and should receive periodic laboratory tests for the levels of protein in their urine (PROTEINURIA) and the level of CREATININE. These two indicators are markers of kidney function, and when minimally abnormal, they may indicate very early kidney disease. Some other tests may be added when the physician wants to pursue a more complete evaluation, such as hemoglobin level, serum protein electrophoresis, calcium, phosphorus, renal ultrasound, 24-hour urine collection to measure creatinine and protein, and other tests as needed.

Three Primary Paths to Diabetic Nephropathy

When individuals develop diabetic nephropathy, it is generally caused by one or more of three primary pathways leading to kidney disease, including HYPERGLYCEMIA (high blood glucose), hypertension and DYSLIPIDEMIA, which is an abnormality of blood lipids (good CHOLESTEROL, bad cholesterol, and TRIGLYCERIDES). With hyperglycemia, the kidney undergoes physiological and then physical changes that ultimately lead to an increased permeability of the blood capillaries (the glomeruli) of the kidney. This allows proteins such as albumin to seep through the kidneys and into the urine. Proteinuria (protein in the urine) is an indication of kidney disease.

Hyperglycemia causes kidney disease though elevated levels of Protein Kinase c, leading to increased vasodilating substances such as endothelin and increased cytokines such as TGF-beta and VEG-f. Chronic hyperglycemia also causes physiological kidney damage as the excessive levels of glucose lead to AGEs (Advanced Glycosylation End products) that damage the kidneys.

The person with both diabetes and hypertension experiences damage to the kidney caused by increased pressures within the kidneys, which eventually increase the capillaries' permeability and cause proteinuria. It is extremely important to treat the person who has both diabetes and hypertension aggressively, because of their high risk for the development of diabetic kidney disease.

According to Kevin Abbott and colleagues in their article in the *Journal of Clinical Pharmacology* on blood pressure control among patients with diabetes and hypertension, they note that only about 11 percent of those being treated for diabetic nephropathy actually achieve a blood pressure goal of less than 130 mm HG, which is likely a key reason why their illness progresses further and may proceed to the need for dialysis. The authors also described the importance of using medications such as ACE inhibitors (angiotensin converting enzyme inhibitors), angiotensin receptor blockers (ARBs), and other medications as well as combinations of ACE inhibitors/diuretics to bring blood pressure levels down. To attain optimal blood pressure (<130/80) the average patient with diabetes and hypertension requires at least three blood pressure medications.

Dyslipidemia has also been demonstrated to play a role in diabetic nephropathy, although the mechanism for how this damage actually occurs is yet unknown as of this writing.

Signs and Symptoms of Diabetic Kidney Disease

In the progressive course of the five stages of kidney disease, with Stage 1 being the first stage and Stage 5 the most serious stage of kidney disease and one that indicates imminent kidney failure, it should be noted that there may be no signs of kidney disease at all in some people until they reach Stage 5. However, some individuals begin to experience signs of diabetic nephropathy in Stage 3, such as nocturia (night-time urination), anemia, and hypertension.

In Stage 4, individuals with diabetic kidney disease may experience such symptoms as shortness of breath, fatigue, and an intolerance to cold. The signs in Stage 5 may include leg cramps, nausea and vomiting, and very severe itchiness (pruritis), due to excessively high levels of blood urea nitrogen (BUN) and other waste products.

Individuals at High Risk for Diabetic Nephropathy

Some groups of individuals with diabetes have a higher risk for the development of diabetic kidney disease than others; for example, AMERICAN INDIANS and AFRICAN AMERICANS both have a high risk for diabetic kidney disease, at least in part because these groups have a higher risk for the development of diabetes mellitus than individuals of other races and ethnicities. Some Native American tribes, such as the PIMA INDIANS of Arizona, have an extremely high rate of diabetic nephropathy, and more than a third of diabetic Pima Indians will develop end-stage renal disease, necessitating either dialysis or a kidney transplant in order to survive.

Individuals with a family history of diabetic kidney disease have an elevated risk for the development of diabetic nephropathy. Researchers have found that the siblings of individuals with both diabetes and kidney disease have an estimated five times greater risk of also developing nephropathy themselves.

Modifiable and Non-modifiable Risk Factors for Kidney Disease

Some risk factors for kidney disease are modifiable and others are not; for example, age and race/ethnicity are not modifiable risk factors, but SMOKING is modifiable because people can work with their physicians to end their smoking habit. In fact, smoking is a major risk factor for the initial development of diabetic nephropathy, as is poor glycemic control. Other important risk factors are older age, a low socioeconomic status, and a low birth weight. Individuals with some diseases and disorders also have an increased risk for the development of diabetic nephropathy, such as those with polycystic kidney disease, urinary stones, and obstructions of the lower urinary tract.

After kidney disease has begun, the risk for the further escalation of the disease is directly affected by such factors as continued smoking, uncontrolled hypertension, and poor glycemic control, as well as continued obesity. These are all modifiable risk factors, and by working with

TABLE 1: MODIFIABLE AND NON-MODIFIABLE RISK FACTORS FOR KIDNEY DISEASE

Modifiable Risk Factors	How They Can be Modified	Non-modifiable Risk Factors
Smoking	End smoking habit	Age
Obesity	Lose weight	Race and ethnicity
Hyperglycemia	Bring high blood sugar into better control	Family history
Dyslipidemia	Medications to improve blood cholesterol levels, dietary changes, exercise, weight loss	Low birth weight
Hypertension	Medications, exercise, weight loss	The presence of other diseases such as kidney stones or diabetes or anatomic abnormalities of the kidneys

their physicians, most people can bring these factors under significantly better control; however, some people continue to fail to take needed actions, and consequently, their disease will progress until kidney failure ultimately results.

Some studies have indicated that the presence of chronic kidney disease (CKD) is a risk factor for an elevated risk for death among patients with Type 1 diabetes. In a study of 4,201 diabetic adults from the Finnish Diabetic Nephropathy study by Per-Henrik Groop, M.D., and colleagues, published in *Diabetes* in 2009, the researchers found that there was a direct association between mortality (death) and the presence and severity of chronic kidney disease. There were 291 deaths over a seven-year follow-up, which was a 3.6 times greater death rate than among the general population of the same age and gender.

With the worsening of the CKD came an increased risk for death compared to the general population; for example, the presence of microalbuminuria (greater or equal to 30 mg/dL albumin per G of creatinine) was associated with a 2.8 times greater death risk compared to the general population. The presence of macroalbuminuria (greater than 300 mg/dL albumin per G of creatinine), indicating a worse stage of CKD, was linked to a 9.2 times greater risk for death. The presence of end-stage renal disease was associated with an 18.3 times greater risk for death among the subjects.

In addition, individuals with impaired kidney function as measured by the glomerular filtration rate had an increased risk of death.

Other Finnish researchers have found that high levels of uric acid in the blood of patients with Type 1 diabetes were predictive for the development of diabetic nephropathy, based on a study of 263 patients by Peter Hovind and colleagues and published in *Diabetes* in 2009. The uric acid levels of the subjects were measured three years after the onset of Type 1 diabetes and before the development of microalbuminuria. They found that among subjects with uric acid levels in the top quartile (25 percent), 22.3 percent developed persistent macroalbuminuria, compared to only 9.5 percent who had lower uric acid levels and who subsequently developed macroalbuminuria.

Most experts feel that excess uric acid is a marker and not a cause of the nephropathy or vascular dysfunction. The elevated levels are usually treated only if the patients have gout, uric acid kidney stones, or very high levels (greater than 10 mg/dL) of uric acid.

Lack of Awareness of Chronic Kidney Disease Is a Major Problem

A major problem in the United States is that many people with diabetes who have chronic kidney disease (CKD) are unaware that they have the problem and thus fail to take any actions that could slow the disease progression. According to research reported by Adam Whaley-Connell and colleagues in the *American Journal of Kidney Diseases* in 2009, an analysis of patients with diabetes and CKD found that of those who were aware that they had CKD,

29.6 percent were being followed by nephrologists, while among those who were not aware that they had CKD, only 2.7 percent were being treated by nephrologists.

The researchers concluded, "The present report extends earlier observations and suggests that in diabetic KEEP [Kidney Early Evaluation Program] participants with CKD, systolic blood pressure, obesity, and triglyceride levels are higher than for nondiabetic participants. In addition, in unaware diabetic participants, those with comorbid hypertension, obesity, or a family history of diabetes are less likely than those without these conditions to reach optimal blood glucose levels."

Being treated by a nephrologist is associated with a better outcome for patients with kidney disease, according to research. For example, a study by Chin-Lin Tseng and colleagues of more than 39,000 patients that was published in 2008 in the *Archives of Internal Medicine* showed that patients with both diabetes and moderately severe to severe chronic kidney disease who were treated by a NEPHROLOGIST had a lower death rate than patients treated by other types of physicians.

The authors said, "It has been demonstrated previously that earlier referral to a nephrologist is associated with lower mortality and morbidity in patients starting dialysis, particularly those with diabetes. The present study extends previous findings in that outpatient nephrologic care in patients with diabetes and CKD [chronic kidney disease] is associated with lower mortality, not only at the onset of ESRD [end-stage renal disease] but also in patients with CKD not receiving dialysis."

Nephropathy with Type 1 and Type 2 Diabetes Mellitus

In general, when it develops, diabetic nephropathy may occur within 10 to 15 years of the diagnosis of Type 1 diabetes. However, individuals with Type 2 diabetes may receive the diagnosis of diabetic nephropathy at the same time as they are diagnosed with diabetes because many people have Type 2 diabetes for many years before they are finally diagnosed with the disease. However, people with Type 1 diabetes are clearly and obviously ill from the onset of their illness because of their need for insulin.

The American Diabetes Association recommends that patients who have Type 1 diabetes should be tested for MICROALBUMINURIA within about five years after their diagnosis and then every year afterwards. However, patients who are diagnosed with Type 2 diabetes should immediately be screened for the presence of diabetic nephropathy. If the tests are negative in the person with Type 2 diabetes, then the screening for diabetic nephropathy should recur on an annual basis.

Other Problems That May Accompany Diabetic Nephropathy

Many patients with diabetic nephropathy have been diagnosed with DIABETIC RETINOPATHY as well. In fact, if a patient is diagnosed with this severe eye disease, he or she should also be evaluated for kidney disease. In a study by Lori D. Bash and colleagues on 1,871 patients with diabetes who were followed up for 11 years, the researchers found that the diagnosis of diabetic retinopathy was a risk factor for diabetic nephropathy, as was albuminuria. (See DIABETIC EYE DISEASES.)

The researchers said, "In this population-based setting, approximately one-third of CKD [chronic kidney disease] incidence occurred in the presence of both albuminuria and retinopathy and one-third occurred in the absence of both conditions. These data suggest that glycemic control is an important modifiable risk factor in the pathology of kidney disease in individuals with DM [diabetes mellitus], both in the presence and absence of other microvascular damage. These results also suggest that urinary albumin screening alone may not be adequate for CKD detection in individuals with Type 2 DM."

Treatment of Diabetes, Hypertension, and Dyslipidemia in Patients with Diabetic Kidney Disease

It is vital for patients with diabetic nephropathy to maintain a tight glycemic control as much as possible, in order to delay or halt the further progression of the illness to a higher and more dangerous stage of kidney disease. This control can be often be achieved with medications as well as with key lifestyle changes that patients can make. In addition, existing hypertension must be managed and the blood pressure should be lowered to as close to normal as is possible. Dyslipidemia must be managed as well, to avoid hastening of the kidney disease to a worse stage.

Medications Individuals with Type 2 diabetes need medication to help them attain better control of their hyperglycemia. Many patients take METFORMIN, a medication in the BIGUANIDE class of diabetes drugs, and which is also a medication that has been shown to be protective against some forms of cancer, such as lung cancer, colorectal cancer, or breast cancer, based on research published in *Diabetes Care* in 2009 by Gillian Libby and colleagues. The Food and Drug Administration (FDA) recommendation is that this medication not be used if the creatinine is 1.5 mg/dL or greater in men or 1.4 mg/dL in women. This remains a very controversial issue. There is supposedly an increased risk for the development of lactic acidosis when metformin is used in those with renal insufficiency, but much of the data and experience worldwide fails to support this notion. Nonetheless the recommendation has remained intact.

Tight glycemic control (keeping blood glucose levels as close to normal as possible) is advocated as long as the patient is safe from severe HYPOGLYCEMIA. Many medications used in patients with nephropathy need dose adjustments, as many are metabolized in part or wholly by the kidney. Patients may also need to take medications in the SULFONYLUREA class of diabetes drugs, the MEGLITINIDE class, or THIAZOLIDINEDIONE medications.

For individuals with hypertension in addition to their diabetes diagnosis, medications such as angiotensin converting enzyme inhibitors (ACE inhibitors) or ANGIOTENSIN II RECEPTOR BLOCKERS (ARBs) are the drugs of first choice if they are tolerated by the patient. Both classes are well tolerated except for occasional cough in those taking ACE drugs. Often a thiazide diuretic at a very low dose is added to magnify the effect of the ACE or ARB.

In general, the rate of renal function decline slows regardless of the agent used as long as the blood pressure is lowered. Having said that, metanalyses have shown that ACE drugs are superior to beta blockers, calcium channel blockers, and diuretics in reducing protein loss in the urine. ACE drugs have been shown to also slow the rate of progression of diabetic retinopathy, which as noted above often occurs simultaneously with the nephropathy. The RENNAL (Reduction of Endpoints in NIDDM with the Angiotensin II Antagonist Losartan) study and the IDNT (Irbesartan Diabetic Nephropathy Trial) study showed that ARBs are superior to standard antihypertensive therapy and that calcium channel blockers specifically are effective at slowing the progression of nephropathy.

Individuals with dyslipidemia in addition to diabetes may be treated with medications to improve their cholesterol levels, such as medications in the HMNB-CoA reductase inhibitor class.

Lifestyle changes Patients with diabetic nephropathy need to limit their consumption of carbohydrates and also to adopt a diet that is low in protein content. When hypertension is present as well, a low salt diet is also important to the individual with diabetic kidney disease. Individuals with hypertension and diabetes may wish to follow the Dietary Approach to Stop Hypertension (DASH) diet or alternatively, the DASH-sodium diet, which requires an even lower consumption of red meat.

Weight loss is another very important lifestyle change among those who are overweight or obese and have diabetic kidney disease. Often excessive weight is linked to the adaptation of a sedentary lifestyle as well as an overconsumption of foods that are very high in carbohydrates. The sedentary lifestyle can be remedied by increased exercise, and even walking for an increasingly longer period each day can significantly improve the individual's obesity problem.

Obesity itself may increase the direct pressure on the kidneys, and weight loss will then decrease this pressure.

It is absolutely essential for individuals who smoke and who have diabetic nephropathy to end their smoking habit. Continued smoking portends a greatly increased risk for a poor outcome for people with diabetic kidney disease, such as kidney failure.

Individuals with dyslipidemia as well as diabetic kidney disease need to significantly decrease their intake of monounsaturated fats. Often they also are advised to consult with a dietitian to determine the foods that are best for them to eat and to avoid eating.

See also EMERGENCY ISSUES IN DIABETES; END-STAGE RENAL DISEASE; METABOLIC SYNDROME; OBESITY.

Abbott, Kevin, Emad Basta, and George L. Bakris. "Blood Pressure Control and Nephroprotection in Diabetes." *Journal of Clinical Pharmacology* 44 (2004): 431–438.

Bash, Lori D., et al. "Poor Glycemic Control in Diabetes and the Risk of Incident Chronic Kidney Disease Even in the Absence of Albuminuria and Retinopathy: Atherosclerosis Risk in Communities (ARIC) Study." *Archives of Internal Medicine* 168, no. 22 (December 8/22, 2008): 2,440–2,447.

Groop, Per-Henrik, et al. "The Presence and Severity of Chronic Kidney Disease Predicts All-Cause Mortality in Type 1 Diabetes." *Diabetes* 58, no. 7 (2009): 1,651–1,658.

Hite, Pamela F., and Heather F. DeBellis. "Diabetic Kidney Disease: A Renin-Angiotensin-Aldosterone System Focused Review." *Journal of Pharmacy Practice* 22, no. 6 (2009): 560–570.

Hovind, Peter, et al. "Serum Uric Acid as a Predictor for Development of Diabetic Nephropathy in Type 1 Diabetes: An Inception Cohort Study." *Diabetes* 58, no. 7 (2009): 1,668–1,671.

Libby, Gillian, et al. "New Users of Metformin Are at Low Risk of Incident Cancer." *Diabetes Care* 32 (2009): 1,620–1,625.

Tseng, Chin-Lin, et al., "Survival Benefit of Nephrologic Care in Patients with Diabetes Mellitus and Chronic Kidney Disease." *Archives of Internal Medicine* 168, no. 1 (January 14, 2008): 55–62.

Whaley-Connell, Adam, et al. "Diabetes Mellitus and CKD Awareness: The Kidney Early Evaluation Program (KEEP) and National Health and Nutrition Examination Survey (NHANES)." *American Journal of Kidney Diseases* 53, no. 4, Supp. 4 (2009): S11–S21.

diabetic neuropathy Refers to nerve damage that is directly caused by diabetes. The Centers for Disease Control and Prevention (CDC) reports that 60–70 percent of individuals with diabetes in the United States have mild to severe nervous system damage. According to Ezekiel Fink, M.D., and Anne Louise Oaklander, M.D., in their article for *Pain Management Rounds* in 2005, diabetic neuropathy is more common in individuals with Type 2 diabetes, and the risk for its development increases with the severity of diabetes as well as with the length of time that the person has had diabetes. (The longer the duration, then the greater the risk for the development of diabetic neuropathy.)

Almost any part of the nervous system can be affected by neuropathy, although it is generally rare for the brain and spinal cord to be involved. Clinically, diabetic neuropathy is usually classified by the type of the nerve affected and the clinical effects or distribution of symptoms; for example a PERIPHERAL NEUROPATHY, an AUTONOMIC NEUROPATHY, a focal neuropathy, or a proximal neuropathy. Some individuals have *polyneuropathies,* or multiple forms of neuropathic damage.

Diabetic neuropathy may result in a variety of ailments. The most common clinically is peripheral sensory neuropathy, i.e., neuropathy affecting peripheral nerves (away from the spine) and causing sensory symptoms. One example of peripheral sensory neuropathy is a loss of feeling in the feet or hands. Impaired sensation neuropathy may eventually (as with repeated trauma to an area that is not felt by the patient leading to ulceration) lead to a lower-extremity AMPUTATION of a foot or leg, although regular examinations of the feet are good preventive means to avoid such an outcome. (See FOOT CARE.) The delayed digestion of food (GASTROPARESIS DIABETICORUM), ERECTILE DYSFUNCTION, and many other medical problems are also examples of diabetic neuropathies.

Causes of Diabetic Neuropathy

Nerve damage that is associated with diabetes often has many different causes. Some causes are linked to inherited family risks for a susceptibility to nerve disease, especially among individuals with a family history of diabetes. Smoking and alcohol use can compound the neuropathy. Hyperglycemia, poor blood supply (microvascular effects), abnormal levels of growth factors and autoimmune factors may trigger an inflammation of the nerves and complicate the picture. Other damage may be caused by mechanical injuries to the nerves, as with such disorders as carpal tunnel syndrome, a painful problem that occurs in the fingers, or with tarsal tunnel syndrome, a problem similar to carpal tunnel syndrome but located in the toes. In other words, the causation of neuropathy is complex and multifactorial, but the clinician and the patient are left to interpret the symptoms and try to treat the known causative and exacerbating factors. Some individuals experience more than one factor, such as a genetic history and an autoimmune factor, as well as other possible combinations of risk factors.

There are risk factors that cannot be changed, such as one's age (with increasing age being associated with an elevated risk for diabetic neuropathy) as well as the length of time that the person has had diabetes (the longer the time, then the greater the risk for the development of diabetic neuropathy). There are also apparent racial and ethnic risks for the development of diabetic neuropathy; for example, AFRICAN AMERICANS and AMERICAN INDIANS have a greater rate of diabetes and also have a higher rate of nerve damage that is associated with diabetes than do WHITES/CAUCASIANS.

It is important to note that diabetic neuropathy is not an inevitable occurrence in individuals with diabetes, and preventive actions can (and should) be taken by individuals with diabetes. For example, there are modifiable risk factors for diabetic neuropathy, such as maintaining tight glycemic control, limiting alcohol consumption (See ALCOHOL ABUSE/ALCOHOLISM) and not SMOKING. Ending the abuse or dependence on alcohol and nicotine decreases the risk for diabetic neuropathy.

Symptoms of Diabetic Neuropathy

According to the National Institute of Diabetes and Digestive and Kidney Diseases (NIDDK) in the United States, some symptoms of diabetic neuropathy may include the following:

- wasting of the muscles of the feet or hands
- numbness, tingling, or pain in the toes, feet, legs, hands, arms, and fingers
- nausea and vomiting and/or indigestion
- erectile dysfunction in males and vaginal dryness in females
- difficulties with urination
- weakness

Some symptoms that are *not* directly caused by diabetic neuropathy but which often may appear with it include DEPRESSION and an unintended weight loss. Anxiety is another possible symptom, particularly if the patient is distressed by unrelieved chronic and severe pain from diabetic neuropathy.

It should be noted that diabetes is not the only cause of painful neuropathies. If individuals with poor glucose control bring their glucose under good control, but there is still no relief of the pain, then another medical problem may be present. According to Dan Ziegler, M.D., in his article on painful diabetic neuropathy, physicians should consider other possible causes of neuropathy when some symptoms are present.

Ziegler says, "The following findings should alert the physician to consider causes of neuropathy other than diabetes and referral for a detailed neurological workup:

- Pronounced asymmetry of the neurological deficits [usually deficits appear on both sides]
- Predominant motor deficits, mononeuropathy [only one form of neuropathy], and cranial nerve involvement
- Rapid development or progression of the neuropathic impairments
- Progression of the neuropathy despite optimal glycemic control
- Development of symptoms and deficits only in the upper limbs
- Family history of nondiabetic neuropathy
- Diagnosis of neuropathy cannot be ascertained by clinical examination."

Zieger also notes that neuropathies can be caused by a vitamin B_{12} deficiency, cancer, peripheral arterial disease, inflammatory and infectious diseases, and neurotoxic medications.

Peripheral Neuropathy

Peripheral neuropathy may be painful. This nerve condition affecting the arms, feet, and legs may affect as many as half or more of all individuals with Type 1 and Type 2 diabetes. It is also associated with problems with foot ulcers and an increased risk for lower extremity amputations. Peripheral sensory neuropathy is the most common form of diabetic neuropathy. Individuals with peripheral neuropathy often have pain or numbness in their toes, feet, legs, arms, and/or hands. Typically symptoms first arise in the toes, as these nerves are the farthest from the spinal cord, and thus it is more difficult for the body to repair damage done there.

Peripheral neuropathy may lead to a loss of coordination and balance, and the person with this condition may also be extremely sensitive to even a very light touch from others. Foot deformities may develop, as may blisters and sores that the individual has not noticed if he or she has failed to perform regular (preferably, daily) inspections of their feet. This is why it is so important for diabetics to inspect their own feet every day and to have the doctor check their feet too. One tip: When seeing the physician, remove the shoes and socks before the doctor enters the room, to help him or her remember to inspect the feet.

One common form of peripheral neuropathy that is caused by diabetes is *distal sensory polyneuropathy* (DSPN), according to Fink and Oaklander. This is a disorder that presents in a "glove/stocking" type of distribution; i.e., the symptoms of DSPN occur primarily in the hands and feet. Early in the disorder, symptoms primarily occur in the evening, and later, they become more constant. Say Fink and Oaklander, "Typical symptoms include spontaneous pain, allodynia (pain due to a stimulus that is not normally painful), and sensitivity to cold temperatures." Diabetic foot ulcers may also be caused by DSPN.

Although diabetes is the primary cause of DSPN, there are also other causes of this condition, such as hypothyroidism, toxic exposures to medication, inflammatory diseases such as sarcoidosis, and autoimmune disorders such as lupus. Of course a person with diabetes may also have hypothyroidism or another disorder that is associated with DSPN.

DSPN is generally treated with antidepressants, antiseizure medications, and a variety of other medications. Duloxetine (Cymbalta), an antidepressant that is a serotonin norepinephrine reuptake inhibitor (SNRI), is specifically approved by the Food and Drug Administration (FDA) to treat diabetic neuropathy. At times several medications are used in combination. However, sometimes the pain is so severe that it can be relieved only with opioid narcotics.

Autonomic Neuropathy

The disorder of autonomic neuropathy affects the nerves of the digestive system as well as the urinary tract. In addition, it can also affect the nerves associated with the heart and the blood vessels, the sweat glands, eyes, lungs, and sexual organs. Autonomic neuropathy sometimes may lead to HYPOGLYCEMIC UNAWARENESS, a condition in which the individual's blood sugar drops dangerously low, but the person does not experience any advance warning signs of hypoglycemia, such as shakiness, palpitations, or sweating. This can become a very dangerous and emergency situation.

The heart According to Martin Schönauer and colleagues in their 2008 article for *Diabetes and Vascular Disease Research, cardiovascular autonomic neuropathy* is a common complication of diabetes, and heart rate variability (HRV) is an early symptom. The authors note, however, that some medications that a patient may take can have the effect of giving either a false positive or false negative for HRV; for example, antiarrhythmic medications, tricyclic antidepressants and clonidine can all give false positives. (This means that they may indicate a heart rate variability problem when there really is no problem with the heart.) In contrast, medications such as angiotensin converting enzyme (ACE) inhibitors, digitalis, and beta blockers can all give false negatives, masking a real problem with the heart rate.

ORTHOSTATIC HYPOTENSION, which is blood pressure which suddenly drops when a person changes from a lying to a sitting or a sitting to a standing position, is a form of autonomic neuropathy. Typically, these patients are chronically slightly dehydrated and their sympathetic nervous system and adrenal glands do not respond appropriately to position changes. Normally when one goes from lying to standing the body releases adrenalin/noradrenalin to increase the heart rate and to constrict blood vessels to help maintain a normal blood pressure. The person may feel very light-headed and may actually faint. Among individuals with this problem, it may help to raise the head of the bed so that the position change will not be so drastic when the person sits up from lying down. Often compression stockings are used, though it is best if they are actually waist high. A form of a steroid known as 9-flurohydrocortisone (Florinef) is used to help retain salt and water and cause some constriction of blood vessels, but by the time it works the patient has to tolerate swelling in his or her lower extremities.

Strangely enough, some people improve from orthostatic hypotension with medications for high blood pressure, such as propranolol and clonidine, but these must be used extremely cautiously by a physician well versed in their use in this situation. A drug known as Midodrine is used to cause blood vessels to constrict. A more severe and less common form of orthostatic hypotension occurs after eating and may respond to octreotide. The down side to all these therapies is that a patient may need to have HYPERTENSION when supine to allow for adequate blood pressure when they are sitting or standing.

The digestive system Autonomic neuropathy that damages the digestive system usually causes constipation, and can also lead to gastroparesis, or slowed stomach emptying. Extreme gastroparesis may cause nausea and vomiting, bloating, and a loss of appetite. The esophagus (the food tube) may also become damaged by autonomic neuropathy, making it difficult for the individual to swallow his or her food. These problems may lead to an unintentional weight loss. Eating small frequent meals and avoiding fatty foods may help individuals with digestive problems. Metoclopramide and erythromycin are also used though they have significant side effects.

The urinary tract When autonomic neuropathy affects the urinary bladder, it may prevent the bladder from emptying completely, and the retained urine can subsequently lead to infections of the bladder and/or the kidneys. The person may also develop urinary incontinence, or a lack of control of the release of the urine. Medications such as bethanechol and doxazosin are used and on occasion patients need to learn to self-catheterize their bladders.

The sexual organs If the male or female sexual organs are affected by autonomic neuropathy, this can cause a serious problem; for example, a man may have erectile dysfunction or he could have an orgasm without any ejaculation or ejaculation backwards into the bladder, which is a problem if the man is hoping to conceive a child. A woman whose sexual organs are affected by diabetic neuropathy may experience difficulty with arousal and orgasm, as well as with the lubrication of the vaginal area.

The sweat glands When the nerves in the sweat glands are affected by autonomic neuropathy, the body temperature is not properly regulated by perspiration. As a result, the person may perspire excessively at night or during a meal, when the body does not need to be cooled down by sweat.

The eyesight Autonomic neuropathy can also affect the eyes and the ability of the pupil to react to ambient light conditions. It may cause severe problems with night vision, making it impossible for the individual to drive at night anymore.

Proximal Motor Neuropathy

Proximal motor neuropathy is a form of diabetic neuropathy that affects the legs, thighs, buttocks, and hips. It also often leads to weakness in the legs. Proximal neuropathy is a condition that is sometimes referred to as *femoral neuropathy, diabetic amyotrophy,* or *lumbosacral plexus neuropathy.* This condition more commonly appears among older people who have been diagnosed with Type 2 diabetes. The cause is unknown, and patients often become cachectic and appear to have a disease such as cancer. It often remits on its own within six to 24 months. There is no known specific therapy, though many medications including immunotherapies have been tried.

Focal Neuropathy

Focal neuropathy can occur with any nerve in the body and refers to a sudden weakness or pain that is caused by nerve damage. It most frequently affects the eyes, ears, pelvis and lower back, abdomen, legs, feet, thighs, chest, or facial muscles. Focal neuropathy is the most common form of neuropathy among older people with diabetes.

Patients with diabetes are more commonly affected than nondiabetics by compression neuropathies, such as carpal tunnel syndrome and tarsal tunnel syndrome. This may be due to the deposit of carbohydrates and proteinlike material

in the canals where the damaged nerves run. It may also be due to an increased level of advanced glycosylation endproducts (AGE) in the tissues as well as abnormal blood flow problems.

Damage to the peroneal nerve in the foot can lead to "foot drop," which is the inability of the individual to dorsiflex the foot (point their toes up), thus causing the foot to drag when they walk.

When the nerves of the face are affected by neuropathy, this is called a *cranial mononeuropathy.* This condition can mimic the symptoms of a stroke, and it may also cause a facial droop that is similar to that found in Bell's palsy. It may also cause an eyelid droop. These types of neuropathies are caused by "nerve attacks," or a sudden blockage of blood flow to the nerve that is similar to what happens in the heart and brain during a heart attack or a stroke. Cranial mononeuropathies often resolve on their own within weeks to months and rarely persist longer than six months.

Radiculopathies

A radiculopathy is a painful form of diabetic neuropathy in which a nerve root of a nerve is affected. If the nerve root that is supplying the nerve is located just below the right lower ribs of the body, then this can cause severe pain that can mimic the symptoms of a gallbladder attack. If it is a lower back nerve root that is supplying the legs, then this condition can cause sciatica, or severe low back pain that radiates down into one or both legs. The type of drugs used to treat peripheral sensory neuropathy are also used in this situation.

Pain with Neuropathy

The various forms of diabetic neuropathies may cause chronic and sometimes severe pain, and people with diabetes may need oral medications and/or analgesic creams to better tolerate the pain. Many clinicians prescribe antiseizure medications off-label to treat the pain of neuropathy, including such medications as gabapentin (Gabarone, Neurontin) or lamotrigine (Lamictal).

(Off-label means that a medication is not specifically approved to treat the condition by the FDA; however, physicians may still prescribe the medication.)

The antiseizure drug pregabalin (Lyrica) is approved by the FDA to treat pain caused by diabetic neuropathy, although as mentioned, other antiseizure drugs are also used in an off-label manner to treat this condition. The most common side effects with pregabalin are dizziness, sleepiness, peripheral edema, headache, and weight gain.

In addition, the antidepressant duloxetine (Cymbalta) has also been approved by the FDA to treat pain stemming from diabetic neuropathy, based on studies proving its pain efficaciousness. Duloxetine is a serotonin norepinephrine reuptake inhibitor, although individuals with neuropathy need not be clinically depressed to obtain significant pain relief from this medication. Ziegler says, "Pain severity, rather than variables related to diabetes or neuropathy, predicts the effects of duloxetine in diabetic peripheral neuropathic pain. Patients with higher pain intensity tend to respond better than those with lower pain levels." As with all medications, there are possible side effects that may occur with duloxetine, and the most common are nausea, somnolence (sleepiness), dizziness, constipation, dry mouth, and reduced appetite. However, these side effects are usually mild and disappear with continued use. Duloxetine may also cause a slight increase in the fasting blood glucose level, according to Ziegler.

Doctors also often prescribe antidepressants off-label to help treat chronic pain, including such antidepressants as amitriptyline (Elavil), desipramine (Norpramin, Pertofrane), bupropion (Wellbutrin, Wellbutrin XL), paroxetine (Paxil), or citalopram (Celexa). Zieger notes that tricyclics can be effective in treating both burning pain and shooting pain. Tricyclics can be sedating and they often cause dry mouth. They should be avoided in patients who have had a heart attack within the past six months or who have other heart disease.

Selective serotonin reuptake inhibitors (SSRIs) are sometimes used to treat pain caused by diabetic neuropathy. Some studies have shown pain relief with paroxetine (Paxil) and citalopram (Celexa); however, studies have not shown pain relief from diabetic neuropathy with the SSRI fluoxetine (Prozac). With regard to side effects, SSRIs may increase the risk for gastrointestinal bleeding similar to that caused by low-dose ibuprofen, according to Ziegler. The use of SSRIs and nonsteroidal anti-inflammatory drugs (NSAIDs) significantly increases the risk of gastrointestinal bleeding.

Narcotic analgesics are sometimes used if the pain cannot be controlled with milder painkillers, and controlled-release oxycodone (OxyContin) or tramadol (Ultram) may be prescribed in such cases. The risk for drug dependence is much lower with tramadol than with oxycodone. Narcotics can cause nausea and constipation.

Prescribed transdermal lidocaine patches (Lidoderm) that are applied to the painful areas may bring some temporary pain relief. (This is an off-label use of the medication.) There appear to be few risks and side effects with this analgesic medication, which provides transient pain relief.

Topical creams that are rubbed onto the painful area can provide some pain relief, particularly those that include capsaicin. Capsaicin is derived from the red pepper. It depletes the nerve of Substance P, a compound that induces pain. It must be applied multiple times and often the pain is at first worsened before it improves.

Some people find relief from the pain of their diabetic neuropathy with acupuncture, biofeedback or other alternative remedies.

See also ALTERNATIVE MEDICINE/COMPLEMENTARY MEDICINE; COMPLICATIONS OF DIABETES AND ASSOCIATED DISORDERS; DIABETIC EYE DISEASES; DIABETIC NEPHROPATHY.

Abrams, Paris J. "Pharmacologic Treatments for Pain Associated with Diabetic Peripheral Neuropathies." *Journal of Pharmacy Practice* 20 (2007): 103–109.

Fink, Ezekiel, M.D., and Anne Louise Oaklander, M.D. "Diabetic Neuropathy." *Pain Management Rounds* 2, no. 3 (2005): 1–6.

Rolim, Luiz Clemente de Souza Pereira, et al. "Diabetic Cardiovascular Autonomic Neuropathy: Risk Factors, Clinical Impact and Early Diagnosis." *Arquivos Brasileiros de Cardiologia* 90, no. 4 (2008): 323–331.

Schönauer, Martin, et al. "Cardiac Autonomic Diabetic Neuropathy." *Diabetes and Vascular Disease Research* 5 (2008): 336–344.

Ziegler, Dan, M.D. "Painful Diabetic Neuropathy: Advantage of Novel Drugs over Old Drugs?" *Diabetes Care* 32, Supp. 2 (2009): S414–S419.

diabetic retinopathy Damage to the blood vessels of the retina, stemming from diabetes. Diabetic retinopathy is the most common eye disease complication that is experienced by people with diabetes, and it is also the leading cause of adult-onset blindness. This eye disease is at least partially caused by high levels of glucose that result in varying levels of harm to the blood vessels in the retina. Retinopathy progresses in typical fashion; first small aneurysms of the retinal blood vessels are seen (microaneurysms), followed by occlusion of some vessels and leakage of fats and proteins from the blood vessels.

When an area of the retina is deprived of normal blood flow and oxygen, the retina sends out signals to the body via chemicals and hormones that cause new vessels to grow (neoproliferation). These new vessels are often abnormal and stray from the back of the eye forward, thus having less stability than healthy vessels. When they rupture/leak, the blood fills the anterior part of the eye and causes at least temporary blindness in that eye. Leakage of fluids into the macula can cause MACULAR EDEMA, which is usually seen when proliferative retinopathy is present, although it can occur during earlier stages of retinopathy. Other factors such as a genetic predisposition to eye disease or the presence of HYPERTENSION, HYPERLIPIDEMIA, and renal insufficiency may exacerbate the retinopathy. SMOKING may also significantly increase the risk for retinopathy.

According to Seema Garg, M.D., and Richard M. Davis, M.D., in their 2009 article for *Clinical Diabetes,* 20 years after a diagnosis of diabetes, more than 90 percent of individuals with Type 1 diabetes and 60 percent of individuals with Type 2 diabetes will have some level of diabetic retinopathy. The primary risk factors are the severity of the hyperglycemia and the length of time (duration) that the person has had diabetes. Hypertension and high serum lipid levels are also risk factors for the exacerbation of diabetic retinopathy. Yet, when the retinopathy is identified in sufficient time, the risk of severe vision loss or blindness is reduced by more than 90 percent, according to Garg and Davis. For this reason, it is important for adults with diabetes to have an annual dilated eye examination; however, according to the Centers for Disease Control and Prevention (CDC), only about 72 percent of adults with diabetes received such an examination in 2007.

Most insurances including MEDICARE and MEDICAID will cover an annual exam for patients with diabetes. Contact the Medicare office for further information.

Women with diabetes who become pregnant should be seen as soon as possible by their eye specialist as the hormonal and fluid conditions that exist during PREGNANCY may exacerbate or provoke retinopathy.

Symptoms and Diagnostic Path

There are few or no symptoms of early diabetic retinopathy that are detectable to the patient, and that is why screening examinations are critical. When there are symptoms, often they may be mistakenly ignored as minor problems or as a sign of aging. Some early symptoms that may appear are a worsening of the peripheral (side) vision, worsening color vision, or the appearance of multiple floaters. A dilated eye examination performed by an ophthalmologist should reveal the problem.

Diabetic retinopathy is usually identified with a dilated eye examination. The eye care expert puts special drops in the eyes so that the pupils will enlarge. This enables the examiner to see the back of the eye easier and to notice any signs of disease. Experts say that the dilated eye examination gives the examiner a clear view of the retina, much like looking through an open door. Without the dilated eye examination, it is like trying to see by peering through the shuttered windows of a house. If macular edema is suspected, the ophthalmologist may perform a fluorescein angiogram, where a special dye is injected into a peripheral vein and photos of the retina are taken.

If a physician other than an ophthalmologist/optometrist performs the examination, a device called an ophthalmoscope is usually used. Endocrinologists and other physicians can screen their patients in the office with these hand-held devices. However, several studies have shown that even experienced examiners generally only detect approximately 30–50 percent of the pathology that is present. This is why dilated exams by the ophthalmologists and optometrists are critical.

Eye professionals use the ophthalmoscope as well but usually they will also use a device called a slit lamp. This device will allow the expert to look at the retina with both eyes simultaneously, i.e., with depth perception. In contrast, the lack of depth perception that is missing when a physician uses a hand-held ophthalmoscope makes the early diagnosis of macular edema very difficult. The device used by the ophthalmologist provides binocular views of the eye.

According to Garg and Davis, the ideal means for diagnosing diabetic retinopathy is the use of 30-degree stereoscopic photography. The authors say, "This has a sensitivity and specificity for the detection of diabetic retinopathy that is superior to direct and indirect ophthalmoscopy by ophthalmologists." The problem with this tool is that it necessitates the use of expensive equipment that is not readily available, and it also must be used by trained retinal photographers and readers.

The authors also say, "Although retinal imaging programs are important in improving access to care and identifying patients who need further evaluation, they do not replace comprehensive eye exams by ophthalmologists. A full evaluation is required when a screening retinal photograph is unreadable and for follow-up of abnormalities detected by the screening system. In addition, non-diabetes-related ocular conditions such as cataract, hypertensive retinopathy, and glaucoma are optimally evaluated during a comprehensive eye exam."

Treatment Options and Outlook

If the retinopathy is in the early stages, the patient may be able to improve his or her condition with tight glycemic control. The best "medicine" is to maintain good glucose control. The key reason for this is that often HYPERGLYCEMIA causes and also escalates the retinopathy.

If the retinopathy is advanced, then laser surgery, also known as photocoagulation, may be recommended. The physician will use a laser to make tiny burns over the surface of the retina in order to destroy blood vessels growing over the surface of the eye or stop leakage from retinal vessels.

Lasers have been the mainstay treatment of diabetic retinopathy since the 1970s. Laser photocoagulation reduces the risk of blindness in people with diabetes by approximately 50 percent. The laser makes burns in the eye area exactly where the doctor directs the instrument. The advantages of laser therapy are that no surgical incision is required and also that it is a procedure that can be performed on an outpatient basis. Many times multiple sessions are required.

The laser therapy can slightly reduce peripheral vision, night vision, and color vision but it will prevent blindness, which is the goal of the therapy. It is best done when eyesight is still normal or near normal. Macular edema is often treated with laser therapy in focal areas of the retina to diminish or stop the leakage of fluid. On occasion, steroids are injected into the eye. Current research also involves the use of drugs that inhibit the growth of new vessels

Sometimes surgery requiring an incision must be performed when proliferative diabetic retinopathy (growth of new vessels) has led to bleeding into the globe of the eye. A vitrectomy is a surgical procedure that removes old blood and scar tissue from within the eye. The old blood and debris is replaced by a clear saltwater solution that allows the patient to see again. The doctor may also need to reattach the retina if there has been a detachment, which often accompanies these so-called vitreous hemorrhages.

Risk Factors and Preventive Measures

AFRICAN AMERICANS with Type 1 diabetes are particularly at risk for developing diabetic retinopathy. HISPANICS with diabetes, especially Mexican Americans, are also at a high risk for developing retinopathy. In addition, it is also possible for children who have diabetes to suffer from diabetic retinopathy, although the risk appears to be low, especially prior to puberty.

The people with diabetes who are the most likely to suffer from diabetic retinopathy include those who have one or more features of the following profile:

- did not control their diabetes in the first years after diagnosis
- have had diabetes for 17 or more years
- experience high blood pressure
- are African American, AMERICAN INDIAN, or Hispanic
- have high cholesterol levels
- have had GESTATIONAL DIABETES
- are smokers
- abuse alcohol
- have other illnesses, such as kidney disease
- have a genetic risk for eye disease

Patients with diabetes are well advised to take the following preventive actions:

- strictly control their glucose levels, to as close to normal levels as possible
- control hypertension. High blood pressure contributes to eye problems. The goal is 120/80 or less.
- stop smoking

- see an ophthalmologist if pregnant or hoping to become pregnant, to detect any early indications of eye problems
- go to the ophthalmologist if vision is blurred, they have double vision, or they feel pressure in the eye. Other indicators of possible problems with the eyes are diminished peripheral (side) vision or lines that seem wavy to the patient when they are actually straight.

Exercise Precautions for People with Diabetic Retinopathy

According to the American Diabetes Association, there are some physical activities that should be discouraged among patients with moderate to severe diabetic retinopathy. Some examples are power lifting, boxing, weight lifting, jogging, high-impact aerobics, and racquet sports (tennis/badminton/squash/racquetball). Trumpet playing (or playing of similar instruments) should also be avoided.

Some activities that are recommended, even for those diagnosed with severe diabetic retinopathy, are swimming, walking, stationary cycling, and low-impact aerobics. Activities that create less pressure on the vessels leading into the eye or create less up and down motion are also recommended.

Screening Children with Diabetes for Diabetic Retinopathy

Children with Type 1 diabetes and no symptoms of eye disease should receive an eye examination within the first year of diagnosis of diabetes and then at three- to five-year intervals thereafter for children who are over the age of nine years. If an adolescent is diagnosed with Type 2 diabetes, he or she should receive a comprehensive eye examination.

See also BLINDNESS; BLURRED VISION; CATARACT; DIABETIC EYE DISEASES; GLAUCOMA.

Garg, Seema, M.D., and Richard M. Davis, M.D. "Diabetic Retinopathy Screening Update." *Clinical Diabetes* 27, no. 4 (2009): 140–145.

dialysis See END-STAGE RENAL DISEASE (ESRD).

diastolic blood pressure Blood pressure maintained by the heart between heart contractions and the lower number or denominator when blood pressure results are reported. In contrast, systolic pressure is the peak pressure generated by the left ventricle as the heart contracts and is the numerator or top number that is reported. The heart spends about ⅔ of its time in diastole and ⅓ in systole.

Individuals with both Type 1 and Type 2 diabetes are at high risk for developing high levels of both diastolic and systolic blood pressure, or HYPERTENSION. When combined with diabetes, hypertension can often lead to severe COMPLICATIONS, such as BLINDNESS, DIABETIC (kidney disease), STROKE, and even DEATH.

See also SYSTOLIC BLOOD PRESSURE.

diet Planned intake of food. May also refer to patterns of foods eaten by an individual, such as a low-fat diet, a high carbohydrate diet, and so forth. There is no one diet for people with diabetes because people vary greatly in their nutritional needs, depending on size, age, and many other factors. As a result, people with diabetes need to work with a registered dietitian to plan a diet that would work best for them to keep their glucose levels as close to normal as possible.

The daily diet is an extremely important aspect of the lives of most people with diabetes because their diet is a key factor in helping to improve (or worsen) their GLYCEMIC CONTROL. In the early stages of Type 2 diabetes, careful attention to diet alone may often be sufficient to keep the illness in check. People with Type 1 diabetes, however, require insulin to remain alive, and they also need to carefully monitor their diets.

Although it is no longer considered necessary for a person with diabetes to give up all sweets forever, it's a good idea to restrict their consumption, not only to keep glucose levels as close to normal as possible, but also to limit the risk of OBESITY, which in itself creates more problems. However, many patients with diabetes report that they resent it when others snatch high-calorie or sugary food away from them because such foods are considered "bad." It's important for the person with diabetes to control his or her own diet to the greatest extent possible.

As a result, dietitians and diabetes experts have created listings or exchanges for the grams of carbohydrates and fats in a wide variety of foods, so that a person with diabetes can make personal choices. This means that if the individual wishes to have a small piece of cake, then he or she would avoid another carbohydrate, such as rice or potato.

Typical meal plans or diets for patients with diabetes contain less than 30 percent of their calories from fat, 50–60 percent from carbohydrates, and 10–20 percent of calories from protein.

For further information, contact:

American Dietetic Association
216 West Jackson Boulevard
Suite 800
Chicago, IL 60606
(312) 899-0040 or (800) 366-1655
(Consumer Nutrition Hotline from 9 A.M.–4 P.M. Central Time, Monday–Friday only)

See also CARBOHYDRATES AND MEAL PLANNING; HYPOGLYCEMIA; NUTRITION.

dietitian Person who is registered in and an expert on nutrition and can advise on healthy eating habits. Upon diagnosis, people with diabetes should receive their health care from a team of experts, including a dietitian. Dietitians can help the patients with meal planning and weight control, and may also assist with any problematic eating patterns. They help patients develop a meal/nutrition plan that they can live with and one that is adapted to an individual's needs and special circumstances. Annual referrals to a dietitian may be advisable, depending on the individual and his or her ability to adapt to the illness.

People with diabetes should look for RDs, or registered dietitians, and, if possible, for one who is also a certified diabetes educator or C.D.E.

Many insurance plans will now cover some consultation on a yearly basis with a registered dietitian. Patients are advised to resubmit claims if they are denied or to appeal the denial, backed up with an accompanying letter from their medical doctor that this education will improve control, prevent complications, and will also save money.

DIGAMI Study   Refers to the Diabetes Mellitus Insulin Glucose Infusion in Acute Myocardial Infarction (DIGAMI) study. Diabetes patients have a two to four times greater risk for death from a myocardial infarction than nondiabetics. The DIGAMI study group looked at the impact of very tight glucose control on the patients' subsequent cardiac history and the researchers found that a significant impact resulted from intensive control.

In this study, 620 Swedish patients with diabetes and an acute myocardial mellitus syndrome were divided into two groups. The first group, 306 patients, received standard intravenous glucose and insulin infusions followed by insulin injection therapy, and the remaining 314 patients received standard diabetes care, mainly the use of oral diabetes medications. These patients were followed by an average of 3.4 years, The insulin-treated group had a 33 percent mortality, and the control group had a 44 percent mortality—an absolute decrease of 11 percent and a relative decrease of 25 percent. Despite this impressive result, experts in the United States disagree about whether it was the early and intensive sulfonylureas medications in the treatment group or another factor that resulted in the difference.

Cummings, Jennifer, M.D., et al. "A Review of the DIGAMI Study: Intensive Insulin Therapy During and After Myocardial Infarctions in Diabetic Patients," from *Diabetes Spectrum* 12, no. 2 (1999), in *Annual Review of Diabetes 2000*. Alexandria, Va American Diabetes Association, 2000.

digestive disorders   This includes dysfunctions of the various parts of the digestive system, primarily including the oral cavity, the esophagus, the stomach, the small intestine, and the colon. In addition, diabetes may predispose to disorders of the pancreas and the gallbladder, such as pancreatitis or cholecystitis. In general, individuals with diabetes, particularly those who have had long-term diabetes, are at an elevated risk for a variety of digestive disorders. Although many people believe that it is only people with Type 1 diabetes who have digestive disorders, numerous studies have revealed that many people with Type 2 diabetes also experience gastrointestinal problems, ranging from mild to very severe ailments. In fact, as many as 75 percent of all patients with diabetes eventually develop some form of digestive disorder. Patients with Type 1 diabetes have a higher than normal risk of celiac sprue as well as Hashimoto's thyroiditis and must be screened for both as possible causes or exacerbators of gastrointestinal problems.

According to Doctors Wolosin and Edelman, in their article on digestive disorders in a 2000 issue of *Clinical Diabetes*,

> The entire GI tract can be affected by diabetes from the oral cavity and esophagus to the large bowel and anorectal region. Thus, the symptom complex that may be experienced can vary widely. Common complaints may include dysphagia [difficulty swallowing, possibly due to a narrowed esophagus], early satiety [fullness], reflux [gastroesophageal reflux disease/GERD], also known as chronic heartburn], constipation, abdominal pain, nausea, vomiting, and diarrhea. Many patients go undiagnosed and undertreated because the GI tract has not been traditionally associated with diabetes and its complications.

The most commonly seen digestive disorders among people with diabetes are

- slow stomach emptying (GASTROPARESIS)
- constipation (colonic dysmotility)
- diabetic diarrhea (often nocturnal and uncontrolled)
- candida esophagitis (yeast infection of the esophagus)

Some other digestive problems that patients with diabetes may experience are the following:

- yeast infections in the gastrointestinal tract and mouth
- abdominal pain and bloating
- pancreatic dysfunction and pancreatitis
- gallbladder disorders such as cholecystitis
- fatty liver (also called NASH—nonalcoholic steatohepatitis)

Often AUTONOMIC NEUROPATHY is the cause for digestive disorders, although medications for diabetes may be implicated as well.

Gastroparesis and Diabetes

Up to 50 percent of individuals with diabetes may have some degree of gastroparesis (very slow stomach emptying). There are many other possible causes of gastroparesis including, but not limited to, the following: post-viral syndromes; prior surgeries on the stomach or vagus nerve; medications, particularly anti-cholinergics and narcotics (these drugs slow stomach and intestinal emptying); anorexia nervosa; hypothyroidism, severe gastroesophageal reflux disease (rarely); amyloidosis; scleroderma; Parkinson's disease; bacterial overgrowth; and abdominal migraine.

According to Juan-R. Malagelada, M.D., in his chapter in *Contemporary Diabetes* on gastrointestinal syndromes that are caused by diabetes mellitus, gastroparesis itself may lead to or be associated with other medical problems such as severe chronic heartburn/GERD, and these conditions together may make glycemic control very erratic and difficult for the diabetic person.

For example, when the person has gastroparesis, the food is moved forward and digested at a significantly slower or more sporadic rate. Thus the slower introduction of calories into the bloodstream may lead to the development of hypoglycemia in concert with the use of both insulin and oral diabetic medications.

An overproduction of prostaglandins in the smooth muscles of the stomach may cause gastroparesis, while acute hyperglycemia may exacerbate the condition and its severity. Other diseases such as chronic pancreatitis and celiac disease may also be implicated in gastroparesis.

Signs and symptoms of diabetic gastroparesis include: abdominal bloating, heartburn, nausea, spasms of the stomach wall that on occasion lead to pain, vomiting of undigested food, a premature feeling of fullness when eating, gastroesophageal reflux (GERD), erratic blood glucose levels, and a lack of appetite, leading to weight loss.

Patents with diabetic gastroparesis are often first advised to eat multiple small meals and snacks and to minimize their fiber intake, if gastric emptying is the primary symptom. They are also advised to eat a low-fat diet, as fat content in general slows gastric emptying. Patients are counseled to maintain their blood glucose levels as near normal as safely possible since hyperglycemia can further delay gastric emptying and symptoms. Maintenance of glycemic control is important.

Metoclopramide and cisapride have been shown to be effective but the latter has been withdrawn from the market due to other adverse effects. Domperidone has been shown to be effective in some patients, although probably no more so than metoclopramide, and has never been released in the United States. Erythromycin has been used intravenously, as a liquid or suppository, and has temporarily aided some patients. Erythromycin seems to act via the motilin receptor.

Surgical intervention has been used in the form of the insertion of a jejunostomy tube into the poorly emptying stomach to bypass the stomach and send nutrients directly to the small intestine. As of this writing, gastric pacemakers have resulted in partial and inconsistent results in small trials.

In clinical studies, gastroparesis has been treated with botulinum toxin, injected directly into the pylorus of the stomach. Very small studies with eight subjects, such as a study performed by Brian E. Lacey, M.D., and colleagues and reported in 2004 in *Diabetes Care,* have indicated some good results with this treatment, although larger-scale studies are needed before this treatment could be widely used.

Problems with Constipation and Diarrhea

Enteropathy is the term that is used to describe problems with either the small intestine (the duodenum, jejunum, and ileum) or the large intestine (colon). Constipation is another very common digestive problem, found in about 25 percent of patients with diabetes. When it becomes severe, fecal matter may become impacted and medical attention is required.

Changes in bowel function, constipation, diarrhea, bloating, and gas may be due to abnormal emptying, leading to bacterial overgrowth. This condition is treated with a two to four week course of antibiotics, often metronidazole, sulfamethoxazole-trimethoprim, or erythromycin, though many others have been used. Bloating and gas and abnormal emptying can also be due to an abnormal physiology of bile salts, and the bile salt seqestrants such as cholestyramine are helpful (primary indication for the use of this drug is actually to lower cholesterol levels).

Diarrhea is also a problem that is experienced by about 20 percent of people with diabetes. On occasion, narcotics can be used to slow emptying. Typically medications such as diphenoxylate and atropine are used, although close clinical observation and caution must be used to avoid severe constipation leading to toxic megacolon. Diarrhea may result from bacterial overgrowth, malabsorption, and other problems stemming from diabetic neuropathy.

Many people with diabetes suffer from intermittent bouts of both constipation and diarrhea. They may have a typical irritable bowel syndrome (IBS), although IBS does not appear to be more common among patients with diabetes than among those in the general population.

In general, constipation is treated with the recommendation for increasing fiber consumption, although the addition of acarbose (Precose) or metformin (Glucophage) may also improve constipation (both have loose stools as an adverse effect), according to Malagelada.

Diarrhea is treated similarly to the diarrhea experienced by nondiabetic individuals, such as with antidiarrheal medications. Some research indicates that metformin (Glucophage, Glucophage XR) may increase the risk for diarrhea in some individuals with diabetes.

Some patients with diabetes suffer from fecal incontinence (involuntary loss of stools); this is a form of neuropathy involving the anal sphincter and can best be approached with behavioral training, although in special instances, surgical procedures may help. Fecal incontinence is more commonly seen among elderly individuals. Fecal impaction (hard stools that are not passed) can increase the risk for fecal incontinence. Good glycemic control and adequate hydration can decrease the risk for fecal impaction.

Poor Glycemic Control May Be a Risk Factor in Digestive Disorders

Individuals with diabetes who have poor GLYCEMIC CONTROL and/or diabetic neuropathy are more likely to experience digestive disorders than others, although some studies indicate that even good glycemic control may not improve existing digestive disorders. Chronic hyperglycemia may lead to and exacerbate autonomic neuropathy, which causes the stomach to empty at a slower than normal rate. This delayed emptying is initially a problem in just the digestion of solid foods but it can later deteriorate to include a slowed digestion of liquids as well. If solid foods remain in the stomach for too long, they may develop into *bezoars,* which is compacted solid food that can cause gastric obstruction.

It is known that improved glycemic control can improve such conditions as fecal incontinence.

Acute Digestive Problems

Sometimes diabetes can lead to acute digestive problems that may be life-threatening and thus require emergency medical attention. Doctors Mesiya and Minocha say, in their 1998/1999 article for *Clinical Reviews,* "Acute problems include acute stress gastritis during ketoacidosis, acute pancreatitis and acute cholecystitis [gallbladder inflammation]. Most problems, are however chronic, and may manifest with remissions and relapses."

Patients with DIABETIC KETOACIDOSIS (DKA) often suffer from upper abdominal (epigastric) pain of an unclear etiology but that apparently clears up when the DKA itself improves. This condition is often mistaken for an ulcer or pancreatitis. The illness may stem from abnormal movements in the gut with the subsequent stretching of the bowel and stimulation of nerve fibers that transmit pain. It may also stem from the direct effects of elevated glucose levels or directly from the ketoacids.

To treat the digestive disorder, prescribed or over-the-counter medications may also be used, depending on the specific digestive problem, its severity, and the health of the patient. In rare cases, surgery may be required.

Lifestyle Changes Often Help

To help resolve or improve their digestive problems, many doctors recommend that patients with diabetes institute a diet that is high in fiber (unless they have severe gastroparesis), and they further recommend that patients eat small and frequent meals (five or six meals per day) rather than consuming "three square meals" per day. However, some experts caution that very high amounts of fiber may actually create more problems in some individuals with diabetes, particularly among those who suffer from

gastroparesis. As a result, each person with diabetes should be sure to carefully consult with his or her own physician in order to determine whether extra fiber is best in their own particular case or not.

In their article for *Diabetes Spectrum* published in 2007, dietitians Carol Lee Parrish and Joyce Green Pastors offer many helpful suggestions for diabetic individuals who suffer from gastroparesis; for example, they advise against eating before bedtime and they also caution against chewing gum, which can increase air swallowing and thus may aggravate gastroparesis. These experts also advise diabetics with gastroparesis against consuming substances containing caffeine, peppermint, chocolate, or alcohol, which can all considerably exacerbate the symptoms of gastroparesis.

Diabetic patients with GERD should consider raising the head of their bed and should avoid eating any food before going to bed or taking a nap.

Doctors strongly advise their patients who smoke to stop as soon as possible, especially when they have both diabetes and digestive problems. Smoking further aggravates many digestive disorders. In addition, smoking is a leading cause of many serious medical problems that directly cause or contribute to death.

It is also advisable for individuals with diabetes to limit the consumption of alcohol, which has empty calories and which may lead to alcohol abuse or alcohol dependence in some individuals, considerably decreasing the likelihood of good glycemic control and increasing the risk for digestive diseases as well as many other medical problems related to diabetes and to the general health of the individual.

See also CARBOHYDRATES AND MEAL PLANNING; DIABETIC NEUROPATHY; OBESITY.

Lacey, Brian E., M.D., et al. "The Treatment of Diabetic Gastroparesis with Botulinum Toxin Injections of the Pylorus." *Diabetes Care* 27, no. 10 (2004): 2,341–2,347.

Malagelada, Juan R., M.D. "Gastrointestinal Syndromes Due to Diabetes Mellitus." In *Contemporary*

Diabetes: Diabetic Neuropathy: Clinical Management, edited by A. Veves and R. Malik, 433–451. 2nd ed. Totowa, N.J.: Human Press, Inc., 2007.

Mesiya, Sikander, M.D., and Anil Minocha, M.D. "Gastrointestinal Disease in Diabetes Mellitus." *Southern Medical Journal* (1998/1999): 33–38.

Minocha, Anil, M.D., and Christine Adamec. *The Encyclopedia of the Digestive System and Digestive Disorders.* New York: Facts On File, 2011.

Noel, Rebecca A., et al. "Increased Risk of Acute Pancreatitis and Biliary Disease Observed in Patients with Type 2 Diabetes." *Diabetes Care* 32, no. 4 (2009): 834–838.

Parrish, Carol Lee, and Joyce Green Pastors. "Nutritional Management of Gastroparesis in People with Diabetes." *Diabetes Spectrum* 20, no. 4 (2007): 231–234.

Sikander A. Mesiya, M.D., and Anil Minocha, M.D. "Gastrointestinal Disease in Diabetes Mellitus." *Clinical Reviews* (Winter 1998/1999): 33–38.

Vinik, Aaron, M.D., et al. "Gastrointestinal, Genitourinary, and Neurovascular Disturbances in Diabetes." *Diabetes Reviews* 7, no. 4 (1999): 346–366.

Vinik, Aaron, M.D., Carolina Casellini, M.D., Abhijeet Nakave, and Chhaya Patel. *Diabetic Neuropathies.* Available online. URL: http://diabetesmanager.pbworks.com/Diabetic-Neuropathies#Gastropathy. Accessed August 1, 2009.

Wolosin, James D., M.D., and Steven V. Edelman, M.D. "Diabetes and the Gastrointestinal Tract." *Clinical Diabetes* 18, no. 4 (Fall 2000): 148–151.

dipeptidyl peptidase-4 (DPP-4) inhibitors See MEDICATIONS FOR TREATMENT OF TYPE 2 DIABETES.

disability/disability benefits A disability is a medical problem that makes it difficult or impossible for a person to perform tasks that others of about the same age and abilities could perform without difficulty. Disability benefits are the financial or medical benefits received by such a person from the federal or state government or from a private employer.

According to the CENTERS FOR DISEASE CONTROL AND PREVENTION (CDC), people with diabetes have a higher rate of disability than nondiabetics. About half of those diagnosed with diabetes (4.1 million) reported a disability that limited their activities in 1996. Of these 4.1 million people, 65 percent said they were limited because of their diabetes.

In 1996, people with diabetes averaged about 36 days per year when they had to restrict their activities. Of these 36 days, 17 days were spent in bed. On average, black patients had a greater number of restricted activity and bed days than whites. When considering gender, females had a greater number of restricted activity and bed days than males.

Disability Benefits

The illness may have been caused by the job or it may be completely independent of work, such as with the development of diabetes or other ailments. The individual who is disabled may be able to collect short-term or long-term disability from an employer, depending on many different factors.

The federal government also has several disability programs. Social Security Administration Disability is one major program and was created for people who have worked for a sufficient time in the past. Another program is the Supplemental Security Insurance (SSI) program for disabled children and adults who have either never worked or who have not worked for enough time.

The person alleging disability must obtain medical documentation on the existence of the disability, how long it is expected to last or if it is considered indefinite, and other related issues. It may take months or even years before the federal government adjudicates the disability.

In the case of a disability approved and acknowledged as valid by the Social Security Administration, the amount paid will date back to the date of application. However, in many cases of SSA disability, the claimant will have contracted with an attorney to document and prove his or her case. At the time of adjudication, the attorney is then entitled to some percentage of the lump sum payment that dates back to the point of application.

For further information, contact:

Disability Rights Education and Defense Fund, Inc.
2212 6th Street
Berkeley, CA 94710
(510) 644-2555 or (800) 466-4232 (Toll-free)

See also AMERICANS WITH DISABILITIES ACT; EMPLOYMENT; FAMILY AND MEDICAL LEAVE ACT; SSI.

Gregg, Edward W., et al. "Diabetes and Physical Disability Among Older U.S. Adults," *Diabetes Care* 23, no. 10 (October 2000): 1,272–1,277.

diuretics Also known as "water pills," these are medications that are taken to rid the body of excess fluids and sodium by increasing the amount of urine excreted by the kidneys. Diuretics may be extremely helpful for those who have CORONARY HEART DISEASE (CHD), HYPERTENSION, or congestive heart failure.

Such medications generally cause a loss of salt and water and may be helpful in low doses to treat patients with edema. However, they can also cause decreased levels of insulin secretion and worsen hyperglycemia. Most people with diabetes can take diuretic medications if they are used judiciously and under the watchful care of a physician who is knowledgeable about diabetes.

Studies such as the Systolic Hypertension in the Elderly Program (SHEP) have proven that diuretic medications can reduce the risk of STROKE among patients with diabetes. Because people with Type 2 diabetes have from two to three times the risk of death from CARDIOVASCULAR DISEASE compared to the general population, a diuretic may be a lifesaving drug for such patients.

Fagan, Timothy C., M.D., and James Sowers, M.D. "Type 2 Diabetes Mellitus. Greater Cardiovascular Risks and Greater Benefits of Therapy." *Archives of Internal Medicine* 159, no. 10 (May 24, 1999): 1,033–1,034.

driving issues Legally operating a motor vehicle. Most adults with diabetes drive without incident; however, if the individual becomes dehydrated, excessively hungry, or overly tired, he or she is more likely to be impaired. It is very important for the person in such a case to pull over and treat himself or herself and also to assess possible indications of HYPOGLYCEMIA.

Some people with diabetes have been denied a commercial driver's license because of the stated or unstated fear that the person might have a severe attack of hypoglycemia and, consequently, could become disoriented or even unconscious. This apparently rarely happens, and most people with diabetes recognize hypoglycemic symptoms that indicate that their glucose levels are out of control, and they are able to act immediately. There are, however, a small but significant number of people who have HYPOGLYCEMIC UNAWARENESS, which means that they have no prior symptoms before severe hypoglycemia suddenly occurs. Such people often have repeated bouts of severe hypoglycemia.

A study from the Netherlands published in 2007 involved 24 patients with Type 1 diabetes with normal awareness of hypoglycemia (Group 1N), 21 patients with Type 1 diabetes with abnormal awareness of hypoglycemia (Group 1A), and 20 patients with Type 2 diabetes and also with normal awareness of hypoglycemia (Group 2N). These patients were tested to see if they made good decisions concerning their ability to drive. They were subjected to evaluation with a normal glucose of 90 mg/dL and a low blood glucose of 49 mg/dL and asked to decide whether they felt it was safe for them to drive. They did not know what their glucose levels were.

- 2 patients (4.2 percent) in 1N felt they could drive with a low glucose
- 9 patients (42.9 percent) in 1A felt they could drive with a low glucose
- 5 patients (25 percent) in 2N felt they could drive with a low glucose

- Thus a significant number of both patients with Type 1 DM and hypoglycemic unawareness and (surprisingly) patients with Type 2 DM and so-called NORMAL hypoglycemic awareness made bad decisions about whether they should drive. Those with Type 2 DM on oral hypoglycemia drugs fared the worst.

- Thus diabetes education about checking glucose PRIOR to driving is critical information to be reinforced with patients, so they can make a decision to test and make appropriate therapeutic changes if needed before they drive.

Confusing Hypoglycemia with Alcohol Intoxication

In some cases, a person with diabetes who is suffering from hypoglycemia may be mistaken for a drunk driver by a police officer. There have been reported cases in which people with diabetes were placed in jail and not given the medical treatment they needed because of the appearance of drunkenness. For this reason, a medical identification bracelet is very important for all individuals who have diabetes. Of course, everyone with diabetes should have a plan for what to do should their blood glucose levels swing dangerously out of control.

Some actions that can be taken are to keep a fluid with sugar that doesn't spoil quickly, such as apple juice, in the car. Some individuals prefer to use candy or gel packs of glucose. If the individual with Type 1 diabetes begins to feel that his or her blood sugar is low, then he or she should pull over immediately. Testing equipment should be readily accessible (not in the trunk of the car).

If a blood glucose problem is identified, the individual with a low blood glucose problem should wait until blood glucose levels are normal and also feel completely recovered before returning to the road. This may take 20 to 45 minutes.

After treatment with juice, candy, or glucose gels, it is important to follow up with more food containing protein and/or fat, in addition to carbohydrates such as crackers, milk, or sandwiches, as soon as possible to prevent the recurrence of low blood sugar, particularly if the individual is on a long drive.

Some Continuing Problems with Laws

The American Diabetes Association worked for many years to eliminate the blanket ban on people with diabetes obtaining a commercial driver's license (CDL). The U.S. Department of Transportation through the Federal Motor Carrier Safety Administration (FMCSA) began a system of individual assessment in 2003 called the Diabetes Exemption Program. Thus each potential driver could be assessed based on how his or her diabetes affected their ability to drive. Unfortunately it also required those on insulin to prove that they had a safe-driving record for three years while on insulin before an exemption could be granted. Many were not able to be licensed in the first place in order to obtain the requisite three-years experience.

In 2005 the Safe, Accountable, Flexible, Efficient Transportation Equity Act: A Legacy of Users (SAFETEA-LU) was signed into law, and it required that FMCSA amend the exemption program to eliminate the three-year requirement and institute the recommendations of the Expert Medical Panel. FMCSA did eliminate the three-year requirement but at the same time released a notice that it would only allow those patients with a hemoglobin HgbA1c between 7 percent and 10 percent to obtain an exemption. In 2006 FMSCA proposed that those with diabetes on insulin could perhaps qualify for a CDL without the three-year exemption based on physical qualifications. That debate is not yet settled. Many states have specific requirements for exemptions to drive with a CDL or noncommercial driver's license (NCDL) that should be researched from each individual state's department of motor vehicles or department of transportation.

The Web site for the American Diabetes Association at www.diabetes.org allows individuals to access their brochure about driving with diabetes for adults and children and for those specifically on insulin, as well as to search for specific issues in each state about the obtaining and maintenance of an NCDL.

Halpern, Kriss. "Diabetes and Driving Responsibilities." *Diabetes Health* (1999). Available online. URL: http://www.diabeteshealth.com/read/1999/10/01/1645.html. Accessed March 10, 2009.
Stork, A. D., T. W. van Haeften, and T. F. Veneman. "The Decision Not to Drive During Hypoglycemia in Patients with Type 1 and Type 2 Diabetes According to Hypoglycemia Awareness. *Diabetes Care* 30, no. 11 (2007): 2,822–2,826.

drug interactions   See MEDICATION INTERACTIONS.

dry skin (xerosis)   An extremely common problem experienced by people with diabetes. Dry skin may be treated with a variety of creams and lotions. These are available either over the counter or by prescription. Dry skin may also become itchy and inflamed and could also become infected. Sometimes as a result of DIABETIC NEUROPATHY, the patient may experience no sweating (anhidrosis), which further increases the problem of dry skin.

Many individuals with diabetes have a problem with dry skin on their feet which leads to cracks in the skin, especially in the heels, predisposing the patients to pain and infection.

As a result, it is very important, especially for those with Type 1 diabetes, to keep the feet clean and moisturized, except between the toes, which should be kept dry to avoid maceration of skin tissue leading to fungal infections and skin breakdown. Thus, daily vigilance to foot care cannot be overemphasized. Patients should also use super-fatted soaps.

See also SKIN PROBLEMS.

dyslipidemia   An imbalance of serum lipoproteins, such as high density lipoprotein cholesterol (HDL) and low density lipoprotein cholesterol (LDL). Dyslipidemia can lead to ATHEROSCLEROSIS, STROKE, and other serious ailments. People with Type 2 diabetes are more prone to suffering from dyslipidemia than nondiabetics. They are especially prone to high triglyceride levels and lower HDL cholesterol levels.

When dyslipidemia is combined with other risk factors (such as OBESITY or SMOKING), the risk for severe disease is further accelerated.

American Diabetes Association, "Position Statement: Management of Dyslipidemia in Adults with Diabetes." *Diabetes Care* 24, Supp. 1 (2001): S58–S61.
Jellinger, Paul S., M.D., "The American Association of Clinical Endocrinologists Medical Guidelines for Clinical Practice for the Diagnosis and Treatment of Dyslipidemia and Prevention of Atherogenesis." *Endocrine Practice* 6, no. 2 (March/April 2000): 162–213.

early detection The diagnosis of diabetes in an early stage of the disease before the onset of complications caused by the disease. This is very important because when detected in the early stages, diabetes is far more manageable and far less likely to cause the severe damage that late-diagnosed diabetes may have already and irreversibly caused, such as diseases of the kidney or other organs.

The UNITED KINGDOM PROSPECTIVE DIABETES STUDY definitively showed that at the point of diagnosis with Type 2 diabetes, most patients had already lost half their ability to secrete insulin, and they were likely to have metabolic abnormalities that had been present for five to seven years prior to diagnosis. Thus, looking at risk factors and screening appropriate populations of individuals at risk for diabetes is critically important. The American Diabetes Association has a diabetes Alert Day every year in March to continue to try and teach the public about risk factors and to push those with significant risk to have screening tests.

It seems clear that the Oral Glucose Tolerance Test (OGTT) and also screening for postprandial (after a meal) hyperglycemia may allow physicians to diagnose diabetes sooner than if they relied upon measuring fasting plasma glucose levels. The older that patients are, the more true that this becomes, that is, they are more likely to have isolated postprandial hyperglycemia.

Some physicians believe that an early detection of TYPE 1 DIABETES may enable physicians to extend the HONEYMOON PHASE, or that time during which there is still some insulin produced by the pancreas.

The DIABETES PREVENTION TRIALS, studies being performed by the National Institutes of Health (NIH), seek to determine what actions may delay the onset of diabetes in individuals who show indications of developing Type 1 diabetes.

Damage That May Occur without Early Detection

Sometimes, by the time a person is diagnosed, very serious damage has occurred, such as the onset of DIABETIC RETINOPATHY. In addition, the female patient may have had frequent vaginal infections and the male patient may have had many urological infections (especially Candida balanitis).

eating disorders Abnormal eating patterns, usually either eating too little or nothing at all (anorexia) or overeating and then inducing vomiting (bulimia). Many studies indicate that people with diabetes, particularly adolescent girls who have Type 1 diabetes, may be at an increased risk for developing eating disorders, including anorexia and bulimia. Eating disorders are associated with poor GLYCEMIC CONTROL. Some adolescent girls purposely withhold their insulin to try to manipulate their weight.

Adolescents with diabetes who seek tight glycemic control are at risk for gaining weight, which is one reason why some may develop eating disorders. Of the adolescents who were part of the DIABETES CONTROL AND COMPLICATIONS TRIAL (DCCT), nearly half (48 percent) gained enough weight to be considered overweight or obese, compared to only 28 percent of adolescents who became overweight while on conventional therapy.

According to Patricia Colton and her colleagues, authors of an article that appeared in a 1999 issue of *Psychiatric Annals*, eating disorder problems among adolescents with diabetes were first reported in the 1970s. Some researchers reporting on adolescents with Type 1 diabetes in 2001 challenge whether adolescent girls with diabetes are at greater risk for having eating disorders, finding few cases of such problems in their study. They did recommend, however, that adolescent females and young adults be screened for eating disorders.

Manipulation of Body Weight through Manipulation of Insulin

One eating disorder-related problem that is unique to girls who have diabetes, and which distresses the medical community, is either purposefully withholding their insulin or decreasing their prescribed insulin dose. This is done in order to lose weight. Adolescents often control their own insulin intake, with variable levels of supervision. As a result, it is possible for them to limit or altogether fail to take their medication, unbeknownst to adults in the adolescent's family or to their physicians—until they come in the doctor's office with significant weight loss or a very high hemoglobin HgbA1c (indicating hyperglycemia).

Of course, sometimes adolescents fail to take their insulin for reasons other than a desire for weight loss. For example, they may be in DENIAL about their illness or may have a fear of low blood sugars (HYPOGLYCEMIA). They may also dislike or fear glucose testing or self-injections. Teenagers may also check their blood glucose levels less frequently than suggested by their physician or fail to check them at all. They may also simply forget or delay taking their insulin. Adolescents have a characteristically poor record with regard to testing their blood as often as they should and recording and acting upon the information.

A study reported in a 2000 issue of the *British Medical Journal* compared 356 adolescent girls in Canada between the ages of 12 and 19 years who had Type 1 diabetes to 1,098 nondiabetic girls in the same age group to determine the level of eating disorders in each group.

The researchers found that about 10 percent of the diabetic adolescents had an eating disorder problem versus only about 4 percent of the nondiabetic girls. They also found that about 11 percent of the girls with diabetes reported taking a below-normal dose of insulin as a weight loss remedy. (Some girls used this method intermittently in order to lose weight.) As might be expected, the mean blood HgbA1c level was higher in the girls with diabetes who had an eating disorder than it was in the diabetic girls who did not have an eating disorder.

The researchers also found a higher percentage (14 percent) of the girls with diabetes who had a "subthreshhold" eating disorder. This is an abnormal eating pattern that meets some, but not all, of the criteria for a diagnosable disorder. About 8 percent of the nondiabetic girls had a subthreshhold eating disorder.

The worsening in glycemic control during adolescence may be attributed to hormonal changes. However, as mentioned earlier in this essay, it is also purposeful for some girls. The authors said in the *Psychiatric Annals* article,

> A subset of adolescent girls tend to be less compliant with a strict diabetic treatment regimen because of their body dissatisfaction, drive for thinness, and associated dietary dysregulation. Indeed 45–80 percent of adolescent girls with DM [diabetes mellitus] admit to binge eating, and 13 percent to 36 percent regularly omit or decrease their prescribed insulin dose in an attempt to control their weight and to compensate for binge eating. By decreasing or omitting their insulin dosage, individuals with DM cause their circulating blood sugar levels to rise, and a large number of calories, in the form of sugar [glucose], are lost in the urine. The frequency of this behavior is surprising and disturbing in view of the extensive education these individuals receive about the serious adverse health consequences of poor blood sugar control.

The authors pointed out circumstances in which purposeful insulin dosage manipulation should be suspected in an adolescent who may have an undiagnosed eating disorder that needs treatment. Some possible indicators they listed are:

- an unexplained high blood glucose level
- recurrent incidents of diabetic ketoacidosis (DKA) or hospitalizations
- frequent cases of hypoglycemia
- delayed growth and/or delayed puberty

Another study of adolescents with eating disorders concentrated on adolescents with diabetes and sought to determine whether eating disorders were linked to poor glycemic control (reported in a 2001 issue of *Diabetes Care*). The researchers studied 152 adolescents ages 11–19 years old. In general, the researchers did not find a pattern of eating disorders among adolescents with diabetes and found that some adolescents had more body satisfaction than a control group of nondiabetic adolescents. When they did find eating disorders, however, they also found poor glycemic control.

The researchers found a subset of teenagers who were at risk for eating disorders especially bulimia: females ages 13–14. There were also several other predictors for an eating disorder, such as a higher BODY MASS INDEX (BMI). Length of disease was also a predictor, with overweight adolescents who had had the illness for years at greater risk than newly diagnosed adolescents.

The researchers said,

> It is interesting to note that male subjects did not report clinically significant symptoms of bulimia in any of the age-groups studied. Clearly, females seem to have more difficulty adapting to hormonal and physical changes associated with puberty and the onset of adolescence.

A Chronology of the Problem

When a young woman who is very slender due to undiagnosed diabetes is then placed on insulin therapy, she may begin to regain the lost weight because she has better blood glucose levels. There is no longer a loss of a considerable amount of calories in her urine and the patient goes from a breakdown type metabolism (catabolic) to a build up state (anabolic). This means her body is now able to store amino acids in protein, fatty acids into triglycerides, and glucose into glycogen.

In addition, the patient's appetite may improve when she is less ill, leading to a larger caloric intake. The increased weight may cause great consternation to a female adolescent, who may now find herself heavier than her friends (in contrast to prediagnosis, when she was probably thinner than average).

To attempt to regain her former weight, an adolescent may radically reduce the amount of food she eats, or she may manipulate her insulin dosages to cause a weight loss. Some adolescents with diabetes binge on food and then purge, although such behavior does not appear to be characteristic for the adolescent with diabetes, perhaps because, as experts speculate, she can manipulate her weight through withholding her insulin.

As a result, it is up to parents or guardians to challenge a sudden weight loss, or the presence of one or more of the previously mentioned indicators of a possible eating disorder. The short- and long-term consequences of eating disorders can be very serious for the adolescent, up to and including death.

Treatment of Eating Disorders

Individuals with eating disorders need help from experienced clinicians, usually a team that includes a mental health professional, registered dietitian, certified diabetes educator, and medical doctor. People with eating disorders may also need day treatment in a hospital or even need to be admitted to a hospital. The individual may also benefit from receiving cognitive-behavioral psychotherapy from a trained psychologist or therapist, who teaches the patient how to challenge unreasonable and unrealistic ideas, such as the importance of attaining a perfect body, and the idea that someone who is not slender is therefore a worthless person.

Can Diabetes Itself Trigger an Eating Disorder?

Some psychiatrists have speculated that the dietary and glycemic management that individuals with Type 1 diabetes need to practice may trigger an eating disorder. They further report that an intense emphasis on tight glycemic control might exacerbate the problem even further because such people may become extremely preoccupied with food and their body. Such individuals need to learn to manage their diabetes without becoming obsessed with the illness or with food, and that is why a trained and experienced diabetes care team is the best choice for an adolescent who has an eating disorder.

See also ADOLESCENTS WITH DIABETES; OBESITY.

Colton, Patricia A., M.D., et al. "Eating Disturbances in Young Women with Type 1 Diabetes Mellitus: Mechanisms and Consequences." *Psychiatric Annals* 29, no. 4 (April 1, 1999): 213–218.

Javonovic, Lois, M.D. "Diabetes in Women Introduction." *Diabetes Spectrum* 10, no. 2 (1997): 178–180.

Jones, Jennifer M., et al. "Eating Disorders in Adolescent Females with and without Type 1 Diabetes: Cross Sectional Study." *British Medical Journal* 320, no. 7249 (June 2000): 1,563–1,566.

Meltzer, Lisa J., et al. "Disordered Eating, Body Mass, and Glycemic Control in Adolescents with Type 1 Diabetes." *Diabetes Care* 24, no. 4 (2001): 678–682.

education about diabetes   Teaching individuals with diabetes and their families about the disease and what is needed to cope with it. Ideally, the person with diabetes would receive education from the team managing his or her case, including such team members as a physician, nurse, and dietitian.

Most diabetes experts believe that education is extremely important for individuals with diabetes and their families as well as for the general public. A key reason for educating the public is that many people (at least half of all those with Type 2 diabetes in the United States) have not yet been diagnosed with the illness. Education and awareness of the symptoms of diabetes can lead people with the illness to their doctors and result in an earlier diagnosis and treatment. Early diagnosis and treatment is best because individuals may avoid developing complications of diabetes that are caused by nontreatment in the early stages of the disease.

Education of the general public is also important even for those who do not have or do not develop diabetes. For example, many people have a distorted view of the severity of diabetes and may regard a person with diabetes as an invalid. Yet, few people with diabetes require constant bed rest or frequent hospitalization (although people with diabetes are hospitalized more frequently—for brief periods—than non-diabetics). Instead, most people with diabetes are active individuals who are employed, have spouses and children, and lead full lives. Members of the general public should also be aware of HYPOGLYCEMIA and its treatment, so that they do not mistake the symptoms of hypoglycemia for intoxication or drug use.

Despite the importance of education about diabetes, researchers have found that less than half (45 percent) of the people who are actually diagnosed with diabetes have received education about their disease. As a result, these individuals are less likely to take actions necessary to control their disease effectively and to minimize the risk for COMPLICATIONS. They may not realize that taking such actions as performing regular foot examinations, having dilated eye examinations, and undergoing annual dental examinations can all screen for early signs of complications.

One of the "Healthy People 2010" federal government goals is that 60 percent of people with diabetes will receive education about their illness. Of course, 100 percent would be better, but that is not a feasible goal at this time.

According to the information provided in the table, both blacks and whites are about equally ill-informed about diabetes, although Hispanics with diabetes have an even lower percentage

(34 percent). Females (49 percent) are more likely to be educated than males (42 percent), but the majority of women do not receive diabetes education. Formal education is clearly related to diabetes education, and people with diabetes who have had at least some college education are the most likely (56 percent) to have received diabetes education. People in urban settings (49 percent) are more likely to receive diabetes education than people in rural settings (37 percent).

Sadly, as people age, they are less likely to receive diabetes education. Those who are ages 18–44 have the highest rate (48 percent) and the rate declined to 40 percent of those who are ages 65–74 and only 27 percent of those who are 75 years or older. Yet, it is older people who are most at risk for the complications of diabetes.

Most states now require insurance companies to pay for both initial and ongoing education for people with diabetes.

De Alva, Maria L. "Education: A Liberating Tool." *Diabetes Spectrum* 12, no. 3 (1999): 132.

elderly People who are age 65 years and older, although some organizations have a younger cutoff of "elderly," such as age 55 or 60 years. Older individuals may have Type 1 diabetes, although older people are much more likely to develop or already to have Type 2 diabetes than younger individuals. As individuals continue to age, the probability of being diagnosed with Type 2 diabetes increases each year. In addition, the likelihood increases that the individual may suffer from other diseases as well, complicating medication treatment. Undiagnosed elderly people are more likely than younger individuals to be diagnosed with diabetes after they have been hospitalized for a complication of their untreated diabetes, such as a STROKE or heart attack.

Who among the Elderly Has Diabetes

About 12.2 million people ages 60 years and older, or 23.1 percent of everyone in this age group, have diabetes but an estimated 25 percent have not yet been diagnosed with the disease, according to the American Diabetes Association. This is disturbing because there are many complications and risks that are associated with diabetes, and if individuals are not treated for their diabetes, then their risks for complications are escalated.

According to Helaine E. Resnick and colleagues in their article on diabetes mellitus among patients in nursing homes, published in *Diabetes Care* in 2008, about 25 percent of 13,507 nursing home residents nationwide had diabetes in 2004. The rate of diabetes among white residents was 22.5 percent, and it was 35.6 percent among nonwhite residents. The diabetic residents had a 39 percent greater risk than nondiabetics of having hospital emergency room visits in the past 90 days. The researchers also found that diabetic nursing home residents were younger (81.7 years) than nondiabetic residents (84.9 years).

Diabetes Is Not "Normal" for Older People

Although many older people have diabetes, diabetes is not an inevitable consequence of aging. In addition, of those older people who do have diabetes, there are many positive actions that an individual (or caregivers) can take to limit the often severe complications stemming from diabetes. Good GLYCEMIC CONTROL (keeping the blood sugar as close to normal as possible), a nutritious diet, and regular exercise are as important to the person who is 80 years old (or older) as they are for the person who is 20 or 40 years old. (Of course, exercise must be tailored to the individual capabilities of the individual.)

Atypical Symptoms of Diabetes among Older People

Elderly people with undiagnosed diabetes may have symptoms that are different from younger people with diabetes, in addition to the usual symptoms of thirst, frequent urination, and so forth. For example, because most discussions and written materials on Type 2 diabetes repeatedly state that OBESITY can lead to Type 2 diabetes (which is true) and also urge obese people to lose weight, many people mistakenly conclude that individuals of a normal weight or those who are thin cannot develop diabetes. However, experts say that among older individuals, obesity should not be the primary criteria for determining whether diagnostic testing should occur, because even slender people who are elderly may have Type 2 diabetes. (Some experts believe that when diabetes occurs among thin elderly people, it is a form of the illness that actually falls somewhere between Type 1 and Type 2 diabetes.)

Other atypical symptoms of diabetes that may occur among the elderly include the following:

- anorexia (lack of appetite)
- incontinence (usually urinary incontinence)
- falls
- behavioral or cognitive changes
- diminished sensation in fingers and feet

Some individuals have none of the typical or atypical symptoms of diabetes; however, most people do have some symptoms.

Hypoglycemia in Elderly Diabetics

In their article for pharmacists on improving care to elderly diabetics published in a 2009 issue of the *Journal of Pharmacy Practice,* authors Amy S. Nicholas and colleagues discuss the issue of HYPOGLYCEMIA, among other issues. They note that the key presenting symptoms among elderly diabetics with hypoglycemia may be neurologic, such as dizziness, confusion, and delirium. They also note that these patients may be misdiagnosed with epilepsy, stroke, or a transient ischemic attack (TIA). They also state that it may take longer for older diabetics to recover from hypoglycemia.

Hypoglycemia among hospitalized elderly diabetics is very serious and may lead to a poor prognosis or even to death.

Medication Considerations for Older Diabetics

Nicholas and colleagues note that thiazolidinediones (TZD), medications such as rosiglitazone and pioglitazone, should be avoided in patients with symptoms of heart failure or in those with evidence of active liver disease. Sulfonylurea medications may cause hypoglycemia and weight gain, and about 1–2 percent of older individuals using these drugs suffer from severe hypoglycemia, as defined by hospitalization, hospital emergency room admission, or death. This is especially true for glyburide, which has a long half-life and active metabolites.

Metformin, which is considered the first-line medication for diabetics who are obese, should not be used in elderly individuals with blood creatinine levels above 1.3 mg/dL in women and 1.4 mg/dL in men. As creatinine may not provide an accurate estimate of kidney function, especially in the elderly with diminished muscle mass, their kidney function levels should be monitored at least yearly in individuals who do use metformin.

Nicholas and colleagues concluded that

care of the older person with diabetes is confounded by concurrent chronic conditions, polypharmacy [the use of many medications], age-related changes in physiology, and diversity of functional status. Attention to blood pressure control and cholesterol management are the elements that largely affect the patient's development or worsening of cardiovascular disease. And, a minimum goal in antihyperglycemic agent use in this population is to achieve a level of glucose control that avoids acute complications of diabetes, disadvantageous effects, and worsening quality of life. Drug-induced hypoglycemia has been the chief consideration as the most serious potential complication. In addition, many agents pose perils for older patients because of reduced renal function and common comorbidities [other diseases].

Complications of Diabetes among Older Diabetics

In a study of diabetics age 65 years and older and their complications, researchers Frank A. Sloan and colleagues reported data from three separate periods, including 1994, 1999, and 2003. They also compared diabetics in these three time frames with results from nondiabetic elderly individuals.

The researchers found a greater number of problems among newly diagnosed diabetics compared to nondiabetics. In addition, they found that among those patients newly diagnosed with diabetes in 2003, there were more problems in some areas than in previous years. For example, the level of kidney diseases was up. In 2003, the rates of diabetic nephropathy were 106 per 1,000 residents in 2003, compared to 81 per 1,000 residents in 1999, and only 54 residents per 1,000 in 1994.

In comparison, the rate of kidney disease among nondiabetics was sharply lower; for example, in 2003, only four out of 1,000 non-diabetic elderly individuals had end-stage renal disease (ESRD), compared to 20 out of 1,000 of the diabetic subjects.

The researchers also found a high rate of cardiovascular disease among the elderly diabetics in 2003, or 298 per 1,000 individuals. In contrast, the nondiabetic elderly subjects had a cardiovascular disease rate of 124 per 1,000 people, or less than half the rate found among the diabetic subjects. The researchers noted that about 40 percent of the diabetic subjects were diagnosed with coronary heart failure (CHF), compared to about 20 percent for the subjects in the control groups. In addition, the rate of myocardial infarction (heart attack) among the diabetics was almost twice that of the nondiabetics.

The researchers noted that new criteria for diagnosing diabetes were employed in 1997, lowering the fasting glucose threshold for diagnosis, and this caused more elderly people to be diagnosed earlier. This would seemingly decrease the risk for complications, since older people could be diagnosed and treated sooner, but those results did not materialize, for unknown reasons.

The researchers concluded, "Overall, our findings emphasize the overwhelming burden of diabetes, including the near 90% prevalence of an adverse outcome and many serious and resource-consuming outcomes such as CHF, MI [myocardial infarction], and stroke. Although other studies have shown improvements with time in surrogate markers for diabetes complications, such as lower low-density lipoprotein cholesterol concentration and hemoglobin A1c level reduction, these findings come primarily from National Health and Nutrition Examination Surveys (NHANES). Although NHANES is nationally representative, it does not focus on the elderly." They also noted, "With population aging and increased incidence of diabetes, demand for medical care will almost surely increase, both for general monitoring of diabetes and for treating its sequelae."

Exercise

Exercise need not be strenuous to be effective. Exercise that is as simple as walking can be very beneficial to older people with diabetes. Most experts recommend low-impact aerobic exercise for senior citizens. All older individuals should check with their doctors before initiating any exercise program. It is also good to test glucose levels before exercising, in case a snack is needed beforehand.

Treatment for Elderly Individuals with Diabetes

Older individuals with diabetes can show considerable improvements with some medications. For example, such studies as the Systolic Hypertension in the Elderly Program (SHEP) study demonstrated that among older individuals with both hypertension and diabetes, those who use DIURETICS dramatically reduced their risk for stroke. In addition, the Heart Outcomes Prevention Evaluation (HOPE) study demonstrated that angiotensin converting enzyme (ACE) inhibitor medications could reduce the risk of complications and death among elderly individuals with diabetes.

See also AFRICAN AMERICANS WITH DIABETES; ALZHEIMER'S DISEASE; ASSISTED LIVING FACILITIES; DEATH; DEPRESSION AND DIABETES; SKILLED NURSING FACILITIES.

Nicholas, Amy S., et al. "Treatment Considerations for Diabetes: A Pharmacist's Guide to Improving Care in the Elderly." *Journal of Pharmacy Practice* 22, no. 6 (2009): 575–587.

Resnick, Helaine, et al. "Diabetes in Nursing Homes, 2004." *Diabetes Care* 31, no. 3 (2008): 287–288.

Sloan, Frank A., et al. "The Growing Burden of Diabetes Mellitus in the US Elderly Population." *Archives of Internal Medicine* 168, no. 2 (2008): 192–199.

electrolytes Chemicals needed to maintain the normal fluid balance and cellular function of the body. Typically, measured electrolytes are sodium, potassium bicarbonate, chloride, magnesium, and calcium. If a person with diabetes becomes dehydrated, this chemical balance may spin out of control. Electrolytes may be depleted when any individual has severe diarrhea and vomiting leading to dehydration. The problem is further magnified in the person with diabetes.

The individual's condition becomes particularly at risk if insulin levels are deficient and the person suffers from DIABETIC KETOACIDOSIS (DKA). In that case, the person requires hospitalization in order to receive adequate dosages of insulin as well as receive replacement of needed lost fluids and electrolyte levels. Such fluid and insulin replacements are accomplished through intravenous feeding.

In some minor cases of DEHYDRATION, consumption of electrolyte-rich fluids such as Gatorade may help.

emergency issues in diabetes Severe to life-threatening complications that require urgent medical attention in individuals with diabetes mellitus, such as DIABETIC KETOACIDOSIS (DKA), which is a condition of severe HYPERGLYCEMIA combined with acidosis. According to Pulin B. Koul in his article on DKA in 2009 for *Clinical Pediatrics*, DKA represents the cause of up to 29 percent of all hospital admissions for patients with diabetes. Individuals with Type 1 diabetes, particularly children and adolescents, may be diagnosed with diabetes for the first time when they are in an emergency state of DKA.

Individuals with diabetes may also suffer from HYPOGLYCEMIA, which can devolve into a severe and dangerously low level of blood glucose in the diabetic person. Emergency treatment is needed and hospitalization may also be required, necessitating the consumption (orally or intravenously) of some form of glucose or an injection of glucagon. Some patients experience repeated bouts of hypoglycemia but they cannot recognize the signs and symptoms of this problem, placing them in serious danger. This condition is referred to as HYPOGLYCEMIC UNAWARENESS.

The HYPEROSMOLAR COMA is another emergency condition that may occur to individuals with Type 2 diabetes.

DKA and Risk Factors

According to Arleta Rewers, M.D., and colleagues in their 2008 article for *Pediatrics*, in a study of 3,666 patients in the United States who had their first onset of diabetes in childhood or adolescence over the period 2002–04, 54 percent of the patients were diagnosed with diabetes when they were hospitalized. Of these subjects, 25.5 percent had diabetic ketoacidosis (DKA). The prevalence of DKA at diagnosis decreased with age, and the researchers found that the prevalence was 37.3 percent for those ages 0–4 years and steadily decreased to 14.7 percent among those ages 15–19 years.

The researchers also found that the presence of DKA at the time of diagnosis was much more common among those with Type 1 diabetes (29.4 percent) than among those with Type 2 diabetes (9.7 percent). In addition, the researchers found that DKA at diagnosis was significantly correlated with low family income, low parental education, and less desirable health insurance coverage.

DKA may also occur among adults with diabetes, particularly among those with poor GLYCEMIC CONTROL and/or who are ill. Some diabetics believe that they do not need to pay attention to their diabetes when they are ill with infections or other diseases, but this is not true, and infections often precipitate DKA.

Symptoms and signs of DKA The key signs and symptoms of DKA are rapid and deep breathing, dry skin, flushed face, a fruity-smelling breath (due to the presence of a ketone or ketoacid, acetone in the blood stream) and nausea and vomiting. Other signs may include frequent urination, fatigue, and decreased appetite, as well as headache. If the DKA progresses even further, the individual may lose consciousness, and the condition may proceed to a state of coma. The individual with DKA may also suffer from complications, such as a heart attack or kidney failure.

Treatment of DKA The person with DKA is stabilized by the administration of insulin. He or she will also need fluid replacement, as there is usually some dehydration as well as electrolyte imbalance. This may occur due to fluid loss caused by nausea and vomiting as well as by the individual's failure to eat enough or drink sufficient fluids. Other causes may be infection or the failure to monitor glucose levels because of sickness. It is also very important to try to determine the cause of the DKA so that the problem will be less likely to recur.

Severe Hypoglycemia

Hypoglycemia can often be treated by regular checking of blood glucose and by taking extra carbohydrates and averting a crisis. The problem arises when hypoglycemia becomes so severe that the person can no longer manage it, and the individual then requires emergency treatment in a hospital emergency department and/or admission to the hospital.

Risk factors Experts report that risk factors for medication-induced hypoglycemic emergencies with insulin are those patients using higher dosages of insulin, a longer duration of diabetes, and a past history of hypoglycemia. Some medications may also increase the risk for the development of severe hypoglycemia.

Medications and hypoglycemic hospitalizations Sometimes medications can overcorrect hyper-

glycemia, causing the blood glucose levels to plummet too low and too rapidly. In a study by Adit A. Ginde, M.D., and colleagues of 436 cases of patients who were seen with hypoglycemia at hospital emergency departments, published in the *Diabetes Educator* in 2008, confirmed cases of hypoglycemia were associated with the use of insulin alone in 286 patients (65 percent) and with the use of SULFONYLUREA medications in 78 cases (16 percent). Note that all patients with Type 1 diabetes take insulin, although some patients with long-term or very insulin resistant Type 2 diabetes will also require insulin.

When the patients in the study were discharged, 27 percent of them were given medication adjustments. Some of the patients (41 percent) were hospitalized, and hospitalization was correlated with older age and with the use of sulfonylureas.

Identifying the cause of hypoglycemia As with DKA, it is important for doctors to try to identify the cause of the hypoglycemia so that this cause can be treated and further episodes avoided. The researchers said, "Half of the charts indicated a missed meal or a change in diabetes medication as the documented cause of hypoglycemia. These are amenable to education and intervention to reduce the risk of recurrent hypoglycemia."

They also stated that the discussion of glucagon emergency kits with severely hypoglycemic patients is an important issue to cover before their discharge, but noted that this was rarely done. They said, "These devices are recommended for any patient with an episode of severe hypoglycemia, in the same way that home epinephrine kits are recommended for patients with severe allergic reactions."

The researchers also found that when hypoglycemia was a secondary diagnosis rather than the primary diagnosis, the odds of hospital admission were 4.7 times greater, leading the researchers to believe that hypoglycemia can be triggered by other more serious conditions such as infection, renal insufficiency, or trauma.

The researchers also said that the level of hypoglycemia that they identified in their study would equal about 450,000 emergency room visits nationwide in the United States.

According to Kimberly L. Tackett and C. Scott Lancaster in their article on diabetes-related medication-induced hypoglycemia, which was published in 2009 in the *Journal of Pharmacy Practice,* problems with insulin are most frequently reported as the cause of hypoglycemia. They say, "Severe hypoglycemia, which is associated with coma or requiring assistance of a third person for reversal, occurs at least once per year in 10% of patients treated with insulin. It is also listed as the cause or contributing factor for death in 3% to 6% of patients with diabetes."

When sulfonylureas are associated with severe hypoglycemia, Tackett and Lancaster say that some key associated risk factors that should be considered are the metabolism, renal insufficiency, possible liver disease, and older age. These drugs are metabolized by the liver and excreted through the kidneys, and some produce active metabolites that will also increase the risk of hypoglycemia.

According to Tackett and Lancaster, other types of medications may also be problematic for those who have had hypoglycemia in the past; for example, beta blockers may delay the recovery from hypoglycemia and may also diminish or prevent the signs and symptoms of hypoglycemia from occurring. In addition, it is important for individuals with diabetes who take beta blocker medications to monitor their blood glucose frequently. Some antibiotics that are given to treat infections may induce hypoglycemia, particularly antibiotics in the following classes of drugs: fluoroquinolones, sulfamethoxazole, and pentamindine. They also note that octreotide, a long-acting somatostatin analog, can be dangerous when it is used by diabetic patients who are taking insulin.

Although few people in the United States suffer from malaria, it is interesting to note that quinine, used to treat it, may lead to hypoglycemia in some patients.

Also important, alcohol itself can induce hypoglycemia, particularly when the diabetic person drinks to excess. Yet the staggering gait or mental confusion that may accompany severe hypoglycemia may be misinterpreted by others, including medical and law enforcement personnel, as a case of intoxication and thus emergency treatment is not sought. (See ALCOHOL ABUSE/ALCOHOLISM.) For this reason, individuals who have had episodes of hypoglycemia should wear a medical bracelet that reveals the condition and provides emergency information.

Lithium, a medication that is sometimes used to treat individuals who have bipolar disorder (a psychiatric disorder that was formerly known as manic depression), can lead to hypoglycemia.

Treatment of hypoglycemia When an individual realizes in time that he or she is hypoglycemic, self-treatment can be administered in the form of oral glucose, and typically 15–30 grams of carbohydrates will work. In 15–20 minutes the glucose level should be retested and the treatment repeated if the glucose is not at an adequate level. (This varies from patient to patient but is somewhere in the 80–14 mg/dL range). Mental symptoms may lag behind the glucose level recovery. In severe cases when oral supplement cannot be used, intramuscular glucagon can be administered by another person, typically 1 mg for adults and doses ranging from 0.2 to 1 mg in children, depending upon their size. If this is unsuccessful, emergency treatment is required and intravenous glucose is utilized.

According to Kimberly L. Tackett and C. Scott Lancaster, "Patients who are unable to take an oral form of carbohydrate require parenteral administration of either dextrose or glucagon. Glucagon administered either intramuscularly or subcutaneously is an effective treatment in the hospital or ambulatory care setting. It is the treatment of choice outside the hospital for those patients unable or unwilling to use oral treatment."

Hyperosmolar Coma

Hyperosmolar nonketotic state (HNS) is an emergency state in which the glucose level is very high but there are no ketones in either the blood or the urine. It is an acute metabolic complication of diabetes mellitus (DM) which is characterized by impaired mental status (MS) and elevated plasma osmolality in a patient with hyperglycemia.

If not treated, this dangerous condition can lead to hyperosmolar coma and then death. It is most likely to occur among elderly diabetics who are ill with other illnesses, and it may be triggered by an infection as well as by dehydration. Hospitalization is required. The individual may experience nausea and vomiting as well as extreme thirst, although the very ill person may be nonresponsive and unable to report symptoms.

In one case of hyperosmolar coma, the disorder was apparently triggered by an extreme overdose of echinacea, an herbal remedy, as reported by Susan C. Smolinske in the *Journal of Pharmacy Practice* in 2005. An apparently healthy, nondiabetic 19-year-old man had reported to his friends that he had not been feeling well, and emergency medical personnel found 20 empty bottles of echinacea capsules. The patient had reportedly been taking massive doses of the herb to boost his immune system. Although he did not die, the young man failed to recover and remained in a permanent vegetative state. (See ALTERNATIVE MEDICINE/COMPLEMENTARY MEDICINE.)

Treatment of HNS involves mainly rehydration and discovery of the underlying cause of the problem, so that cause can be remedied and rectified.

Problems with Insulin Pumps

Some individuals with diabetes, primarily those with Type 1 diabetes, rely upon subcutaneous insulin pumps to deliver their needed dosage of insulin. (See INSULIN PUMP.) This choice can be far more convenient than injecting oneself frequently with repeated subcutaneous injections, and it can be much more efficient as well. Rarely, however, the pump itself fails or other problems with the pump may develop, and this situation can develop into a medical emergency if the individual is unaware of the resultant escalating hyperglycemia.

In an article in *Diabetes Educator* in 2008, Stephen W. Ponder and colleagues discuss the occurrence of unexplained hyperglycemia with insulin pumps. They found some problems occurred with the pump itself, while others occurred with the catheter site, the tubing, and other issues.

The authors first discussed the benefits of the insulin pump, and they said, "The use of continuous subcutaneous insulin infusion (CSII) and insulin analogs can provide a near-physiologic replacement of insulin in patients with diabetes." They also noted that about 160,000–200,000 individuals with Type 1 diabetes in the United States use insulin pumps.

Problems can arise when the patient changes an infusion site to another area, although patients may be unaware that they need to measure their blood glucose two hours after the change. They say, "Accidental air in the infusion line may occur, leaving the patient without insulin, and within a few hours will cause development of hyperglycemia and ketosis if not identified. In addition, the pump as well as the infusion tubing and infusion site should be inspected. Incorrect basal rate programming, air bubbles in the infusion tubing, and a dislodged or improperly inserted infusion catheter are all possible explanations for unexplained hyperglycemia and ketosis. Other possible reasons include outdated or temperature-damaged insulin, incorrect time set on the pump's internal clock, dead batteries, or even an internal pump malfunction."

As a result, patients who are using insulin pumps should be aware of all the signs of hyperglycemia, which knowledge should also alert them to when they need to test their blood glucose. If the blood level exceeds 250 mg/dL, then the person should also check for possible ketosis with a urine ketone assessment test. If the individual notes that a state of DKA has begun, the injection of rapid or fast-acting insulin with a syringe may be all that is needed in order to avert a major hyperglycemic crisis. However, oral fluids should be increased to avoid dehydration. The patient may also wish to move the injection site. It is also a very good idea to contact the physician.

Other Research

In a study of individuals with diabetes mellitus or asthma who were hospitalized for severe conditions, reported in 2004 in *Medical Care Research and Review,* researcher Elaine J. Yuen divided adult patients into different stages of illness; for example, patients in Stage 2 included those who were hospitalized for such conditions as DIABETIC RETINOPATHY, DIABETIC NEUROPATHY, urinary tract infection, and other conditions. Stage 3 diabetic hospitalizations included those individuals who were hospitalized because of DKA, those with diabetes with hyperosmolar state, and patients with kidney failure, coma, hyperosmolar coma, septicemia, necrotizing papillitis, and shock.

Based on these classifications laid out by the researcher, about a third of the 4,982 diabetes hospitalizations were categorized as Stage 3. Yuen also found differences between races and ages; for example, she discovered that diabetic blacks had a higher level of Stage 3 hospitalizations, or 42.3 percent of blacks compared to 29.4 percent of whites. Interestingly, she found that although diabetics ages 18–44 years had the lowest hospitalization rate, they represented the greatest percentage of Stage 3 diabetes hospitalizations, or 57.7 percent.

Yuen also noted that many high-severity hospitalizations could be avoided if the patients received adequate outpatient care and that hospitalization for coma and diabetic shock should occur only rarely when diabetes is well controlled.

See also COMPLICATIONS OF DIABETES AND ASSOCIATED DISORDERS.

Ginde, Adit A., M.D., Daniel J. Pallin, M.D., and Carlos A. Camargo, Jr., M.D. "Hospitalization and Discharge Education of Emergency Department Patients with Hypoglycemia." *Diabetes Educator* 34 (2008): 683–691.

Koul, Pulin B. "Diabetic Ketoacidosis: A Current Appraisal of Pathophysiology and Management." *Clinical Pediatrics* 48, no. 2 (2009): 135–144.

Ponder, Stephen W., M.D., et al. "Unexplained Hyperglycemia in Continuous Subcutaneous Insulin Infusion: Evaluation and Treatment." *Diabetes Educator* 34 (2008): 327–333.

Rewers, Arleta, et al. "Presence of Diabetic Ketoacidosis at Diagnosis of Diabetes Mellitus in Youth: The Search for Diabetes in Youth Study." *Pediatrics* 121, no. 5 (2008): e1,258–e1,266. Available online. URL: http://www.pediatrics.org/cgi/content/full/121/5/e1258. Accessed October 3, 2009.

Smolinske, Susan C. "Herbal Product Contamination and Toxicity." *Journal of Pharmacy Practice* 18 (2005): 188–208.

Tackett, Kimberly L., and C. Scott Lancaster. "Diabetes-Related Medication-Induced Hypoglycemia." *Journal of Pharmacy Practice* 22, no. 6 (2009): 553–559.

Yuen, Elaine J. "Severity of Illness and Ambulatory Care-Sensitive Conditions." *Medical Care Research and Review* 61, no. 3 (2004): 376–391.

emergency medical identification   Usually a wearable device that makes it possible to identify a person who cannot provide his name or address or information on a medical condition that he or she has. In general, emergency medical identification refers to an emergency bracelet, necklace, anklet, or other item worn on the body that identifies the individual as a person who has diabetes. An emergency medical ID could also include a tattoo, as long as it is easily visible when the person is fully clothed.

Some people carry emergency medical identification cards in their wallets but these are far less likely to be seen than an emergency bracelet, necklace, or anklet, and as a result, they are far less useful in a medical emergency.

Emergency medical identification is very important because in the event of an emergency and a loss of consciousness, HYPOGLYCEMIA, or a COMA, others who know about the diabetes may not be present or they may be too rattled to report the illness to emergency medical staff.

employment   Work for which the individual receives some form of payment.

The ability to work is important to many people in our society; however, sometimes people with diabetes report that they experience difficulties and even discrimination in the workplace. Some studies indicate that people with diabetes may also earn a lower wage than that earned by nondiabetics. According to a 2000 report on diabetes from the National Academy on an Aging Society, the median monthly earnings of people with diabetes for employees ages 18–64 years is $796. In contrast, the median monthly earnings for the same age group for nondiabetics is $1,677, more than double the earnings of the workers with diabetes.

Of course, one major reason for the lower income may be due at least in part to missed workdays. Research indicates that of workers with diabetes who are ages 18–64, 13 percent reported missing work. Nondiabetics in the same age group reported missing work only 6 percent of the time.

Not all studies have found that people with diabetes earn lower wages. In a 1999 study reported in *Diabetes Care* that contrasted 1,502 people with diabetes to 20,405 people without diabetes (all over age 25), the researchers did not find any significant difference in hourly wages. They did find, however, that the people with diabetes had a few more days of lost work per year than the nondiabetics. For example, men with diabetes lost 5.9 days per year versus the 3.9 days lost per year by nondiabetic men. Women with diabetes lost 5.4 days of work per year versus 3.8 days for nondiabetic women.

Fear of Diabetes Status Being Found Out

Sometimes people with diabetes feel that they have to hide their illness from employers. In a study reported in a 1999 issue of *Diabetes Care*, 16 percent of 129 subjects with Type 1 diabetes said that they hid their diabetes from employers because of fear of rejection or discrimination or because of financial concerns. This study also revealed that the support of the supervisor was very important to the worker with diabetes. Since some people take great pains to hide their diabetes from supervisors, it appears that they may be depriving themselves of a happier work relationship.

On the other hand, people with diabetes who wonder about revealing their illness to an employer may be right about the possible negative ramifications of disclosure. Because of some employers' limited experience with people with diabetes—or perhaps because of past experience with a person who had severe complications from diabetes—some supervisors may overreact to the news that a worker has diabetes. They may not realize that today most working age people can readily cope with their blood testing and medication needs, whether they have Type 1 or Type 2 diabetes.

Employers need to stop assuming that all people with diabetes are alike in their problems, any more than all people with arthritis are alike or all people who are African American or Asian are alike. It was hoped that the AMERICANS WITH DISABILITIES ACT would eliminate all or most discrimination against people with diabetes and other medical problems; however, incidents continue to occur and lawsuits are filed and adjudicated.

Some people with diabetes have experienced difficulty with discrimination at work, especially if they have Type 1 diabetes and must take insulin injections. The American Diabetes Association once provided a "friend of the court" brief on a case in which a police officer in San Antonio, Texas, who had been previously employed in police work was denied a job solely because he had Type 1 diabetes. His individual situation was disregarded because of a blanket policy against any person who needed insulin. The case was litigated for more than eight years until Kapche prevailed (*Kapche v. City of San Antonio*).

The court ruled for the man with diabetes, but a higher court ruled against him. The U.S. Supreme Court reversed the lower court, thus the man prevailed.

People with diabetes need to work with their diabetes care team to adjust to night shifts or to erratic work schedules. Workers who travel frequently also need specific help with their meal and medication planning.

Workers should know that sharing information about diabetes with their coworkers and employers can help everyone learn more about diabetes. They can also help others with hypo-glycemia symptoms.

The FAMILY AND MEDICAL LEAVE ACT allows workers up to 12 weeks of unpaid leave each year to care for their own serious illness or the illness of a person in their family. Absences may be taken all at once or in smaller increments of time.

See also DISABILITY/DISABILITY BENEFITS.

Mayfield, Jennifer A., M.D., et al. "Work Disability and Diabetes." *Diabetes Care* 22, no. 7 (July 1999): 1,105–1,109.
Padgett, Deborah L., et al. "Managing Diabetes in the Workplace: Critical Factors." *Diabetes Spectrum* 9, no. 1 (1996): 13–20.
Shirey, Lee, et al. "Diabetes: A Drain on U.S. Resources." *Challenges for the 21st Century: Chronic and Disabling Conditions* 1, no. 6 (April 2000): 1–6.
Trief, Paula M., et al. "Impact of the Work Environment on Glycemic Control and Adaptation to Diabetes." *Diabetes Care* 22, no. 4 (1999): 569–574.

endocrinologist Physician who is expert in treating endocrine (hormonal) diseases such as diabetes, thyroid ailments, and adrenal difficulties. Most physicians who monitor the health care of persons with diabetes are family practitioners or internists who are not endocrinologists; however, it can be difficult for these doctors to stay up to date on the latest treatments and medications for diabetes care or to provide the latest lifestyle advice and recommendations.

Endocrinologists with a major interest in diabetes belong to the AMERICAN DIABETES ASSOCIATION as professional members and may also be members of the American Association of Clinical Endocrinologists (AACE). Fellowship training for endocrinology takes two to three years, following a three-year residency in internal medicine or pediatrics.

Studies indicate that it is significantly more cost-effective for patients and health care companies when endocrinologists are the doctors who see patients with diabetes. One study on the outcomes of hospitalized patients diagnosed with DIABETIC KETOACIDOSIS (DKA), a very dangerous and life-threatening disease, revealed a significant difference in the length of time spent in the hospital and hospital costs, depending on whether the patient was seen by a general practitioner or an endocrinologist.

The study, reported by Dr. Levetan and colleagues in a 1999 issue of *Diabetes Care,* looked at 260 patients hospitalized over a three and a half year period in Washington Hospital, a large hospital in Washington, D.C. The researchers found that although the severity of the illness was about the same for patients, the patients who were seen by general practitioners spent 4.9 days in the hospital versus 3.3 days for the patients of the endocrinologists. The mean general cost for the practitioners' patients was almost double, at about $10,000. The endrocrinologists' patients incurred an average hospitalization cost of about $5,500.

Note: these dollar figures may be higher or lower in later years, but what is significant is the ratio of almost two to one in costs, when comparing internists and endocrinologists. The increased number of days in the hospital when under the care of non-endocrinologists also continues to be significant.

One of the reasons for the much higher cost of the practitioners' patients was that they were much more likely to order many tests. For example, only 24 percent of the patients of the endocrinologist had one or more tests during their hospital stay, compared to 49 percent of the general practitioners' patients. The authors said,

> Because endocrinologists have additional training in and familiarity with the management of DKA, they may be more confident than generalists in their medical management and may not need to order as many diagnostic procedures. For example, patients with DKA commonly present with symptoms that mimic an acute abdomen. For these patients, physicians who are less familiar with DKA may be more likely to include more comprehensive testing such as abdominal computer tomography or ultrasonography in the initial battery of tests . . . Additionally, endocrinologists may be more

comfortable discharging patients earlier and caring for recently hospitalized diabetic patients in an outpatient setting.

It is not clear whether the savings in time and dollars in the hospital can also be extrapolated to general outpatient services, but it would appear to be a logical deduction that it could be.

Levetan, Claresa S., M.D., et al. "Effect of Physician Specialty on Outcomes in Diabetic Ketoacidosis." *Diabetes Care* 22, no. 11 (November 1999): 1,790–1,795.

end-stage renal disease (ESRD) Kidney failure. The stage in chronic kidney disease in which either kidney dialysis (artificial purification of the blood) or the transplantation of a kidney from a recently deceased person or from a live donor is necessary for the person with ESRD to continue to live. People with diabetes have about a 25 times greater risk of developing ESRD than nondiabetics. However, according to the Centers for Disease Control and Prevention (CDC), improvements in blood glucose levels could reduce kidney failures by half.

There were 111,000 new cases of ESRD diagnosed in 2007 in the United States. The most common cause of kidney failure was diabetes, which represented the cause in 48,871 cases, or 44.0 percent of all cases of ESRD for 2007, according to the U.S. Renal Data System (USRDS), a federal agency that provides annual reporting on ESRD statistical data. (See Table 1.)

HYPERTENSION is the second leading cause of ESRD and represented 27.6 percent of all cases of ESRD in 2007. Since many people with diabetes also suffer from hypertension, this means that people who have both diabetes and hypertension are at an even higher risk for kidney failure.

Symptoms and Diagnostic Path

There are five stages from the beginning of kidney disease to end-stage renal disease. Unfor-

TABLE 1: INCIDENCE OF NEW CASES OF ESRD IN 2007 IN THE U.S.: COUNT, PERCENTAGE AND ADJUSTED RATE

	Count	Percent
Age		
0–19	1,304	1.2
20–44	13,831	12.5
45–64	42,184	38.0
65–74	25,446	22.9
75+	28,234	25.4
Race		
White	72,668	65.5
African American	31,561	28.4
American Indian	1,254	1.1
Asian/Pacific Islander	5,106	4.6
Ethnicity		
Hispanic	15,057	13.6
Non-Hispanic	95,943	86.4
Gender		
Male	62,239	56.1
Female	48,758	43.9
Primary diagnosis		
Diabetes	48,871	44.0
Hypertension	30,657	27.6
Glomerulonephritis	7,571	6.8
Cystic kidney disease	2,633	2.4
Urologic disease	1,554	1.4
All	111,000	

Adapted from: *United States Renal Data System: The Concise 2009 Annual Data Report.* Available online. URL: http://www.usrds.org/2009/usrds_booklet_09.pdf. Page 7. Accessed November 13, 2009.

tunately, there are few or no symptoms in the early stage, although diagnostic testing, such as a urine test of microalbumin or protein or a blood test for creatinine can often determine people who are at risk so that they can be treated early in the disease. Early detection and treatment of kidney disease can be lifesaving.

In Stage I, the blood flow through the kidneys is greater than normal and the kidneys become enlarged. Because there are no symptoms, the patient will not complain to the doctor at this point. If the creatinine clearance is measured at this time, it is above normal and thus is an early marker of kidney disease.

In Stage II, the blood vessels within the kidney (glomeruli) that filter the waste and extra water from the blood start to show wear and tear from the disease. Tiny amounts of albumin can be found in the urine (microalbuminuria), and this is another early indicator of kidney disease. There are still no symptoms that are apparent to the patient or physician at this point. As the rate of albuminuria increases, however, the albumin may be detected with laboratory tests such as a urinalysis or a 24-hour collection of urine to measure creatinine clearance and the loss of protein.

In Stage III of kidney disease, the albumin and other proteins increase even more and they will show up in simple urine tests. At this point, patients who do not already have hypertension may develop it, which harms the kidneys further. Hypertension is both a cause and the result of kidney disease.

In Stage IV, the person is in a state of "advanced clinical nephropathy," and the blood levels of creatinine begin to rise (as kidney function worsens, blood creatinine increases, and creatinine clearance decreases). Large amounts of protein can also be detected in the urine (proteinuria). At this point, patients are not feeling well and they may feel fatigued and have decreased endurance. They may also retain fluid, develop puffy ankles, and have generalized malaise. Yet they may still not be diagnosed because they have not seen a doctor or the doctor has not tested them for kidney disease.

The last stage of kidney disease, Stage V, is renal failure, also known as end-stage renal disease. At this point, the patient is experiencing extreme fatigue and malaise, as well as itching and nausea. Increased levels of proteinuria can lead to further swelling (edema) and to a lack of appetite (anorexia). Patients with ESRD at this stage may lose weight due to malnutrition or they may actually gain weight as a result of fluid retention (edema). At this point, the person is clearly ill, and if he or she has not yet been diagnosed, the person will probably see a physician; however, it is too late for the doctor to reverse the process.

In general, people with Type 1 diabetes may go from Stage I to Stage V in about 10 to 20 years, although the disease could progress more rapidly or slower, depending on the individual circumstances.

At Stage V, patients either will require dialysis or will need a kidney transplant from a recently deceased or live donor. Eventually, nearly all patients on dialysis will require a kidney transplant to avoid death.

When patients receive hemodialysis, they travel to a dialysis center three times a week to have a machine filter their blood of its impurities for three to four hours. Patients may also have peritoneal dialysis performed at home, where fluid is placed in the abdominal cavity and then it is drained. This can be done either continuously or overnight. Most people with kidney failure who receive dialysis go to the dialysis center.

The subject of kidney transplantation is very complex. Many individuals have to go on a waiting list to receive a kidney, and many die before a kidney becomes available. However, if a family member or friend is willing to donate a kidney, if the kidney is found to be a match, then the individual avoids the waiting list altogether.

Treatment Options and Outlook

If kidney disease is diagnosed and treated prior to the stage of ESRD, it can often be slowed or even reversed; however, by the time the person is in the final stages of chronic kidney disease, it cannot be reversed. Patients on dialysis require a great deal of medical care. Individuals who receive kidney transplants also require medical care; for example, they must take immunosuppressive medications to prevent their bodies from rejecting the kidney. These drugs also leave the individual open to catching infections that he or she would not otherwise contract when their immune system was not being suppressed.

Risk Factors and Preventive Measures

People with diabetes have an elevated risk for the development of ESRD. Males have a greater risk for ESRD than females. Older people have a greater risk for ESRD than younger people. In terms of sheer numbers, however, whites have the greatest number of new cases or 65.5 percent of all new ESRD cases in 2007. In considering the adjusted rate that takes into account the population size of race and ethnicity, African Americans have the highest rate and whites have the lowest rate.

In a study by Chi-yuan Hsu, M.D., and colleagues with the goal of finding risk factors for ESRD, the researchers analyzed 177,570 individuals starting in 1964–73 and following them through the year 2000. Their findings were published in the *Archives of Internal Medicine* in 2009.

The researchers found that some factors were significantly predictive for the development of kidney failure, such as male sex, older age, African-American race, proteinuria, and a diagnosis of diabetes mellitus. Other factors that were also predictive for ESRD were a lower educational attainment, higher blood pressure, and a higher body mass index. The researchers noted that the two most powerful predictive factors were proteinuria and obesity. The researchers also identified other predictive factors of kidney failure, such as higher serum uric acid levels, lower hemoglobin levels, a self-reported history of nocturia (having to urinate frequently at night), and a family history of kidney disease.

This does not mean that everyone with any one of these symptoms or signs will develop kidney failure; for example, having to urinate at night could indicate a dysfunction of the bladder in men or women or of the prostate gland in men. However, individuals with these symptoms or signs should be evaluated for kidney disease.

Preventing or delaying ESRD It may not be possible to avoid ESRD altogether, but it is certainly possible for many people with diabetes to delay the disease by maintaining excellent glycemic control, keeping their blood pressure as close to normal as possible and being careful with their diet, especially avoiding a high intake of protein.

Studies such as the DIABETES CONTROL AND COMPLICATIONS TRIAL (DCCT) and the UNITED KINGDOM PROSPECTIVE DIABETES STUDY (UKPDS) have definitively demonstrated that tight glycemic control can prevent or delay kidney failure among people with Type 1 diabetes and Type 2 diabetes.

Blood pressure lowering is the most important factor when trying to preserve kidney function in patients with diabetes. The degree of blood pressure lowering is more important than the specific medication utilized, although drugs that impact the renin-angiotensin system (ACE and ARB drugs) are more effective at preventing the progression of nephropathy as well as cardiovascular problems and thus are the preferred starting agents, unless there is a specific contraindication. Often a low dose diuretic is added to the mix. Based on the RENAAL (Reduction of Endpoints in NIDDM [non-insulin-dependent diabetes mellitus] with the Angiotensin II Antagonist Losartan) trial and the Irbesartan Diabetic Nephropathy Trial (IDNT), the American Diabetes Association has recommended ACE inhibitors as first-line therapy for patients with Type 1 diabetes and nephropathy and ARBs for Type 2 patients with nephropathy. On average, the person with diabetes and hypertension may need three to four drugs to reach goal blood pressure of less than 130/80 mm Hg. There are many choices, and therapy must be individualized in each case.

If a patient with diabetes consumes a diet with excessively high protein content, then he or she is more likely to develop kidney abnormalities. Several studies have shown that restriction of protein and phosphate in the diet can slow the decline in renal function. Currently, patients with diabetes are taught to eat no more than 0.8 g/kg/day of protein. Lowering their protein intake even further to less than 0.6 g/kg/day may place less strain on their kidneys and may slow the development of kidney disease. A meta-analysis showed this to be true; however, many patients find these dietary changes very difficult to maintain and impractical.

See also DIABETES MELLITUS.

Hsu, Chi-yuan, M.D., et al. "Risk Factors for End-Stage Renal Disease." *Archives of Internal Medicine* 169, no. 4 (2009): 342–350.

Pedrini, M. T., A. S. Levey, J. Lau, and T. C. Chalmers. "The Effect of Dietary Protein Restriction on the Progression of Diabetic and Nondiabetic Renal Disease: A Meta-Analysis." *Annals of Internal Medicine* 124, no. 7 (April 1, 1996): 627–632.

United States Renal Data System: The Concise 2009 Annual Data Report. 2009. Available online. URL: http://www.usrds.org/2009/usrds_booklet_09.pdf. Accessed November 13, 2009.

Erb's palsy Tremors and weaknesses that have occurred as the result of an injury to a newborn infant as the consequence of a birthing crisis. This medical problem may be found in infants who are very large (macrosomic) at the time of delivery. Women with diabetes diagnosed prior to pregnancy or who have GESTATIONAL DIABETES have a greater risk of delivering very large babies, particularly when their glucose levels are not under control.

Erb's palsy is the result of harm to the fourth and fifth nerve roots in the baby, which usually occurs because the baby cannot move its arm and shoulder correctly while being delivered. SHOULDER DYSTOCIA is a common cause of the problem but it can also occur without shoulder dystocia.

According to author Barbara Apgar in an article for *American Family Physician,* 80 percent of the cases of Erb's palsy resolve within three to six months and only 1–5 percent are unresolved after a one-year period. In a two-year study, 126 incidents of shoulder dystocia were found among 9,071 children born of vaginal deliveries. Of these, 40 children had Erb's palsy and it is estimated that the risk of the infant having Erb's palsy with shoulder dystocia is 18.3 percent.

When children with Erb's palsy did *not* have shoulder dystocia, they were generally not as large as the babies that did have shoulder dystocia and were within the normal range of birth weights. The babies that did not have shoulder dystocia were more likely to have experienced fractures of the clavicle. These children generally took longer to recover.

See also PREGNANCY.

Apgar, Barbara. "Spontaneous Vaginal Delivery and Risk of Erb's Palsy." *American Family Physician* 58, no. 4 (1998): 973–976.

erectile dysfunction (ED) An inability to attain or maintain an erection that is satisfactory for sexual intercourse. Also commonly referred to as impotence. Men with diabetes have a greater risk for ED than nondiabetic men.

Erectile dysfunction does *not* refer to an occasional inability to attain or maintain an erection, nor does it include diminished libido (sex drive), premature ejaculation, or the inability to ejaculate or reach orgasm. Many men have intermittent sexual difficulties, and this is normal. It is when the problem becomes frequent or constant that the diagnosis may be one of erectile dysfunction. Erectile dysfunction is usually not a sudden problem but is rather a more gradual one. That is, the man may have some difficulty maintaining an erection but it is still possible. Then the instances of difficulty gradually increase to a point where he may not be able to attain an erection at all.

Who Has Erectile Dysfunction

Erectile dysfunction is a common problem for an estimated 10–15 million men in the United States, and the rate of ED increases with age. About 5 percent of all men who are age 40 have problems with impotence. This percentage rises to about 15–25 percent of men at the age of 65.

It is estimated that 50–60 percent of men with diabetes who are over age 50 have problems with erectile dysfunction. In addition, ED becomes a problem for men with diabetes about 10 to 15 years earlier than when it becomes a problem for nondiabetic males.

Major Causes of ED

In general, erectile dysfunction may be caused by diseases or injuries or may be due to a side effect of other medications that the man is taking. Any problem that affects the blood flow or nerve connections to the penis can cause ED.

Smoking can cause ED because it can affect the blood flow to the arteries and veins.

Hormonal causes may also be a factor in causing erectile dysfunction, such as a low amount of the male hormone, testosterone. Sometimes replacement therapy with supplemental testosterone can resolve the problem; however, this is rarely the cause of ED. Instead, low testosterone levels generally cause men to have low libido with intact erectile function.

Many medications can cause a temporary problem with erectile dysfunction and experts estimate that up to 25 percent of all cases of ED are related to medications. Some examples of particular categories of drugs which have such a side effect are: hypertension medications (especially beta-blockers and diuretics), antihistamines, tranquilizers, and most antidepressants. Even a common over-the-counter drug such as Tagamet, taken for stomach upset or heartburn, can impair the ability to have an erection. Illegal drugs such as anabolic steroids that are taken for weightlifting and marijuana, cocaine, heroin, or any narcotic may also cause or contribute to ED.

Surgery on the prostate gland or in the pelvis or genitourinary tract in general may also cause ED. In most cases, if the entire prostate gland is removed (usually because of cancer), the man will develop ED. However, some specialty urologists seek to maintain the nerve connections, even with removal of the entire gland, so that the man can still achieve erections.

Diabetes and Erectile Dysfunction

ED in men with diabetes is often multifactorial. Poor glycemic control will damage both nerves (DIABETIC NEUROPATHY) and blood vessels (ATHEROSCLEROSIS). Medications used to treat HYPERTENSION or DIABETIC NEPHROPATHY also can lead to ED.

When men with diabetes are heavy consumers of ALCOHOL (two to three drinks per day or more), they increase their risk of ED. ALCOHOL ABUSE can also subvert sexual relationships.

Emotional Issues Related to Erectile Dysfunction

Sometimes emotional or psychological concerns can be involved in ED. Interestingly, as recently as 20 to 30 years ago, it was thought that the majority of ED cases were caused by psychological or emotional problems. At that time, most experts believed that only in a minority of cases was there an underlying physical cause for the ED. Now it is known that the reverse is true and that most ED actually stems from physical problems rather than psychological ones.

Despite this, it is undeniable that an inability to achieve or sustain an erection may cause great anxiety in a man and that anxiety can further contribute to his difficulties with erection. Ironically, he may become so worried about whether or not he can achieve an erection that the very worry itself contributes or causes him to be unable to have one. It is also true that the man may not be worried about his sexuality but instead be very stressed about other problems such as at work or with other issues. Stress definitely contributes to ED.

Diagnosing Erectile Dysfunction

Most cases of ED in the United States are first evaluated by the patient's primary care provider, internist or family practitioner, or endocrinologist. The patient may also be referred to a urologist for further evaluation and treatment. Often the urologist will wish to question both the man and his sexual partner, to obtain an understanding of the full extent of the problem. The physician will make a diagnosis based on the man's medical history, a physical examination, and a limited number of laboratory tests. Some laboratory tests that the doctor may order for a man with diabetes are:

- HgbA1c
- free testosterone
- thyroid function

- prolactin levels
- kidney function
- liver function

Important areas of the physical exam are an assessment of the following:

- secondary sexual characteristics (scalp, axillary, pubic hair, muscle mass, pitch of voice)
- arterial pulses
- size and shape of the penis and testicles

The doctor will also examine the penis itself for any abnormalities and will often order a urinalysis to determine if there may be an infection that is contributing to the problem.

Treating Erectile Dysfunction

There are a variety of different treatments for ED, including medications, devices, and surgery. The most commonly known remedy is sildenafil (Viagra).

Viagra and erectile dysfunction Viagra (sildenafil) was approved by the FDA in 1998 and was immediately a very popular drug. It raises the nitric oxide in the blood vessels in the penis, allowing them to stay distended and trapping the blood in place in order to maintain the erection. Viagra has proven successful in about 56 percent of men with diabetes who have erectile dysfunction. (The success rate for nondiabetic men is about 70 percent.) Viagra is taken an hour or two before intercourse is planned. Viagra must be absorbed and delivered by the bloodstream to the appropriate blood vessels. The standard starting dosage is 50 mg.

Sexual stimulation is still necessary to attain an erection when taking Viagra. According to an article by Drs. Neelima V. Chu and Steven V. Edelman in the winter 2001 issue of *Clinical Diabetes,* a patient complained to physicians that Viagra did not work at all for him. Doctors later learned that the man took the pill and then he sat on the couch and read a book about how to grow tomatoes. This did not sexually stimulate him; hence, Viagra had no effect.

Viagra should only be prescribed for men who have problems with ED since it has no effect on sexual desire or the ability to ejaculate/come to orgasm. Men who note that Viagra greatly improves their sex lives almost always had erectile dysfunction problems. Viagra is not intended to be used by men with normal erectile function because it will not improve their erectile function to a significant degree. If a man says that Viagra dramatically improved his sexual performance, then he may have had ED prior to taking Viagra.

Most doctors suggest that their patients use the 50 mg dose a minimum of three times with limited or no success before increasing the medication to the 100 mg dose. Many managed care plans will now cover a limited number of Viagra tablets monthly, generally between five and 10.

Side effects of Viagra There are side effects to using Viagra, for some men. Facial or body flushing (reddening) is a common side effect. About 10–15 percent of men experience headaches, and nasal congestion is seen in 5–10 percent of men. One side effect reported by some men is having a transient change in color vision, so that they feel like they are wearing blue sunglasses for several hours. This is because the drug affects enzyme levels in the retina.

Viagra must never be used by a man who is taking any form of nitroglycerin, whether it is an oral tablet, sublingual tablet, spray, topical patch or paste. The combination of Viagra and nitrates can cause the blood pressure to drop suddenly and cause fatal hypotension (low blood pressure).

If a man with ED uses Viagra and then he develops chest pain (angina) during or within 24–48 hours after intercourse occurs, then he *absolutely* cannot use nitrates. He must also immediately proceed to the nearest hospital facility to obtain relief of symptoms with another type of analgesic such as morphine. Of course, he must also inform the ER staff that he has taken Viagra.

Other drugs Viagra is not the only medication for erectile dysfunction. Other drugs can be injected directly into the penis in order to dilate the blood vessels. Caverject (alprostadil) and Genabid (papaverine) have been used in this manner, with a success rate of over 70 percent. The patient is trained to self-inject the drug about 10–15 minutes prior to planned intercourse. Patients have reported that the injection is not painful.

An insertable pellet is another drug that may succeed. Muse (alprostadil) is a pellet, inserted into the urethra, and used 5–10 minutes before intercourse. It should not be used to have intercourse with a pregnant woman because it could be dangerous to the woman and/or the fetus.

Nondrug treatments Other nondrug treatments for erectile dysfunction are also available. For example, there are mechanical vacuum devices that force blood into the penis and they are reported to succeed for about 67 percent of men with erectile dysfunction.

Surgical solutions Surgery may be the answer for some men. The doctor may implant a device called a prosthesis, which can restore erection. The prosthesis may be an implant or a rod that is inserted into the penis and which the man can manually adjust. There are also inflatable implants. According to experts, the primary problem with surgery is postoperative infection, which may be difficult to treat because of the location of the infection. Also, if the patient does have surgery, the other options, such as oral medications or vacuum devices, will no longer work.

The problem that is causing impotence is rarely an internal blockage; however, if a blockage is present, it can be surgically corrected.

See also MEN WITH DIABETES.

estrogen replacement therapy See HORMONE REPLACEMENT THERAPY.

euglycemia/normoglycemia A level of blood glucose that is within the normal range. This level can vary, depending on whether the blood is measured from a finger stick (capillary) or a venipuncture (vein), or it is taken arterially. Normalcy also depends on whether the blood test is taken when a person is fasting or after a meal. Typically, the normal fasting range is 65–109 mg/dL.

The person with diabetes (both Type 1 and Type 2 diabetes) uses HOME BLOOD GLUCOSE MONITORING to try to reach or approach this goal of glycemic normalcy or to be as close as possible to the normal glucose levels. By doing so successfully, he or she greatly reduces the risk of serious medical COMPLICATIONS in the future, as proven by clinical studies, most notably the DIABETES CONTROL AND COMPLICATIONS TRIAL (DCCT) on people with Type 1 diabetes and also the UNITED KINGDOM PROSPECTIVE DIABETES STUDY on people with Type 2 diabetes.

See also GLYCEMIC CONTROL.

exercise Planned and often repetitive physical activity with the goal of improving physical fitness and overall health. Regular exercise is very important for people who have diabetes because it reduces the risk of HYPERTENSION, OBESITY, DEPRESSION, joint disorders, and other ailments. At the same time, people with Type 1 diabetes need to carefully monitor their glucose levels as a routine part of their exercise regimens, because they could become either hyperglycemic or hypoglycemic as a result of exercise. Monitoring their blood levels will let them know, for example, if a glucose snack is indicated or if more insulin is needed.

People with Type 2 diabetes usually have fewer problems with exercise causing hypoglycemia and it often will improve their glucose levels, moving them toward the normal range.

Exercise need not be complicated or intense, and moderate exercise can reap very large rewards for people with diabetes. For example, researchers of one study that was reported in the *Archives of Internal Medicine* evaluated about 5,000 British men with Type 2 diabetes who were between the ages of 40–59 years. These men had no family history of cardiac problems. The study found a direct and inverse relationship between exercise and cardiac problems: the more physical activity that the men engaged in, the less their risk for a heart attack.

It can also be risky to pursue extremely active physical activities after living a sedentary life. According to the 1996 Surgeon General's report, physical activity should not be excessive because it

> can sometimes cause persons with diabetes (particularly those who take insulin for blood glucose control) to experience detrimental effects, such as worsening of hyperglycemia and ketosis from poorly controlled diabetes, hypoglycemia (insulin-reaction) either during vigorous physical activity or—more commonly—several hours after prolonged physical activity, complications from proliferative retinopathy (e.g. detached retina), complications from superficial foot injuries, and a risk of myocardial infarction and sudden death, particularly among older people with NIDDM [Type 2 diabetes] and advanced, but silent, coronary atherosclerosis. These risks can be minimized by a pre-exercise medical evaluation and by taking proper precautions.

This does not, however, mean that people with diabetes must always restrict themselves to only moderate exercise. If the physician agrees, individuals with diabetes can engage in very active exercise. Swimmer Gary Hall, Jr. has diabetes and it did not hold him back from winning an Olympic gold medal in Australia in 2000.

Exercise Can Prevent or Delay Diabetes

Regular exercise among people who do not have diabetes generally decreases the probability that they will later develop Type 2 diabetes, particularly when the primary problem is INSULIN RESISTANCE, or the body's inability to effectively use all the insulin that is produced.

In a study of male physicians who were at high risk for later developing Type 2 diabetes (due to a family history of diabetes, their own hypertension, and other factors), researchers found an inverse relationship between physical activity and the onset of diabetes. The more that the men exercised, the less likely they were to develop diabetes.

Regular exercise also decreases the risks for developing STROKE, OSTEOPOROSIS, and other serious medical problems that are more commonly found among sedentary individuals, including some forms of cancer, such as colon cancer.

Exercise Precautions for People with Diabetes

Any person with diabetes who plans to engage in an exercise program after an inactive period should have a physical examination. They should be sure to have their eyes, kidneys, heart, and nervous system checked by the doctor and should also discuss the type of exercise they plan to engage in, so that the doctor can offer advice.

Some people with diabetes should also have an exercise stress test before undergoing a moderate or intensive exercise program in order to rule out CARDIOVASCULAR DISEASE. According to the American Diabetes Association in their 2001 Position Statement on exercise, people who fit the following categories are most likely to need a stress test before undertaking moderate or high intensity exercise. Those who:

- are over age 35
- have had Type 2 diabetes for more than 10 years
- have had Type 1 diabetes for more than 15 years
- have any microvascular diseases, such as nephropathy (kidney disease) or proliferative retinopathy
- have peripheral vascular disease
- have autonomic neuropathy
- have any other risk factors for coronary artery disease (hypertension, hyperlipidemia, family history)

Precautions on Types of Exercise

The type of exercise they choose to perform is also very important for people with diabetes, particularly if they have any diabetic complications. For example, according to the American

Diabetes Association, a person with diabetic retinopathy should avoid weight lifting, jogging, racquet sports, and high impact aerobic exercise, because such types of exercise could worsen their condition. Instead, better choices would be low-impact activities such as walking, swimming, and stationary cycling.

A person with some loss of sensations, such as neuropathy that affects the feet, should avoid jogging, using the treadmill or prolonged walking. Instead, swimming, bicycling, and other nonweight-bearing exercises would be preferable. Of course, whatever exercise the person chooses should be performed wearing well-fitted and well-made athletic shoes and socks. Shoes and socks should be changed after exercising.

How Much Exercise Is Enough?

According to the Surgeon General's 1996 report on physical activity, individuals over the age of two years should engage in 30 minutes of endurance-type physical activity that is moderately intense on all or most days of the week—with the warning that people with diabetes, cardiovascular diseases, and other chronic health problems would first consult with their doctor before starting an exercise program. In addition, all previously inactive men who are over age 40 or previously inactive women over age 50 should discuss their new fitness plans with their doctor first.

Older Individuals and Exercise

People who are over age 65 and have diabetes as well as other ailments can still benefit from exercise but they also need to make adaptations. For example, if they lift weights, older indi-

viduals should lift lighter weights than younger individuals. They also will probably do fewer repetitions of exercises and may need special shoes and other items. Dr. Robert Petrella said in his 1999 article for *Physician & Sportsmedicine:*

> Exercise is an effective adjunctive treatment for patients who have Type 2 diabetes, especially for those who are older. Patients should be instructed on how to integrate diet and hydration management with workouts and glucose monitoring, use of proper footwear, and adequate warm-up and cool-down routines. Patients may want to consult a podiatrist or athletic trainer with expertise in footwear. Timing high-energy snacks with workouts and balanced fluids should facilitate a euglycemic exercise.

American Diabetes Association. "Diabetes Mellitus and Exercise." *Diabetes Care* 24, Supp. 1 (2001): S51–S55.

Petrella, Robert J., M.D. "Exercise for Older Patients with Chronic Disease." *Physician & Sportsmedicine* 27, no. 11 (October 15, 1999). Available online. URL: www.physsports.med.comissues/1999/10_15_99/petrella.htm.

U.S. Department of Health and Human Services. *Physical Activity and Health: A Report of the Surgeon General.* Atlanta, Ga.: U.S. Department of Health and Human Services, Centers for Disease Control and Prevention, National Center for Chronic Disease Prevention and Health Promotion, 1996.

Wannamethee, S. Goya, et al. "Physical Activity, Metabolic Factors, and the Incidence of Coronary Heart Disease and Type 2 Diabetes." *Archives of Internal Medicine* 160, no. 14 (2000): 2,108–2,116.

eye diseases See DIABETIC EYE DISEASES.

family, the impact of diabetes on   The effect of family members on a person with diabetes and his or her effect on them. The family of the person with diabetes has a major role in his or her life and can provide enormous care and support. Children and adolescents with diabetes need their parents and other family members to assist them in monitoring and controlling their symptoms. Adults with diabetes should educate other family members, including children, on their needs and possible dangerous symptoms, such as indicators of possible HYPOGLYCEMIA. Family members will also need to know how to inject GLUCAGON for severe hypoglycemia, if needed.

See also FAMILY AND MEDICAL LEAVE ACT.

Fisher, Lawrence, et al. "The Family and Disease Management in Hispanic and European-American Patients with Type 2 Diabetes." *Diabetes Care* 23, no. 3 (2000): 267–272.

Family and Medical Leave Act (FMLA)   A law in the United States that allows leave from work in relation to the illness of an employee or family members.

Enacted by the U.S. Congress in 1993, the Family and Medical Leave Act went into effect on August 5, 1993 and the final regulations took effect on April 6, 1995. The law requires most employers in the United States to allow employees who have worked for them for at least a year (and have met other provisions of the law) to take up to 12 weeks of *unpaid* leave per year.

There are two primary reasons for leave: a serious health condition in oneself or in another family member who needs an employee's care

and assistance. A serious health condition is defined as "an illness, injury, impairment, or physical or mental condition that involves inpatient care or continuing treatment by a health care provider." As a result, if a person was hospitalized and then needed to recuperate at home for some period, the FMLA would generally apply.

The FMLA specifically lists diabetes under the law in 29 C.F.R. § 825.114 (a)(1), (2), where it is one of five situations under "continuing treatment by a health care provider." That situation is defined as follows: "any period of incapacity or treatment due to a chronic serious health condition requiring periodic visits for treatment, including episodic conditions such as asthma, diabetes, and epilepsy."

Thus, if a person with diabetes becomes seriously ill or a family member becomes seriously ill with complications from diabetes or other illnesses that fit the parameters, then the provisions of the FMLA could be used.

The person may also take time off under the FMLA to take care of a new baby or newly adopted child (whether ill or not) or to care for a parent with a serious health condition.

The leave can be taken for 12 consecutive weeks or may be split up into smaller increments, according to the Department of Labor. The Department of Labor enforces violations of the FMLA.

Many people do not use the entire 12 weeks because the leave is unpaid and most people can only afford to take a few unpaid weeks off. The person may also combine paid sick leave from work with FMLA leave.

The employee has certain responsibilities under the law. For example, the employer must be notified about what the serious health condition is, although this can be done confidentially.

While on leave under the provisions of the FMLA, any health insurance benefits that the employee previously held before the leave will continue, as long as the employee pays the premium expense. When the leave is over, the employer must allow the worker to come back to the same job or to a comparable job.

To learn more about the FMLA, the employer's human resources office should be able to provide needed information. For background information on the FMLA and the Americans with Disabilities Act, the following Web site is useful: www.eeoc.gov/docs/fmlaada.html.

See also AMERICANS WITH DISABILITIES ACT; EMPLOYMENT.

fasting plasma glucose (FPG) test   See DIABETES MELLITUS.

fats   See CHOLESTEROL; HDL; LDL; TRIGLYCERIDE.

federal government   See GOVERNMENT, FEDERAL.

fertility   The ability to create a pregnancy. There are some indications that fertility may be impaired among people who have Type 2 diabetes.

In 2000, scientists reporting their results in *Nature* revealed that insulin receptor substrate-2 (IRS-2), a special cellular protein that is needed for a normal response to insulin, was also needed by mice to avoid obesity and infertility. Apparently, the lack of IRS-2 caused the mice to develop Type 2 diabetes and also to become infertile and obese. Scientists speculate that if IRS-2 should act in the same way in humans, then its lack could be the reason for Type 2 diabetes, as well as excessive eating and problems with fertility.

Because of the increasingly prevalent problem of OBESITY that is found in people in the United States as well as in other Western countries, this research finding may have profound implications, particularly if scientists can find a way to correct the genetic deficiency. Women with insulin resistance syndrome/polycystic ovarian syndrome often have irregular periods and anovulation leading to infertility that can be treated with METFORMIN, rosiglitazone, or pioglitazone (all non-FDA-approved for this indication.)

Burks, D. J., et al. "IRS-2 Pathways Integrate Female Reproduction and Energy Homeostasis." *Nature* 407 (September 2000): 377–382.

fiber   Material from plant cell walls that cannot be digested by the stomach but which the body can use to aid in the healthy functioning of the gastrointestinal tract. Many physicians recommend a diet that is high in fiber as a preventive to a broad array of medical problems. A high fiber diet has also been proven to benefit many people with diabetes. There are some indications that individuals with diabetes may consume even less fiber than the average American. Some studies have also indicated that eating WHOLE GRAIN FOODS may act as a factor to prevent the development of Type 2 diabetes.

Note: people with diabetes who also suffer from GASTROPARESIS (slow stomach emptying) or from colon dysmotility should consult with their physicians before increasing their fiber levels, because fiber can make these conditions worse.

Water insoluble fiber comes from wheat, wheat bran, and some fruits and vegetables. Water soluble fiber is found in oats, beans, peas, and some fruits and vegetables, and it may help lower blood lipid levels.

Some researchers believe that diets that are high in natural dietary fiber are very beneficial for individuals with both Type 1 and Type 2 diabetes because such a diet has the effect of both improving GLYCEMIC CONTROL and lowering CHOLESTEROL levels. High fiber diets that are recommended by experts include many servings of fruits and vegetables, generally far more helpings than are consumed by the average American. Some individuals increase their fiber intake by ingesting fiber powder that is mixed with water or by eating high fiber wafers.

In a 2000 article in the *New England Journal of Medicine,* researchers studied 12 men and one woman with Type 2 diabetes who had greatly increased their consumption of fiber to about 50 grams per week. This is roughly triple what the average American consumes in fiber every week and is approximately double what is recommended by the American Diabetes Association, as of this writing.

Subjects were placed on either a high fiber diet for six weeks or the American Diabetes Association (ADA) diet for six weeks. At the end of the six weeks, subjects switched to the other diet.

The results: the glucose levels for the high fiber group improved significantly. Other improvements were also found. For example, the high fiber diet lowered the subjects' total cholesterol concentrations by nearly 7 percent. In addition, this diet resulted in cutting back triglyceride concentration by about 10 percent and also in reducing very low-density lipoprotein cholesterol concentrations ("bad" cholesterol) by 12.5 percent.

The researchers concluded that dietary guidelines for individuals with Type 2 diabetes "should emphasize an overall increase in dietary fiber through the consumption of unfortified foods, rather than the use of fiber supplements."

The researchers said their subjects had excellent compliance with the high fiber diet. However, others have stated that they would have great difficulty in convincing patients that they should eat twice as much fiber as the level recommended by the American Diabetes Association. The researchers themselves speculated that it would be difficult to convince most patients to increase their fiber intake so greatly.

In another study of 63 patients with Type 1 diabetes, 32 subjects were placed on a high fiber diet (about 30 grams per day) and 31 on a low fiber diet for 24 weeks. It should be noted that the percentage of fiber given to these subjects was lower in this study than in the *New England Journal of Medicine* study.

Researchers reported that about 83 percent of the subjects were compliant with the high fiber diet. Of those who did comply, individuals on the high fiber diet significantly improved their glucose control and they had less incidences of hypoglycemia. The high fiber diet group experienced more incidents of mild gastrointestinal complaints.

Fruits that are especially high in fiber content are: apples, blueberries, avocados, blackberries, oranges, and pears. Vegetables that are high in fiber content are: peas, Brussels sprouts, carrots, green beans, and tomatoes.

In the EURODIAB IDDM Complications Study, an increased fiber intake led to lower LDL and increased HDL in men and women with Type 1 diabetes.

See also NUTRITION.

Chandalia, Manisha, M.D., et al. "Beneficial Effects of High Dietary Fiber Intake in Patients with Type 2 Diabetes Mellitus." *The New England Journal of Medicine* 342 (May 11, 2000): 1,392–1,398.

Giacco, Rosalba, M.D., et al. "Long-Term Dietary Treatment with Increased Amounts of Fiber-Rich Low-Glycemic Index Natural Foods Improves Blood Glucose Control and Reduces the Number of Hypoglycemic Events in Type 1 Diabetic Patients." *Diabetes Care* 23, no. 10 (October 2000): 1,461–1,466.

Toeller, M., et al. "Fiber Intake, Serum Cholesterol Levels, and Cardiovascular Disease in European Individuals with Type 1 Diabetes: The EURODIAB IDDM Complication Study Group." *Diabetes Care* 22 (1999): B21–B28.

flu   See IMMUNIZATIONS.

foot care   For people with Type 1 or Type 2 diabetes mellitus, careful attention to and care of their feet is very important because diabetes overlays an escalated risk for the development of foot ulcers and infections. Individuals with diabetes also risk the subsequent loss of a foot or even a leg by AMPUTATION as a result of problems with their feet.

Research has shown that among diabetics, nearly 85 percent of all their amputations were preceded by a foot ulcer. The majority of all amputations for any reason (about 60 percent) occur to people with diabetes, according to the Centers for Disease Control and Prevention (CDC). In addition, there were 71,000 hospital discharges for nontraumatic (not caused by an accident, such as a car crash) lower extremity amputations among diabetics in 2005 in the United States. Yet it is estimated that more than half of all diabetic foot complications are preventable.

Because people with diabetes often experience a loss of sensation in their feet, an actual examination of their feet is necessary, since the pain that would normally alert another person to an ulcer or infection or other damage may be absent. According to Andrew J. M. Boulton, M.D., and colleagues in their 2008 article for *Diabetes Care*, the lifetime risk for foot ulcers in a person with diabetes may be up to 25 percent, compared to the annual incidence of about 2 percent in nondiabetics.

General Foot Care Recommendations

Foot care includes at least annual examinations of the feet by a physician and/or a podiatrist, as well as the regular cleaning and drying of the feet and careful trimming of toenails, whether this care is performed by the person with diabetes or someone else. The feet should also be examined for any sores, cuts, or other damage during the annual foot examination. (Among high-risk individuals who have had foot ulcers or infections in the past, the foot examination should be performed every six months.)

In addition, people with diabetes should check their own feet every day, and they should *never* go barefoot (even inside their homes). In addition, they should always wear shoes that are chosen more for comfort than for stylish-

ness; thus, high heels are not recommended for females with diabetes, no matter how stylish they may be at the time.

According to the National Diabetes Education Program (NDEP), podiatrists should assess the health of the foot by considering the presence of neuropathy, vasculopathy, dermatological conditions, musculoskeletal conditions, and the patient's lifestyle and family medical history. For example, neuropathy is the presence of a feeling of burning, tingling, or numbness in the foot, which may indicate that peripheral sensory neuropathy is a problem. This condition can be detected with the use of special monofilaments. The NDEP offers these filaments as well as a description of how to perform a foot examination in a free kit that is available at http://www.ndep.nih.gov/diabetes/pubs/Feet_Kit_Eng.pdf.

Claudication (vasculopathy) is a general term meaning that there is a problem with the blood vessels. It refers to the cramping of the calf muscles during walking, which requires the person to take frequent rest periods. This condition may be caused by an insufficient blood supply to the area under the knee, which further indicates an early or moderate occlusion of the arteries (peripheral arterial disease or PAD). Patients may also experience intense aching and cramping in their toes at night that is relieved only by either hanging their feet over the side of the bed or by walking around. (This condition is referred to by doctors as rest claudication or neuropathy.)

Dermatological conditions refer to dryness (a form of neuropathy and the inability to sweat) and corns and calluses in the feet. They often occur before blisters or ulcerations develop. The presence of corns and calluses can also indicate that the patient has sensory neuropathy. Fungal infections are another issue of concern because they may lead to the development of secondary bacterial infections.

The foot examination will also show the presence of musculoskeletal symptoms, such as the presence of flat feet, bunions, high-arched feet, or hammertoes, all of which conditions cause irritation to the feet.

The family history of the diabetic is also important. If there is a family history for coronary artery disease or cerebrovascular accidents, this may indicate an increased risk for lower-extremity arterial complications.

Three Primary Types of Foot Care Problems Among Diabetics

There are three primary types of foot problems that people with diabetes may experience: peripheral neuropathy, peripheral vascular disease, and infection. In addition, foot ulcers are a serious problem.

Peripheral neuropathy of the foot When a person has *peripheral sensory neuropathy,* this means that they still may feel some pain, but that the pain itself is not always a reliable indicator of the severity of a foot injury. Typically, the loss of sensation is the most worrisome type of neuropathy because it can mask a significant acute injury as well as mask repetitive minor traumas that can subsequently lead to an ulceration. This loss of sensation of feedback from the feet can also hide problems that are caused by poorly fitting footwear. The loss of sensation is also why people with diabetes need to visually inspect their feet every day.

Warren Clayton, Jr., M.D., and Tom A. Elasy, M.D., further explain the need for the examination of the feet in a 2009 issue of *Clinical Diabetes.* "The loss of sensation as a part of peripheral neuropathy exacerbates the development of ulcerations. As trauma occurs at the affected site, patients are often unable to detect the insult to their lower extremities. As a result, many wounds go unnoticed and progressively worsen as the affected area is continuously subjected to repetitive pressure and shear forces from ambulation [moving about] and weight bearing."

Peripheral vascular disease in the foot Another form of foot damage is *peripheral vascular disease* (PVD or PAD), a circulation disorder that can cause severe cramping with activity (claudication) and that may cause the affected foot to become very red. People with diabetes who are diagnosed with peripheral vascular disease are at risk for infection and even for the development of gangrene. They may need special (therapeutic) shoes. If they are unable to examine the bottoms of their own feet, then they need someone else to check their feet, including the soles, or they need to use mirrors to check their feet for injuries or damage. PVD leads to intermittent claudication, which is pain in the buttocks, thighs, calves, or the feet. It indicates a poor blood flow to the affected area.

Foot infections Any infection of the foot can contribute to foot damage. When such infections are combined with hyperglycemia, then a foot injury takes longer to heal, and the infection could spread to the bone and even lead to the necessity for the amputation of limbs. After a study of 1,666 diabetic patients who were followed for two years for foot care infections, Lawrence A. Lavery and colleagues discussed their results in a 2006 issue of *Diabetes Care.* The researchers found that of 151 subjects evaluated over two years, 9.1 percent developed 199 foot infections, and nearly all of these infections involved either a wound or a penetrating injury.

The patients who developed a foot infection had a 55.7 times greater risk of hospitalization than those without foot infections, and they also experienced a rate of amputation that was 154.5 times greater than those without foot infections. The authors said, "Foot infections occur relatively frequently in individuals with diabetes, almost always follow trauma, and dramatically increase the risk of hospitalization and amputation. Efforts to prevent infections should be targeted at people with traumatic foot wounds, especially those that are chronic, deep, recurrent, or associated with peripheral vascular disease."

Foot Ulcers

Individuals with diabetes are more likely to suffer from foot ulcers than are nondiabetics. According to Warren Clayton, Jr., M.D., and Tom A. Elasy, M.D., in their article on foot ulcers in diabetic patients for *Clinical Diabetes* in 2009, the reported incidence of foot ulcers in the United States and the United Kingdom (UK) is as high as 10 percent. They report that diabetic foot ulcers often have multiple causes. About 60 percent of all foot ulcers are caused by DIABETIC NEUROPATHY, or nerve damage that is caused by diabetes. This neuropathy causes an imbalance between the extension and flexion of the foot and leads to foot deformities that in turn lead to abnormal pressure points and bony prominences. Autonomic neuropathy causes a decrease in sweating, and thus the foot is not moisturized, and the skin becomes dry and can become more easily cracked and damaged.

In their chapter in *Joslin's Diabetes Deskbook: A Guide for Primary Care Providers,* authors Richard S. Beaser, M.D., and John M. Giurini report that 15 percent of individuals with diabetes develop foot ulcers, and 50 percent of those with foot ulcers will have a recurrence of the problem within two years. In addition, they report that 20 percent of patients with foot ulcers must undergo an amputation.

Treatment of foot ulcers According to Clayton, Jr., and Elasy, offloading and debridement are two vital treatment aspects of foot ulcers. Offloading refers to taking the weight off the foot ulcers, and this task can be accomplished in a variety of ways: with a total cast of the foot or with cast walkers, half shoes, crutches or even with requiring the patient to use a wheelchair. Each choice has advantages and disadvantages, which the physician should explain to the patient.

Debridement refers to the removal of dead or unhealthy skin tissue. This will rid the area of dangerous bacteria. The doctor may, on occasion, also wish to culture the wound to determine what pathogens are infecting the foot, if any. Typically these wounds are polymicrobial, involving many types of bacteria.

Clayton, Jr., and Elasy say that the most common microbes that are likely to infect diabetic feet are gram-positive cocci, although the person may also be infected with gram-negative rods or anaerobic bacteria. However, some patients are infected with pathogens that are resistant to antibiotics, such as methicillin-resistant staphylococcus aureus (MRSA). This is a situation that is more likely to occur among patients who were recently treated with antibiotics, were hospitalized, or who reside in a long-term care facility, such as a nursing home. Patients with severe infections need to be hospitalized and to receive intravenous mediation.

Some patients with foot ulcers are treated with hyperbaric oxygen therapy (HBOT). This involves placing the patient in an environment that delivers oxygen at higher than normal atmospheric pressures. This is a controversial therapy for foot ulcers as of this writing, although the Centers for Medicare & Medicaid Services (CMS) offers reimbursement for HBOT for the treatment of diabetic ulcers, as of this writing.

Foot ulcers and amputation Studies have revealed disturbing statistics surrounding problems with foot ulceration among people with diabetes. In a study of 449 patients with foot ulcers, reported in 2006 in *Diabetes Care* by researchers William J. Jeffcoate and colleagues, the researchers analyzed patients referred to a foot care clinic and studied the outcome of one foot ulcer in each patient. Of those patients whose foot ulcers healed, the healing time was an average 78 days.

The researchers found that of the 449 patients, less than half (45.0 percent) were alive and foot ulcer–free after 12 months. About 11 percent of the patients had experienced amputation and about 17 percent had died. These grim statistics are reminders that, even with the care of a foot clinic, the outcome can be serious, and it is likely that without foot care, the risk for amputations and death would be even greater. The researchers said, "These data illustrate the extent to which ulcer-related outcomes may underestimate the true morbidity [disease] and mortality [death] associated with diabetic foot disease."

Foot Deformities Caused by Diabetes

Charcot's foot (also called Charcot's joint or CHARCOT'S ARTHROPATHY) is another serious medical problem experienced by people with diabetes. It is also one that should be treated immediately because the joints can self-destruct within weeks of the onset of the disease. Charcot's foot is due to a loss of sensation in the joint and bones, which causes bone destruction and drastic changes in the shape of the feet. If patients develop warm and swollen joints in their feet, they should seek immediate medical attention. Often there is only slight pain, so pain is not an indicator of the severity of the problem. Charcot's foot is often misdiagnosed as an infection.

Other foot deformities experienced by people with diabetes are bunions, corns, calluses, and blisters. Of course, people who do not have diabetes may experience these foot problems; however, when the person also has a lack of feeling in the foot, he or she often goes untreated. As a result, these foot problems, which may start out as minor medical problems can escalate rapidly to serious and even life-threatening conditions.

Important Specific Aspects of Foot Care

According to the National Institute on Diabetes Information Clearinghouse, individuals with diabetes should clean and inspect their feet every day, keeping in mind the following points:

- Use warm, not hot, water and mild soap. Use a soft towel to dry the feet and also between the toes.
- Inspect the feet and toes daily for cuts, blisters, redness, swelling, calluses, or any other problems.
- Use lotion to moisturize the feet but do not get the lotion between the toes.
- File down corns and calluses gently with a pumice stone after a bath or shower.
- Cut the toenails to the shape of the toes and file the edges with an emery board each week or as needed.
- Always wear shoes or slippers to protect the feet from injury. Thick seamless socks may prevent skin irritation. Never go barefoot, even inside the house.

- Wear shoes that fit well and that also allow the toes to move around. Wear new shoes for only an hour at a time to break them in.
- Footwear should be adjustable with laces, Velcro, or buckles.
- Before putting on any shoes, check them carefully. Feel the insides to make sure there are no sharp edges, tears, or objects that could harm the feet.

Other suggestions by experts include the following for patients with diabetes who are at high risk for foot problems because of such factors as the loss of protective sensation, absent pedal (foot) pulses, a foot deformity, a history of a foot ulcer, and a prior amputation. Others who may be considered at high risk have uncontrolled glucose levels, hypertension, hyperlipidemia, and/or a continuation of the SMOKING habit.

- Clear the areas where the person with diabetes walks of any dangerous objects. Minor foot trauma caused by bumping into objects often leads to foot ulcers.
- Be sure that night lights are present so that the person with diabetes does not bump into or trip over objects when using the bathroom at night.
- Do not soak the feet. The diabetic person may have dry feet and impaired sweat glands and soaking could lead to cracking of the skin of the feet.
- Avoid scalding the feet at bath time by checking the temperature of bath water with the hand first or, if hand sensations are impaired, by using a thermometer.
- Immediately report all infections, ulcers, and cuts that do not heal after three days to the physician for evaluation. Deep cuts or wounds with dark discoloration should be reported to the physician the same day.
- High-risk feet should be checked at least twice a year, rather than annually.

Richard S. Beaser, M.D., and John M. Giurini have specific recommendations for different foot problems suffered by diabetics. For example, they advise that the diabetic person with sensory neuropathy should wear socks to keep moisture away from the skin and socks with extra padding can be helpful. They should also change socks frequently. For those with diabetic neuropathy, patients should wear athletic shoes or well-cushioned shoes to reduce the pressure. Soft orthotic devices may also be helpful but rigid devices should be avoided.

Other issues Some patients with diabetes will need to wear specially made shoes. If they are receiving Medicare, they may qualify for such shoes under the Medicare Therapeutic Shoe Act. They can receive a prescription for therapeutic shoes from their medical doctors. Medicare beneficiaries pay 20 percent of the Medicare-approved amount after meeting their annual Part B deductible.

It is also important for people with diabetes to make lifestyle changes. For example, they will need to adjust their patterns of exercise, going on shorter walks or exercising using stationary equipment rather than taking mile-long hikes. Individuals with diabetes should consult with their physicians for the best approach to preserve the health of their feet.

According to the American Diabetes Association, individuals with impaired or lost sensations in the feet should avoid any exercise that involves the treadmill, step exercises, jogging, and extended walking. Instead, the preferred exercise activities are swimming, bicycling, and rowing.

Smoking and Its Relation to the Feet

Smoking increases the risk for problems with the feet and also increases the risk for amputation of a lower limb. People with diabetes who smoke should stop immediately because according to the National Diabetes Education Program, those who smoke are four times more likely than are nondiabetic smokers to develop lower-extremity vascular disease.

Podiatry Care Is Important

Patients with diabetes who are at risk for feet problems should receive podiatric care because such care has been associated with a markedly reduced risk for lower extremity amputation as well as a decreased risk in ulceration rates. The podiatrist can also assist the diabetic patient in choosing appropriate footwear as needed. Some patients may need orthotics, or custom-molded shoes. The podiatrist can also evaluate the level of pain, if any, that the patient experiences and make recommendations to resolve or improve the pain.

See also DIABETES MELLITUS.

Beaser, Richard S., M.D., and John M. Giurini. "The Foot: Clinical Care and Problem Prevention." In *Joslin's Diabetes Deskbook: A Guide for Primary Care Providers,* 2nd edition, edited by Richard S. Beaser, M.D., and the Staff of Joslin Diabetes Center, Boston, Mass.: Joslin Diabetes Center, 2007, pp. 505–519.

Boulton, Andrew J. M., M.D., et al. "Comprehensive Foot Examination and Risk Assessment." *Diabetes Care* 31, no. 8 (2008): 1,679–1,685.

Clayton, Warren, Jr., M.D., and Tom A. Elasy, M.D. "A Review of the Pathophysiology, Classification, and Treatment of Foot Ulcers in Diabetic Patients." *Clinical Diabetes* 27, no. 2 (2009): 52–58.

Ghanassia, Edouard, M.D., et al. "Long-Term Outcome and Disability of Diabetic Patients Hospitalized for Diabetic Foot Ulcers." *Diabetes Care* 31, no. 7 (2008): 1,288–1,292.

Jeffcoate, William J., et al. "Assessing the Outcome of the Management of Diabetic Foot Ulcers Using Ulcer-Related and Person-Related Measures." *Diabetes Care* 29, no. 8 (2006): 1,784–1,787.

Lavery, Lawrence A., et al. "Risk Factors for Foot Infections in Individuals with Diabetes." *Diabetes Care* 29, no. 6 (2006): 1,288–1,293.

Working Together to Manage Diabetes: A Guide for Pharmacy, Podiatry, Optometry, and Dental Professionals. Washington, D.C.: National Diabetes Education Program, May 2007.

gangrene Death of body tissues that is usually caused by inadequate or no blood supply, followed by or accompanied with a very severe infection. This condition will lead to a loss of life if the affected body part is not amputated. People with diabetes are far more prone to developing gangrene because of their greater tendency to have circulatory difficulties (ATHEROSCLEROSIS) and nerve problems (DIABETIC NEUROPATHY), both of which can be exacerbated by poor glycemic control.

Around 1921 in North America (and before the discovery of insulin), many physicians did not treat gangrene with amputation because they felt that people with diabetes would not heal after the surgery. As a result, individuals who were affected had to suffer as the gangrene spread and wait until they died from the infection.

Amputation is still the common therapy for gangrene today, although physicians seek to prevent this infection by encouraging appropriate FOOT CARE. On occasion, an area of gangrene such as a toe is left to "auto-amputate" (essentially dries up and falls off due to complete lack of blood flow) but most of the time, the surgeon amputates the dead tissue and will save as much living tissue as possible.

Diabetes is not the only cause of gangrene. Injuries sustained during wartime were also responsible for cases of gangrene. For example, many people became aware of gangrene during the Civil War in the United States, when many soldiers were severely wounded in the leg or arm. Because of the lack of sanitation or antibiotics, infection and gangrene quickly set in. Doctors amputated the limb to save the soldier's life. An estimated 60,000 soldiers had limbs amputated during the Civil War, and few if any of them had diabetes.

gastroesophageal reflux disease (GERD) Chronic disease in which gastric acid backs up from the stomach into the esophagus. Also known as "acid reflux" disease or "heartburn." People with diabetes have a greater risk for developing GERD than nondiabetics.

According to a 1997 issue of *Diabetes Forecast,* as many as 75 percent of people with diabetes have problems with "motility," or the movement of the food along the esophagus. This problem can lead to GERD, in which acid "refluxes" or backs up, sometimes leading to regurgitation. This illness may be more common among individuals with diabetes, in part because of the presence of GASTROPARESIS, or a slower rate of stomach emptying than normal. Gastroparesis occurs largely because of nerve damage.

Some medications can lead to the development of GERD; for example, some medications prescribed for the treatment of hypertension can slow the action of the stomach and, subsequently, cause acid reflux. The primary medication culprits are aspirin and nonsteroidal anti-inflammatory drugs (NSAIDs). Medications known as COX-2 inhibitors are less likely to cause GERD or esophagitis, but may still do so.

Other illnesses contribute to or are associated with GERD; for example, OBESITY and untreated hypothyroidism are associated with acid reflux disease.

Symptoms and Diagnostic Path

The symptoms vary, but in general they include: heartburn, chronic cough, hoarseness, and difficulty swallowing. The individual with GERD may also have chest pains that are not cardiac in nature (if a heart attack has been ruled out). Some less common symptoms of GERD are: GINGIVITIS (gum disease), a constant sore throat, and the frequent clearing of the throat. GERD is also associated with asthma, although medical experts disagree on whether GERD results from asthma or GERD causes asthma. Many experts also believe that GERD causes a chronic cough and vocal cord dysfunction that may mimic asthma.

GERD symptoms are frequently ignored and the disease may go undiagnosed because it is not brought to a physician's attention until the individual has difficulty swallowing due to narrowing of the esophagus (stricture) or heartburn symptoms have become extremely severe, leading to esophagitis (erosion of the esophagus) and other ailments. Untreated GERD can lead to a precancerous condition known as "Barrett's esophagus."

Another symptom is the constant consumption of over-the-counter antacids. Some patients take as many as 20 or more antacids per day before asking a physician for help.

Treatment Options and Outlook

This illness may need to be treated by a gastroenterologist, a physician who is an expert in gastrointestinal diseases, but it is usually treated by internists and other primary care physicians.

Medications known as "proton pump inhibitors" or "H2 blockers" (histamine-2 blockers), usually taken as pills, are given to many people diagnosed with acid reflux disease. These medications can suppress the production of acid and enable the esophagus to heal. Some individuals may also need a prescribed dose of an antacid medication, because of a problem known as "nocturnal breakthrough" of GERD that can occur in the evening. In severe cases, surgery may be necessary.

Lifestyle changes recommended   Physicians generally recommend lifestyle changes for people who have been diagnosed with GERD, such as raising the head of the bed, taking smaller and more frequent meals (five small meals as opposed to three large ones), and avoiding eating a large meal at night. Some activities aggravate GERD, such as weightlifting, extensive bicycling, and jogging.

People with GERD should avoid SMOKING, which can exacerbate the illness. They should also restrict their consumption of ALCOHOL, caffeine, and fatty foods.

Obese individuals should lose weight because excessive weight can exacerbate heartburn symptoms.

Risk Factors and Preventive Measures

In addition to diabetes being a risk factor for GERD, other associated risk factors are smoking, alcohol consumption, an overall sedentary life, and obesity.

Elderly people, particularly those residing in skilled nursing facilities (SNFs, formerly known as "nursing homes"), are at high risk for developing GERD, largely because of two factors. SNF patients who must lie down most of the time and who get very little exercise are at risk for GERD. In addition, acid reflux may also be found in elderly individuals who have had acid reflux problems for years but symptoms were not recognized and the illness was not treated. The elderly person may complain less of heartburn than about the more atypical symptoms, which can in turn inhibit proper diagnosis.

See also DIGESTIVE DISORDERS; EXERCISE.

Minocha, A., M.D., and Christine Adamec. *How to Stop Heartburn: Simple Ways to Heal Heartburn & Acid Reflux.* New York: John Wiley & Sons, 2001.

gastroparesis diabeticorum   Refers to a delayed emptying of the stomach, due to nerve damage (AUTONOMIC NEUROPATHY) caused by diabetes. Gastroparesis may also be a consequence of medications that the patient takes that have a side effect of slowing down digestion, such as some antidepressants, tranquilizers, calcium channel–blocker medications, and other drugs.

As many as half of all patients with Type 1 and Type 2 diabetes have some level of gastroparesis. In some patients, the problem is so severe that the patient may require gastric surgery.

In the earlier stages of gastroparesis, the individual has a problem with the stomach's delay in digesting solids. If the condition deteriorates, then there is also a delay in the emptying of liquids as well. Patients with gastroparesis need to monitor their glucose levels to avoid hypoglycemia, especially if they are taking insulin. A new diagnosis of gastroparesis warrants referral to a diabetes care team.

Gastroparesis can make it very difficult for the person with diabetes to control glucose levels, including controlling them through both dietary and medication controls. Gastroparesis also often leads to GASTROESOPHAGEAL REFLUX DISEASE (GERD).

Symptoms and Diagnostic Path

Some individuals who have gastroparesis have no symptoms while others have problems with nausea, vomiting, anorexia, early satiety (feeling full very quickly), bloating, and abdominal pain. Acid reflux commonly accompanies gastroparesis.

Treatment Options and Outlook

Lifestyle changes are usually recommended for patients who have mild-to-moderate cases of gastroparesis, including a *low* fiber diet (because fiber may exacerbate the condition), and five or six small meals per day rather than three large meals. Some patients are placed on a liquid diet.

As of this writing, few medications are considered effective at treating gastroparesis. In the United States, metoclopramide is the only drug that is specifically approved for treatment of this condition; however, metoclopramide has serious potential side effects because of its action on the central nervous system, causing tremors and Parkinsonian effects. Domperidone is useful, as

are anti-emetic agents. Some physicians have also used erythromycin to treat gastroparesis. Cisapride was an effective medication for gastroparesis but because of its side effects, the Food and Drug Administration (FDA) decreed that it be prescribed on an individual basis only in the United States.

Medical procedures may be required in very severe cases. Some physicians have reported success with the endoscopic insertion of a percutaneous endoscopic jejunostomy (PEJ), although this procedure would not be used except in advanced cases. In this procedure, a tube is placed into the small bowel, bypassing the stomach.

Risk Factors and Preventive Measures

Risk factors for gastroparesis among diabetic individuals include prior stomach surgery and post-viral syndromes as well as some medications, such as narcotics. In addition, individuals with hypothyroidism, amyloidosis, Parkinson's disease, and gastroesophageal reflux disease (GERD) are at risk for gastroparesis.

It is also true that often there is little correlation between the patients' symptoms and objective measures of gastroparesis.

Preventive measures include eating multiple small meals rather than three large meals each day and also to minimize the intake of fiber if the main problem is delayed gastric emptying. A low-fat diet may also improve symptoms. It is also important to maintain blood glucose levels as close to normal as reasonably possible.

Smoking is also known to worsen gastroparesis, and consequently smokers with gastroparesis are urged to stop smoking before the problem worsens. Even if a smoker does not yet have gastroparesis, it is advisable to stop smoking before the condition occurs.

See also DIGESTIVE DISORDERS.

genetic manipulation/gene therapy Changing genetic material to achieve a desired result. Based on genetic mapping information, medical researchers hope that in the future, they will be able to interfere with genetic processes that lead to diseases such as diabetes. For example, gene therapy could theoretically interrupt the process that leads to the damage and death of beta cells in the pancreas and that ultimately causes Type 1 diabetes. As of this writing, this genetic research is in its early stages.

Several genes that lead to a predisposition to diabetes for both Type 1 and 2 diabetes have been identified by researchers. Perhaps as these findings become clearer, physicians will be better able to ascertain a patient's risk for developing diabetes. Those patients could then be approached more aggressively in terms of nutrition, exercise, and medications.

Concerns about Genetic Manipulation

As attractive as it is to think that diabetes could be eliminated through genetic manipulation, there are several potential disadvantages of having this individual genetic information. Some people may not want to know that they are at a serious risk for a medical illness, especially if they have a low risk. Other people worry that genetic information in the wrong hands could lead to profiling (being singled out in a negative way), larger insurance premiums, and other forms of social and business prejudice. They worry about being turned down for jobs, promotions, insurance, or other opportunities.

It is also true that a genetic predisposition does not mean that the person will always develop the disease. It usually means that the probability is higher for the person to develop the disease than for others without the genetic predisposition. But it rarely means that it is a certainty.

Another issue to consider with regard to genetic manipulation is that people react differently to the news of genetic predispositions. For example, some people who learn that they have a genetic risk for diabetes (or cancer or another disease) may take appropriate actions to decrease the risk. The person at risk for diabetes might exercise, eat a healthy diet, and avoid drinking and smoking. If genetic manipulation is available as an option, they will take advantage of it.

However, there are some people who think more fatalistically and mistakenly assume that they are doomed to develop a disease. Such people are less likely to take appropriate actions, because they wrongly assume that there is no point in doing so. They are also less likely to accept genetic manipulation. Some people may fear that it is wrong or even sinful to do so.

Appropriate genetic study and manipulation may lead to new therapies, including vaccines. However, it also remains a complex social, religious, and scientific area that is yet unresolved.

genetic risks Inherited predispositions to develop diseases. One genetic risk is the possibility that people may carry a gene predisposing them to develop diabetes; for example, children born to parents with Type 2 diabetes are more likely to develop Type 2 diabetes, as are the siblings of those who have Type 2 diabetes. Often, however, the genetic predisposition alone is not enough to cause the development of diabetes. An environmental trigger is also necessary. Thus, without an environmental or other trigger, a person may not develop diabetes but could pass on the predisposition to develop the disease to their biological children.

Some researchers have found that the gene, calpain 10, is significantly linked to the development of Type 2 diabetes among the PIMA INDIANS, Mexican Americans, and people from a Northern European lineage. Not all Pima Indians, however, develop diabetes. The Pima Indians in Mexico have a markedly reduced rate of diabetes compared to the Pima Indians in the United States.

In a study for genetic markers for Type 2 diabetes, described in a 2000 issue of the *American Journal of Human Genetics,* researchers looked for actual genetic markers for diabetes among 835 whites, 591 Mexican Americans, 229 blacks, and 128 Japanese Americans. They found such markers, although they were in different chromosomal places, depending on race and ethnicity. Thus, there is not just one gene that makes people develop diabetes but a group of genes that lead to a predisposition or susceptibility. Research must continue before scientists can provide more predictability of diabetes than exists at present.

Ongoing research since 1946 by Dr. Elliott Joslin, founder of the JOSLIN DIABETES CENTER, and other physicians who have followed him, have determined some general genetic risks. For example, if a parent or sibling has Type 1 diabetes, the risk for other individuals in the immediate family is greater than the risk of other families. The risk is higher for a child if the father rather than the mother has Type 1 diabetes.

In general, Type 2 diabetes is more highly heritable than Type 1 diabetes. For example, in identical twin studies, where the twins are raised in the same environment, if one twin develops Type 1 diabetes, then the other twin has a risk of 30–50 percent of also developing Type 1 diabetes. However, when twins who are raised together have one member with Type 2 diabetes, the risk for the other twin developing Type 2 diabetes is 60–80 percent.

The HLA DR3 and DR4 genes are highly linked with Type 1 diabetes. For Type 2 diabetes, researchers have also located a gene for a protein called PL-1, which affects the insulin receptor and causes insulin resistance.

Ehm, Margaret Gelder, et al. "Genomewide Search for Type 2 Diabetes Susceptibility Genes in Four American Populations." *American Journal of Human Genetics* 66 (2000): 1,871–1,881.

Josefson, Deborah. "New Gene Implicated in Type 2 Diabetes." *British Medical Journal* 321 (2000): 854.

gestational diabetes mellitus (GDM) Diabetes that has its onset during pregnancy and which usually ends after childbirth; however, women with gestational diabetes (GDM) are significantly more likely to experience the problem again with any subsequent pregnancies, and they also have an increased risk for developing TYPE 2 DIABETES later in life: 40 to 60 percent of women who have had gestational diabetes will ultimately develop Type 2 diabetes within five to 10 years. According to the American Diabetes Association, all pregnant women should have a 75 g oral glucose tolerance test for diabetes between the 24th and 28th weeks of pregnancy.

Women with fasting hyperglycemia, those with pre-existing glucose intolerance and with GDM that is diagnosed before 24 weeks, and those with impaired glucose tolerance (IGT) at six to eight weeks postpartum, all have an even higher risk for developing permanent Type 2 diabetes. In addition, within five years from their diagnosis with GDM, up to four out of five women from a high risk ethnic group (Hispanics, Native Americans, Pacific Islanders, and African Americans) with postpartum IGT will develop full-blown Type 2 DM. Those in a high risk group should be targeted for preventive measures in advance, including making dietary changes and performing exercises that lead to weight loss. As the infant is also at risk for IGT, the child's nutrition and activity should also be considered.

According to the National Diabetes Information Clearinghouse, two to 14 of every 100 pregnant women in the United States will develop gestational diabetes. The wide variation is due to the much higher prevalence of GDM that is seen among certain ethnic groups.

Research has shown that the first trimester of pregnancy is likely the most crucial time for the elevated risk of the development of gestational diabetes and that those women who gained more weight than recommended by the Institute of Medicine (IOM) had a 50 percent greater risk of developing gestational diabetes when compared with women whose weight gain was either at or below the IOM guidelines. This research was based on a study lasting over the course of three years comparing 800 pregnant women who did not have gestational diabetes and 345 women who did have GDM. Researchers M. Hedderson, E. Gunderson, and A. Ferrara published their findings in 2010 in *Obstetrics & Gynecology.* Said the researchers, "Gestational weight gain during early pregnancy may represent a modifiable risk factor for GDM and needs more attention from health care providers."

According to *The Healthy Woman,* published by the federal Office on Women's Health in 2008, women with GDM who wish to get pregnant again should have a blood glucose test up to three months *before* they wish to become pregnant in order to ensure that their glucose levels are normal, since hyperglycemia in the early pregnancy increases the risk for birth defects in a child.

Medications including metformin (Glucophage), pioglitazone (Actos), and rosiglitazone (Avandia) are being tested as of this writing to determine if they will prevent the onset of Type 2 DM among women who have had gestational diabetes, but these drugs are not yet approved by the Food and Drug Administration (FDA) for the prevention of diabetes or for the treatment of GDM.

The American Diabetes Association (ADA) and the Fourth International Workshop-Conference on GDM have chosen to accept the criteria developed by Doctors Carpenter and Coustan for the diagnosis of GDM. As a result, both the ADA and the American College of Obstetricians and Gynecologists recommend routine screening for GDM among all pregnant women, but the United States Preventive Medicine Task Force does not recommend such screening.

In addition to their diabetes, another problem faced by many women with GDM, as well as women with pre-pregnancy diabetes, is that they have an increased risk for suffering from depression compared to women with no form of diabetes, based on research by K. B. Kozhimannil and colleagues and published in the *Journal of the American Medical Association* in 2009. These researchers found that of 11,024 low-income women who were enrolled in Medicaid in New Jersey and who gave birth from 2004–06, 15.2 percent of the women with either pre-pregnancy diabetes or with GDM were clinically depressed,

compared to 8.5 percent of pregnant women who were depressed but did not have either pre-pregnancy diabetes or GDM. As a result, depression should be considered as a possibility among women with GDM or who had diabetes prior to their pregnancy.

Screening for GDM

The key recommendations for screening for diabetes have now been divided into three groups: those of low, average, and high risk for developing GDM. Low-risk women must meet all of the following criteria: younger than 25 years old, of a normal weight pre-pregnancy, belonging to a low-prevalence GDM ethnic group, having no first-degree relatives with diabetes, having no prior history of IGT, and having no history of bearing macrosomic (large) babies or of poor obstetrical outcomes. Individuals who fit all the criteria in this group require no formal testing for GDM.

Women at High or Average Risk for GDM The high risk group for GDM includes those who are obese (a body mass index greater than 30), a prior history of GDM or of having a large baby, glucose in the urine (glucosuria), or a strong family history of diabetes. The average risk status group includes being older than age 25, being a little overweight, having one relative with diabetes, and so forth.

If a woman has a fasting glucose level that is greater than 125 mg/dL or a random non-fasting (post-prandial) glucose greater than 200, she has GDM and no further screening is necessary.

The high-risk woman should be given the 50 gram glucose challenge (Glucola) or go directly to the 100 gram oral glucose challenge as soon as they begin prenatal care. It is important to not wait until weeks 24–28. If the initial testing is normal, the high-risk woman can be rechecked at 24–28 weeks. The average risk group receives the 50 gram glucose challenge between weeks 24 and 28 and if this test is abnormal, proceeds to the three-hour 100 gram glucose challenge.

The 50 gram glucose challenge may be done at any time of day without regard to meals or fasting. A glucose level (serum) is obtained (a venipuncture is preferred over a fingerstick) exactly 60 minutes after the glucose is administered.

Several cut-off values are employed depending upon the sensitivity and specificity the doctor wishes to obtain. A one-hour glucose level of greater than 140 mg/dL will identify about 80 percent of those with GDM, but about 15–20 percent of those who are screened will fail the test and require the three-hour glucose 100 gram challenge. If a cut-off of >130 mg/dL is chosen, then 90 percent of those with GDM will be identified but an additional 5–10 percent more women will need to proceed to the three-hour glucose challenge (a total of about 25 percent will fail the one-hour test).

The three-hour 100 gram glucose challenge is performed on a day the woman is fasting after three days of an unlimited carbohydrate diet. To be considered positive for GDM, two of the four values must be abnormal. If only one glucose level is abnormal, then the test should be repeated in four weeks, as about 33 percent of these women will eventually develop full-blown GDM.

The criteria for a positive three-hour oral glucose challenge (the oral glucose tolerance test [OGTT]) are as follows: a fasting glucose greater than 95 mg/dL, a one-hour glucose greater than 180 mg/dL, a two-hour glucose level greater than 155 mg/dL, and a three-hour glucose level greater than 140 mg/dL. As previously mentioned, if the woman's fasting glucose is greater than 125 mg/dL, then the patient has GDM and the test can be stopped before the administration of the oral glucose.

In addition, if the laboratory values are known during the course of the test, many physicians will choose to diagnose GDM, and they will stop the test if either the one-hour or two-hour glucose level exceeds 200 mg/dL. A fasting plasma glucose level of 126 mg/dL or greater indicates the diagnosis of GDM.

Routine screening for GDM In his chapter on screening for GDM in *The Diabetes in Pregnancy Dilemma*, Langer says that certain individuals fit the criteria for a low risk of developing GDM.

However, despite this, Langer says that most physicians do ultimately screen for GDM, based on a survey of physicians that was performed in 2003. He says, "A recent survey reported that routine screening for GDM is a common practice and is used by 96% of obstetricians in the US; 95.2% used a 50-gm glucose challenge test. Furthermore, in 1987, only 83.8% of ACOG [American College of Obstetricians and Gynecologists] members used universal screening and this increased to 96% in 2003."

Many doctors check all pregnant women in the third trimester Many doctors check all pregnant women for GDM in the third trimester as well as in the first trimester as a precaution. Some studies have revealed small numbers of cases of women who fit no criteria at all for developing GDM and yet, when they are checked, they *do* have gestational diabetes. For example, in one study of nearly 3,000 pregnant Australian women who were screened in their third trimester, 573 were considered low-risk for having GDM. Yet of these women, about 3 percent tested positive for GDM. Since the consequences of untreated GDM can be very dire, testing for diabetes, which is easy and inexpensive, seems like a reasonable precaution.

TABLE 1: ABOVE-NORMAL RESULTS FOR THE ORAL GLUCOSE TOLERANCE TEST IN PREGNANT WOMEN

Fasting	95 or higher
At 1 hour	180 or higher
At 2 hours	155 or higher
At 3 hours	140 or higher

Note: Some labs use other numbers for this test. These numbers are for a test using a drink with 100 grams of glucose.

Source: Adapted from the National Institute of Diabetes and Digestive and Kidney Diseases (NIDDK). "What I Need to Know about Gestational Diabetes." Available online. URL: http://diabetes.niddk.nih.gov/dm/pubs/gestational. April 2006. Accessed December 26, 2008.

Potential outcomes with GDM When treated by competent specialist physicians and when patients closely follow the medical advice received from their obstetricians (and often a team made of a dietician, endocrinologist, and others) about medications, nutrition, exercise, and other medical matters, most women and their babies do well; however, women with GDM are at increased risk for preeclampsia, polyhydramnios (excessive amniotic fluid), and HYPERTENSION, as well as the need for a cesarean delivery because the baby is large, a condition known as macrosomia.

Research continues to provide new information on the risks and causes of GDM as well as actions that women with GDM and their physicians should take.

If Symptoms Occur

If symptoms of GDM occur, they may include thirst, increased urination and increased appetite, as well as weight loss and nocturia (urinating at night more than usual). However, these symptoms are often missed or they are seen as normal in pregnancy, which is why testing for GDM is so important. Other possible symptoms of GDM may include blurred vision, fatigue, and nausea and vomiting.

Possible Causes and Risks of GDM

GDM is caused by abnormalities in the mother's ability to secrete adequate insulin, increased resistance to the effects of insulin, and an overproduction of glucose by the liver. These same abnormalities are seen in classic Type 2 diabetes mellitus, although in GDM, there are additional hormones that are major contributors to these defects. Thus the hypothesis has been that GDM may well "unmask" underlying Type 2 diabetes mellitus. During pregnancy, both human placental lactogen and placental growth hormone contribute to the insulin resistance which is worst during the third trimester.

Hormones named tumor necrosis factor–alpha (TNF alpha) and leptin are also increased, while adiponectin is decreased and may play a role in the development of GDM. Women without GDM compensate for these hormonal changes during pregnancy by secreting a much greater amount of insulin; thus, those who develop GDM have inadequate beta cell (the cells in the

ISLETS OF LANGERHANS in the pancreas that specifically synthesize and secrete insulin) reserve in the pancreas (likely a genetically acquired defect). There are complex changes in muscle cells that likely also contribute to the decreased effectiveness of insulin (insulin resistance) during a woman's pregnancy. In addition, as in those with obesity and/or traditional Type 2 diabetes mellitus, the levels of free fatty acids are increased in those who develop GDM, and these fats contribute to the insulin resistance.

Risks to the fetus and newborn child from GDM It is important to identify GDM in susceptible women because both the fetus and newborn baby as well as the woman with GDM herself are at risk for serious medical problems. In the case of the fetus and newborn, the child may have HYPOGLYCEMIA (below-normal levels of glucose in the blood), hypocalcemia (below-normal levels of calcium in the blood), and hyperbilirubinemia (excessive levels of bilirubin in the blood).

Because the mother with GDM is also at risk for having an oversized baby (macrosomia), the baby may be difficult to deliver vaginally and a cesarean section may be required. The baby is also at risk for premature birth and respiratory distress syndrome (RDS), and some premature babies need care in a neonatal intensive care unit.

Some studies have found that the risk of perinatal mortality (fetal death) is four times greater in cases of untreated GDM versus the rate found among pregnant women with normal glucose levels.

Other risks to the child born to the woman with GDM are SHOULDER DYSTOCIA, ERB'S PALSY, collar bone fractures, low APGAR scores, and birth asphyxia (suffocation), conditions that result from a difficult birth of a large infant. Polyhydramnios (excessive amniotic fluid) can be seen leading to preterm labor. Hypoglycemia may be a major problem for the newborn, and the child may need glucose intravenously after delivery. The child of the mother with GDM is likely also at risk for the development of adolescent obesity and Type 2 diabetes. Childhood Type 2 diabetes is 20 times higher in the children of mothers with GDM than among those children whose mothers had normal glucose levels during their pregnancies. (See CHILDREN OF DIABETIC MOTHERS.)

To determine the periodic status of the fetus, physicians may monitor the 28+-week fetus with "kick counts," or the number of times that the fetus kicks when the mother lies on her side about an hour after a meal. About 10 kicks within one hour after eating are considered normal. The proportion of head to abdomen is also measured. The abdominal circumference of the fetus is a good predictor for large babies.

Fetal weight can be predicted and if a large (macrosomic) fetus is detected, then an elective cesarean section can be considered by mother and obstetrician. It is not inevitable, however, that GDM leads to cesarean births. A study performed in Australia by Moses et al. (described by Kripke in a 1999 issue of *American Family Physician*) compared 216 women with GDM to 216 women without GDM. The researchers found no significant differences in the rate of cesarean sections in the two groups.

Ultrasound and other tests may also help monitor the status as well as the size of the fetus.

Risks to the mother with GDM Women with GDM are at risk for *preeclampsia* (about 25 percent of women with GDM), which is a form of hypertension that is induced by pregnancy. Some symptoms of preeclampsia are swelling in the hands and face, heartburnlike pain, blurred vision, and headache. If the condition is severe, hospitalization may become necessary.

According to the American Diabetes Association in their book *Gestational Diabetes: What to Expect,* women with GDM may have a greater risk for developing urinary tract infections, which are treatable with antibiotics. Symptoms of a urinary tract infection are urgency, frequency of urination, and burning and pain with urination.

The woman with GDM may also develop excessive amounts of acidic substances that are known as *ketones* (or ketoacids or ketone bodies), and even moderate amounts of ketones can be harmful to the fetus. In general, the production of excessive ketones leading to ketonuria occurs when the woman is not eating enough. (Ketonuria refers to ketones in the urine, and they are easily monitored with a urine dipstick test.) Thus the dietitian often will recommend a bedtime snack to avoid this problem. Ketonuria can also be prevented by keeping the blood glucose levels under tight control by having the pregnant woman monitor her own blood levels and then act on the information that she receives; for example, if the glucose levels drop to below normal, she needs to increase her glucose intake. If the glucose levels are too high, then she needs to adjust her dietary intake and insulin (if she is using insulin).

If GDM Is Untreated

Women with untreated gestational diabetes face the risk of severe hyperglycemia that could lead to COMA. Other risks are hypertension, DYSLIPIDEMIA, and DIABETIC RETINOPATHY. According to Catherine Davis et al., in a 1999 article for the *Journal of Diabetes Complications,* women who have had gestational diabetes are also at increased risk for the later development of coronary heart disease and atherosclerosis.

Treatment of even mild GDM is important. A study reported at the Society for Maternal-Fetal Medicine meeting on February 3, 2009 by Mark Landon, M.D., on the National Institute of Child Health and Human Development Maternal-Fetal Medicine Units Network revealed that in comparing women with mild GDM who were treated and not treated, the treated group were less likely to have large babies, and the treated mothers gained less weight during pregnancy and had a lower body mass index at delivery. However, there were still similarities in the rate of small-for-gestational-age babies, preterm delivery, admission to the neonatal intensive care unit, and other factors. Landon said that the study supports treatment of mild GDM.

Glycemic Control Is Crucial with GDM

Many experts recommend that the woman with gestational diabetes should check her blood at least three to four times per day, using a blood glucose meter. There are various times when the glucose should be tested. These times often include just before meals, one or two hours after meals, and at bedtime. (In patients with pre-existing Type 1 diabetes as compared to GDM, women may check their blood levels as frequently as seven to eight times per day, before and after each meal, at bedtime and at 2–3 A.M.) Many women with GDM are asked to check their blood levels after each meal and at bedtime, although the regimen is often individualized. The woman will need a thorough education on how to check her blood and on what actions she will need to take, based on these daily findings. For example, she may need to adjust her food intake or the timing of meals. As soon as a pregnant woman is diagnosed with GDM, she should be referred to the diabetes care team within 48 hours.

TABLE 2: BLOOD GLUCOSE TARGETS FOR MOST WOMEN WITH GESTATIONAL DIABETES

On awakening	Not above 95
1 hour after a meal	Not above 140
2 hours after a meal	Not above 120

Source: The National Institute of Diabetes and Digestive and Kidney Diseases (NIDDK). "What I Need to Know about Gestational Diabetes." Available online. URL: http://diabetes.niddk.nih.gov/dm/pubs/gestational. April 2006. Accessed December 26, 2008.

Insulin may be needed   Sometimes women with GDM may need to take INSULIN if diet and exercise cannot control the diabetes. Between 30 and 60 percent of women with GDM will need insulin. If insulin is required, human insulin is recommended during pregnancy. As the pregnancy progresses, women may need higher doses of insulin, particularly in the case of obese women. Some women who have not previously required insulin at all will need it as their pregnancies progress.

Some experts say that hormonal measurements may be used to determine if insulin ther-

apy should be initiated. According to Langer in his 2000 article in *Clinical Obstetrics and Gynecology*, some physicians have used amniotic fluid taken at the 28th week of pregnancy to test for maternal hyperglycemia and fetal hyperinsulinemia. The results can help predict the risk for fetal death. This is however, an invasive test, and consequently, most medical doctors rely instead on glucose measurements and the size of the fetus.

Typically, NPH insulin twice per day or pre-meal, or rapid-acting insulin such as lispro (Humalog), aspart (NovoLog), or glulisine (Apidra) may be used in addition to bedtime NPH. The newer longer-acting insulins such as glargine (Lantus) and detemir (Levemir) are not currently approved for use in pregnancy. There are some theoretical concerns about the former binding to growth hormonelike receptors and possibly causing birth defects, although there has been absolutely no evidence of this to date.

There are indications that some women may be able to take the oral medication glyburide to control their diabetes rather than needing to use insulin. Apparently minimal to no glyburide crosses the human placenta, in contrast to other oral medications for diabetes. According to a study in a 2000 issue of the *New England Journal of Medicine*, researchers studied 404 women with gestational diabetes who were divided into glyburide-treated or insulin-treated groups. The women in the glyburide group appeared to fare as well or better than the insulin group; for example, they had fewer incidents of hypoglycemia. The two groups did not differ significantly in the outcome of their pregnancies. In this study no glyburide was detected in the placental blood. Further analysis is clearly needed before considering glyburide as a primary first-line therapy in GDM.

In some foreign countries, metformin is also used. Metformin is often used pre-pregnancy, and in women with polycystic ovarian syndrome and a history of first-trimester pregnancy loss the metformin is often continued until the end of the first trimester. This therapy appears to decrease the risk of first-trimester fetal loss. Metformin is not FDA-approved for this use in the United States, although it is a commonly used regimen and is near to a standard of care in specific cases. A study reported in 2009 in *Obstetrics and Gynecology* by W. Nicholson and colleagues found no benefit in using insulin compared to oral diabetic agents. However, in the United States, *only* insulin (specific types) is approved for use in GDM.

Diet and Exercise Are Important in Women with GDM

If gestational diabetes is diagnosed, the treatment usually includes an emphasis on a very careful monitoring of the woman's food intake. In general, women are encouraged to eat three meals and three snacks per day, eating a small breakfast in order to avoid midmorning hyperglycemia. Some physicians recommend the complete avoidance of carbohydrates at breakfast because a person's glucose tolerance is lower upon arising. The woman with GDM should be advised to consult with a diabetes care team. All weight gain of the pregnant woman with GDM is very carefully monitored.

The physician may also prescribe a regular exercise plan with such non-weight-bearing exercise as walking or bicycling. Contraindications to exercise are a risk of premature labor or the existence of cardiac, pulmonary, or thyroid disease, among other risk factors. Each woman should consult with her own obstetrician and diabetes care team about what exercise is appropriate in her case.

Delivery of the Baby

Physicians may recommend the induction of labor when the child is full term if there are no indications that labor is starting. The reason for induction is to avert delivery of a very large infant. Sometimes pediatricians and neonatologists are on "standby" or are in the delivery room, should the newborn experience any distress.

The newborn baby is carefully checked, especially for indications of hypoglycemia and respiratory distress. If the baby weighs more than nine pounds at delivery, calcium and magnesium levels are also checked to determine if the infant needs supplemental calcium or magnesium.

After Delivery

Only about 10–15 percent of women with GDM have overt diabetes immediately after the birth of their children. After the child is born and the placenta is delivered, if the mother was receiving insulin during her pregnancy, her doctor may decide to cut the mother's insulin dose by as much as half or may stop it altogether; however, medical experts warn that women who have just had gestational diabetes should continue to monitor their blood glucose levels for at least several weeks after being discharged from the hospital.

Breast-feeding after GDM

BREAST-FEEDING is generally encouraged for the woman who has GDM. In addition to the many known benefits of breast-feeding to both the mother and child, breast-feeding may also improve the mother's insulin status. In addition, it may help her to lose weight and further decrease her susceptibility to developing Type 2 diabetes.

Attitudes of Pregnant Women Diagnosed with GDM

Women who have been notified of their gestational diabetes may find it difficult to accept and may even deny the condition. The woman may experience no symptoms of diabetes, thus increasing the difficulty of acceptance. It is important for women with gestational diabetes to understand the potentially dire consequences of ignoring the illness.

Home glucose monitoring is essential not only to verify the problem to newly diagnosed women with gestational diabetes but also to provide them with a feeling of some control and a realization that their own actions are important. Blood glucose monitoring provides immediate feedback to the mother and clearly shows her the role of specific items in changing her blood levels.

Research on Gestational Diabetes

Even mild hyperglycemia can be problematic for the pregnant woman and her child. In a study of 23,316 pregnant women in nine countries, discussed by the HAPO Study Cooperative Research Group in a 2008 issue of the *New England Journal of Medicine*, the researchers studied pregnant women with glucose levels not high enough for diabetes mellitus but still high enough to be associated with adverse pregnancy outcomes. The researchers found that insulin resistance was associated with an increased birth weight of the child as well as with increased cord-blood serum C-peptide levels.

Said the researchers, "Questions have been raised regarding the benefits of treating 'mild' gestational diabetes mellitus. However, one recently published randomized clinical trial, the Australian Carbohydrate Intolerance Study in Pregnant Women (ACHOIS), found reduced perinatal morbidity and mortality when standard contemporary treatment of gestational diabetes mellitus was compared with no intervention."

A study of 498 women in Norway who had experienced gestational diabetes, reported in a 2000 issue of the *British Medical Journal* by Egeland et al., looked at the characteristics of these women when they were infants. The researchers found that women born to mothers who had GDM during their pregnancies were in turn more likely to themselves have GDM when they later became pregnant. They also found that women who were born at a low birth weight were more likely to develop GDM when they became pregnant.

The researchers also found other factors that related to gestational diabetes; for example, the prevalence of the disease increased with the age of the mother, with the lowest risk to women who were age 20 and under and the highest risks to women who were age 30 and over. "Parity," or the number of children that the women had previously borne, was another significant

factor related to the development of GDM, and the risk of having gestational diabetes increased with each pregnancy.

Some experts believe that a thiamine vitamin deficiency (vitamin B_1) may lead to gestational diabetes, although further study on this issue is needed. This is the contention of Bakker et al., in their article in a 2000 issue of *Medical Hypotheses*. These researchers contend that the average nonpregnant woman is barely at an adequate level of thiamine and that a thiamine deficiency resulting from the additional strain on the body caused by pregnancy could trigger hyperglycemia in some women, presumably due to effects on carbohydrate metabolism.

Some women who are diagnosed with gestational diabetes actually had undiagnosed diabetes prior to their pregnancy. An estimated 10–15 percent of the women who are diagnosed with gestational diabetes had Type 2 diabetes before their pregnancies. However, the majority of women diagnosed with GDM were nondiabetic before pregnancy and become nondiabetic again after delivery for years, until another pregnancy or a later onset of diabetes.

Preventing Type 2 Diabetes Later in Life

According to the National Institute of Diabetes and Digestive and Kidney Diseases (NIDDK), women who have had GDM can reduce their risks of developing Type 2 diabetes later in their lives by avoiding obesity. Even a weight loss of 10 to 14 pounds in a 200-pound woman can significantly reduce the risk of diabetes.

In their later life, women who have a history of GDM should also walk, swim, and perform other exercises because staying active can reduce the risk for the onset of Type 2 diabetes.

See also DIABETES MELLITUS; PREGNANCY; TYPE 1 DIABETES.

American Diabetes Association. *Gestational Diabetes: What to Expect.* 5th ed. American Diabetes Association: Alexandria, Va., 2005.

Bakker, S. J. L., et al. "Thiamine Supplementation to Prevent Induction of Low Birth Weight by Conventional Therapy for Gestational Diabetes Mellitus." *Medical Hypotheses* (July 2000): 88–90.

Barbour, Linda A., and Jacob E. Friedman. MANAGEMENT OF DIABETES IN PREGNANCY, Endo. text.com pp. 1–40. Available online. URL: http://diabetesmanager.pbwiki.com/Management-of-Diabetes-in-Pregnancy. Accessed March 5, 2009.

Coustan, D. R., and M. W. Carpenter. "The Diagnosis of Gestational Diabetes." *Diabetes Care* 21, Supp. 2 (1998): B5–B8.

Diabetes Mellitus: A Guide to Patient Care. Ambler, Pa.: Lippincott, Williams and Wilkins, 2007.

Egeland, Grace M., et al. "Birth Characteristics of Women Who Develop Gestational Diabetes: Population Based Study." *British Medical Journal* 321, no. 7250 (September 2000): 546–547.

Gao, X. L., Yang, H. X., and Zhao, Y. "Variations of Tumor Necrosis Factor–alpha, Leptin and Adiponectin in Mid-trimester of Gestational Diabetes Mellitus." *Chinese Medical Journal* (Engl). 121, no. 8 (2008): 701–705.

HAPO Study Cooperative Research Group. "Hyperglycemia and Adverse Pregnancy Outcomes." *New England Journal of Medicine* 358, no. 19 (May 8, 2008): 1,991–2,002.

The Healthy Woman: A Complete Guide for All Ages. Washington, D.C.: Office on Women's Health, U.S. Department of Health and Human Services, 2008.

Hedderson, M. M., E. P. Gunderson, and F. Ferrara. "Gestational Weight: Gain and Risk of Gestational Diabetes Mellitus." *Obstetrics & Gynecology* 115, no. 3 (2010): 597–604.

Jensen, D. M., et al. "Maternal and Perinatal Outcomes in 143 Danish Women with Gestational Diabetes Mellitus and 143 Controls with a Similar Risk Profile." *Diabetes Medicine* 17, no. 4 (April 2000): 281–286.

Kozhimannil, K. B., M. A. Pereira, and B. L. Harlow. "Association between Diabetes and Perinatal Depression among Low-Income Mothers." *Journal of the American Medical Association* 301, no. 8 (2009): 842–847.

Langer, Oded. "Screening for Gestational Diabetes." In *The Diabetes in Pregnancy Dilemma: Leading Change with Proven Solutions,* edited by Oded Langer. Lanham, Md.: University Press of America, 2006, pp. 432–443.

Moses, Robert G. "Gestational Diabetes: Is a Higher Cesarean Section Rate Inevitable?" *Diabetes Care* 23, no. 1 (January 2000): 15–17.

Neale, Todd. "SMFM: Clinical Benefits Found from Treating Mild Gestational Diabetes." Available online. URL: http://www.medpagetoday.com/MeetingCoverage/SMFM/12726. Accessed March 7, 2009.

Nicholson, W., et al. "Benefits and Risks of Oral Diabetes Agents Compared with Insulin in Women with Gestational Diabetes: A Systematic Review." *Obstetrics & Gynecology* 113, no. 1 (2009): 193–205.

Petit, William, Jr., M.D. "Management of Diabetes Mellitus during Pregnancy." In *Self-Assessment Profile in Endocrinology and Metabolism,* edited by Pasquale J. Palumbo, M.D., 102–107. Washington, D.C.: The American Association of Clinical Endocrinologists and The American College of Endocrinology, 2001.

gingivitis   Serious gum inflammation and infection. Gingivitis is an early stage of PERIODONTAL DISEASE and people with diabetes have a higher risk of gingivitis than nondiabetics. In addition, sometimes diabetes is undiagnosed until the individual's dentist suspects the presence of diabetes because of oral diseases, according to Jonathan Ship in his article for the *Journal of the American Dental Association.* Ship also points out that GLYCEMIC CONTROL worsens when the patient has an untreated infection, as with severe gingivitis. The patient who is acutely insulin-deficient and hyperglycemic may have a "fruity" breath, according to Ship (due to excess ketone bodies, which are breakdown products of fats circulating in excessive concentration in the bloodstream).

A study reported in a 2000 issue of *Diabetes Care* compared "dentate adults" (people with at least some teeth of their own) with and without diabetes. The researchers found that people with diabetes were less likely to have seen a dentist than nondiabetics. About 66 percent had seen a dentist in the past year, compared to 73 percent of those who did not have diabetes.

Some other oral manifestations of diabetes are xerostomia (severe dry mouth) related to salivary dysfunction, gingivitis, periodontitis, taste dysfunction, and an oral yeast infection (candidiasis, commonly called thrush). Individuals with diabetes are also more prone to dental cavities.

If left untreated, gingivitis may lead to periodontitis, which can cause bone and tooth loss. All cases of periodontitis start out as gingivitis, although not all cases of gingivitis deteriorate to the point of periodontitis.

Symptoms and Diagnostic Path

The key symptoms of gingivitis are painful, bleeding, or puffy gums with or without sores, persistently bad breath, itchy gums, bad taste (dysgeusia) in the mouth, and gum recession, although symptoms are often minor and unnoticeable to the average person.

Medications may be another cause of gingivitis, and thus the medications the patient takes should be explored; for example, many medications have a side effect of creating chronic dry mouth, which can increase the risk for gingivitis. A final reason why people with diabetes may be more likely to have dental problems is that they do not go to the dentist frequently enough.

Treatment Options and Outlook

Gingivitis is easily diagnosed by a dentist, who will then recommend treatment for the problem. The usual treatment is scaling to remove the plaque and tartar and often an antimicrobial mouth rinse along with overall good dental hygiene, including at least twice daily tooth brushing (with a soft or electric brush), and flossing. Regular dental checkups for teeth cleaning at least two times per year and often three or times per year are important until the problem is well controlled. These same steps will also prevent gingivitis. Some dentists recommend vitamin C, cranberries, and even grapefruit seed extract applied to your toothbrush. Grapefruit seed extract can interfere with many medicines so it should not be used unless discussed thoroughly with both the dentist and medical doctor.

If the disease progresses to periodontitis, then gum surgery may be needed. The outlook is positive if the patient maintains good control of glucose levels and sees a dentist on a regular basis.

Risk Factors and Preventive Measures

In the study published in *Diabetes Care*, the researchers found that there were racial differences between people with diabetes who had seen a dentist and those who had not. For example, only about half of Hispanics with diabetes saw a dentist, versus 58 percent of African Americans, and 70 percent of Caucasians with diabetes.

In addition, those with more education were more likely to see a dentist. Only about 48 percent of subjects with diabetes who had less than a high school diploma had seen a dentist in the past year. The percentage increased dramatically to 66 percent of high school graduates and further to 73 percent of those with some education beyond high school.

People with diabetes who had more education may have seen a dentist more often because they had enough money to afford to pay the dentist or they had dental insurance. This likelihood is further underlined by the fact that when looking at income alone, the percentage that saw a dentist increased as income increased.

Only about 41 percent of people with diabetes earning $10,000 or less per year saw a dentist. This figure steadily increased with income, with 55 percent of people with diabetes earning $15,000–$19,999 and 68 percent earning $25,000–$34,999 seeing dentists. Those who earned $50,000 or more per year had a rate of 82 percent for seeing a dentist in the past year.

However, when asked why they had not seen a dentist in the past year, the main reason respondents gave was that they believed there was no need for them to see the dentist. Other reasons for not seeing a dentist were cost, followed by fear and anxiety about seeing a dentist. The researchers said, "The lower use of dental services among people with diabetes suggests a need for promotion of appropriate dental preventive and treatment services in that group. However, the finding that the leading reason for not seeing a dentist within the preceding 12 months was a lack of a perceived need, regardless of diabetic status, suggests the need for the general promotion of regular preventive dental visits. Adults may not yet appreciate the interrelationship between oral health and general health."

People with diabetes who smoke should quit smoking to improve their oral health, as should people who do not have diabetes, as far as they know. People with diabetes should have a dental cleaning every four to six months. They should brush their teeth twice each day and floss once daily. A dentist should be called if any of the following is observed:

- bleeding gums
- puffy, swollen, tender gums
- persistent bad breath
- gums appear to recess from teeth
- a change in the fit of dentures

See also DIABETES MELLITUS; TYPE 1 DIABETES; TYPE 2 DIABETES.

Ship, Jonathan A. "Diabetes and Oral Health: An Overview." *Journal of the American Dental Association* 134 (2003): 4S–10S.
Tomar, Scott L., and Arlene Lester. "Dental and Other Health Care Visits among U.S. Adults with Diabetes." *Diabetes Care* 23, no. 10 (October 2000): 1,505–1,510.

glaucoma Eye disease in which the fluid pressure inside the eye increases and may damage the optic nerve of the eye. People with diabetes have nearly twice the risk for developing glaucoma as those with normal glucose tolerance. Glaucoma is highly treatable when diagnosed in an annual eye examination. People with diabetes who receive Medicare are entitled to an annual eye examination.

According to the Glaucoma Research Foundation, about 4 million Americans have glaucoma but only about half have been diagnosed with the disease. About 120,000 Americans have gone blind from glaucoma. Glaucoma is also the biggest cause of blindness among African Americans. Glaucoma becomes increasingly likely to occur with aging and is most common among African Americans, those over age 60, and people with a history of glaucoma in their family. Even when treated, about 10 percent of those with glaucoma eventually do go blind; however, diagnosis and treatment is clearly indicated, since the vast majority (90 percent) of those who are treated retain their eyesight.

There are two types of glaucoma: closed angle and open angle glaucoma. Open angle glaucoma is more common, and people with diabetes are also more likely to have open angle glaucoma. Open angle glaucoma leads to painless progressive visual loss. Because it does not hurt the patient, it is often easily ignored, which is why an annual eye examination is so important.

Closed angle glaucoma refers to a narrowing of the angle of the eye such that the aqueous fluid does not flow properly. It is painful to the patient, and it must be treated immediately.

Symptoms and Diagnostic Path

There are few or no symptoms of glaucoma in the early stages, although an eye professional such as an OPHTHALMOLOGIST or an optometrist could detect the disease with special equipment used in an annual eye examination. The diagnosis of glaucoma involves the measurement of intraocular pressure as well as a determination of visual fields. Unfortunately, some people with diabetes do not have these examinations. The consequences of not diagnosing and treating glaucoma can be very grim. The increased pressure in the eye from glaucoma can cause damage to the optic nerve and result in vision impairment, abnormal visual fields, and even BLINDNESS.

As the disease progresses, the person may notice a worsening of peripheral (side) vision. Some other symptoms of open angle glaucoma may be difficulty seeing well enough to drive at night and difficulty seeing in the dark. Some symptoms of closed angle glaucoma are pain, headache, and nausea/vomiting.

Neovascular glaucoma is rare but diabetes is a risk factor. It occurs when vessels grow from the retina to the iris (colored part of the eye). It can be treated with laser therapy or on occasion implants to allow drainage.

Treatment Options and Outlook

If open angle glaucoma is diagnosed, the treatment is usually prescribed eye drops. For closed angle glaucoma, the pain is likely to require surgery or laser treatment of the afflicted eye.

Risk Factors and Preventive Measures

Elderly people with diabetes have a high risk for glaucoma and should have annual eye examinations so that the condition can be identified and treated if it is present.

African Americans older than age 40 have a high risk of developing glaucoma. Mexican Americans older than 60 years have an elevated risk for the development of glaucoma, according to the National Eye Institute (NEI). Individuals with a family history for glaucoma have an increased risk for developing the disease.

An annual dilated eye examination is recommended for people with diabetes to determine the presence of glaucoma, CATARACTS, DIABETIC RETINOPATHY, macular edema/degeneration, or other eye diseases. (See DIABETIC EYE DISEASES.) If the patient has diabetes, he or she should be sure to tell the ophthalmologist or an optometrist, so that the eye professional can be even more aware of potential problems to look for.

glucagon   A polypeptide (protein) hormone that is secreted by the alpha cells of the pancreas. The hormone is administered to a person with diabetes in the event of severe HYPOGLYCEMIA and an inability to eat or drink. These cells lie within the ISLETS OF LANGERHANS of the pancreas. Glucagon acts to increase the glucose level of the blood by stimulating glycogen that is stored in the liver to break down (glycogenolysis). Thus, if a person has no stored glucose, the glucagon cannot work, for example, in the cases of severe alcoholism or starvation.

Interestingly, after five years of Type 1 diabetes, although glucagon remains present in the alpha cells, it can no longer be secreted in response to hypoglycemia. This response is a counterregulatory mechanism that the body has made in an attempt to maintain the glucose level within the normal range.

Glucagon is also available in an emergency kit to be injected intramuscularly into a patient with severe hypoglycemia who is unable to correct the low blood glucose level by eating and drinking. Someone must do this injection other than the patient, because they are often incoherent or unconscious when their glucose is low enough to require an injection of glucagon. The injection will work within 10–20 minutes to increase blood glucose level. The most common side effect is nausea. Adults are generally given 1 mg and children 0.25 mg–1.0 mg.

The standard procedure away from the hospital when someone is thought to be experiencing severe hypoglycemia would be to: 1) call 911; 2) mix the diluent provided in the kit with the glucagon that is kept in a separate vial as a powder; 3) draw the mixed glucagon into the syringe to be used for injection; 4) inject the glucagon intramuscularly into a large muscle group such as the thigh or shoulder. Thus, when a person has episodes of severe hypoglycemia it is critical for them to have access to glucagon and, more importantly, for their spouse, parent, child, friend, or roommate to be capable of injecting it properly. If glucagon is premixed it is only stable for about 48 hours. When the diluent and the glucagon powder are kept separate they are stable for about two years. Patients should check the expiration date.

Glucophage   See METFORMIN.

glucose   A simple (monosaccharide) sugar that is found in the blood and that is required for energy. It is the only fuel used by the brain during usual living conditions. People with diabetes should carefully monitor their own blood glucose levels because the body is unable to do so, either because of low or no insulin (Type 1 diabetes) or because of INSULIN RESISTANCE (Type 2 diabetes). If levels are high or low, changes to diet and medication are needed.

Other forms of sugar are dextrose, fructose (fruit sugar), lactose (milk sugar), galactose, sucrose (table sugar), sorghum, corn syrup, maple syrup, and carob powder.

Many people mistakenly believe that people with diabetes must or should forego consumption of all sugar forever, but this is not true. Instead, most experts recommend moderation in the consumption of sugar and advise people with diabetes to practice carbohydrate counting.

See also GLYCEMIC CONTROL.

glucose intolerance The physiological phase between normal glucose levels and diabetes mellitus. It is formally defined by the two-hour ORAL GLUCOSE TOLERANCE TEST (OGTT), in which the one- and two-hour glucoses are greater than 140 but less than 199 or more mg/dL. It is typically associated with the insulin resistance syndrome and thus these patients often have OBESITY, HYPERTENSION, DYSLIPIDEMIA, polycystic ovarian syndrome, and premature coronary artery disease.

Many patients are relieved to find that they do not have diabetes, but it is a mistake for them or for their medical doctors to believe that IMPAIRED GLUCOSE TOLERANCE is a benign syndrome.

It is important to note that not all patients with impaired glucose tolerance (IGT) progress to diabetes, although it is a risk factor. The risk varies with ethnic groups; for example, Pima Indians with IGT have a higher risk of developing diabetes.

In the Paris Police Study, individuals with IGT and impaired fasting glucose levels had the highest risk of developing diabetes.

A variety of studies have shown that IGT is associated with a greatly increased risk of cardiovascular disease. It is likely that it is not only the level of glycemia but also concomitant risk factors that greatly increase the risk (obesity, hyper-lipidemia, hypertension, etc.). Some people have multiple risk factors. The seven-and-a-half-year risk of cardiovascular death was double among those with IGT in the Whitehall Study.

See also CARDIOVASCULAR DISEASE.

Fuller, J. H., et al. "Coronary Heart Disease Risk and Impaired Glucose Tolerance: The Whitehall Study." *The Lancet* 1373 (1980): 1.
Saad, M. F., et al. "The Natural History of Impaired Glucose Tolerance in the Pima Indians." *New England Journal of Medicine* 1500 (1988): 319.

glycemic control A description of overall blood glucose control. A favorable level of glycemic control depends on the ability of a person with diabetes (or others who provide care, when the person with diabetes needs help) to keep glucose levels as close to normal as possible. Attaining good or excellent glycemic control is the critical goal to attain and the key concept to grasp for every person who has diabetes.

Tight glycemic control is the key to decreasing risks for many severe short-term and long-term complications, which experts believe are avoidable. It may also increase an individual's life span, adding years to the person's life compared to inadequate glycemic control.

It is not mere speculation that glycemic control enhances the lives of people with diabetes. Studies such as the DIABETES CONTROL AND COMPLICATIONS TRIAL, on individuals with Type 1 diabetes and the UNITED KINGDOM PROSPECTIVE DIABETES STUDY, on individuals with Type 2 diabetes, have clearly and definitively illustrated that tight glycemic control can greatly reduce the risk of serious complications from diabetes.

Some medical problems/complications of diabetes that can be prevented or delayed with good glycemic control include:

- diabetic neuropathy
- diabetic retinopathy
- diabetic ketoacidosis/hyperosmolar state
- diabetic nephropathy/kidney failure

- amputation of limbs
- erectile dysfunction
- cardiovascular disease
- problem pregnancies/large babies
- periodontal disease
- yeast (Candida) vaginitis/balanitis

Key Elements of Glycemic Control

Glycemic control is maintained through a combination of medication, good nutrition, exercise, and frequent blood glucose testing with an appropriate response to those test results (modification of diet, exercise, oral medication, and/or the insulin dose). This requires education and involvement with a diabetes care team. Yet sadly, many people with diabetes do not attend to each of these key proponents of glycemic control—and some people ignore all of them, to their physical and emotional detriment as well as their families'.

The problem may lie in their denial of the existence of their illness and its severity. It may also be due to a lack of education. A third cause of poor glycemic control is fear or dislike of pain, including the brief pain of blood testing and the pain of injecting medication. Some people may also dislike the additional burden of time and money that their illness brings.

Improvements in Blood Testing and Monitoring

Until the latter part of the 20th century, it was difficult or impossible for most people with diabetes to monitor their glucose blood levels. The creation of glucose meters that can be easily used at home resolved this issue. Still, many people dislike having to pierce their skin to extract a drop of blood for evaluation.

As a result, less painful micro-lancet equipment such as pen devices were developed, as well as devices which could extract the blood from the forearm or other body parts with less sensitive nerve endings than the fingertip.

Another aspect of glycemic control disliked by most people with diabetes is the injection of medication, which is a must for all those with Type 1 diabetes and for some people with Type 2 diabetes. Since they don't want to give themselves shots, they may skip testing their blood altogether and ignore their illness. New breakthroughs may make the taking of medication painless and thus, more people will work on glycemic control.

For example, inhaled insulin is another emerging 21st century option for people with Type 1 diabetes. Experts report that early results on this painless product are very promising. Other methods of medication delivery are being researched. Several companies are teaming together to work on insulin that can be given under the tongue much like a nitroglycerin tablet.

Glycemic Control Is Spotty or Inadequate among Many Groups

According to 1998 statistics provided by the Centers for Disease Control and Prevention (CDC), only 42 percent of individuals with diabetes in the United States test their blood at least once a day. Native American and Alaska Natives were the most likely (53 percent) to perform daily glucose testing, followed by Caucasians (43 percent), African Americans (40 percent), Hispanics or Latinos (36 percent), and Asian or Pacific Islanders (30 percent).

This finding appears to be backed up by another study reported by Maureen Harris in a 2001 issue of *Diabetes Care*. This study looked at the self-monitoring of patients with Type 2 diabetes, some of whom used oral agents while others used insulin. According to this study, 29 percent of those who treated their diabetes with insulin had either never monitored their blood glucose or they monitored it only once a month or less. Among those who treated their diabetes with oral medications, 65 percent never or only once a month or less had monitored their blood levels. Among patients who treated their diabetes with diet only, 80 percent had never or only once a month or less monitored their blood glucose levels.

These are discouraging findings because most physicians expect patients to perform daily blood monitoring so that they can make adjustments to their diet and medication and report extreme changes to their physician.

Dietary control Few people enjoy having to think critically about what they should or should not eat and how and why it may affect their blood glucose levels. Yet this is another essential aspect of good glycemic control for people with both Type 1 and Type 2 diabetes. Thus nutritional education is critical as well as support from family and friends.

Lifestyle changes Another aspect of good glycemic control is for the person with diabetes to make basic lifestyle changes in order to avoid behaviors that can worsen glucose levels. For example, SMOKING is known to cause many severe problems for people with diabetes. However, since people with diabetes have a higher risk than the general population without diabetes for developing HYPERTENSION, STROKE, CARDIOVASCULAR DISEASE, and many other blood vessel–related diseases that are aggravated by smoking, it is critical and lifesaving for anyone who has diabetes to stop smoking as soon as possible.

OBESITY is a risk factor for the development of Type 2 diabetes and after diagnosis will increase insulin resistance and thus worsen overall glycemic control. Most people with IMPAIRED GLUCOSE TOLERANCE or Type 2 diabetes or hypertension or HYPERLIPIDEMIA (or any combination of those problems) will improve their condition by losing weight.

Regular daily exercise is another way for people with diabetes to maintain healthy glycemic control.

See also BLOOD GLUCOSE MONITORING, NUTRITION.

Harris, Maureen I. "Frequency of Blood Glucose Monitoring in Relation to Glycemic Control in Patients with Type 2 Diabetes." *Diabetes Care* 24, no. 6 (June 2001): 979–982.

Hunt, Linda M., et al. "How Patients Adapt Diabetes Self-Care Recommendations to Everyday Life." *Journal of Family Practice* 46, no. 3 (March 1998): 207–216.

glycogen Stored glucose within the body, found primarily in the liver and the muscles. When needed by the body, it is transformed through glycogenolysis, back into glucose. Conversely, glycogenesis is the process by which glucose is converted into glycogen.

Glycogen can be thought of as stored glucose. It is comprised of strands that are bound end to end in a branching form, much like the branches on a Christmas tree. Two enzymes are important in this process. Glycogen synthase controls synthesis and glycogen phosphorylase controls breakdown of glycogen. Working together, these enzymes control the glucose balance.

During times between meals when glucose is needed, the body breaks down stored glycogen to normalize the blood glucose level. At one time, it was thought that an excessive breakdown of liver glycogen was the major determinant of the fasting blood glucose level in patients with Type 2 diabetes. However, special liver studies (in vivo nuclear magnetic resonance spectroscopy) have determined that the predominant contributor to the increase in fasting glucose is due to gluconeogenesis; that is the formation of new glucose.

The average person has about 18 hours of glycogen stores in the liver before the body needs to begin making new glucose or burning fat (i.e., ketosis).

glycosuria/glucosuria Glucose in the urine, which is an abnormal sign, and an indicator of diabetes. People with undiagnosed diabetes have a typically sweet taste to their urine, attractive to insects and which has been noted since ancient times.

Generally, glucose will "spill over" into the urine in this condition, if the glucose blood levels are greater than 180 mg/dL. In people who have diabetes, their kidneys adapt and glucose may not show up in the urine until levels are greater than 250–300 mg/dL. As a result relying on urine testing only is an inadequate method of screening for and monitoring diabetes.

Occasionally, people without diabetes have a lower than normal renal glucose threshold and it will spill glucose into the urine even when the person has normal blood glucose levels.

government, federal   The U.S. government and its role in diabetes research, treatment, and payment.

The federal government performs or pays for research on diabetes, primarily through the National Institutes of Health and based on funds that are provided by Congress. Federal agencies also provide information to individuals with diabetes and their families.

The key federal organizations involved in diabetes are the Centers for Disease Control and Prevention, the National Diabetes Information Clearinghouse, and the National Institute of Diabetes and Digestive and Kidney Diseases (NIDDK).

There are also several programs important to many people with diabetes, including MEDICARE and MEDICAID. MEDICARE is a federal medical program that is primarily oriented to people over age 65 and that also includes many younger disabled people. Medicaid is a program that receives some federal funds but that is managed by the states. It provides medical care to indigent people of all ages.

Medicare provides coverage for IMMUNIZATIONS for flu and pneumonia, which are important for people with diabetes. Medicare recipients also receive coverage of syringes and related material that are needed by individuals with diabetes. Medicare also covers some limited HOME HEALTH CARE services and very limited (30 days after hospitalization, as of this writing) SKILLED NURSING care services. Medicare also pays for therapeutic shoes for some patients who need them.

government, state   Governments at the state level and their role in research, treatment, and payment for diabetes programs.

All state governments have an agency that is dedicated in part or solely to the subject of diabetes. Some states place this responsibility within their state health department while others place it under other offices. Some states have more active programs than others and this may also vary from year to year.

State governments administer the MEDICAID program, receiving some federal money as well. Medicaid is a program for indigent people who are eligible for assistance because of old age, disability, or other reasons.

growth hormone   A substance that is naturally produced by the anterior pituitary gland in response to stimulation by growth hormone-releasing hormone (GHRH) produced by the hypothalamus. In growing children, growth hormone is released in a pulsatile fashion mainly at night, and it stimulates growth and development via an array of intermediary hormones.

Growth hormone is also released in response to HYPOGLYCEMIA, although its metabolic effects are slow and most people's recovery from hypoglycemia is mainly mediated via adrenaline and noradrenaline.

Natural levels of growth hormone tend to be slightly higher in overweight patients with Type 2 diabetes. Excessive growth hormone production in children can cause gigantism and excessive levels of growth hormone in adults can result in ACROMEGALY.

Growth Hormone as Treatment

Growth hormone that was created from recombinant processes is administered to children with documented growth hormone deficiency due to pituitary tumor or trauma. Females with Turner's syndrome may also be given growth hormone to help them grow taller.

Growth hormone may be administered to adults to increase their lean body mass, increase strength, and improve their quality of life. Typically, growth hormone is given only to adults with documented growth hormone deficiency.

When they are stronger and have less fat, most people feel better. They are also less likely to fall and become injured and more likely to be able to lift and exercise. Currently ongoing studies are looking at whether or not the use of an oral GHRH, which will increase endogenous growth hormone secretion, will benefit the "pre-frail elderly."

A disadvantage to administered growth hormone is that it may induce diabetes or impaired glucose tolerance in susceptible children, especially if the dose is excessive. Experts recommend that before administering any growth hormone to children (or adults), their blood glucose levels should be checked first to verify that they are within the normal range.

According to an article in a 2000 issue of *The Lancet* by Cutfield et al., the researchers found that although the risk was very low, children who were given growth hormone had a six times greater rate of developing Type 2 diabetes than children who did not receive the hormone.

It is possible that the children would have developed diabetes anyway without receiving the growth hormone. Further research is needed on this topic before conclusions can be drawn.

It was also interesting to note that the children who received growth hormone and, subsequently, developed Type 2 diabetes were *not* obese, in contrast to the majority of children and adolescents with Type 2 diabetes, 80 percent of whom are obese. It is not clear why this was true.

Cutfield, Wayne S., et al. "Incidence of Diabetes Mellitus and Impaired Glucose Tolerance in Children and Adolescents Receiving Growth-Hormone Treatment." *The Lancet* 355, no. 9204 (February 2000): 610–613.

Fukui, Michiaki, et al. "Growth-Hormone Treatment and Risk of Diabetes." *The Lancet* 355, no. 9218 (May 2000): 1,912–1,913.

gum disease   See GINGIVITIS.

HDL A fatty lipid protein that circulates in the blood and is found throughout the body. High density lipoprotein (HDL) cholesterol, is often referred to as "good" cholesterol because high levels of HDL decrease a person's risk for having a heart attack or stroke. HDL is responsible for removing cholesterol from blood vessels and back to the liver, a process also known as "reverse cholesterol transport."

If a person has a low level of HDL, it is possible to increase the levels by as much as 10 percent through exercise, weight loss, and smoking cessation.

Because people with diabetes have a higher risk than nondiabetics for both heart attack and stroke, it's important for physicians to run periodic testing on blood levels of HDL and LDL. (Low density lipoproteins are considered "bad" cholesterol and high levels of LDL increase the risk for heart attack or stroke because the LDL stays within the arteries and builds up.)

See also ATHEROSCLEROSIS/ARTERIOSCLEROSIS; CHOLESTEROL, LDL; TRIGLYCERIDE.

hepatitis C virus (HCV) A type of hepatitis virus, an infectious agent. There is an apparent association between the hepatitis C virus and Type 2 diabetes, based on a study reported in a 2000 issue of the *Annals of Internal Medicine*.

Researchers studied 9,841 people with HCV infection and noted that 8.4 percent of the subjects had Type 2 diabetes. They also found that subjects who were age 40 or older were more than three times more likely to have Type 2 diabetes. Type 2 diabetes was also found more frequently among subjects who were nonwhite, had low socioeconomic status, and had high BODY MASS INDEX ratings. It is not clear if HCV may in some way cause or trigger Type 2 diabetes.

Mehta, Shruti H., et al. "Prevalence of Type 2 Diabetes Mellitus among Persons with Hepatitis C Virus Infection in the United States." *Annals of Internal Medicine* 133 (2000): 592–599.

HHNS See HYPEROSMOLAR COMA.

Hispanics/Latinos People of Latin origin in the United States, including Mexican Americans, Puerto Ricans, Central and South Americans, and Cuban Americans, as well as individuals of mixed ethnicities of one or more of these groups. Hispanics in the United States, particularly those who are Mexican American, have a higher risk of developing Type 2 diabetes than do non-Hispanic whites.

Diabetes is the fifth leading cause of death among Hispanics in the United States, and it is also a leading cause of kidney disease, BLINDNESS, STROKE, AMPUTATION, and heart disease among this group.

According to the Centers for Disease Control and Prevention (CDC), an analysis of Hispanics in six areas with high levels of Hispanics (California, Florida, Illinois, New York and New Jersey combined, Texas, and Puerto Rico) over the period 1998–2002 found that 7.4 percent of Hispanics had diabetes. The CDC also noted that diabetes is diagnosed in Hispanics at younger ages than it is among white non-Hispanics; for example, in California, 3.2 percent of Hispanics ages 18–44 had been diagnosed with diabetes compared to 1.3 percent of non-Hispanic whites. In considering the entire Hispanic population in the United States, the CDC noted that the overall prevalence of diabetes among Hispanics was 9.8 percent compared to 5.0 percent for non-Hispanic whites.

The CDC also noted that diabetes rates more than doubled for obese Hispanics; for example, among those with a BODY MASS INDEX (BMI) of 25 or less (normal weight), 7.0 percent reported a diagnosis of diabetes. In contrast, among those with a BMI of 30 or greater (overweight to obese), 15.3 percent of Hispanics had been diagnosed with diabetes. The CDC also reported that diabetes decreased with education; for example, among Hispanics with less than a high school education, 11.8 percent had diabetes, while among those with a college education, only 7.0 percent had diabetes.

The CDC also looked at the lifetime risk of developing diabetes among Hispanics and found that Hispanic females who were born in 2000 had a 52.5 percent risk of ever developing diabetes, while Hispanic males had a 45.4 percent risk. This is in contrast to non-Hispanic white females, among whom the lifetime risk for developing diabetes was 31.2 percent, while the lifetime risk for developing diabetes among non-Hispanic white males was 26.7 percent. (See Table 1.)

TABLE 1: LIFETIME RISK OF DEVELOPING DIABETES FOR THOSE BORN IN 2000

Race/ethnicity and Gender	Lifetime Risk, by Percent
Hispanic females	52.5
Hispanic males	45.4
African-American females	40.2
African-American males	40.2
Non-Hispanic white females	31.2
Non-Hispanic white males	26.7

Knowledge about Diabetes

From a study of the prevalence (entire population), incidence (new cases in a year), demographics, and clinical characteristics of diabetes in Hispanics (about 70 percent were Mexican Americans) ages 10–19 years, researchers Jean M. Lawrence and colleagues reported their findings in *Diabetes Care* in 2009. There were 551 subjects with Type 1 diabetes and 127 subjects with Type 2 diabetes.

The researchers found that among youths, Type 1 diabetes was significantly more common than was Type 2 diabetes. They also found that among those with Type 2 diabetes, the incidence was twice as common among females as it was among males for those ages 10–14 years. They also found that among youths in the age range of 15–19 years, the incidence of Type 2 diabetes was greater than that of Type 1 diabetes for females only.

The researchers noted that poor glycemic control was a common issue among Hispanic youths age 15 years and older with either Type 1 or Type 2 diabetes. Overweight was a common problem among those with Type 2 diabetes; however, interestingly, 44 percent of the youths with Type 1 diabetes were either overweight or obese.

In a study on general knowledge about diabetes risks and preventive measures among Hispanics and African Americans, researchers Karen Weber Cullen and Bonnie B. Buzek interviewed 21 students in the ninth and 10th grades and 39 of their parents, reporting their findings in *Diabetes Educator* in 2009. The majority of the parent and child interviewees were overweight.

Most of the interviewees did not know that overweight or obesity was a risk factor for diabetes, although the majority of the adults knew that a family history of diabetes was a risk factor for the development of diabetes. As a result, the researchers were not surprised that the preventive measure of losing weight to avoid diabetes was identified by only 8 percent of the parents and 5 percent of the children.

Variations among Hispanics in Incidence of Diabetes and Hypertension

In the results of a study published in 2010 in the *Journal of General Internal Medicine*, the researchers compared different ethnic groups of more than 31,000 foreign-born Hispanics living in the United States and their incidence of diabetes and hypertension and found considerable disparities between the different groups. For example, the prevalence of diabetes was highest among foreign-born Puerto Ricans or 15 percent for diabetes and 32 percent for those with hypertension. Mexican-Americans had the next highest rate, and the rate was lowest among Cubans, Central/South Americans, and Dominicans, or half or less the rate of Mexican-Americans. This research illustrates that grouping Hispanics together as one group does not provide adequate information on issues such as diabetes and hypertension, where some groups of Hispanics have much higher rates of these diseases than others.

The primary risk factors for Hispanic Americans to develop diabetes are as follows:

- a family history of diabetes
- gestational diabetes
- insulin resistance
- physical inactivity
- obesity
- hyperinsulinemia

Hispanics with Diabetes and Related Disorders

In both the San Antonio Heart Study and in the National Health and Nutrition Examination Survey III (NHANES III, using data from 1988–94), the rate of diabetic retinopathy among Mexican Americans was more than twice that of non-Hispanic white Americans. As with non-Hispanic whites, the severity of the diabetes was indicated by poor glycemic control, the need for INSULIN use, and the length of time with diabetes, all factors that were significantly associated with retinopathy. The San Antonio Heart Study showed more nephropathy, while the San Luis Valley Diabetes Study showed no difference in the rates of nephropathy when compared to non-Hispanic whites. Interestingly, Mexican Americans with diabetes live longer on dialysis than do non-Hispanic whites, although the reasons for this are unknown.

While in general about 50 percent of women with GESTATIONAL DIABETES will eventually develop chronic diabetes, the rate is between 10 and 15 percent per year in the Hispanic population.

Many Hispanics may present with DIABETIC KETOACIDOSIS (DKA), and after receiving acute therapy for this problem, they are then able to be treated with diet and/or oral MEDICATIONS FOR TYPE 2 DIABETES. This particular phenomenon has been referred to as "Prairie diabetes" among Hispanics and as "Flatbush diabetes" when it occurs among African Americans (for Flatbush, New York).

See also AFRICAN AMERICANS WITH DIABETES; AMERICAN INDIANS/ALASKA NATIVES; ASIANS/PACIFIC ISLANDER AMERICANS; ALCOHOL ABUSE/ALCOHOLISM; DEATH; DIABETES MELLITUS; DIABETIC NEPHROPATHY; DIABETIC NEUROPATHY; DIABETIC RETINOPATHY; OBESITY; WHITES/CAUCASIANS.

Burke, James P., et al. "Rapid Rise in the Incidence of Type 2 Diabetes From 1987 to 1996: Results From the San Antonio Heart Study." *Archives of Internal Medicine* 159 (1999): 1,450–1,456.

Lawrence, Jean M., et al. "Diabetes in Hispanic American Youth." *Diabetes Care* 32, Supp. (2009): S123–S132.

Pabon-Nau, Lina P., et al. "Hypertension and Diabetes Prevalence among U.S. Hispanics by Country of Origin: The National Health Interview Survey 2000–2005." *Journal of General Internal Medicine* 25, no. 8 (2010): 847–852.

Rodacki, M., et al. "Diabetes Flatbush—from Ketoacidosis to Non Pharmacological Treatment." *Arquivos Brasileiros de Endocrinologia & Metabologia* 51 (2007): 131–135.

Seaquist, E. R., et al. "Familial Clustering of Diabetic Kidney Disease: Evidence for Genetic Susceptibility to Diabetic Nephropathy." *New England Journal of Medicine* 320 (1989): 1,161–1,165.

Weber Cullen, Karen, and Bonnie B. Buzek. "Knowledge about Type 2 Diabetes Risk and Prevention of
African-American and Hispanic Adults and Adolescents with Family History of Type 2 Diabetes." *Diabetes Educator* 25, no. 5 (2009): 836–841.

**home blood glucose monitoring/self-blood glu-
cose monitoring**   Testing of the levels of the
blood, performed by an individual at home, and
subsequent actions based on the results of the
test. (Such as taking medication, consuming a
snack for low levels of glucose, etc.) Home blood
glucose monitoring is critically important for all
individuals with diabetes because it is not possible for physicians or other medical professionals to provide daily testing.

People diagnosed with both Type 1 and Type
2 diabetes need to keep track of their blood glucose level and watch themselves for any signs
of a surge or sudden drop. This is referred to as
maintaining GLYCEMIC CONTROL.

Very large scale studies, such as the DIABETES
CONTROL AND COMPLICATIONS TRIAL (DCCT), a
10-year, federally funded study of individuals
in North America with Type 1 diabetes, have
validated the importance of self-monitoring and
maintaining tight glucose levels in limiting the
risk of severe future complications of diabetes,
such as AMPUTATION, END-STAGE RENAL DISEASE,
and other complications including an earlier than
necessary death.

In addition, a large-scale study on individuals
with Type 2 diabetes, the UNITED KINGDOM PRO-
SPECTIVE DIABETES STUDY (UKPDS), also revealed
the importance of tight glucose monitoring in
aiding patients with Type 2 diabetes to avoid
severe complications in the future.

A plunge in blood glucose level is an indication of HYPOGLYCEMIA, while elevated levels indicate HYPERGLYCEMIA. Many patients believe that
they can tell what their glucose level is without
performing any monitoring, but this is generally unreliable except when glucose levels are
exceedingly high or low.

Although most people with diabetes are well
aware of the need to monitor blood, sometimes
compliance is lax because the person is ill or
tired or distracted by other activities.

Most individuals with Type 1 diabetes must test
their blood at least several times a day and if they
are complying with an intensive testing regimen,
at least four times per day is considered best. To
achieve tight glycemic control, most people with
Type 1 diabetes need to monitor their blood four
times a day (three times before meals and one
time at bedtime). People on insulin pumps often
monitor themselves seven times a day, including three times a day pre-meal, three times post
meal and once at bedtime. Patients should do
extra tests when they are ill or they suspect they
are hypoglycemic or hyperglycemic. They should
also perform extra tests if they change their diet,
exercise, or activity levels.

Patients with Type 2 diabetes and who do not
require injections of insulin, may test their blood
as infrequently as several times per month or
3–4 times per day. Each patient should consult
with his or her physician and diabetes team to
determine how much monitoring will help to
optimize the individual's glycemic control.

Based on the glucose level readings, the individual can adjust his or her diet or exercise plan.
The person with Type 1 diabetes can also adjust
his or her insulin intake as well as adjust diet
and exercise programs. Some people with Type
2 diabetes also require insulin and must make
adjustments to their intake based on the results
of their blood glucose test.

Excellent glycemic control levels are as follows:

pre-meal: 80–120
pre-bedtime: 100–140

home health care   Health care that is provided
to people within their homes, rather than in hospitals, clinics, or other settings. This may include
injections, special treatments, or any other medical care that is indicated for a home-bound individual. Some people with diabetes need to receive
home health care due to severe kidney disease
or other ailments that are directly or indirectly

related to their diabetes. They may need home health care aides or may need visits from nurses or other medically trained individuals.

MEDICARE has strict rules on what services may be paid for in home health care.

Medicare and Home Health Care

According to the Centers for Medicare and Medicaid Services, formerly the Health Care Financing Administration (HCFA), the organization that determines Medicare payments, there are four conditions that must *all* be met in order for Medicare to approve home health care. They are:

- A physician has determined that home health care is needed and has written a plan for care. This plan must be updated about every two months.
- The patient needs one or more of the following: skilled nursing care, or intermittent nursing care, or physical or speech therapy.
- The patient cannot leave the house except with extreme difficulty and is essentially considered "housebound."
- The home health care agency is approved by the Medicare program.

If the above conditions have been met, Medicare will pay (as of this writing) for the following types of services:

- skilled nursing care that is part time or intermittent and is provided by either a licensed practical nurse or registered nurse (for example, help with taking medications or injections)
- home health aide services provided on a part-time or intermittent basis. Examples of services are help with dressing, bathing, toileting, etc.
- physical therapy
- speech language pathology services
- occupational therapy
- medical social services such as counseling or assistance in locating resources in the patient's area

- assistance with blood glucose monitoring at home and reviews of medications
- some medical supplies such as bandages but not to include prescribed medications
- some medical equipment, which Medicare may pay 80 percent towards, such as a walker or a wheelchair.

Medicaid and Home Health Care

For patients who are indigent and receiving Medicaid services, home health care may be available. In some cases, Medicaid will cover services not paid by Medicare, such as homecare services, and personal care.

See also MEDICAID.

honeymoon phase A time that may occur early after a person with Type 1 diabetes has been diagnosed with the disease. By definition, people with Type 1 diabetes make no insulin and they are thus dependent upon insulin to live. However, early in the disease process, the patient's body may actually still make small amounts of insulin.

The person with new diabetes may also begin to have hypoglycemic episodes that lead the patient and physician to appropriately decrease the insulin dose. Sometimes insulin can be discontinued for a short period, which is generally no more than weeks. However, many endocrinologists prefer to maintain patients on small doses of insulin to avoid giving the patient false hope that the diabetes is cured. Also, some endocrinologists argue that stopping and starting insulin therapy may induce antibody formation and could cause the body to become more resistant to insulin. This could then result in the injected dose to become less effective in the future. In that event, a larger injected dose of insulin would be needed.

HOPE Study Refers to the Heart Outcomes Prevention Evaluation (HOPE) study in Canada, which was performed with subjects who had a high risk for developing cardiovascular disease.

The subjects were about 9,000 patients over age 55 who were also at very high risk for developing cardiac ailments. Of these patients, 1,808 were men and women with diabetes. The average age of the patients studied was 65 years and 58 percent of them had a previous history of HYPERTENSION. Two thirds of the subjects also had a problem with high CHOLESTEROL.

The purpose of the study, which was completed in 1999, was to determine if the administration of a specific angiotensin converting enzyme (ACE) inhibitor medication (ramipril) would reduce the risk of heart disease. The researchers found that treatment with the medication was successful at reducing the overall death rates, dropping the risk for heart attack by 20 percent, and decreasing the incidence of complications related to diabetes by 16 percent. Overall, the risk of death was reduced by 16 percent. The study was ended early because the findings were so promising for the patients receiving the medication. Researchers wanted those patients taking the placebo to have the chance to take an ACE inhibitor drug and gain from its benefits.

Among the diabetic subjects, the researchers found that the medication effectively decreased the risk of serious cardiovascular problems, whether the patients were also taking oral hypoglycemic medications or they were injecting insulin and even if patients had a prior history of cardiovascular ailments. The study also revealed that ramipril decreased the risk of DIABETIC NEPHROPATHY (kidney disease) in patients by about 24 percent.

Jensen, Tonny, et al. "The HOPE Study and Diabetes." *The Lancet* 355, no. 9210 (April 2000): 1,181.
Peters, Anne, M.D. "Landmark Studies: Hope for the Diabetic Heart." *Clinical Diabetes* 18, no. 3 (Summer 2000): 130–131.

hormone replacement therapy (HRT)/estrogen replacement therapy (ERT) Hormones prescribed for women, with and without diabetes, after the onset of menopause or in the transitional period known as the "perimenopause."

This entry covers both estrogen-only therapy and combination therapy (estrogen and progestogen), and umbrellas both therapies under "hormone replacement therapy." It should be noted that most doctors consider only combination therapy as HRT and they call estrogen therapy alone "ERT."

Many physicians recommend medications to replace the hormones that are no longer produced or are produced in diminished quantities by the woman's own body. Doctors may recommend estrogen replacement therapy (ERT) if patients have had a hysterectomy. If the woman still has her uterus, physicians may recommend a combination therapy of estrogen and a progestational agent such as medroxyprogesterone acetate, which will allow the lining of the uterus [endometrium] to cycle and minimize the risk of endometrial cancer. These medications are offered to women with and without diabetes.

Pros and Cons of HRT

As of this writing there are mixed findings on the pros and cons of administering hormone replacement therapy to menopausal women, including women with diabetes. In general, HRT may provide some protection against heart disease, STROKE, ALZHEIMER'S DISEASE, colorectal cancer, tooth loss, age-related macular degeneration, and OSTEOPOROSIS/fractures. These problems are also experienced by many women with diabetes. HRT may also give the woman relief from sleep disorders, improving the quality and duration of sleep. HRT may also improve cognitive function. In addition, women who take HRT may find relief from many other problems such as atrophy of the genitourinary track and vasomotor symptoms, such as hot flashes and temperature intolerance. HRT may also bring relief from emotional problems such as DEPRESSION. Many women with diabetes have high risks for the aforementioned problems.

There are also some negative aspects to taking female hormones. Women who use HRT are more prone to developing gallbladder disease, blood clots (phlebitis, phlebothrombosis, and pulmonary embolism-blood clots from the legs or pelvis that can break off and travel to the lungs). Breast cancer is another risk of HRT, particularly in women with a family history for the disease. In addition, if the woman still has her uterus, HRT may present a greater risk than the woman not taking hormones for causing the development of endometrial (uterine lining) cancer. Added estrogen may also cause breast tenderness, precipitate migraine headaches, and also cause fluid retention and mild weight gain. It can create depression in some women.

Studies on HRT and Heart Disease

There are currently 35 observational studies that show a 50 percent decrease in heart disease in women on HRT. This makes sense given what we know of the effects of estrogen; improved lipid profile, decreased INSULIN RESISTANCE, decreased stickiness of platelets, increased blood flow, as well as an improved ability of the coronary arteries to dilate, better pumping of heart muscle, and decreased plaque formation in blood vessels.

Much of the controversy over HRT in recent years has come up in studies that looked at the potential benefits of HRT in women with known heart disease (which includes many women with diabetes mellitus). For example, the Heart and Estrogen/Progestin Replacement Study (HERS), was a study of 2,763 women with an average age of 66.7 years. The subjects were treated with both 0.625 mg of estrogen and 2.5 mg of medroxyprogesterone acetate for 5 years. A control group received a placebo.

At the end of the study, researchers concluded that there were no major differences between the treated and untreated groups. Of greatest concern, however, was the observation that there was actually an *increased* incidence of heart problems in the first eight months in the women who were treated with HRT. Paradoxically, however, as the study carried on, this trend reversed itself. The women who continued in the study were found to have a greater protection from heart events.

It may be that the initial effects of estrogen tend to lead to an increased risk of clotting and, thus, blockages that are already present in women taking HRT become a problem. Over time, however, as the multiple positive metabolic effects kick in, HRT may offer greater protection and overcome the impact of the clotting effects.

Similar results were reported in the Women's Health Initiative (WHI) study. In the first two years of the study, about 1 percent of the women had heart attacks, strokes, and blood clots in their legs and lungs whether they were on estrogen therapy, combination therapy, or placebo. Again, as in the HERS study, the situation changed after two years and the hormones were shown to be protective.

As a result of these studies, current recommendations are that hormone replacement drugs should not be considered as therapy for secondary prevention for women who already have known heart disease. But in women who do not have heart disease but who are at risk for disease, HRT may be beneficial.

To be effective and safe, it appears that women who use HRT need to start taking hormones prior to the development of problems in the blood vessels in order to allow the medication to continue to protect women. If a woman already has heart problems, it's best to avoid these drugs unless further evidence indicates this group should take them.

Women with Diabetes and HRT

It had long been thought that administering HRT to women with diabetes would worsen their control of glucose levels; however, recent studies have shown that this is generally not the case. All parameters of glucose metabolism, especially insulin resistance and lipid profiles, appear to improve with HRT.

Note: HRT is not the same situation as is found with oral contraceptives (which also have female hormones) prescribed for birth control. The reason for this is that birth control pills may contain a larger dose of estrogen than found in hormone replacement therapy. Consequently, birth control pills are more likely to increase insulin resistance (probably because of the progestational component) than HRT. Thus, women with normal glucose tolerance and with risk factors for diabetes who are taking birth control pills may find that their condition worsens to IMPAIRED GLUCOSE TOLERANCE (IGT), with higher than normal glucose levels but not high enough to be diagnosed with diabetes. Women who already have IGT and who take oral contraceptives may progress to overt diabetes. Women who already have diabetes may require an adjustment in their medication in order to continue to maintain their usual level of glycemic control.

Consulting with gynecologists Because the issue is so complex and so individual for each woman, and because there are many types of medications and dosages, it is best for menopausal women with diabetes who are considering HRT to consult with their own gynecologists on what course of action to take. If the woman is under age 50, it's probably a good idea to request a blood test of estrogen levels (generally, FSH), to avoid unnecessary medication.

Multiple medical professional organizations such as the American Association of Clinical Endocrinologists (AACE), the American College of Obstetricians and Gynecologists (ACOG), and the Association of Professors of Gynecology and Obstetrics (APGO), have published evidence-based guidelines on HRT/ERT that attempt to weigh the benefits and risks of this therapy.

For further information on the Internet, go to the National Women's Health Information Center at www.4woman.gov/faq/hormone.htm. The National Institute on Aging also offers information on the pros and cons of HRT on the following Web site: www.aoa.dhhs.gov/aoa/pages/agepages/hormone.html.

hospitalization Admission to a hospital for treatment of a serious disease. Individuals with diabetes may need hospitalization for a variety of problems, including severe foot problems, extreme HYPOGLYCEMIA or HYPERGLYCEMIA, DIABETIC KETOACIDOSIS (DKA), HYPERTENSION, COMA, and an array of other medical problems. According to the Centers for Disease Control and Prevention (CDC), diabetes was the first diagnosis in 503,000 hospital discharges in 1996. Diabetes was also a factor in thousands of other cases in which it was not the first diagnosis.

Diabetic individuals are also more likely than nondiabetics to need hospitalization; for example, studies indicate that people with diabetes are four times more likely to be hospitalized than nondiabetics, or 24 percent to 6 percent, respectively. People with diabetes in the United States are hospitalized over 3 million days per year and also make over 15 million visits to their physicians on an outpatient basis.

This high rate of hospitalization may be due in part to the fact that 51 percent of the population with diabetes is in fair or poor physical health versus 9 percent of nondiabetics who are in fair to poor health. An estimated 80,000 former workers are permanently disabled because of their diabetes.

In one study of the risks for hospitalization among people with diabetes, reported in a 1999 issue of the *Archives of Internal Medicine*, the researchers found that people with Type 1 diabetes had a greater risk for hospitalization when they had high glycosylated hemoglobin levels or they had hypertension. Among those with Type 2 diabetes, the key factor that predicted hospitalization was high glycosylated hemoglobin levels. As a result, good GLYCEMIC CONTROL was a factor in keeping both Type 1 and Type 2 diabetes patients out of the hospital.

See also EMERGENCY ISSUES IN DIABETES.

Moss, S. E., et al. "Risk Factors for Hospitalization in People with Diabetes." *Archives of Internal Medicine* 159 (1999): 2,053–2,057.
National Academy on an Aging Society. "Diabetes: A Drain on U.S. Resources." *Challenges for the 21st Century: Chronic and Disabling Conditions* 1, no. 6 (April 2000): 1–6.

Humalog A form of insulin lispro trademarked by Eli Lilly & Company and approved by the Food and Drug Administration (FDA) in the

United States in 1996. Humalog is made from manipulated DNA material rather than from beef or pork insulin. Such forms are generally better tolerated by people with diabetes than are forms derived from animal insulin. Humalog is a rapid-acting insulin that starts working within five to 15 minutes from injection. The bulk of its action ends within three to four hours, as opposed to five to eight hours with regular insulin. Humalog is less likely to cause HYPOGLYCEMIA.

Because of the change in the amino acids, Humalog is more rapidly absorbed from subcutaneous fat sites after absorption. It peaks in one hour, which is typically when the body's glucose level peaks, thus creating a good match. Humalog is more convenient and effective than traditional regular insulin.

See also INSULIN.

hyperglycemia   An excessive level of glucose in the bloodstream of an individual and the hallmark feature of diabetes.

The key symptoms of hyperglycemia (and diabetes) are:

- increased urination
- increased thirst
- unexplained weight loss
- blurred vision

Individuals diagnosed with TYPE 1 DIABETES should self-test their blood three to four times per day, and should also use INSULIN as prescribed by their physicians in order to control the hyperglycemia. Individuals with TYPE 2 DIABETES should also do daily blood testing and use oral medications, diet, and exercise to control hyperglycemia. Those with Type 1 and Type 2 diabetes need to monitor their diet carefully and also exercise on a regular basis in order to better control the symptoms and the moderate-to-severe complications that can come with diabetes.

See also GLYCEMIC CONTROL.

hyperinsulinism/hyperinsulinemia   Excessive amounts of insulin in the body. This condition may occur when the body creates large amounts of insulin in an attempt to overcome INSULIN RESISTANCE (the inability to properly use the insulin). Hyperinsulinism results in a lowered blood level of HDL cholesterol ("good" cholesterol) and is also associated with increased levels of TRIGLYCERIDES. This condition may lead to the development of Type 2 diabetes, although it is not inevitable that diabetes will occur. The likelihood of developing diabetes is increased, however, if there are other family members who have a medical history of diabetes.

If a person has HYPERTENSION in addition to hyperinsulinism, this condition can cause DIABETIC NEPHROPATHY, or kidney damage. When hyperinsulinism is associated with hypertension, obesity, DYSLIPIDEMIA, polycystic ovarian syndrome, or premature cardiovascular disease, it is known as Syndrome X. Other names for Syndrome X are Cardiac Dysmetabolic Syndrome and Insulin Resistance Syndrome.

Reaven, G. M. "Role of Insulin Resistance in Human Disease." *Diabetes* 37 (1998): 1,495.

hyperlipidemia   Excessive levels of blood lipids (fats), such as LDL cholesterol and triglycerides. This is a dangerous condition that can lead to serious medical consequences, such as heart attack, STROKE, and other problems. A physician will almost invariably recommend dietary changes and, if the patient is overweight as well, will also recommend weight loss. The doctor may also prescribe medications to lower cholesterol levels. (See CHOLESTEROL, DYSLIPIDEMIA, HDL, LDL, TRIGLYCERIDE.)

hyperosmolar coma   A very serious condition of unconsciousness that occurs in patients with Type 2 diabetes. It is also known as hyperosmolar hyperglycemia non-ketotic coma (HHNC). In about a third of cases, a hyperosmolar coma is the presenting stage of diabetes in a previously undiagnosed person. This syndrome may develop over the course of days to a week.

Symptoms and Diagnostic Path

The primary symptoms are:

- thirst and dry mouth
- decreased sweating
- increased urination initially and then decreased urination
- confusion or increased sleepiness
- sunken eyes and rapid pulse
- weakness and leg cramps

The primary signs are:

- glucose typically greater than 600 mg/dL
- poor skin turgor
- dry mucous membranes
- tachycardia
- blood pH greater than 7.30
- elevated blood urea nitrogen (BUN) levels
- abnormal level of consciousness
- low blood pressure

Treatment Options and Outlook

The person with hyperosmolar coma urgently needs hospitalization. Primary treatment at the hospital is aimed at rehydration with the use of intravenous fluids as well as identifying and correcting the underlying cause of the condition.

Risk Factors and Preventive Measures

Elderly diabetic individuals are at risk for hyperosmolar coma, particularly if they have other coexisting illnesses. The condition may also be precipitated by infections, such as a urinary tract infection or pneumonia. Dehydration may also be a cause, which may have resulted from poor fluid intake, diarrhea, or bleeding. Other individuals at risk for hyperosmolar coma are those who abuse or are dependent on alcohol.

Daily blood testing is a good preventive measure. Daily blood testing will generally alert a person with diabetes to a state of increasing blood levels before reaching the stage of hyperosmolar coma. Close observation of the elderly with diabetes when they are taking fluids poorly or are having a diarrheal illness is also helpful.

hypertension Excessively high levels of blood pressure. Also known as "high blood pressure." Many people with diabetes also suffer from hypertension, which is a dangerous combination of illnesses that significantly increases the risk for kidney disease, CARDIOVASCULAR DISEASE, and other serious illnesses. About 21 percent of those with hypertension in the United States have not yet been diagnosed, and thus they are at serious risk for complications, since they are not being treated for their high blood pressure.

Nearly a third of all American adults (31.3 percent) have hypertension, and almost one half (44.1 percent) of all African-American women ages 20 years and older in the United States have hypertension, followed by 42.2 percent of black males. (See Table 1.) In many cases, hypertension is directly related to the diagnoses of both OBESITY and DIABETES MELLITUS.

Note that individuals taking hypertension medications subsequently may find that their blood pressure readings are close to normal or even normal. This does *not* mean that they can stop taking their medications; instead, it means that the blood pressure medication is working. No one should stop taking hypertension medications without first consulting with the prescribing physician.

In 2004, the National High Blood Pressure Education Program defined hypertension in adults ages 18 and over in their report *The Seventh Report of the Joint National Committee on Prevention, Detection, Evaluation, and Treatment of High Blood Pressure*. According to these experts, normal SYSTOLIC BLOOD PRESSURE (the upper number in the measurement of blood pressure) is less than 120 mm Hg. Normal DIASTOLIC BLOOD

TABLE 1: AGE-ADJUSTED PERCENT OF ADULTS AGED 20 YEARS AND OLDER WITH HYPERTENSION AND/ OR TAKING BLOOD PRESSURE–LOWERING MEDICATION, 2003–2006

Overall:	31.3%
Women	
All women	30.3%
White	28.3%
African American	44.1%
Mexican American	28.6%
Men	
All men	31.8%
White	31.2%
African American	42.2%
Mexican American	24.8%
Poverty status	
Poor	35.0%
Near Poor	34.1%
Non-poor	30.3%

Source: National Center for Health Statistics. Health, United States, 2008, with Chartbook on the Health of Americans. Hyattsville, Md.: National Institutes of Health, 2008. Available online. URL: http://www. cdc.gov/nchs/data/hus/hus08.pdf. Accessed June 15, 2009.

PRESSURE (the lower number) is less than 80 mm Hg. There is also a category known as prehypertension, and there are two stages of hypertension. (See Table 2.)

Symptoms and Diagnostic Path

Headache, nausea, and blurred vision may be symptoms of hypertension, but often there are no symptoms, and high blood pressure is detected

TABLE 2: CLASSIFICATION OF BLOOD PRESSURE FOR ADULTS

Blood Pressure Classification	SBP mmHG	DBP MM HG
Normal	<120	and <80
Prehypertension	120–139	or 80–89
Stage 1 Hypertension	140–159	or 90–99
Stage 2 Hypertension	≥160	or ≥ 100

Source: National High Blood Pressure Education Program, National Heart, Lung, and Blood Institute. The Seventh Report of the Joint National Committee on Prevention, Detection, Evaluation, and Treatment of High Blood Pressure. Bethesda, Md.: National Institutes of Health, September 2004, p. 12.

with a blood pressure reading. Physicians, nurses, staff members, and even a patient can determine blood pressure levels with a blood pressure cuff device. Experts say that devices that take the blood pressure by the insertion of a finger in a cuff are generally not as accurate as the devices that determine the blood pressure that is taken in the arm. It is also important to use the right cuff size because it may be difficult to obtain an accurate measure on a very obese or extremely thin person. Large or small devices may work better, depending on the size of the person.

Before the blood pressure is taken, the person should avoid caffeine for several hours and also should not smoke. Just before the reading is taken, the person should rest for about five minutes and his or her arm should be supported. Knees should be uncrossed.

Laboratory tests may be taken to look for an underlying cause of the hypertension or to determine if any complications are already present. Doctors generally order blood tests that measure levels of hematocrit, serum electrolytes (especially sodium and potassium), blood urea nitrogen (BUN), creatinine and glucose levels, and also plasma lipid levels. The patient's urine may be checked for albumin excretion, and an electrocardiogram may also be ordered to check for any irregularities. A 24-hour urinary protein excretion level can also provide important diagnostic information; for example, the normal range of urinary albumin excretion rate is less than 150 mg/day. Any amount above that level may be indicative of the presence of DIABETIC NEPHROPATHY and other complications.

Treatment Options and Outlook

Treatment of hypertension includes taking medications as well as making lifestyle changes, such as increased exercise, weight loss, and an improved diet.

Lifestyle changes Individuals who smoke should immediately stop smoking. If the person with hypertension consumes alcohol, he or she should stop drinking altogether or severely limit alcohol intake.

Dietary changes can also provide enhanced health benefits to the person who has hypertension. Salt should not be added to foods, and high salt foods should be avoided. Some types of foods should be added while others should be cut back or eliminated. For example, it is important for the person with hypertension to ensure an adequate intake of potassium, which often may be taken care of with diet.

Eating fresh vegetables may provide sufficient potassium. However, sometimes people with hypertension become hypokalemic (low potassium blood levels) because of their medications (particularly diuretics) or for other reasons, and, thus, they may need to take a potassium supplement in addition. Note that people with diabetes should not self-treat with potassium supplements; instead, potassium should be taken only by prescription, because some drugs that are used to treat hypertension can raise potassium levels.

Regular EXERCISE is another important lifestyle component of keeping hypertension within control. Even a brisk walk for 30 to 45 minutes, several days a week, can be sufficient to improve health. Some exercise, however, can be detrimental to the person who has hypertension; for example, heavy weight lifting or other isometric exercises can raise rather than lower the blood pressure, and consequently such activities should be avoided by people with high blood pressure.

Emotional stress can also raise blood pressure. People with hypertension may need to learn relaxation tactics to cope with their reactions to the problems of life. Stress cannot be altogether eliminated from life; however, it is the individual's reaction to stress that may be modified.

Medication Many people who have hypertension need to take one or more medications to lower their blood pressure, and many people with diabetes will need two or three different medications to optimally control their hypertension. The Joint National Committee VII stated that individuals with high-normal blood pressure and diabetes should take medication.

Some medications that are used to control diabetes will also lower blood pressure, such as METFORMIN and drugs in the THIAZOLIDINEDIONE class, but they should not be used solely for this purpose. Medications that are specifically used to treat hypertension include the following classes of drugs: ACE inhibitors, alpha blockers, alpha-2 agonists, alpha-beta blockers, alpha receptor blockers (ARBs), angiotensin II antagonists (also known as angiotensin receptor blockers or ARBs), beta blockers, calcium channel blockers, central nervous system inhibitors, and vasodilators.

Medication may also be needed to bring DYSLIPIDEMIA under control. LDL cholesterol levels should be brought to below 100 mg/dL for patients who have both diabetes and hypertension.

Risk Factors and Preventive Measures

Although people of any age, even children, can be hypertensive, most people with hypertension are middle-aged or older, and the risk for developing hypertension steadily increases with age.

Ethnic factors Another key factor associated with hypertension is ethnicity: African Americans, New Zealand Maoris, and some Native American tribes in the United States, such as the PIMA INDIANS, have higher rates of hypertension and greater risks for cardiovascular disease than do individuals of other ethnicities.

Gender and hypertension Both women and men suffer from hypertension, although WOMEN WITH DIABETES have higher rates of hypertension than either nondiabetic individuals or diabetic men. AFRICAN-AMERICAN women are particularly at risk for high blood pressure, as are AMERICAN INDIAN men and women.

Other factors Smoking is a risk factor for hypertension, and anyone who smokes should stop immediately. Obesity is also a risk factor, and weight loss is recommended, although fad diets are discouraged. Avoid using any herbal remedies or supplements that promise rapid weight loss because such drugs may be dangerous and could also interact with blood pressure medications. Always ask the doctor first before taking any alternative remedy.

Hypertension Is a Chronic Condition

People with hypertension and their families need to realize that this is a chronic and life-long condition. Although lifestyle changes and medication can vastly improve blood pressure measurements, it is still necessary to continue to monitor the condition. Many patients make a classic mistake of taking their medicine and noting their improved blood pressure readings. They may decide they are "cured" and stop taking their medication. The blood pressure will typically go up again and serious medical complications can ensue.

It may be possible to "step down" on medications, taking a lower dose, but only upon the advice of the treating doctor. It may also be advisable to change or add medications, should the physician believe it becomes necessary.

Cardiovascular Risk Factors and Hypertension

When combined with hypertension, diabetes is a major risk factor for the development of cardiovascular diseases. Other risk factors that further exacerbate the risk of cardiovascular diseases among all people with hypertension include:

- smoking
- dyslipidemia (abnormal cholesterol levels: increased levels of LDL and triglycerides and decreased levels of HDL)
- age: over 60 years
- a family history of cardiovascular disease in females over age 65 and in males over age 55

There are also particular organs within the body that are most prone to damage from hypertension. The major types of damage that may occur are

- heart disease (left ventricular hypertrophy [thickening of heart muscle] /angina/myocardial infarction [heart attack] /heart failure)

- stroke or transient ischemic attack (TIA), which is a "mini-stroke"
- renal (kidney) disease, up to and including end-stage renal disease that requires dialysis or a kidney transplant
- ERECTILE DYSFUNCTION
- peripheral arterial disease/claudication
- DIABETIC RETINOPATHY

Major Studies on Hypertension

Several major studies on individuals with hypertension are often cited by experts and researchers. These studies placed subjects in groups with different medications that reduced blood pressure. The researchers worked to intensively reduce blood pressure in one group and achieve a more moderate blood pressure goal in the other group. The researchers then compared the two groups to each other. Invariably, the group who brought their blood pressure down lower fared much better and had far lower rates of later developing serious complications in most categories.

The United Kingdom Prospective Diabetes Study (UKPDS) looked at 1,148 patients with diabetes, comparing the results of the "intensively treated" group to the "conventional" group and then following them for more than eight years. Results: the intensively treated group had 32 percent fewer deaths and 44 percent fewer strokes and also accrued other health benefits. This was true even though the intensively treated group averaged a still high blood pressure of 144/82 mm Hg versus the control group's average blood pressure of 154/87 mm Hg. Thus, the improvement was only a very small 10/5, and yet it meant the difference between life and death for some.

Experts now know, however, that when a person has both diabetes and hypertension, even those with high/normal blood pressures of between 130–139/85–89 will benefit from lifestyle changes as well as from medication therapy. One reason for this is that many people with diabetes do not experience a nocturnal decrease in their blood pressure ("non-dippers"), as do nondiabetics. As a result, the continued higher level of pressure at a "24/7" level, along with the harm that diabetes alone can bring, can be very damaging.

Problems with Medication Adherence

Despite information that is provided to patients about the risks that they face with both hypertension and diabetes, as well as the emphasis upon the necessity to take their medication to decrease these risks, physicians report many problems with nonadherence to their prescribed medication regimen. There are a variety of reasons why people with hypertension and diabetes do not take their medicine.

Some patients do not take their medicine for hypertension regularly (or at all) for the same reason they do not take their medicine for other illnesses. For example, they may forget to take the medicine or may minimize the extent of their problem. Hypertension generally causes no symptoms and is a "silent killer."

Patients may fail to take their medication because they may not like the side effects of medication, or they may not be able to afford the drugs. Note that some pharmaceutical companies offer coupons of $20 or more on their Internet sites which can be printed out. Search for the availability of such coupons by using the brand name of the medication and the name of the drug company.

Researchers have found a unique reason for why some men, especially African Americans, Mexican Americans, or American Indians, refuse to take their medicine. The common belief among such men is that their medication will cause ERECTILE DYSFUNCTION (ED). Yet studies indicate that the incidence of sexual dysfunction with the newer medications for hypertension is low.

"White Coat" Hypertension/ The White Coat Effect

Some individuals have a tendency to experience an elevated blood pressure when they are in a physician's office, presumably as a reflexive act of seeing a doctor. (The white laboratory coat of the doctor is the "white coat": just seeing the doctor temporarily elevates blood pressure in some individuals.)

Such individuals may have normal blood pressure readings when absent of this reflex. For this reason, doctors should take at least several readings that are two minutes or more apart, and should also take readings on different occasions before diagnosing hypertension in a person—unless the blood pressure is so high that it would be dangerous to delay the treatment. White coat hypertension is another reason why doctors advise people with diabetes and hypertension to monitor their blood pressure at home, just as they should monitor their glucose on a schedule recommended by their physicians.

Questions Patients with Hypertension Should Ask Their Physicians

Patients with hypertension should be as aware of their health and their hypertension problem as possible. Some questions to ask the doctor include the following:

- What is my blood pressure reading?
- Is my blood pressure under control? If not, what should my blood pressure be?
- Is my weight affecting my blood pressure? If so, how much should I weigh?
- If I am overweight, can you recommend a diet to help me lose weight?
- Is it safe for me to exercise on a regular basis? If not, why not?
- What is the name of the blood pressure medication you are prescribing (or have prescribed)? Is that the brand name or generic name?
- What are possible side effects of my hypertension medication(s)?
- Should I take my blood pressure medication at a particular time of day?
- Should I take my medication with or without food?
- Are there any foods or beverages that I should avoid while I take this medication?

- What should I do if I forget to take the medication at the regular time? Should I take it as soon as I remember it or wait until the next day?
- Are there any side effects of my medication that I should be sure to report to you?

See also ASPIRIN THERAPY; CARDIOVASCULAR DISEASE; DIABETIC EYE DISEASES; DIABETIC NEPHROPATHY; DIABETIC NEUROPATHY; GLAUCOMA; LIFESTYLE ADAPTATIONS.

National High Blood Pressure Education Program, National Heart, Lung, and Blood Institute. *The Seventh Report of the Joint National Committee on Prevention, Detection, Evaluation, and Treatment of High Blood Pressure.* Bethesda, Md.: National Institutes of Health, September 2004.

hypoglycemia Very low blood glucose (sugar) levels requiring the emergency administration of glucose. Hypoglycemia is the most common complication of diabetes, particularly Type 1 diabetes, although people with Type 2 diabetes may also experience this problem.

People who do not have diabetes at all may also become hypoglycemic, although this occurs far less frequently than was believed in the past. As many as 20 percent of all people with diabetes have at least one experience with hypoglycemia and some people have repeated incidents. Hypoglycemia may also be a problem during PREGNANCY for the woman with diabetes because most women are seeking to attain very tight levels of glycemic control. One risk that accompanies such a goal is hypoglycemia.

Symptoms of Hypoglycemia

If a person exhibits at least several of the following symptoms, he or she should be evaluated as soon as possible for possible hypoglycemia as well as for other illnesses that may be present:

- headaches/nausea
- shakiness

- rapid heartbeat
- paleness
- confusion or drowsiness
- dizziness (not vertigo)
- feeling faint
- agitation/irritability/impatience
- sweating in normal temperatures and without exerting oneself

Those Most at Risk for Developing Hypoglycemia

Any person with diabetes can develop hypoglycemia and if they exhibit symptoms, then they should be tested. Those at risk for developing hypoglycemia include:

- people with a history of hypoglycemia
- males
- people over age 65
- patients on tight glycemic control
- patients using insulin
- patients taking more than five medications
- recently hospitalized patients

The hypoglycemic newborn may have hypoglycemia that stems from the mother's diabetes or from her toxemia. The newborn may also be hypoglycemic for other reasons, such as malnutrition, a hormone deficiency, or a side effect from a medication. In very, very rare cases, the infant may have diabetes.

Adults who abuse ALCOHOL may also become hypoglycemic and alcohol abuse is the second most common reason why people with hypoglycemia present to emergency rooms. If a person with diabetes also abuses alcohol, then the risk for hypoglycemia increases further. Some people do not abuse alcohol but for a variety of reasons, they are prone to bouts of hypoglycemia. The more times that a person has a serious incident of hypoglycemia, the more likely it is that it will happen again and again.

Diagnosis/Failure to Diagnose Hypoglycemia

One key problem experienced by people with hypoglycemia is that they may appear intoxicated, drug-impaired, or even mentally ill to the physician and others. If such mistakes or misdiagnoses are made, then proper treatment is delayed or not performed at all and the person with hypoglycemia will become sicker. This could cause the individual to lapse into a coma and die.

In his article on hypoglycemia for a 2001 issue of *Emergency Medicine Report Archives,* Dr. Brady recommended that emergency room doctors consider hypoglycemia as a possible diagnosis in any patient with any apparent mental abnormality or even seizures, and that they should also perform a bedside glucose analysis to rule out hypoglycemia. He advises doctors not to listen to police officers who insist the person is intoxicated, because the police may be wrong. Instead, the doctor should make the evaluation for himself or herself.

Brady also noted that hypoglycemia may be misdiagnosed as seizure disorder, a brain tumor, psychosis, a cerebrovascular accident, a traumatic head injury, narcolepsy, multiple sclerosis, drug ingestion, depression, hysteria, and an incidence of cardiac arrhythmia.

Phases of Hypoglycemia

Hypoglycemia has two primary phases, including the sympatho-adrenal phase or "fight or flight" phase and the neuroglycopenic phase. In the first phase, most patients have symptoms that alert them to their low glucose levels. Some patients, however, do not have such symptoms, a condition called HYPOGLYCEMIC UNAWARENESS. Often they are individuals who have had repeated incidents of hypoglycemia.

In the second phase of hypoglycemia, it may be difficult or impossible for most people with hypoglycemia to recognize their own symptoms and/or to act on them. This is why it is so important for people who do recognize their symptoms in the first phase to test frequently and act right away, if they feel something is amiss. The risk is that if the problem gets worse and the person goes into a neuroglycopenic phase, he or she may no longer be able to act at that point and can become extremely ill. Hypoglycemia is usually not fatal (although it can be) but the person may sustain irreversible central nervous system damage if hypoglycemia is not treated in time. It is far better to take a little time to attend to symptoms in the first stage and avert a medical crisis.

Causes of Hypoglycemia among People with Diabetes

Individuals who have diabetes may develop hypoglycemia for the following reasons:

- imbalance of insulin/oral medications to the level of glucose
- failure to eat a meal or delayed eating
- overexertion
- excessive alcohol consumption

A combination of the above reasons or other factors beyond those listed here may also cause hypoglycemia. For example, people with diabetes who also take beta-blocker drugs for HYPERTENSION, angina, or migraine headaches may then perform strenuous exercises, leading to hypoglycemia, whose symptoms are masked by the beta-blocker. Tight glycemic control of insulin is also a very common cause of hypoglycemia.

Other causes of hypoglycemia   Some foods may (rarely) cause hypoglycemia, such as the unripe ackee fruit that is found in Jamaica. Adrenal insufficiency (Addison's disease) may cause hypoglycemia. In rare cases, such as children with growth hormone deficiency, this deficiency can also cause hypoglycemia. Individuals with widely metastatic cancer to the liver or adrenal glands may develop hypoglycemia. In addition, people with severe liver or kidney disease are also more susceptible to suffering from hypoglycemia. Chronic alcohol abuse is also a frequent cause of hypoglycemia, in part because the alcoholic may be malnourished and anorexic.

Treatment of Hypoglycemia

Immediate treatment involves restoring the blood glucose level to normal by the patient taking glucose formulations or food that contains sugar, such as apple juice, fruit, or glucose tablets or gels. If the person is conscious, the glucose can be taken orally. If the person is unconscious, it is administered intravenously. In some emergencies, GLUCAGON is injected intramuscularly to treat the hypoglycemia. Solid foods such as candy should not be given unless the person has regained a completely normal mental state. Otherwise, the individual could risk choking on the candy if he or she is semiconscious, thus creating another medical emergency on top of the hypoglycemia.

People who have recurrent bouts of hypoglycemia (and even people who experience intermittent bouts of hypoglycemia) are wise to ensure that both testing equipment and a source of sugar are readily available to them at all times—including in their car, at work, and at school. They should also seek a consultation with an endocrinologist and a diabetes care team, including a registered dietitian, a registered nurse, and a certified diabetes educator, to find out how to effectively deal with this problem.

Treatment also involves identifying and working to resolve the source of the problem. The disease must be better controlled with appropriate adjustments in medication, diet, exercise, and regular physician visits.

If Hypoglycemia Is Not Treated

If the individual with diabetes or others around do not recognize that the person's blood sugar has dropped precipitously, then action may not be taken or it may be delayed. This can be very dangerous and even lead to the person suffering from seizures, coma, and/or death. For this reason, it's very important that the person with diabetes, especially one prone to hypoglycemic attacks, wear some EMERGENCY MEDICAL IDENTIFICATION in the form of an easily visible necklace, bracelet, anklet, or some other form. Emergency medical cards are good to have as well, but they may not be found in a person's purse or wallet in sufficient time to take appropriate medical action.

Complete recovery can be delayed   Another problem with hypoglycemia is that recovery is not immediate upon administration of glucose. Instead, it takes the body time to recover from hypoglycemia, even after treatment. One study of 20 people with diabetes looked at how long it took people who had a hypoglycemic attack to regain their full cognitive function as well as a stable mood. This study was reported by Strachan et al., in a 2000 issue of *Diabetes Care*.

The researchers found that although hypoglycemia did not have long-term effects when it was promptly treated, the test subjects still took about a day and a half to fully recover their cognitive function. Researchers also found that a temporary depressed and anxious state often occurred to the subject after an attack. Individuals who had many bouts with hypoglycemia had even more difficulty recovering.

The researchers said that the results "imply that acute severe hypoglycemia does not have a prolonged effect on cognitive functions, and patients with insulin-treated diabetes may be reassured that performance of activities such as work or driving is not likely to be impaired 36 h [hours] after an episode." As a result, given sufficient time, and adequate treatment, most people recover fully from a bout of hypoglycemia. But because their faculties may be somewhat impaired for a day or so afterwards, they should not engage in any difficult activities or make any important decisions during that time.

See also COMA; DEHYDRATION; GLYCEMIC CONTROL.

Brady, William J., M.D. "Hypoglycemia: Current Strategies for Diagnosis and Management." *Emergency Medicine Reports Archives* (January 15, 2001).

The Diabetes Control and Complications Trial Research Group. "Hypoglycemia in the Diabetes Control and Complications Trials." *Diabetes* 46 (February 1997): 271–286.

Strachan, Mark, et al. "Recovery of Cognitive Function and Mood After Severe Hypoglycemia in

Adults with Insulin-Treated Diabetes." *Diabetes Care* 23, no. 3, (March 2000): 305–312.

Ter Braak, Edith, M.D., et al. "Clinical Characteristics of Type 1 Diabetic Patients with and without Severe Hypoglycemia." *Diabetes Care* 23, no. 10 (October 2000): 1,467–1,471.

hypoglycemic unawareness The condition when a person with diabetes has no symptoms of a low blood glucose level (HYPOGLYCEMIA). Typically, they have lost the first phase when the sympathetic nervous system induces the release of adrenaline and noradrenaline. Thus, they have no nervousness, sweating, rapid heartbeat, and other symptoms to warn them that their glucose level is declining. Patients with well-controlled diabetes will begin to experience symptoms at 55–60 mg/dL.

Hypoglycemic unawareness occurs most commonly in those who try to control their glucose levels very tightly. It is common in pregnant women for this reason. It can also be a late complication of long-standing diabetes (25 to 35 years in duration) due to AUTONOMIC NEUROPATHY.

Abnormal thinking and behavior is one of the first symptoms of hypoglycemic unawareness. At that point, the patient is unable to treat him- or herself and others must provide treatment. Some indications of such abnormal behaviors are

- the person stops an activity and begins staring off into space
- what the person says makes no sense
- there is a sudden change in personality, facial expression, or mood

When patients have hypoglycemic unawareness, the glycemic goals are increased and the patient is asked to aim for slightly higher glucose levels to avoid hypoglycemia. The patient is also advised to monitor glucose levels more frequently, especially ensuring to check blood levels before driving. Patients are also educated about the importance of eating meals on time and avoiding missing meals or delayed meals. Patients are also advised to inform family members as well as friends and coworkers about hypoglycemic unawareness, so that they can look for subtle signs of hypoglycemia.

Hypoglycemic unawareness is reversible unless the cause is a chronic form of autonomic neuropathy.

I

immunizations (flu/influenza, pneumococcal vaccine, and others) Vaccines introduced into the body that cause the creation of antibodies, which are proteins made by B lymphocytes. These antibodies, in turn, protect against the disease. For those who have diabetes, it is very important to obtain flu and pneumonia immunizations, particularly among people who are over age 65. Of course, individuals with diabetes should receive periodic immunizations for tetanus and other immunizations as needed by individuals in his or her area and recommended by their physicians.

According to the Centers for Disease Control and Prevention (CDC), 10,000–30,000 people with diabetes die each year from flu and pneumonia. People with diabetes have nearly triple the risk of dying from flu or pneumonia. In addition, people with diabetes who contract flu are six times more likely to need hospitalization than are nondiabetics. Experts also recommend that family members of individuals with diabetes should be immunized as well. Not only will they be protected from the flu but they will also help their family members with diabetes by avoiding the flu and eliminating the risk of contagion.

Although a flu shot is generally a good idea for most people, individuals should be sure to check with their physicians first before receiving the immunization. Someone who is acutely ill or feverish should not take the vaccine nor should it be taken by anyone who is allergic to eggs or who has had a prior severe systemic reaction to the flu shot.

Yet despite warnings from the medical profession, many people with diabetes fail to obtain immunizations against flu or pneumonia.

According to the federal data reported in *Healthy People 2010,* of those with high risk conditions, only 27 percent of diabetes patients ages 18 to 64 had obtained a flu shot and only 15 percent had received the pneumonia vaccine. Of people over age 65, they were the least likely of older people with high risk conditions of obtaining either a flu or pneumonia vaccination.

Frequency of Immunizations

Influenza is generally a problem between November and April, and pneumonia generally follows the same pattern. Most people who receive these immunizations obtain them sometime between October and mid-November. New flu shots are required each year, although pneumococcal immunizations may only need to be repeated every five to seven years, depending on the patient's physician's advice.

It may take three to four weeks for the body to develop antibodies against the flu. As a result, timing of the injection is important. For example, if a person received an injection on November 5, and then was exposed to the flu on November 11, then he or she could still develop the flu despite having received the injection. The body would not have had enough time to marshal its defenses in that time frame.

Providers and Costs of Immunizations

Flu shots and pneumococcal vaccines are covered by Part B Medicare. If the immunization must be paid for, it is generally low cost. The state health department or local clinic may provide the shot for free or at low cost, or the individual may pay to obtain the immunization from his or her doctor.

Primary Symptoms of Flu and Pneumonia

Not everyone feels the same, but most people experience common symptoms. People with the flu have at least several of these symptoms:

- fever that is greater than 101.5 degrees Fahrenheit
- sore throat (pharyngitis)
- chills
- muscle aches (myalgia)
- headache
- cough, generally dry and nonproductive

Symptoms of pneumonia are:

- fever
- coughing up sputum (generally greenish, brown or blood-tinged and *not* white or clear)
- chest pain, generally sharp

Categories of People Who Should Be Immunized

According to the CDC, an annual flu shot is particularly recommended for people who fall in one or more of the following categories. Those who:

- are over age 50
- live in a long-term care facility, such as a skilled nursing facility
- have a long-term health problem, such as diabetes, heart disease, lung disease, asthma, kidney disease, or anemia
- have a weak immune system because of HIV or medications that weaken the system, such as cancer treatments or steroids
- children ages six months to 18 years on long-term aspirin treatment (and who could develop Reye's syndrome if they caught the flu)
- doctors, nurses, and other health care providers who are likely to come in contact with people at risk of having severe flu

Minor and Major Reactions to Flu/Pneumococcal Injections

Many people have mild reactions to the injection, such as soreness at the injection site or redness. There may be some temporary achiness or slight fever for one or two days as well.

On rare occasions, individuals experience a bad reaction to the immunization. Anyone who experiences a fever of greater than 101.5 degrees F or who exhibits signs of an allergic reaction should obtain immediate medical attention. Some examples of an allergic reaction are:

- hives
- difficulty breathing/shortness of breath
- paleness/pallor
- wheezing
- rapid heartbeat
- light-headedness

A person who experiences such a severe reaction should also ask the doctor to file a Vaccine Adverse Event Reporting System (VAERS) form with the Centers for Disease Control or, upon treatment and recovery, patients may call the VAERS later themselves at 1-800-822-7967.

Emergency treatment may be required   Some individuals who have diabetes and who are ill with flu or pneumonia may need to be taken to see their medical doctor or may need to go to the emergency room or even be hospitalized in order to avoid severe consequences. Circumstances when the sick person with diabetes should see his doctor or, if this is not possible, go to the hospital emergency room are:

- if the individual is too ill to monitor his or her blood glucose levels and has no one to help with monitoring
- if he or she has high ketone levels in his urine
- if the person has severe nausea and vomiting and is unable to keep up with the needed intake of fluids (and there is no one else

available to provide assistance). This could lead to DEHYDRATION

Other Immunizations That Are Needed

Individuals who have diabetes should also obtain diphtheria-tetanus (dT) shots every 10 years. Children should obtain hepatitis B injections, as should adults who are at risk of contracting the disease. Children should also have the hemophilus vaccine.

Smith, Steven A., M.D., and Gregory A. Poland, M.D. "Use of Influenza and Pneumococcal Vaccines in People with Diabetes." *Diabetes Care* 23, no. 1 (January 2000): 95–108.

impaired glucose tolerance (IGT)   A condition in which the blood glucose levels are higher than normal but they are not high enough that the person could be diagnosed with diabetes. Former names of IGT, no longer in use (because they are inaccurate), are "borderline diabetes," "subclinical diabetes," "chemical diabetes," and "latent diabetes."

People with IGT may go on to develop diabetes as well as the microvascular complications that accompany this disease. Studies of the PIMA INDIANS of Arizona, a tribe with an extremely high rate of Type 2 diabetes, have revealed that there is about a three-year period from the development of impaired glucose tolerance to the onset of Type 2 diabetes.

These same studies from the Pima Indians reveal that patients with IGT appear to more likely have HYPERINSULINISM, i.e., they are more insulin resistant and thus need to attempt to overproduce insulin to compensate than those with impaired fasting glucose (IFG). The Pima Indians in these studies who developed IFG appeared to have more beta cell dysfunction, which means that they are less able to secrete enough insulin to normalize the blood glucose. (It is necessary for patients to have both insulin resistance and impaired insulin secretion to develop Type 2 diabetes mellitus.)

IGT seems to be a better predictor of the future development of Type 2 diabetes as well as the development of cardiovascular disease.

The Diabetes Prevention Program is a study that is ongoing in the United States, as of this writing, and seeks to determine if changes made by a person who has impaired glucose tolerance (in lifestyle and medication) can delay or altogether slow down the progression to diabetes. We know from the UNITED KINGDOM PROSPECTIVE DIABETES STUDY (UKPDS) that patients who eventually develop Type 2 diabetes have metabolic abnormalities that can precede the diagnosis by as much as 10 years. As a result, most experts feel that any efforts to slow down the progression to diabetes will have a positive effect in terms of preventing and delaying complications.

In 2001, researchers who studied 522 middle-aged adults with impaired glucose tolerance sought to determine if lifestyle changes could prevent or delay the onset of diabetes. Their findings were reported in the *New England Journal of Medicine*. The researchers definitively proved that lifestyle changes such as weight loss, increased exercise, and dietary changes such as decreased sugar consumption and increased vegetable and fiber consumption, dramatically reduced the risk of diabetes for subjects, even when followed up four years after the study. The "intervention group" that made lifestyle changes had an incidence of diabetes of 11 percent while the control group had an incidence of diabetes of 23 percent.

Davies, M. J., N. T. Raymond, J. L. Day et al. "Impaired Glucose Tolerance and Fasting Hyperglycemia Have Different Characteristics." *Diabetes Medicine* 17 (2000): 433–440.

impotence   See ERECTILE DYSFUNCTION (ED).

infants and preschool children with diabetes
The presence of Type 1 diabetes in babies and preschool children, an uncommon condition.

According to authors Denis Daneman, Marcia Frank, and Kusiel Perlman in their book, *When a Child Has Diabetes,* less than 1 percent of the cases of diabetes are diagnosed in a child's first year and less than 10 percent are diagnosed before the child is age five. When a small child does have diabetes, the illness is often not diagnosed until the child becomes severely ill with DIABETIC KETOACIDOSIS (DKA).

Children can also develop Type 2 diabetes but when it occurs among children, it nearly always develops during or after puberty. Type 2 diabetes is unknown in babies and preschool children.

An infant or toddler with diabetes suffers from the same symptoms as older children or adults with Type 1 diabetes, exhibiting thirst, weight loss, and fatigue. The AMERICAN DIABETES ASSOCIATION advises against tight glycemic control for children under the age of two.

According to Daneman et al., a healthy baby or toddler with controlled diabetes will grow normally and have a normal weight gain. The child will also meet normal developmental milestones for sitting up, crawling, standing, and so forth. There will be no KETONES in the child's urine when diabetes is under control and the child will have good energy levels.

Because babies and small children cannot check their own blood levels or inject insulin, this task must be performed by adult caregivers. Whenever possible, it should be shifted among adults, so that one person does not always have to be the "bad guy." The child's feelings about finger pricks should be acknowledged but they should also not be delayed, because the child's health is at stake.

Alternate site glucose monitoring, by testing the blood in other parts of the body such as the arm, may be preferable in infants and preschool children. Obviously, noninvasive monitoring will be very helpful when it becomes available.

A helpful educational game, "Wizdom Kids," is offered at www.diabetes.org/wizdom.

Some helpful books for parents include the following:

American Diabetes Association Guide to Raising a Child with Diabetes by Linda M. Siminerio, R.N., M.S., C.D.E. and Jean Betschart, R.N., M.N., C.D.E. (NTC Publications Group, 2000).

Sweet Kids: How to Balance Diabetes Control and Good Nutrition with Family Peace by Betty Page Brackenridge, M.S., R.D., C.D.E. and Richard R. Rubin, Ph.D., C.D.E. (NTC Publications Group, 1996).

The Ten Keys to Helping Your Child Grow Up with Diabetes by Tim Wysocki (NTC Publications Group, 1997).

When a Child Has Diabetes by Denis Daneman, M.B., B.Ch., F.R.C.P.C., Marcia Frank, R.N., M.H.Sc., C.D.E., and Kusiel Perlman, M.D., F.R.C.P.C. (New York, N.Y.: Firefly Books, 1999).

infections Bacterial, fungal, or viral invasions of the body. People with diabetes are more prone to contracting a variety of infections than are nondiabetics. They are also at graver risk for contracting and becoming very ill from influenza or pneumonia. The greatest risk is seen in patients with poor glycemic control. High glucose levels prevent the immune system from working well, particularly impairing the abilities of the white blood cells to work at an optimal level to fight off infection. Yet only an estimated 50 percent of those who know they have diabetes obtain an annual flu or pneumonia immunization.

When individuals with diabetes suffer from DIABETIC NEUROPATHY, they are also at a greater risk for developing infections of the foot which, if not treated, may progress to GANGRENE and the necessity for an AMPUTATION of a limb.

Rates of kidney infections (pyelonephritis) are similar in people with and without diabetes; however, patients with diabetes are twice as likely to need hospitalization when they do have a kidney infection. Diabetic neuropathy that leads to a neurogenic bladder tends to significantly increase the number of bladder infections. This problem may also occur after surgery, especially in cases of surgery for cardiac, chest, or abdominal areas. People with good glycemic control and with fewer complications are likely to be discharged from the hospital sooner.

Women with diabetes are susceptible to Candida vaginitis (yeast) and men to Candida balanitis. Candida grows well in warm, moist environments where glucose is plentiful.

See also FOOT CARE; GINGIVITIS; IMMUNIZATIONS; URINARY TRACT INFECTION; VAGINITIS.

Paauw, Douglas S., M.D. "Infectious Emergencies in Patients with Diabetes." *Clinical Diabetes* 18, no. 3 (Summer 2000): 102–106.

injection devices   Devices used to introduce medications into the body. The majority of people with diabetes in the United States and Canada who self-inject insulin use traditional insulin syringes with 29- and 30-gauge needles. There are now "short" needles available for thin patients to avoid inadvertent intramuscular injections. (Insulin should be injected into the subcutaneous fat.) In Europe, most insulin is injected with pen devices with 30- and 31-gauge needles.

All syringes in the United States and Canada are calibrated to U-100 (100 units of insulin/1 cc or mL). Syringes are available in 1/3 cc (30 units), 1/2 cc (50 units) and 1-cc (100 unit) sizes.

There are also insertion aids available that will inject the needles when triggered. Some will also automatically release insulin, while others need to be manually activated after the needle is in place.

Jet injectors that force insulin through the skin via air pressure are available but they are expensive. Since standard needles have become very small and also very sharp, there has been much less demand for these devices. They can also cause some bruising and need to be cleaned regularly.

Multiple devices are also available for the visually impaired. These devices help patients measure the insulin dose and guide and stabilize the needle, while also magnifying the syringe so that they can read the dose correctly.

injection/injection site rotation   Method to deliver medications directly into the body. In most cases, individuals with TYPE 1 DIABETES must inject themselves with insulin at least twice daily and usually on a more frequent basis. As they age, individuals with TYPE 2 DIABETES may have an increasingly impaired insulin secretory system and may also need to self-inject insulin. Insulin is injected into subcutaneous fat, where it is absorbed into small blood vessels.

Because many people dislike not only testing their blood but also injecting insulin, and because this dislike often leads to failure to self-test or to self-inject, scientists have sought other solutions. One such solution is the implantable pump, which provides insulin on a regular basis to the patient. Inhaled insulin is an alternative that is being tested in 2001 and which appears to be a viable alternative to injected insulin for many patients with diabetes.

Some patients actually inject their medicine through their clothes, although there is considerable controversy among physicians as to whether this is an acceptable or safe procedure.

Glucagon, which is administered for severe hypoglycemia, is generally injected into a large muscle, such as the muscle in the shoulder or the thigh.

Injection Site Rotation

Injection site rotation is the practice of giving oneself an injection in different sites of the body so that one particular part of the body doesn't become overly inflamed or harmed. Repeated injections in the same site could result in lumps that are called "lipodystrophies" or "lipohypertrophies." For people with Type 1 diabetes, this is a key reason for rotating the location of the insulin injection.

Most people inject insulin in areas of the body that are easy to reach, such as the outer arm, close to the waist, the upper buttock, and the thigh. Sometimes people give themselves their morning injection in one part of the body and then administer their evening injection in another part. In the future, medical experts hope that many people with diabetes will be able to use bloodless testing, so that they may easily and painlessly monitor their glucose levels.

With the newer pure insulin available today, patients can use one site to inject as long as they move 1-2 finger widths away with each injection. They should follow a pattern of moving from left to right or up and down to rotate within one area.

Absorption of insulin varies from site to site and it is absorbed most quickly and consistently in the abdomen and slowest in the buttocks. Absorption and injection in the arms and thighs provide medium absorption. If the person exercises a leg or arm after an injection, it will increase the speed of absorption.

See also LANCET.

insulin A medication that is used to treat people with diabetes and also the single most important factor enabling many people with diabetes to survive and thrive, particularly those who have Type 1 diabetes. Many people with Type 2 diabetes use oral MEDICATIONS or other types of injectable medications rather than insulin; however, some people with Type 2 diabetes also use insulin, particularly those who are elderly or who have had Type 2 diabetes for many years. In addition, sometimes women with GESTATIONAL DIABETES need to use insulin during their pregnancies. According to the Agency for Healthcare Research and Quality in their 2009 booklet on premixed insulin for individuals with Type 2 diabetes, three out of every 10 people with Type 2 diabetes use insulin.

Insulin Basics

Insulin was first discovered as a treatment for diabetes in 1921 at the University of Toronto in Canada by Dr. Frederick Banting, a Canadian physician, and Charles Best, his medical student assistant. Prior to that time, people with Type 1 diabetes died at young ages or they suffered greatly until their death in young adulthood, becoming very emaciated and ill because of their lack of natural endogenous insulin.

Human insulin is a naturally produced hormone that is made by the beta cells of the islets of Langerhans, which are located in the organ known as the pancreas. The pancreas secretes insulin in order to regulate the levels of glucose (blood sugar) in the bloodstream. Insulin is a polypeptide (protein) hormone that is comprised of two chains and is derived from proinsulin, which has some activity to lower blood glucose levels but is a pro-hormone. The C-peptide (connecting peptide) is removed to create what is known as insulin and which is primarily the substance which the body utilizes. It is this C-peptide fragment that can be measured in the body to determine if a patient's body is still producing insulin.

Individuals with Type 1 diabetes have very low levels of insulin (for the first few years after their diagnosis) or no insulin at all (thereafter), because their illness has destroyed the beta cells of the pancreas. As a result, they need to receive insulin that is injected or is pumped subcutaneously with an insulin pump into the body on a daily basis. In the normal state when the body produces insulin, this insulin is released into the portal vein, and it is first delivered to the liver, where most of the body's gluconeogenesis (synthesis of new glucose) takes place. The route that subcutaneously injected (exogenous insulin) insulin takes is more circuitous than the route that natural insulin produced by the body takes. Subcutaneously injected insulin is absorbed by the capillaries and then returned via the venous circulation to the right side of the heart. It is then pumped out to the lungs, returns to the left side of the heart, and is pumped out to the rest of the body, in particular to the liver and muscles, as well as the rest of the body. In contrast, with insulin produced from the individual's own pancreas, the insulin gets to the liver and muscles much more directly and rapidly via the arterial circulation without having to first pass through the heart and lungs—thus less insulin is degraded or lost to other tissues and consequently, smaller amounts are more effective.

In contrast, people with Type 2 diabetes have a different problem. Although their bodies produce insulin, they suffer from *insulin resistance*, which means that the body still produces insulin, but it produces an inadequate amount to overcome the body's resistance to its effects. A good physiological example is the case of pregnancy, where resistance to the effects of insulin increase by 300–400 percent. Despite this, among the white population, 97 percent of pregnant women are able to produce an abundance of insulin that overcomes the acquired resistance. As a result, their blood glucose levels remain normal.

Insulin may be injected or individuals may use an insulin pump for a continuous delivery of insulin as needed. (See INSULIN PUMP.) There are also insulin pens that may be used, and researchers are working with an inhaled form of insulin that may become commercially available in the future. Pfizer voluntarily withdrew their inhaled insulin, Exubera, from the market due to very poor sales.

The number of daily injections that are needed vary from person to person. Some people who inject their insulin need only one or two injections per day while others need four to seven injections to obtain sufficient physiological insulin for their needs.

Types of Insulin

When insulin was first discovered, there was only one form available. As of this writing, there are seven primary types of insulin, and people who use insulin generally take two of these types or they may take a premixed combination form of insulin that includes two types within the vial or pen cartridge. Most insulin is now U-100, which means that the concentration is 100 units/cc. However, U-500 (500 units/cc) can be special-ordered for the rare case of patients who require very large doses of insulin, such as in the case of patients who are very insulin resistant, usually due to obesity, though there are very rare auto-immune forms of insulin resistance as well.

The Onset, Peak, and Duration of Insulin

Three keys to understanding each type of insulin are its onset of action, the peak time of action, and the duration of effect. The onset of action refers to how soon the insulin begins to lower the blood glucose after it is administered. The peak time of action refers to when the insulin works the hardest (typically when it is at its peak concentration in the bloodstream) to lower blood glucose levels. The duration of effect refers to how long the insulin acts within the body to lower blood glucose.

The onset, peak, and duration of insulin vary according to the type of insulin that is used. For example, rapid-acting insulin starts working within 15 minutes. It peaks at from 30–90 minutes, and then it lasts for about three to five hours from when it was first administered. There are also short-acting forms of insulin, intermediate-acting forms, and long-acting forms. In addition, there are three different forms of premixed insulin, which include a combination of types of insulin; most include a combination of both intermediate-acting and short-acting forms of insulin. Somewhat confusingly, short-acting insulin is referred to as "regular" insulin.

Some forms of insulin are supposed to be clear in appearance (such as insulin aspart, insulin lispro, and insulin glulisine, among other types of insulin), while others are supposed to be cloudy in their appearance, such as intermediate-acting forms of insulin or combinations of insulin. If the insulin is cloudy when it should be clear, it should not be used. See Table 1 for further information on types of insulin, their onsets, peaks, and durations and other data.

All insulin is now made using recombinant genetic DNA technology. Bovine (cow) and porcine (pig) insulin are no longer available.

Factors That Affect Insulin Absorption

If insulin is injected into an arm or leg and then that person exercises that limb, the absorption may be more rapid due to the increased blood flow. This is especially true with regular insulin.

A patient who is insulin resistant and injects a very large dose at one time in one area may see a slower and more variable rate of absorption.

For insulin mixtures and those that include protamine, if the insulin is not properly resuspended prior to injection, there may be variable

TABLE 1: INSULIN FORMS AND THEIR ONSETS, PEAKS, AND DURATIONS

Type of insulin	Brand name	Generic name	Manufacturer	Cloudy or Clear?	Onset	Peak	Duration
Rapid-acting	NovoLog	Insulin aspart	Novo Nordisk, Inc.	Clear	15 minutes	30 to 90 minutes	3 to 5 hours
	Apidra	Insulin glulisine	Sanofi-Aventis	Clear	15 minutes	30 to 90 minutes	3 to 5 hours
	Humalog	Insulin lispro	Eli Lilly and Company	Clear	15 minutes	30 to 90 minutes	3 to 5 hours
Short-acting	Humulin R	Regular (R)	Eli Lilly and Company	Clear	30 to 60 minutes	2 to 4 hours	5 to 8 hours
	Novolin R		Novo Nordisk, Inc.	Clear			
Intermediate-acting	Humulin N	NPH (N)	Eli Lilly and Company	Cloudy	1 to 3 hours	8 hours	12 to 16 hours
	Novolin N		Novo Nordisk, Inc.	Cloudy			
Long-acting	Levemir	Insulin detemir	Novo Nordisk, Inc.	Clear	1 hour	Peakless	20 to 26 hours
	Lantus	Insulin glargine	Sanofi-Aventis	Clear			
Premixed NPH, (intermediate-acting) and regular (short-acting)	Humulin 70/30	70% NPH and 30% regular	Eli Lilly and Company	Cloudy	30 to 60 minutes	Varies	10 to 16 hours
	Novolin 70/30		Novo Nordisk, Inc.	Cloudy			
Premixed insulin lispro protamine suspension (intermediate-acting) and insulin lispro (rapid-acting)	Humalog Mix 75/25	75% insulin lispro protamine and 25% insulin lispro	Eli Lilly and Company	Cloudy	10 to 15 minutes	Varies	10 to 16 hours
	Humalog Mix 50/50	50% insulin lispro protamine and 50% insulin lispro	Eli Lilly and Company	Cloudy	10 to 15 minutes	Varies	10 to 16 hours
Premixed insulin aspart protamine suspension (intermediate-acting) and insulin aspart (rapid-acting)	NovoLog Mix 70/30	70% insulin aspart protamine and 30% insulin aspart	Novo Nordisk, Inc.	Cloudy	5 to 15 minutes	Varies	10 to 16 hours

Source: Adapted from National Institute of Diabetes and Digestive and Kidney Diseases (NIDDK). *What I Need to Know about Diabetes Medicines*. March 2008. Insert C. Available online. URL: http://diabetes.niddk.nih.gov/dm/pubs/medicines_ez/meds.pdf. Downloaded October 10, 2009.

effects in absorption (patients should roll the bottle or cartridge between their hands prior to injection).

Ambient (room or environmental) temperature can affect the absorption of the insulin; for example, when it is very hot and the subcutaneous capillaries are dilated, then the absorption may be more rapid. In contrast, when it is very cold, the absorption may be slower.

Patients who repeatedly inject the same areas over and over again may develop lipohypertrophy, which can slow absorption and make it quite variable.

Proper Care of Insulin

Extra insulin should be stored in the refrigerator and later discarded after its expiration date, if it is not used. **Do not store insulin in the**

freezer. Once opened, insulin can be stored in the refrigerator for up to three months, and then it should be discarded. Insulin glargine (Lantus) should be discarded within 28 days after the vial has been opened.

If it is not refrigerated but is kept at room temperature (55 to 75 degrees F), insulin should be discarded after one month.

Insulin that is available in cartridges for use with insulin pen devices is generally used for seven days after the cartridge is opened at room temperature. Patients should be sure to throw away any insulin in cartridges that seem to be "frosted" in appearance or that have any clumps in them.

If insulin is stored in the refrigerator, it may feel uncomfortably cool to the diabetic person if it is injected right away. As a result, after the appropriate dosage of insulin is drawn up into the syringe, it can then be rolled gently in the hands until it is warm. Do *not* shake the insulin.

Periodic Blood Testing and Acting on Results

Individuals who use insulin must test their blood at least once per day and often more frequently, depending on the advice of their physicians. The blood test results provide information that can be acted upon; for example, if the glucose level is high, then the individual must either adjust his/ her intake of carbohydrates or adjust the dosage of insulin. If it is too low, as with hypoglycemia, then the individual needs to ingest additional carbohydrates to bring the blood glucose up to normal. When faced with a similar situation again, the individual may choose to use less insulin to avoid the hypoglycemia.

Cancer and Insulin

As of this writing, insulin glargine (Lantus) is under further study by the Food and Drug Administration (FDA), because some observational studies in Europe have found a possible increased risk for cancer among diabetes patients who use insulin glargine. However, the FDA does not recommend that patients end their insulin therapy without consulting with a physi-

cian first, because the risks of uncontrolled blood sugar levels can have both immediate and long-term severe adverse effects.

At this time, the European data provide no conclusive evidence of an increased risk of cancer associated with insulin glargine, and thus insulin glargine is still approved for use as of this writing.

Adverse Effects of Insulin

The key adverse effects that are found with insulin include hypoglycemia, weight gain, lypohypertrophy, and an allergy to insulin.

Hypoglycemia   Insulin helps the body utilize glucose, and when the combination of available glucose, insulin, and activity are mismatched hypoglycemia may result.

Weight gain   Insulin is an anabolic hormone that helps utilize and store glucose as glycogen, fatty acids as triglycerides, and amino acids as proteins. Weight gain can occur due to frequent hypoglycemia that then requires snacks to correct the low glucose level. In two very large trials involving Type 1 diabetes (the Diabetes Control and Complications Trial) and Type 2 diabetes (the United Kingdom Prospective Diabetes Study), the average weight gain for those on insulin was nine to 10 pounds over a five to 10 year period. It appears that less weight gain is seen with the newer very long-acting insulin analogues.

Lipohypertrophy   An overgrowth of individual fat cells may develop when insulin is repeatedly injected in the same area over and over again. This will disturb the normal absorption characteristics of any insulin injected in that area. As a result, individuals should rotate the injection sites of the insulin to avoid this problem.

True allergy   An allergy to insulin causes an itchy rash and is most common with insulins that contain a substance known as protamine.

Mistakes Made with Insulin

There are many possible errors that patients can make with the use of insulin, as with the use of all medications. Here are some common patient errors.

- taking an inappropriate dosage of insulin
- using old and outdated insulin
- refusing to test one's blood and/or to act on the information that the blood test provides
- seeing the doctor infrequently
- delaying seeing the doctor when ill
- failing to take medication when ill
- failing to describe problems to the doctor because he/she might change the medication dosage
- leaving newly purchased insulin in a hot car (or outside) in the summertime or hot weather

Taking an inappropriate dosage of insulin Much of what patients do when they are dosing their insulin is based first on the advice that they have received from their endocrinologist/registered dietitian/certified diabetes educator. As they gain experience over time, patients using insulin learn how their body reacts to certain doses of insulin given certain activities and carbohydrate intakes.

Common errors are to underestimate the amount of carbohydrates that were consumed and thus to underdose with insulin. Another common error is to fail to decrease the dose appropriately when the individual is pursuing vigorous activities. As an example, when children attend diabetes summer camps, many camps have a policy of cutting the children's dosages by 50 percent to start, due to the fact that their activity level is so much higher at camp than at home. Sometimes ill patients require more insulin due to the stress of the illness, but because they are not eating well, individuals often take less insulin and their glucose levels climb even higher.

Using old and outdated insulin Some patients may try to stockpile their medications or even use medications beyond their expiration date to save money. Using old medications is a serious error and can be very dangerous, because these medications are not as efficacious as medications that have not reached their "sell-by" date.

Refusing to test blood and/or act on the information the blood test provides Some patients, particularly adolescents and young adults, may decide to skip the blood testing because they feel fine or because they do not want to interrupt their current activities. Without testing their blood, they cannot determine whether they need to cut back on carbohydrates or, in some cases, to increase their carbohydrate level.

Some patients do test their blood but then they fail to act on the information that the test gives them if their blood sugar is high or low. This defeats the entire purpose of testing the blood in the first place, and it is a serious mistake.

Seeing the doctor infrequently Even patients who are very dedicated to maintaining good glycemic levels may decide to cut back on their doctor visits because they do not want to take the time for an office visit or they may not want to or be able to make the copayment (or perhaps they have no health insurance and must pay the full fee for the doctor.) It is important to see the physician on a regular basis, particularly if there are other health problems. Individuals who face financial difficulties may be able to obtain help or medical assistance from the local health department.

Delaying seeing the doctor when ill If very ill, it is important for the diabetic person to consult with his or her physician, especially if there are any symptoms of hyperglycemia or hypoglycemia. In such a case, the insulin dosage may need to be adjusted. At the least, the doctor's office should be called and the information on the patient's condition reported. This may alleviate a later trip to the emergency room of the hospital.

Failing to take medication when ill Some patients mistakenly believe that they do not need to take their insulin when they are ill, as they are often eating poorly. However, sickness itself can take a heavy toll on the body, and it is as important, or even more important, to take insulin when ill, as recommended by the physician.

Failing to describe problems to the doctor because he/she might change the medication dosage Some patients feel that they do not want to "rock the boat," so they fail to tell their doctors about health problems that they are currently experiencing. It is true that the doctor might change the dosage of insulin to accommodate the patient's current symptoms. It is also true that such a dosage change might be extremely necessary and important.

Leaving newly purchased insulin in a hot car (or outside) in the summertime Insulin should never be left in the car for hours while a patient does his or her other shopping or performs other errands, just as a small child should not be left in a closed car in the summer. The temperature within the car can get very high and cause the insulin not to be as effective as it would normally be. In addition, if insulin is purchased through a mail-order pharmacy, arrangements in advance should be made so that the package is not left outside with the hot sun beating down it for hours.

Predictors of Good Adherence with Insulin among Adolescents

Because many teenagers find it difficult to comply with any medication regimen, it is not surprising that some adolescents are lackadaisical about their use of insulin. In a study of 300 adolescents ages 13–17 with Type 1 diabetes in Finland, researcher Hevi A. Kyngäs sought to identify the factors related to good diabetes treatment compliance, reporting on the findings in *Chronic Illness* in 2007. Treatment compliance included such factors as taking their insulin as directed, following dietary advice, and adhering to home-monitoring instructions for their diabetes.

Kyngäs found that 19 percent of the respondents said they complied completely with their treatment regimens, while 75 percent said they performed at a satisfactory level. Six percent said

that they had poor treatment adherence. In considering insulin adherence alone, the researchers found that 81 percent ranked themselves as highly compliant. Home monitoring was not an area of high compliance, and only 25 percent of the subjects said that they complied fully with monitoring their diabetes at home.

Kyngäs found that the most important issue related to treatment adherence was the feeling that diabetes was a threat to the adolescent's mental well-being. Those subjects who felt that diabetes was a threat to their mental well-being were 7.68 times more compliant with their treatment regimens than were those who did not see the disease as a threat. The next most important factor in treatment compliance was receiving support from their physicians, followed by receiving support from nurses and reporting having the motivation, energy, and will power to comply with the regimen.

Kyngäs says, "Threat to mental wellbeing is the most powerful predictor of good adherence. Nevertheless, there is a need to consider seriously how an adolescent with diabetes will cope with their life if they have a long-term burden that causes a threat to their mental as well as physical wellbeing. The effects of this threat on psychological wellbeing should be studied and discussed with adolescents in clinical practice."

See also ADOLESCENTS WITH DIABETES; CARBOHYDRATES AND MEAL PLANNING; EMERGENCY ISSUES IN DIABETES; LIFESTYLE ADAPTATIONS.

Agency for Healthcare Research and Quality. *Premixed Insulin for Type 2 Diabetes: A Guide for Adults.* Washington, D.C.: Agency for Healthcare Research and Quality. March 2009. Available online. URL: http://effectivehealthcare.ahrq.gov/repFiles/Insulin_Consumer_Web.pdf. Downloaded October 16, 2009.

Colhoun, H. M., on behalf of the SDRN Epidemiology Group. 2009. "Use of Insulin Glargine and Cancer Incidence in Scotland: A Study from the Scottish Diabetes Research Network Epidemiology Group. *Diabetologia* 52: 1,755–1,765.

Currie, C. J., C. D. Poole, and E. A. M. Gale. "The Influence of Glucose-lowering Therapies on Cancer Risk in Type 2 Diabetes. *Diabetologia* 52, no. 9 (2009): 1,766–1,777.

The Diabetes Control and Complications Trial Research Group. "The Effect of Intensive Treatment of Diabetes on the Development and Progression of Long-term Complications in Insulin-Dependent Diabetes Mellitus." *New England Journal of Medicine* 329 (1993): 977–986.

Hemkins, L. G., U. Grouven, R. Bender, et al. Risk of Malignancies in Patients with Diabetes Treated with Human Insulin or Insulins Analogues: A Cohort Study. *Diabetologia* 52, no. 9 (2009): 1,732–1,744.

Home, P. D., and P. Lagarenne. "Combined Randomised Controlled Trial Experience of Malignancies in Studies Using Insulin Glargine. *Diabetologia* 52 (2009): 2,499–2,506.

"Insulin." Diabetes Forecast 2008 Resource Guide. Available online. URL: http://www.diabetes.org/uedocuments/df-rg-insulin-0108.pdf. Downloaded October 16, 2009.

Jonasson, J. M., R. Ljung, M. Tälback, et al. "Insulin Glargine Use and Short-term Incidence of Malignancies—a Population-based Follow-up Study in Sweden. *Diabetologia* 52 (2009): 1,745–1,754.

Kyngäs, Helvi A. "Predictors of Good Adherence of Adolescents with Diabetes (Insulin-Dependent Diabetes Mellitus." *Chronic Illness* 3 (2007): 20–28.

National Institute of Diabetes and Digestive and Kidney Diseases (NIDDK). What I Need to Know about Diabetes Medicines. March 2008. Available online. URL: http://diabetes.niddk.nih.gov/dm/pubs/medicines_ez/meds.pdf. Downloaded October 10, 2009.

Rosenstock, J., V. Fonseca, J. B. McGill, et al. "Similar Risk of Malignancy with Insulin Glargine and Neutral Protamine Hagedorn (NPH) Insulin in Patients with Type 2 Diabetes: Findings from a 5 year Randomized, Open-label Study. *Diabetologia* 52 (2009): 1,778–1,788.

United Kingdom Prospective Diabetes Study (UKPDS) Group. "Intensive Blood-glucose Control with Sulphonylureas or Insulin Compared with Conventional Treatment and Risk of Complications in Patients with Type 2 Diabetes (UKPDS 33). *Lancet* 352 (1998): 837–853.

insulin-dependent diabetes mellitus (IDDM)

The former name for Type 1 diabetes. The disease was also called "juvenile onset diabetes" in past years, until researchers realized that not only children but also adolescents and even adults may be diagnosed with this form of diabetes. In addition, sometimes people with what was formerly called "non-insulin dependent diabetes" develop the need to take insulin after many years or during pregnancy or at other times. As a result, for clarity, insulin-dependent diabetes mellitus was renamed Type 1 diabetes.

Note: the Arabic number "1" is used rather than the Roman numeral I for the purposes of clarity. The Arabic number "2" is used for what was formerly called non-insulin dependent diabetes or adult onset diabetes. The reason for this numbering choice was that experts feared that if, for example, they used "Type II," some people would misread it as "Type Eleven." However, there still is some confusion and some people continue to mistakenly use the Roman numerals rather than the correct Arabic numbers.

insulin pump   An insulin pump is a device that delivers continuous background (also called basal rate) insulin to the person with diabetes, usually Type 1 diabetes, although some individuals with insulin-requiring Type 2 diabetes may use an insulin pump. This battery-driven device is used instead of the usual injections of insulin. The individual using the insulin pump needs to give him- or herself insulin (also known as bolus doses) prior to meals and snacks (to cover the food taken in). Insulin pump therapy is also known as *continuous subcutaneous insulin delivery* (CSII) because it delivers a minute amount of insulin on a regular basis, in contrast to the three to six insulin injections given each day to the individual not using the insulin pump.

Software in the pump also enables users to attain better control over their blood sugar; for example, the software may recommend extra insulin if information from blood testing is automatically entered or entered by the user and indicates that more insulin is advisable. This is based on entering information into the pump prior to the meal and includes insulin to carbohydrate ratios, insulin sensitivity factors or corrections, target blood sugar levels, and the insulin action so that the "insulin-on-board" feature can be utilized.

Candidates for Insulin Pumps

Not everyone is a good candidate for the insulin pump, and candidates should be carefully selected. In general, children and adults with Type 1 diabetes and/or people who have a great deal of trouble controlling their diabetes may be good candidates for pump therapy, although this is a decision that should be discussed between the patient and provider (usually an endocrinologist and a certified diabetes educator, who may be an R.N., A.P.R.N. or R.D.) or the parent and the pediatric endocrinologist or provider.

Patients with GASTROPARESIS (slow stomach emptying) may also be candidates for the insulin pump, as many individuals who desire tighter control of their blood sugar levels have been unable to achieve it via their multiple daily injections of insulin.

Patients who must undergo surgery may benefit from the temporary use of the insulin pump while they are in the hospital.

Sometimes WOMEN WITH DIABETES who are pregnant may have difficulty maintaining excellent ("tight") glycemic control, and a pump may be a good solution for them. Children and adolescents with Type 1 diabetes may also find the insulin pump to be a good answer for them, because they will not need to inject themselves daily with insulin, which can cause embarrassment among other students or even disapproval among the teaching staff. However, they will still need to test their blood at regular intervals that are recommended by their diabetes team.

Some adolescents may not be sufficiently mature to handle the insulin pump. According to Gary Scheiner and colleagues in their 2009 article in *Diabetes Educator*, five adolescent deaths were linked to use of the insulin pump, and there were device-related incidents of HYPOGLYCEMIA and hyperglycemia requiring hospitalization. Scheiner et al. noted that the key causes of these adverse events were

"lack of education, unwillingness to perform diabetes self-care activities, and problems during sports or other activities."(See ADOLESCENTS WITH DIABETES.)

Elderly people who do not have dementia or other cognitive difficulties may also benefit from insulin pump therapy. They should not be individuals with severe end-stage complications of diabetes.

Candidates for pump therapy must be motivated enough to monitor their glucose levels as frequently as four to 10 times per day. They must also either continue or learn how to do carbohydrate counting and must also be fastidious in pump preparation.

According to Laurel Messer and colleagues in their 2009 article for *Diabetes Educator*, there are four FDA-approved continuous glucose sensing units for adults age 18 years and older and two continuous glucose sensing devices that are approved for use in children. The units that are approved for adults include the Medtronic MiniMed Guardian REAL-Time System; the Medtronic MiniMed Paradigm REAL-Time System, the DexCom STS; and the Abbott Free Style Navigator. For children, the two units that are FDA-approved continuous glucose sensing devices are the Medtronic MiniMed Paradigm REAL-Time system with a 522K/722 K model pump and the pediatric model of the Medtronic MiniMed Guardian REAL-Time System.

How Insulin Pumps Work

All insulin pumps currently in clinical use in 2010 are external pumps. The Animas One Touch Ping, the Medtronic Minimed Paradigm, the Accu-Check Spirit, and the Omnipod pumps are worn outside the body (clipped to a belt or brassiere or in a pocket), and the insulin is delivered subcutaneously. They weigh between 1.2 and six ounces when they are full of insulin, and they deliver a continuous basal dose of insulin. Bolus (a burst of insulin) units are delivered at mealtime to "cover" the food, and additional insulin may be added to correct a blood sugar level above the target goal or at other times when additional insulin is felt to be needed, such as from stress caused by illness.

There are three basic parts to the pump system, including the pump itself, the infusion set, and the tubing between the pump and the infusion set. The insulin pumps vary in size but are typically about the size of a package of cards and weigh between 1.2 and six ounces when filled with insulin. It can be worn on a belt or in a pocket. The pump and the additional equipment are purchased directly from the manufacturer and needed supplies are generally mailed to the consumer. As of this writing in 2010, the insulin pump costs about $6,000 in the United States, and monthly supplies for the pump cost about $250. Medicare and Medicaid both cover the cost of the pump if their internal medical utilization necessity criteria are met, but copayments may be required. Contact Medicare or Medicaid offices for further information.

In most cases, the pump uses a disposable plastic cartridge as an insulin reservoir, and the needle and plunger are attached by the user to fill the cartridge with insulin from a vial. The needle is then removed and the filled cartridge is inserted into the pump.

Disposable infusion sets that include a needle or small soft tube are inserted just under the skin in a fatty area, such as the abdomen, buttocks, thigh, or upper arm (the same areas where insulin is manually injected by individuals not using an insulin pump). Flexible plastic tubes transport the insulin from the pump to the site where it is infused. An adhesive patch holds the infusion set in place until it is removed every two to three days and replaced because the pump must be relocated to a new site.

See the drawing of a female torso with an insulin pump and an infusion set. In this case, the pump has buttons and a readout screen and

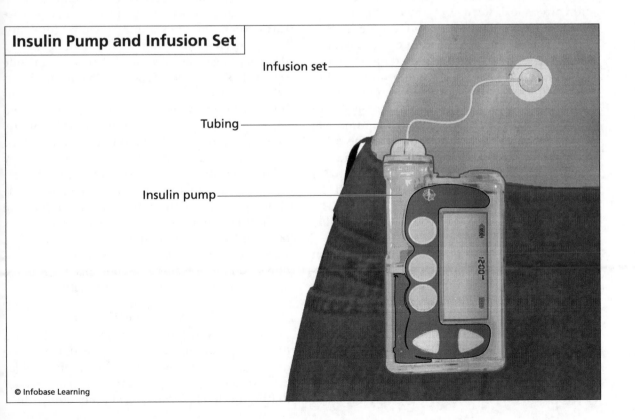

Insulin Pump and Infusion Set

Infusion set

Tubing

Insulin pump

it is clipped to the woman's skirt. Narrow tubing connects the insulin pump to the infusion set that is attached to the abdomen. The infusion set has a round adhesive patch on the skin that covers a cannula that is inserted under the woman's skin.

The pumps may be placed manually, but this is rare and most use an insertion device.

There are several different pumps that may be used and there are some commonalities and variations. The Medtronic MiniMed Paradigm REAL-Time insulin pump 522 and 722 models hold 176 or 300 units of insulin respectively and can integrate the continuous sensor without the use of a second device but require a second insertion device. However, the purchase of the sensors and transmitter is separate when obtaining this pump. The Medtronic pump is water resistant, wirelessly communicates with the One Touch Ultralink meter, and has a bolus wizard calculator that can calculate the bolus for a meal and correction if needed. A remote can be purchased to deliver boluses remotely, if desired.

The Animas One Touch Ping pump is waterproof and comes with a meter remote, which is a One Touch meter that communicates wirelessly with the insulin pump. The meter remote can calculate a bolus and can remotely direct the pump to deliver the bolus. This pump can deliver a smaller basal rate than all of the other pumps, as low as 0.025 units per hour. The reservoir holds 200 units of insulin. It uses an AA alkaline battery or lithium battery, but with the lithium battery, it has a longer battery life. The remote meter can also store the nutritional value of 500 foods.

Both Medtronic and Animas have an "insulin-on-board" feature to prevent over stacking of insulin and the subsequent development of hypoglycemia. Computer software programs are available with a 24-hours per day customer service line for assistance.

The Accu-Chek Spirit pump provides five different freely adjustable basal rate profiles and can deliver boluses in increments as low as 0.1 units per bolus (there are five different bolus dose adjustments available). It has three different user menus. It can be easily used by left-handed and right-handed patients as the illuminated display can be rotated 180 degrees. It operates on an AA battery and uses a simple Luer lock connection. A separate device is used to calculate the appropriate bolus but does not automatically forward this information to the pump at this time.

The first pump that does not require an infusion set with tubing, the Omnipod, delivers insulin wirelessly with a hand-held PDM. It has a built-in Freestyle meter and contains all of the above features, including being waterproof, calculating bolus dosages and corrections, providing a 200-unit reservoir, holding 1,000 common foods items for reference, and also delivering basal rate in increments of 0.05 units per hour. It has the advantage of utilizing additional sites (the back of the arm, leg, and above the buttock), as it is without tubing for delivery of insulin.

According to Scheiner and colleagues, "Features common to all pumps include durability, safety mechanisms, and product support from the manufacturer. Features that vary include reservoir size; screen type/size, basal and bolus delivery increments, compatibility with continuous glucose sensors, the way in which blood sugar testing results are entered into the pump. The Medtronic Minimed pump and the Animas One Touch Ping use a wireless technology to transfer the readings to the pump. SMBG meter(s)/(self monitoring of blood glucose) compatibility with continuous glucose monitoring (CGM) device(s), specificity of bolus calculations or bolus calculators, simplicity of programming, waterproof or water resistance of pumps, data-downloading-uploading options, history reports, and availability of some advance features."

The Decision to Go with the Pump

There are many pros and cons associated with the insulin pump, as illustrated by Table 1. For example, a key benefit is that the pump provides a continuous delivery of insulin versus insulin that is injected at least several times a day; thus, the pump provides a "smoother" and more predictable delivery of insulin to the body, mimicking how the nondiabetic body works. The pump can allow students or athletic adults to engage in many physical activities because it is portable and durable. These are only a few of the advantages of the insulin pump.

On the negative side, however, the person must still test his or her blood and must also act on the information that is provided from the blood testing. In addition, the pump may need new batteries and can also suffer from mechanical failures, necessitating the person to inject insulin as was done before the pump was used. It is also true that the infusion site must be changed every few days, and the change must be made carefully, to ensure that the pump will work correctly and safely.

A continuous glucose monitoring system does measure glucose levels frequently (about every one to five minutes), but it is inserted in interstitial fluid rather than blood, and thus, any critical changes should to be double-checked with a blood sugar test. The reason for this is that there can be time lags between what a sensor records as a glucose reading and a blood sugar test on a meter, and therefore it may not match the blood glucose reading; for example, when the person just ate a snack or a meal or just participated in physical activities.

General Guidelines for Insulin Use with Pumps

Typically, rapid-acting insulin is used in pumps. Typically, patients use about 80 percent of their usual total daily dose (prior to using the pump) and divide it into about 40–50 percent for the basal insulin and 50–60 percent for the bolus insulin. The basal dose is divided by 24 to give an hourly rate and is corrected for activities and hormonal changes throughout the day based on prior experience and testing.

With the help of a certified diabetes educator, the insulin-to-carbohydrate ratios are calculated (the amount of insulin needed to "cover" a gram of carbohydrate), and a correction dose is calculated to correct for glucose levels that are too low or too high. Much of this can be programmed into the pump after it has been calculated and adjusted based on the glucose monitoring that is done.

TABLE 1: PROS AND CONS OF INSULIN PUMPS

Pros	Cons
Pump is portable, lightweight and waterproof or water resistant.	Pump is worn externally and may be seen as a slight bulge by others. Some women believe the pump is unattractive.
Pump provides software that gives increased information on blood levels that can help with daily management of diabetes.	Pumps sometimes fail; the battery may fail, the connection may come loose or other mechanical problems may occur.
The pump provides better glycemic control in patients who have trouble with controlling their glucose levels.	Close attention must be paid to the pump, and the individual must still react to the information that is provided by frequent glucose testing. For example, if blood sugar is high, the individual needs to cut back on carbohydrates. If it is low, the individual needs to consume carbohydrates.
When the individual reports the result of the blood test, the pump software may recommend that additional insulin bolus should be programmed to adjust blood levels.	Individuals with pumps must bring extra batteries with them to school or work, and they also need other supplies to use or maintain the pump. The user manual should also be readily available.
Individuals using the pump can participate in most athletic activities.	If the pump fails, individuals must be ready and able to inject insulin, as needed.
Pregnant women can attain tighter glycemic levels with the pump. Pregnancy often makes it difficult to control blood glucose levels.	Supplies must be purchased by mail order or the Internet and generally are not available locally at pharmacies or medical supply houses.

Research Studies

In a review and meta-analysis of studies on the use of the insulin pump, K. Jeitler and colleagues reported their findings in a 2008 issue of *Diabetologia*. They found that continuous subcutaneous insulin infusion in adults and adolescents with Type 1 diabetes resulted in a lower need for daily insulin as compared to individuals who used multiple daily injections (MDI). However, there appeared to be no advantage among those with Type 2 diabetes who used the system.

See also CARBOHYDRATES AND MEAL PLANNING; INSULIN; LIFESTYLE ADAPTATIONS.

Evert, Allison, et al. "Continuous Glucose Monitoring Technology for Personal Use: An Educational Program that Educates and Supports the Patient." *Diabetes Educator* 35 (2009): 565–580.

Hammond, Peter. "Review: Use of Continuous Subcutaneous Insulin Infusion in Special Populations and Circumstances in Patients with Type 1 Diabetes." *British Journal of Diabetes and Vascular Disease* 8 (2008): S11–S14.

Jeitler, K., et al. "Continuous Subcutaneous Insulin Infusion versus Multiple Daily Insulin Injections in Patients with Diabetes Mellitus: Systematic Review and Meta-Analysis." *Diabetologia* 51 (2008): 941–951.

Marschilok, Catherine. "Insulin Pump Therapy." *NASN School Nurse* 24 (2009): 25–26.

Messer, Laurel, et al. "Educating Families on Real Time Continuous Glucose Monitoring: The DireNet Navigator Pilot Study Experience." *Diabetes Educator* 35 (2009): 124–135.

Scheiner, Gary, et al. "Insulin Pump Therapy: Guidelines for Successful Outcomes." *Diabetes Educator* 34 (2009): 29S–41S.

insulin resistance The impaired ability of the body to efficiently utilize the insulin that is produced by the pancreas. Insulin resistance is a necessary requisite to develop Type 2 diabetes. It is also an intrinsic part of Syndrome X, also known as INSULIN RESISTANCE syndrome.

Insulin resistance may be a problem for years before the insulin resistance and/or diabetes is actually diagnosed. Most insulin resistance occurs in muscle cells. The problem in diabetes is not due to a lack of insulin receptors but rather due to a problem within the cell. It does not allow the insulin "message" to be appropriately transmitted.

Using the analogy of locks and keys, the key is insulin. The locks are the insulin receptors in the muscle cells. These locks must be opened to allow insulin inside the cell to be used for fuel, stored for future use, or converted to another compound. The locks are plentiful in a person with diabetes but, in this analogy, can be considered "rusty." Therefore, they must be forced open. Clinically, one can force these locks open by using more insulin, exercising, eating less and losing weight, or taking oral medications such as THIAZOLIDINEDIONES (TZDs) or METFORMIN.

insurance Medical or life coverage that is provided by private, state, or federal organizations. Such coverage is important to individuals with diabetes, who may otherwise be unable to afford medication and physician visits. Studies indicate that people with health insurance are more likely to have dilated eye examinations, foot examinations, and annual dental examinations, all methods to screen for and prevent COMPLICATIONS of diabetes.

Health Insurance

What is covered by insurance varies; for example, some insurance, such as Medicaid and some private insurance carriers, provide for the coverage of medications, while other insurance, such as Medicare, does not cover medications as of this writing. (There may be a predetermined copayment amount for Medicare patients through some carriers that offer prescription drug coverage.)

In 1998, the federal government began offering Medicare recipients payment of insulin, syringes, and related material that are needed by individuals with diabetes. Prior to that time, they were responsible for this expense on their own unless they qualified for a low income program such as Medicaid. Another relatively new offering for Medicare recipients was coverage for therapeutic shoes.

Racial/ethnic differences in health insurance coverage   Researchers considering data from the Third National Health and Nutrition Examination Survey (NHANES III) looked at the health insurance coverage of people with diabetes among a group of approximately 1,500 adults.

According to author Maureen Harris, there were marked differences in insurance coverage between races. In looking at all patients with diabetes, the researchers found that 93 percent had some form of insurance, and 73 percent were covered by private health insurance, 48 percent were on Medicare, 15 percent were on Medicaid, and 5 percent were on Champus/VA (military-related insurance). About half the people with diabetes had dual coverage.

Of those with no insurance, 4.7 percent were non-Hispanic white, 7 percent were non-Hispanic black and a much higher percentage, 23.2 percent of Mexican Americans, had no health insurance at all.

Non-Hispanic whites were most likely to have private insurance only (40.8 percent), followed by non-Hispanic blacks (35.9 percent). Mexican Americans were *least* likely to have private insurance only (29.9 percent). Non-Hispanic blacks were *most* likely to have government-sponsored insurance only (Medicare or Medicaid), and 37.3 percent of this group had only government insurance. They were followed by Mexican Americans at 32.2 percent.

Non-Hispanic whites, in sharp contrast, had only 14 percent receiving government-sponsored insurance only.

These racial groupings were found to be similar for nondiabetics, with the exception that people with diabetes are more likely to be receiving government health insurance than nondiabetics.

Life and Accident Insurance

Accident and/or life insurance is another form of insurance purchased by individuals with diabetes, and premiums are generally higher for those with Type 1 diabetes. Several researchers studied the mortality and accident rates of people with Type 1 diabetes over three years, including approximately 7,600 members of the Danish Diabetes Association who had purchased group accident insurance. About 6,200 were using insulin and the other individuals were being treated with oral medications or by diet only. The researchers looked at accidents such as falls (the most common injury), as well as sports injuries, and traffic accident injuries.

Although the researchers found that the death rate among diabetics was higher than the nondiabetic population, they did not find a higher rate of accidents. They also looked at permanent injuries and found no difference from what would be expected from the nondiabetic population. In some cases, the numbers of accidents were lower for people with diabetes. For example, the average number of accidents in the two nondiabetic groups were 4.5 and 5.5 per 1,000. The average for the people with diabetes was 0.7 per 1,000 person-years. "Based on the data from control group 1, a total of 102 accidents were expected, while 16 were observed," said the authors.

They further commented on their findings,

This suggests that insurance premiums and conditions have been based on assumptions rather than scientific evidence from actuarial studies. The fact that diabetic patients have an increased mortality and a risk of developing late diabetic complications (neuropathy, retinopathy, macroangiopathy, etc.) has led to the assumption that the diabetic individual has an increased risk of experiencing an accident and that the degree of permanent injury after an accident may be higher in a diabetic than in a nondiabetic individual.

The authors suggest that insurance companies look at facts rather than relying on perceptions only.

See also MEDICAID; MEDICARE; SSI.

Harris, Maureen I. "Racial and Ethnic Differences in Health Insurance Coverage for Adults with

Diabetes." *Diabetes Care* 22, no. 10 (October 1999): 1,679–1,682.

Mathiesen, Brent, M.D., and Knut Borch-Johnsen, M.D. "Diabetes and Accident Insurance." *Diabetes Care* 20, no. 11 (November 1997): 1,781–1,784.

Islet Neogenesis Associated Protein (INGAP)
One of a family of recently discovered naturally occurring proteins that has been synthesized in the laboratory. It can stimulate the growth of the insulin-producing beta cells in the pancreas. In initial animal studies, INGAP has increased insulin levels and has apparently cured the diabetes in these animals, at least for the short term.

As of this writing, INGAP is being tested in 62 human patients. Theoretically, INGAP has the potential to cure Type 1 diabetes because it stimulates the individual's own pancreas to produce new beta cells that make insulin.

The only cure for Type 1 diabetes available as of this writing is the transplantation of an entire pancreas or the transplantation of beta cells from organ donors. Two pancreases are required for each beta cell transplantation in order to obtain an adequate number of cells, and insufficient numbers of pancreases are available. In addition, the transplantation recipients will need to take antirejection drugs for their lifetime. Hopefully, this problem will not occur if INGAP is successful as a treatment.

islets of Langerhans A structure within the pancreas that contains alpha, beta and delta cells. Together these cells produce and secrete hormones that aid in the digestion of food and the maintenance of normal glucose levels. In a person with Type 1 diabetes, the beta cells cease to function. Supplemental doses of insulin, either through injection or pump, are needed as a substitute.

In 1999, physicians using the "Edmonton Protocol" successfully transplanted islet cells from the pancreases of recently deceased individuals into eight patients with Type 1 diabetes. In 2001, the patients continued to do well and did not need any insulin or other medications for diabetes.

ketones Chemicals that the liver derives from fat and that may accumulate rapidly in the blood when the body has insufficient insulin and thus, it must consequently break down body fat rather than use carbohydrates for energy.

There are two types of ketones: acetoacetate and B-hydroxybutyrate. Standard REAGENT STRIPS for the urine only measure acetoacetate. There is now a reagent strip that will measure B-hydroxybutyrate in the blood. It is probably best used in physician offices.

"Ketosis" is the state in which fat is being broken down and accumulates in excessive amounts in the bloodstream. This may become a problem for people with diabetes when they become ill with an intercurrent illness such as flu, thus increasing both stress on the body and resistance to insulin and consequently, throwing the body out of balance. It can also become a problem if they undergo a rigorous or special diet or fasting. Anyone may develop mild fasting ketosis after an overnight fast. This is not considered a pathological condition.

People with diabetes may become extremely ill when they enter DIABETIC KETOACIDOSIS (DKA), a life-threatening condition that requires immediate emergency medical treatment.

Contrary to popular belief, if a person with diabetes is unable to eat because of nausea or vomiting, this does *not* mean that it is all right to ignore glucose levels. Quite the contrary: the person who takes insulin may need even more insulin. An imbalance of ketones is also the reason why people with diabetes need to learn SICK DAY RULES, so that they will know what to do when they become ill.

kidney disease See DIABETIC NEPHROPATHY.

Kumamoto Study A small controlled study that was performed at the Kumamoto University School of Medicine on 110 Japanese men with Type 2 diabetes and was reported in 1995. The subjects were leaner than their American counterparts who have diabetes; however, this study definitively proved that improved GLYCEMIC CONTROL of multiple injections of insulin significantly decreased the risk of the complications of diabetes. For example, a 2 percent decrease in the HgbA1c of the subjects resulted in the dramatic reduction of 68 percent fewer incidences of DIABETIC RETINOPATHY and 70 percent fewer incidences of DIABETIC NEPHROPATHY.

Intensive therapy also reduced the deterioration to microalbuminuria by 57 percent.

See also CLINICAL STUDIES/RESEARCH.

L

lancet The sharp needle-like device used by people with diabetes (or physicians, or laboratory workers) to prick the finger in order to obtain a droplet of blood that will be tested for glucose levels. Pricking the side of the finger is much less painful than pricking the finger tip as there are far fewer pain receptors present at that location. Newer devices enable the user to obtain a blood drop from alternate sites of the body with even fewer pain receptors than the fingertip or side of the finger.

There are a number of lancing devices with accompanying meters that allow for lancing alternate sites such as the forearm. There are also devices that will allow the patient to individualize the force of the automatic lancing action as well as the depth of penetration, thus making the process much more comfortable.

lawsuits Litigation filed by individuals who believe they have been wronged in some way. Because of problems with perceived discrimination against individuals with diabetes in the workplace, school, and other environments, individuals with diabetes have filed many lawsuits. Many people hoped that the AMERICANS WITH DISABILITIES ACT would correct many of the problems faced by individuals with disabilities; however, apparent inequities continue.

Organizations such as the American Diabetes Association (ADA) have found it necessary to assist individuals in cases where their rights were violated. For example, in some cases, schools have refused to provide testing for children with diabetes or to allow school-age children to test their own blood. In some cases, schools or even laws have required that a physician perform the testing, and thus a conflict occurs between clashing federal laws and the needs of children.

The ADA prevailed in a lawsuit in which a day-care center denied admission to a child solely because of her Type 1 diabetes and need for testing and medication.

See also DISABILITY/DISABILITY BENEFITS.

LDL Refers to low density lipoprotein cholesterol, which, in contrast to high density cholesterol (HDL), is often called "bad" cholesterol. People with diabetes have a greater than normal risk for heart attacks and strokes. Because high levels of LDL can increase the probability of either a heart attack or stroke, it's important for people with diabetes to work at lowering their LDL levels through diet, EXERCISE, and other lifestyle changes, such as losing weight and quitting smoking.

LDL levels should be lower than 100 mg/dL. Studies are ongoing to determine if even lower levels will be advantageous to people with diabetes. LDL should be measured in the fasting state and can be calculated if total cholesterol, triglyceride level, and HDL are also measured. It can also be measured directly, which is preferable in patients with diabetes.

See also CHOLESTEROL; HDL.

leprechaunism A very rare disease caused by a genetic mutation that also causes HYPERGLYCEMIA and INSULIN RESISTANCE. It is characterized by severe mental and physical retardation and causes the progressive wasting away and death of the afflicted infants. These children are very small but leprechaunism should not be confused with dwarfism, which is a general term for all people of short stature.

According to the *Encyclopedia of Genetic Disorders and Birth Defects,*

> The nasal bridge is flat, nostrils flared, the ears low-set. Infants may have excessive facial hair (hirsutism). The features are quite coarse, not cute as the leprechaun label might suggest. Excessive skin folds, lack of subcutaneous tissue and low birth weight give infants an emaciated appearance. Breast enlargement is common in males and females, as are penile and clitoral enlargement. The hands and feet are also large. The striking physical appearance is usually sufficient for diagnosis.

Wynbrandt, James, and Mark D. Ludman, M.D. *The Encyclopedia of Genetic Disorders and Birth Defects.* 2nd ed. New York: Facts On File, Inc., 2000.

leptin A hormone that is secreted by fat cells and that acts on cells in the brain and tissues to regulate food consumption and overall energy levels.

Some researchers have found, as of this writing, a genetic link between obesity and diabetes, based on testing with rats. Further research may indicate that manipulation among human subjects can control the serious problem of OBESITY.

Researchers have also found a link between DIABETIC RETINOPATHY and high levels of leptin in the eye.

Circulating leptin levels may be related to INSULIN RESISTANCE. In patients with HYPERTENSION, leptin may also be increased.

Agata, J., et al. "High Plasma Immunoreactive Leptin Level in Essential Hypertension." *American Journal of Hypertension* 10, no. 10, part 1 (1997): 1,171–1,174.

Segal, K. L., et al. "Relationship between Insulin Sensitivity and Plasma Leptin Concentrations in Lean and Obese Men." *Diabetes* 45, no. 7 (1996): 988–991.

lifestyle adaptations The diagnosis of DIABETES MELLITUS requires a considerable number of time-consuming adjustments, adaptations, and lifestyle modifications for most people with diabetes. These adaptations must be continued for the rest of their lives, whether the individual is diagnosed with Type 1 diabetes or Type 2 diabetes. In both forms of diabetes, the blood must be tested on a regular basis, and the blood results acted upon; for example, if the blood sugar is too high, then the person needs to cut back on carbohydrates or adjust an insulin dosage, while conversely, if the sugar is too low, as with HYPOGLYCEMIA, then carbohydrates need to be consumed to raise the blood glucose level to normal levels.

Other actions must be taken as well by those with diabetes, such as careful meal planning (a subject that is covered in more detail in CARBOHYDRATES AND MEAL PLANNING), regular checks of the feet (see FOOT CARE), and at least annual eye examinations (covered in DIABETIC EYE DISEASES), particularly among older diabetics. There are other actions that need to be taken to maintain or attain as good health as possible among diabetics and to avoid or at least limit in severity the many COMPLICATIONS OF DIABETES.

Testing Blood Sugar

Whether their blood sugar is tested once or twice a day or on a more frequent schedule, most patients with diabetes should check their blood sugar every day on a schedule recommended by their physician. Even individuals with continuous glucose monitoring systems linked to an insulin pump need to test their blood, because there is a time lag in the information reported from these systems, and a blood test yields more current information. It also serves as a "calibration test" of the sensor. Blood should also be tested when the person with diabetes is ill; in fact, it is particularly important at such times because the blood sugar may ascend to dangerously high levels or fall to severely low levels (hypoglycemia).

In past years, blood sugar testing was far more cumbersome and involved dipsticks and various paraphernalia, but today, individuals with diabetes can use a glucometer, not only to extract the blood, but also to provide the individual with nearly instant information on blood sugar levels, as well as trend data with regard to recent past blood levels. If the individual is a child, however, an adult must usually test the blood for the child until he or she reaches an age at which they can manage the testing and interpretation of results on their own.

There are also many more helpful gadgets for diabetics than in past years. In fact, as of 2010, there is a product called the Glucophone, which enables the user to test his or her blood and then send the immediate data as well as trend data out over the Internet to others, including their physicians. This product is a phone with text messaging capabilities, manufactured by Genesis Technologies. As with all blood testing, it is important for the individual to act on the information from the blood test. If the blood glucose level is within normal ranges, then in most cases, no action is required. If it is high or low, then action may be needed.

Considering information provided from the blood test The target blood glucose levels for most meals is somewhere between the range of 70–130 before meals and less than 180 one to two hours after the start of a meal.

Some basic questions that individuals with diabetes should ask themselves when they test their blood and discover that their blood sugar is higher or lower than normal but not abnormally high or low (for example, when it is less than 300 and higher than 70) are the following:

1. Did you just eat a meal or a snack? This can raise blood sugar.
2. Did you just exercise vigorously? This can lower blood sugar.
3. Are you under extreme stress for some reason? This can affect your blood sugar.
4. Are you ill? You may not have been eating normally and may have failed to take your medications. (Medications are still needed even when individuals with diabetes are sick.)

Useful Devices for Diabetics

Many useful devices available today for people with diabetes can make self-management of diabetes far less cumbersome than in the past. For example, in addition to the glucometer, which tests the blood and provides instant data as well as trend data, individuals using insulin may inject their medication with insulin pens, including either a disposable pen or a refillable pen.

Some individuals who must use insulin, mostly individuals with Type 1 diabetes, but some who have Type 2 diabetes, are phobic about injecting themselves, and in such cases, automatic insulin injectors can considerably ease this task for them. These devices use high pressure air to inject the insulin without a needle. They must be cleaned frequently to avoid any bacterial contamination. However over the past 10 to 15 years the needles attached to insulin syringes have become so fine, sharp, and smooth that it is quite rare for those on insulin to use the "needleless" devices.

There are also safety devices to avoid scalding the skin in the bathtub, such as devices to measure the temperature before stepping in, including rubber ducks with alarm warnings for children with diabetes. There are also extendable mirrors, enabling individuals with diabetes to check their feet daily with ease and without the need to crouch or otherwise contort the body.

Making Lifestyle Changes

People with diabetes can significantly improve their health by making some basic changes, such as losing weight if they are obese, stopping smoking if they smoke, and giving up all or significantly limiting consumption of alcoholic beverages. These actions will extend the diabetic's life and reduce the risk of complications caused by DIABETIC NEUROPATHY (nerve damage that is caused by diabetes). Taking these actions will also reduce the risk for kidney disease and particularly for kidney failure (END-STAGE RENAL DISEASE).

Losing weight About 25 percent of adults in the United States are obese, and for some individuals, this obesity ultimately will lead to the development of Type 2 diabetes. Among adult diabetics as a group, about half of them are obese, according to the Centers for Disease Control and Prevention (CDC). Yet weight loss among the obese can dramatically improve a diabetic person's blood sugar level, and in some cases of Type 2 diabetes, weight loss may reverse the diabetes altogether. Even a loss of five to 10 pounds can make a significant difference and improvement in a person's life.

Generally, over-the-counter diet pills do not work effectively, and they may also be harmful, especially those drugs which are primarily either laxatives or diuretics. In addition, a minimal weight loss may occur with prescribed weight-loss medications, such as sibutramine (Meridia) or orlistat (Xenical). Note that orlistat is available as Alli, an over-the-counter (OTC) medication.

Some individuals have experienced a major weight loss from bariatric surgery, which is surgery that limits the intake of food by the stomach and small intestines through a surgical intervention, although this weight loss is not always sustained. In general, eating less food and exercising more is the seemingly boring yet valid formula for achieving and maintaining a sustained weight loss.

Ending a smoking habit   People with diabetes who smoke cigarettes should stop smoking as soon as possible. Smoking is the most preventable cause of many major diseases, and smoking increases the risk of CARDIOVASCULAR DISEASE, DIABETIC NEPHROPATHY (kidney disease), diabetic neuropathy, and many other diseases and disorders, including cancer. Smoking also accelerates the risk for kidney failure and the need for dialysis or kidney transplantation. Most physicians will gladly assist diabetic patients who wish to give up smoking by recommending a smoking cessation medication.

Giving up alcohol or cutting back consumption considerably   Many adults in the United States consume alcoholic beverages, but for those with diabetes, females should limit their alcohol consumption to no more than one drink per day and males should limit themselves to no more than two drinks per day. Alcohol contains empty calories, and it can markedly increase the risk for some complications among people with diabetes, whether they have Type 1 diabetes or Type 2 diabetes.

In addition, individuals who drink heavily and become intoxicated are more likely to fail to test their blood sugar levels and to take appropriate actions based on the blood test results, such as cutting back on carbohydrates, or in the case of hypoglycemia (low blood sugar), consuming some carbohydrates.

According to authors Susan E. Ramsey and Patricia A. Engler in their 2009 article for *Substance Abuse Research and Treatment*, alcohol abuse and dependence is a problem among many diabetic adults. For example, some research indicates that 28 percent of diabetic adults meet the lifetime criteria for alcohol abuse (having been an alcohol abuser at some point in their lives) and 13 percent meet the lifetime criteria for alcoholism (alcohol dependence). The rates of alcohol disorders were even higher among adults who have both diabetes and hypertension, or a 35 percent rate for lifetime alcohol abuse and a 12 percent lifetime risk for a diagnosis of alcohol dependence. The authors said, "During the course of one study of veterans receiving medical treatment, 17.8% of patients treated for diabetes also received treatment for alcohol dependence. High rates of co-morbid diabetes and alcohol problems have also been found among adolescents."

The authors also noted that alcohol may have a hazardous interaction with diabetes medications, and it also may increase the risk for hypoglycemia among diabetic individuals who are taking sulfonylurea medications.

The authors noted that adherence to treatment regimens is poor among individuals who abuse or are dependent on alcohol. They state, "For instance, alcohol use may decrease one's food intake or reduce patients' willingness to adhere to dietary regimens. Further, researchers argue that because alcohol impairs judgment, it interferes with one's attention to diet and medication and may adversely affect other self-care behaviors such as exercise and glucose self-monitoring.

Heavy drinkers have been shown to have poorer insulin treatment adherence and reduced motivation to adhere to their treatment regimen. Poor treatment adherence has also been demonstrated among those who drink moderately."

Research has also shown that heavy drinkers are less likely to have annual eye examinations than nondrinkers, and even moderate drinkers are less likely than abstainers to see their physicians.

Some research has found that alcohol abuse is an even greater problem than estimated by Ramsey and Engler; for example, a study by A. T. Ahmed and colleagues in 2006 and reported in *Diabetes Medicine* found that the extent of alcohol consumption was inversely related to adherence to diabetes self-care behaviors. This means that with increasing levels of alcohol consumption came decreasing levels of treatment adherence.

The researchers found that more than half of diabetic patients said they currently used alco-

hol. They also found that heavy drinkers had the greatest risk for complications such as peripheral neuropathy. Diabetic self-care was significantly poorer among those with greater use of alcohol.

Having regular checkups   Adults with diabetes need to have their feet inspected by a physician on at least an annual basis, whether they have Type 1 or Type 2 diabetes. The diabetic adult should also have annual eye examinations, particularly as they age and have an increased risk for the development of DIABETIC RETINOPATHY, CATARACTS, GLAUCOMA, and MACULAR EDEMA.

Increasing exercise levels   Although most people with diabetes do not expect to achieve a "ripped" muscular body of a bodybuilder, it is best for nearly everyone with diabetes to exercise on a regular basis, based on the prior approval of their physicians. Even a simple daily walk around the neighborhood can burn extra calories and improve health. The National Insti-

CHART: A SAMPLE WALKING PROGRAM			
Warm-up Time	Fast-walk Time	Cool-down Time	Total Time
Week 1			
Walk slowly 5 minutes	Walk briskly 5 minutes	Walk slowly 5 minutes	15 minutes
Week 2			
Walk slowly 5 minutes	Walk briskly 8 minutes	Walk slowly 5 minutes	18 minutes
Week 3			
Walk slowly 5 minutes	Walk briskly 11 minutes	Walk slowly 5 minutes	21 minutes
Week 4			
Walk slowly 5 minutes	Walk briskly 14 minutes	Walk slowly 5 minutes	24 minutes
Week 5			
Walk slowly 5 minutes	Walk briskly 17 minutes	Walk slowly 5 minutes	27 minutes
Week 6			
Walk slowly 5 minutes	Walk briskly 20 minutes	Walk slowly 5 minutes	30 minutes
Week 7			
Walk slowly 5 minutes	Walk briskly 23 minutes	Walk slowly 5 minutes	33 minutes
Week 8			
Walk slowly 5 minutes	Walk briskly 26 minutes	Walk slowly 5 minutes	36 minutes
Week 9 and Beyond			
Walk slowly 5 minutes	Walk briskly 30 minutes	Walk slowly 5 minutes	40 minutes

Source: National Institute for Diabetes and Digestive and Kidney Diseases (NIDDK). "Walking . . . A Step in the Right Direction." Bethesda, Md.: National Institutes of Health, March 2007.

tute of Diabetes and Digestive and Kidney Diseases (NIDDK) offers a walking program that is easy to follow. (Individuals with diabetes should check with their physicians before implementing this program.)

Dealing with emergencies Although many people with diabetes do not face constant emergencies, an emergency situation can happen, and is especially likely to occur among some groups. Some individuals who are at risk for diabetic emergencies are

- those whose blood glucose fluctuates wildly or is not managed adequately
- adolescents or children who fail to comply with the recommended regimens of their physicians
- older people who may forget to comply with medication regimens or may choose not to follow them
- individuals who have had hypoglycemic emergencies in the past or episodes of DIABETIC KETOACIDOSIS (DKA) in the past

Blood glucose fluctuation management Some people with diabetes have major difficulty managing their diabetes. They may not be trying sufficiently to manage their diet and their medications, or they may struggle to control their glycemic levels, yet are not making progress. For such individuals, an INSULIN PUMP may be an answer only if they are willing to test their blood glucose frequently, count their carbohydrate intake, and adjust their insulin according to plans agreed upon by themselves, their physician, and their diabetes educator. The pump is NOT a panacea if patients are unwilling to do the necessary work.

Failure to comply among adolescents or children In some cases, children and adolescents fail to keep track of their blood sugar, and they may even eat recklessly like their nondiabetic friends. They may tell themselves that it is unfair that they have diabetes, that they are not really sick, or other such fictions. This can be danger-

ous because the child or adolescent risks serious hyperglycemia as well as hypoglycemia. A talk with the school nurse may help, as well as discussion with the physician.

Some studies indicate that if children and adolescents with diabetes meet and interact with others of their age who also have diabetes, then they may become more comfortable in accepting their disease and the accommodations that they must make. For this reason, a diabetes summer camp may be a good answer.

Failure to comply among older people As with younger people, elderly people sometimes may fail to adhere to taking their diabetes medications, testing their blood, or paying attention to what they eat. They may fail despite normal cognitive abilities or they may fail because they have impaired abilities. It is important for those who care about the older person to try to determine which issue (or another issue) is causing the medication and treatment nonadherence. Sometimes the problem may be linked to confusion or forgetfulness, and it can help when an adult child accompanies a parent or other older relative to the physician's office and works together with the older person and the physician to attempt to resolve adherence issues.

Recent past diabetic emergencies In general, those who have had recent hypoglycemic or hyperglycemic emergencies, particularly those individuals who required hospitalization, should be seen by their diabetes educators and physician to determine as best as possible what the genesis of the problem is. It is important for these patients to closely monitor their blood glucose levels, and it is also a good idea for those who have had severe episodes of hypoglycemia or DKA to wear emergency medical identification bracelets, so that if they should lapse into unconsciousness, others will know who to call and what to do.

Explaining Diabetes to Others

One issue with diabetes is that it can seem difficult for many diabetics to talk to others about their diabetes. They may fear that others will consider them disabled or "weird," or be concerned that telling others at work about diabetes may make them seem more disabled than they are or could prevent them from getting promoted. CHILDREN WITH DIABETES have reported a reticence to talk about diabetes with their teachers, and this problem is likely to be more apparent among adolescents with diabetes, since teenagers are acutely sensitive over many different issues and often actively seek to be like their peers (but most of their peers do not have diabetes).

Some people prefer not to discuss their diabetes with others unless it becomes absolutely necessary, while others are far more open and matter-of-fact about their illness and its requirements.

Keeping Physicians Informed

Doctors need not be called on a diabetic patient's "speed dial," but health changes should be reported promptly to the physician, and the diabetic person should have an annual physical examination with their primary care physician. Diabetic patients are typically seen three to four times per year by their endocrinologist or primary care provider (PCP). When they run into treatment difficulties, they may be seen monthly or even weekly by the diabetes team (medical doctor, dietitian, and educator) until the problem is stabilized and they are again "safe." The frequency of visits is thus determined by the level of control the patient is able to obtain, how often they have intercurrent problems with their diabetes, and how often they have intercurrent illnesses. The better educated patients are about their diabetes, then the less often they typically need to be seen by diabetes professionals.

Adaptations to Make When Illnesses Intrude

One major problem that faces many people with diabetes is that when they become ill, it can be very difficult to comply with their normal dietary regimens and to adhere to the prescribed medications plan that the doctor has created. Even a severe cold can make testing of the blood glucose level seem to be an unimportant task (but it *is* still important), and a more serious illness can make compliance with normal routines to manage diabetes very difficult. Requesting help from others may become necessary at such times. In addition, sometimes pushing oneself to perform daily blood tests and to consider what the results mean are needed actions. (See SICK DAY RULES.)

See also EMERGENCY ISSUES IN DIABETES.

Ahmed, A. T., A. J. Karter, and J. Liu. "Alcohol Consumption Is Inversely Associated with Adherence to Diabetes Self-Care Behaviours." *Diabetic Medicine* 23 (2006): 795–802.

Brown, Anne W. "Clinicians' Guide to Diabetes Gadgets and Gizmos." *Clinical Diabetes* 26, no. 2 (2008): 66–71.

Ramsey, Susan E., and Patricia A. Engler. "At-Risk Drinking among Diabetic Patients." *Substance Abuse Research and Treatment* 3 (2009): 15–23.

macrovascular/microvascular disease A general term that refers to damage to the large (macrovascular) or smaller (microvascular) blood vessels. This damage results from a build up of fat, blood clots, and oxidation to the endothelium (the lining of the blood vessels). Macrovascular disease is the most common cause of death among individuals with Type 1 and Type 2 diabetes.

Macrovascular Diseases

Macrovascular diseases include coronary artery disease, cerebrovascular disease, and peripheral vascular disease. Some complications of macrovascular disease are ischemic heart disease, heart attack (myocardial infarction), intermittent claudication, lower extremity ulcer, and STROKE.

Microvascular Diseases

Some complications of microvascular diseases are DIABETIC NEPHROPATHY, DIABETIC NEUROPATHY, and DIABETIC RETINOPATHY.

Microvascular diseases harm the small blood vessels and can occur in people who have had diabetes for many years.

The Diabetes Control and Complications Trial Research Group. "Effect of Intensive Diabetes Management on Macrovascular Events and Risk Factors in the Diabetes Control and Complications Trial." *The American Journal of Cardiology* 75 (May 1, 1995): 36–51.

macular edema A swelling in part of the retina known as the "macula," and also a frequently seen complication of DIABETIC RETINOPATHY. This generally occurs due to formation of many microaneurysms that lead to leaking of retinal capillaries. It is diagnosed by an examination with a device called a slit lamp and by fluorescing angiography (a procedure in which a colored dye is injected into an arm vein and special photos of the retina are taken). The macula provides fine central vision or reading vision. There are about 75,000 new cases of diabetic macular edema each year.

See also BLINDNESS; DIABETIC EYE DISEASES.

maturity onset diabetes of the young (MODY) An uncommon to rare subset of Type 2 diabetes in which the diagnosis is typically made prior to the age of 25. MODY is generally found in slender African-American adolescents, and is rarely found in white adolescents. This type of diabetes runs in families, and more than 50 percent of these patients have an abnormal glucokinase enzyme (a protein in the beta cells of the pancreatic islets that senses the glucose level in the blood). Other genetic abnormalities have also been found. Inheritance is often autosomal dominant.

Typically the patients are not insulin dependent and do not develop ketosis, although they may require insulin for the glucose control.

Scott, Carla R., M.D., et al. "Characteristics of Youth-onset Noninsulin-Dependent Diabetes Mellitus and Insulin-dependent Diabetes Mellitus at Diagnosis." *Pediatrics* 100, no. 1 (July 1997): 84–90.

meals, timing of Planning for when and what to eat, based on factors affecting a person with diabetes.

People with diabetes need to be careful about not only *what* they eat but also *when* they eat. For example, if an extended period occurs between meals, the person's blood sugar levels may drop to a dangerous level. Timing of meals also affects the choice of the type of insulin one uses, and whether the person uses a rapid, short-acting, intermediate, or long-acting insulin—or some combination of these various types of insulin preparations.

Blood testing results are also affected by the timing of meals. Studies indicate that postprandial (after a meal) testing provides a far better indicator of the individual's health than does a blood test that is administered before a meal.

See also CARBOHYDRATES AND MEAL PLANNING; DIET; GLYCEMIC CONTROL; NUTRITION.

Medicaid Refers to the medical insurance program under Title IX of the Social Security Act, which was first enacted in 1965. This program is both federally and state funded in its mission to provide medical benefits to indigent individuals who are disabled and who are also often ineligible for other federal or private programs. At the federal level, Medicaid (and also MEDICARE) is overseen by the Centers for Medicare and Medicaid Services (CMS), formerly known as the Health Care Financing Administration (HCFA). Medicaid affects many people with diabetes who are elderly, disabled, and who earn a low income.

To qualify for Medicaid, people must be "categorically eligible" for Medicaid, which means that being poor is not sufficient by itself to guarantee eligibility. Instead, the person must also receive Temporary Aid to Needy Families (TANF) payments or receive Supplemental Security payment benefits (SSI) due to a disability or qualify in some other category of public assistance. Some other categories of individuals who are also eligible for Medicaid, include the following groups:

- children under age six whose family income is at or below 133 percent of the federal poverty level

- pregnant women whose family income is at or below 133 percent of the federal poverty level

- recipients of foster care assistance or adoption assistance under Title IV of the Social Security Act

- some Medicare beneficiaries who are indigent

Some states extend Medicaid coverage to more groups, depending on their state plan.

Types of services Medicaid provides coverage for the following forms of medical services:

- inpatient hospital care
- outpatient physician care
- prenatal care
- medications
- vaccines for children
- laboratory and x-ray services
- family planning services
- skilled nursing facility services

Some states also provide dental and optometric care in their Medicaid plans, as well as other services. Another option chosen by many states is a form of managed care or HMO coverage for Medicaid enrollees, in which a particular physician or group will be the one(s) to provide care. This service has proven to be cost-effective for states and the federal government because it diverts individuals on Medicaid from seeking their routine medical care at hospital emergency rooms.

See also DISABILITY/DISABILITY BENEFITS.

Shatin, Deborah, et al., "Health Care Utilization by Children with Chronic Illnesses: A Comparison of Medicaid and Employer Insured Managed Care." *Pediatrics* 102, no. 4 (October 1998): 102–106.

Social Security Administration, Office of Policy, Office of Research, Evaluation and Statistics. *Annual Statistical Supplement 2000 to the Social Security Bulletin.* Baltimore, Md.: Social Security Administration, 2000.

Medicare A massive federal medical program for individuals who are eligible for monthly checks in relation to their retirement or disability benefits, not including Supplemental Security Insurance (SSI). Medicare provides medical coverage for 95 percent of the aged population in the United States and also provides medical coverage for many disabled adults. As of 1999, Medicare payments totaled $213 billion for the year. Contrary to the SSI program, individuals receiving Medicare benefits need not be indigent as a requirement of eligibility. Instead, they must meet age or disability requirements, among other conditions of eligibility.

The Centers for Medicare and Medicaid Services (CMS), formerly known as the Health Care Financing Administration (HCFA), is the federal organization that oversees the Medicare program, including the care of an estimated 40 percent of all Americans with diabetes (more than 4 million individuals). CMS also administers the End-Stage Renal Disease Program to pay for dialysis and kidney transplants in Medicare patients whose kidneys fail them.

At the outset of the program, Medicare was part of the Social Security Amendments of 1965, under Title XVIII of the Social Security Act. The program originally covered only eligible people who were ages 65 and older. In 1973, the program was amended to include people under age 65 who were entitled to either Social Security disability benefits or Railroad Retirement disability benefits. At that time, most people with END-STAGE RENAL DISEASE (ESRD) were also added to the program, which is still a feature of the program today. This is important for many people with diabetes whose DIABETIC NEPHROPATHY devolves into renal failure.

Parts of Medicare

Medicare has four basic parts, including Part A, Part B, Part C (which not everyone uses), and Part D, the prescription drug benefit. Medicare Part A covers inpatient hospital care, hospice care, and some home health care. It also covers very limited periods of SKILLED NURSING CARE.

Part B primarily covers outpatient (doctor) visits, as well as some home health care and some preventive services, such as flu shots and screening for colorectal cancer. In addition, Part B covers diabetes screening for individuals with existing risk factors such as hypertension, abnormal cholesterol levels, obesity, or a history of hyperglycemia. It also covers self-management training for individuals newly diagnosed with diabetes. Part B covers diabetes supplies such as blood sugar test strips, lancet devices, lancets, and insulin that is used with an INSULIN PUMP. (Self-injected insulin may be covered under Part D.) Individuals pay 20 percent of the Medicare-approved fees unless they have "Medigap" coverage for this 20 percent through another payer or Medicaid. Glaucoma testing is covered by Part B for individuals with diabetes, with the individual paying 20 percent of the Medicare-approved cost. Medical nutrition therapy for individuals with diabetes is also covered by Part B. Smoking cessation is also covered by Part B for individuals whose illness is complicated by the use of tobacco. (Individuals with diabetes who smoke are urged to stop smoking to improve their health status.)

There is also a third part of Medicare known as the Medicare Choice Program, which allows some individuals to participate in private health plans. Part C, also known as Medicare Advantage Plans, encompasses both Parts A and B and usually offers prescription drug coverage, according to the Centers for Medicare and Medicaid Services.

Part D covers prescription drugs in a program administered by private companies that are approved by and under contract with Medicare. According to the CMS, greater than 2 million people qualify for help with prescription benefits but they do not know it. As of this writing in late 2010, there are two options under Part D, including Medicare Prescription Drug Plans, which add additional coverage for medications to the original Medicare plan, and also Medicare Advantage Plans, which are drug plans under health maintenance organization (HMO) or preferred provider organization (PPO).

Individuals must apply for Part D. A monthly premium fee is charged and the fee varies. There is also a yearly deductible of an amount that the patient pays before the plan starts to pay part of the medication cost. In addition, there are copayments that patients pay for each medication. Most Part D plans have a coverage gap in which, after both the patient and the drug plan has paid a given amount of money for drugs, then the cost of any more medications needed in that year must be paid for by the patient. However, there are low-income subsidies available to individuals whose income does not exceed an amount stipulated by Medicare for that year. Individuals who receive Medicaid or Supplemental Security Income (SSI) automatically qualify for this additional help.

For more detailed information, contact Medicare at 1-800-MEDICARE, which is also 1-800-633-4227.

Supplies and Equipment Covered and Not Covered by Medicare

Medicare also pays for some HOME HEALTH CARE, as well as some approved medical equipment, such as wheelchairs, prosthetic devices, and oxygen equipment.

Coverage for devices such as syringes, needles, supplies, and meters that are needed by some individuals with diabetes, particularly those with Type 1 diabetes who must self-inject insulin, are partly covered under Medicare. To receive coverage, the patient's doctor must fill out a form every six months. Medicare may cover special shoes as well, if needed. In general, the individual must pay for 20 percent of the Medicare-approved amount.

Paying for Noncovered Items

Because Medicare does not cover all medical needs as of this writing, most seniors purchase what is called "Medigap" insurance, to pay for such items as medications and chiropractic care. Some Medigap insurers provide prescription coverage. Medigap insurance also covers the copay for Medicare recipients. If a retired person has health insurance from a private company, usually that insurance company pays for medical costs first and then, if there are still costs remaining, Medicare will consider paying some of the balance.

For more information on Medicare, contact the local Social Security Administration office or contact CMS at:

Centers for Medicare and Medicaid Services
7500 Security Boulevard, C2-26-112
Baltimore, MD 21244
(800) 444-4606
www.medicare.gov

National Diabetes Information Clearinghouse
National Institute of Diabetes and Digestive and Kidney Diseases (NIDDK)
1 Information Way
Bethesda, MD 20892-3560
(800) 860-8747 or (301) 654-3327
www.niddk.nih.gov/health/diabetes/ndic.htm

See also DISABILITY/DISABILITY BENEFITS; ELDERLY; MEDICARE THERAPEUTIC SHOE ACT.

Levetan, Claresa, M.D., "Mastering Diabetes at Medicare." *Clinical Diabetes* 18, no. 2 (Spring 2000): 74–79.
Social Security Administration, Office of Policy, Office of Research, Evaluation and Statistics. *Annual Statistical Supplement 2000 to the Social Security Bulletin,* Baltimore, Md., Social Security Administration, 2000.

Medicare Therapeutic Shoe Act Passed in 1993, this act allows for the coverage of special protective shoes and/or inserts or shoe modifications for some people who have diabetes along with certain other medical problems, such as PERIPHERAL NEUROPATHY, a history of foot ulcers, a severe foot deformity, impaired circulation or prior amputation of part or all of a foot.

Medicare recipients must obtain a prescription for such shoes from the physician who is treating them for diabetes, and an approved podiatrist or other approved foot expert must fit the shoes. As of this writing, Medicare will pay for 80 percent of the reasonable charge for the shoes or shoe modifications.

Experts say that many patients with diabetes are not taking advantage of this benefit. According to Michael S. Pinzur, M.D., a study of about 400 long-term patients with diabetes, who were an average of 62 years old, revealed that only a minority (about 12 percent) of patients wore special shoes.

See also FOOT CARE; MEDICARE.

"Letters: American Orthopaedic Foot Ankle Society Diabetic Shoe Survey." *Diabetes Care* 22, no. 12 (December 1999): 2,099.

medication adherence/compliance Refers to a patient following a physician's orders for the timing and amount of medication. Medication nonadherence is a very serious problem for people who have diabetes for a variety of reasons; for example, it results in worse control of glucose and blood pressure. Over the long-term, failure to take medications prescribed by physicians can lead to eye, kidney, cardiac, and other diseases, as well as an earlier death that would not have occurred if the medication were taken as ordered by the physician.

Reasons for Nonadherence

Some reasons why people with and without diabetes do not follow their doctor's orders for taking their medication are:

- not understanding the physician's instructions
- deciding after a few doses that they are not "really sick" and thus, no longer need medicine
- confusing one medication with another and consequently taking the wrong one
- becoming confused because the patient takes many medications. The patient may skip a medicine if she isn't sure she took it. Or she may take it anyway, possibly administering an unwitting second dose

- forgetting to take the medicine
- losing the medicine
- other individuals administering the medicine fail to provide it on time, because they forget or lose the medicine or don't think the person needs it
- not taking medication because of side effects it causes
- being unable to afford medications

Nonadherence among People with Diabetes

Several recent studies indicate that noncompliance is a very serious problem among those with diabetes, particularly with individuals diagnosed with Type 2 diabetes, who may not take the illness as seriously as they should.

A study reported at the American Diabetes Association's 60th Annual Scientific Sessions provided data on individuals with diabetes in Scotland and gave insight on medication adherence problems. Medical records were studied on 400,000 residents over three years, including 3,000 individuals who were diagnosed with diabetes.

Only about one third of the individuals taking sulfonylureas or metformin refilled their prescriptions sufficiently to maintain acceptable blood glucose levels. When individuals were prescribed both drugs, only 13 percent complied.

Adherence to the medication plan varied with the number of pills that were prescribed. Patients who only had to take one pill per day had a higher compliance rate than those who had to take two or more pills daily. Researchers found a 22 percent decrease in compliance with each additional drug that was added to the medication regimen.

In another study reported in Belgium in 1999 for the period 1991–97, researchers found very poor rates of compliance among people with Type 2 diabetes. About half the patients taking acarbose did not refill their prescription within a one-year period. In addition, about one third of those taking metformin apparently discontinued the drug altogether.

Failure to take their medications did have a serious impact on the subjects with diabetes. Researchers in the Belgium study found that the patients who stopped taking their oral antidiabetic medications were nearly twice as likely to require emergency hospital treatment.

Nonadherence among adolescents According to researchers in Scotland who reported their findings in a 1997 issue of *The Lancet,* it is likely that adolescents and young adults with Type 1 diabetes who suffer from complications are not taking their insulin as directed. They found that among 89 patients, 16 patients (18 percent) had been hospitalized 37 times over the period 1993–1994. Of these, 36 of the 37 hospital admissions were for acute complications stemming from their diabetes, including 15 with DIABETIC KETOACIDOSIS (DKA) and 21 with HYPOGLYCEMIA. Some of the patients had failed to take any insulin at all. The authors said,

> The reasons for failing to take insulin are complex, but may include deliberate failure as part of a weight-loss strategy, manipulation, recklessness, error, or simple fatigue in the day-to-day effort of managing diabetes. Overall adherence were excellent before puberty and improved again in the adult years; we maintain this is related to behavioural factors. Parents will supervise the treatment regimen for their children, and this may explain the positive adherence index.

Improving Medication Adherence

Because medication compliance is so critically important for individuals with diabetes and other illnesses, doctors try to make compliance as easy as possible. Some ways that doctors simplify the drug regimen, whenever possible, are the following:

- They order time-release medications that can be used once a day.
- Medication is ordered to be taken at meals or upon arising or before bed.

- When possible, combination medications are ordered.
- Doctors review the medication regimen, each time they see the patient.
- Medications given in calendar blister packs may be easier for patients to comply with.
- Medication is put into containers (with one section for "Monday," "Tuesday," and so forth) that are set up in advance by the patient or visiting nurse or family members.

Medication Packaging Can Help

In a study reported in a 2000 issue of *Diabetes Care,* researchers sought to find if individuals with diabetes were more likely to take their medication at the proper time and in the designated dose if a calendar blister pack were provided.

The researchers ran the test for eight months on 68 patients with diabetes in New Zealand. About half the patients took three or more medications per day. Their patients using the calendar blister pack were given both their oral antidiabetic medication and antihypertensive medicine. The results: researchers found that both the glucose levels and the hypertension levels of those who were using the calendar blister pack dropped significantly versus the levels for the control group subjects who did not receive the blister pack.

Probably the key problem with blister packing multiple medications is that many individuals take medications produced by different pharmaceutical companies and would require some means of cooperation between sometimes heavily competitive companies. For example, to illustrate just one problem, would the packaging be done at Pharmaceutical Company A's plant or Pharmaceutical Company B's plant? Of course, if one pharmaceutical company produced both the antidiabetic medicine and the antihypertensive, this would not present the same problem.

All patients with diabetes should carry a list of their medications, both prescribed and nonprescribed medications. The list should also include all vitamins, herbs, and other supplements the person may take, as well as dosages of each drug. This information should be provided to all health care providers that they see.

Patients with diabetes should also attempt to obtain all their medications and supplements from one pharmacy only, in order to minimize errors and drug to drug interactions that may occur. The patients should be sure to tell the pharmacist about supplements they plan to use, so that he or she can enter the information into the computer.

See also ADOLESCENTS WITH DIABETES; GLYCE-MIC CONTROL.

Dey, Jayant, M.D., et al. "Factors Influencing Patient Acceptability of Diabetes Treatment Regimens." *Clinical Diabetes* 18, no. 2, (Spring 2000): 61–67.

Morris, Andrew, et al. "Adherence to Insulin Treatment, Glycaemic Control, and Ketoacidosis in Insulin-Dependent Diabetes Mellitus." *The Lancet* 350, no. 9090 (November 22, 1997): 1,505–1,510.

Simmons, D., M.D., et al. "Can Medication Packing Improve Glycemic Control and Blood Pressure in Type 2 Diabetes?" *Diabetes Care* 23, no. 2 (2000): 153–156.

medication interactions The effect that medications may have on each other when taken by a person at about the same time or together. Some medications may boost ("potentiate") the impact of other drugs. They may also lower the efficacy of other medications. Some medications, when taken together, can result in medical problems that would not occur if they were not combined.

Medication interactions are a potential problem for any person who takes any medicines, including over-the-counter drugs. Even alternative remedies can cause a problem, for example, ginkgo biloba can cause blood thinning and boost the impact of other blood thinners such as warfarin (Coumadin). If a physician did not know a patient was taking an herbal remedy, then he could not provide a warning. Many individuals, particularly older people who have diabetes, are likely to be on more than two or three medications for chronic conditions such as hypertension, cardiac problems, and other

ailments. It's a good idea for patients to use just one pharmacy, if possible, so that the pharmacist can help track possible drug interactions. It's also a good idea for patients to keep a complete list of all medications and supplements, so that this information can be provided to new physicians or to pharmacists.

See also MEDICATION ADHERENCE/COMPLIANCE; MEDICATIONS FOR TREATMENT OF TYPE 2 DIABETES.

medications for treatment of Type 2 diabetes
Most individuals with Type 2 diabetes need to take one or more medications in order to keep their glucose levels in control and as close to normal as possible. Most individuals with Type 2 diabetes take prescribed oral medications; however, sometimes individuals with long-term and/or severe Type 2 diabetes also need to take INSULIN. Some physicians refer to all diabetes medications in general as anti-diabetes medications. In the past, all medications that were prescribed for patients with Type 2 diabetes were often referred to as "oral agents." However, some patients with Type 2 diabetes also need insulin, and newer medications for Type 2 diabetes that accompany insulin use, such as amylin mimetics, are injected rather than taken orally. This overview covers non-insulin medications for diabetes.

The Action to Control Cardiovascular Risk in Diabetes (ACCORD) study analyzed the results of 5,518 patients with diabetes at high risk for cardiovascular disease who took a combination of fenofibrate and simvastatin to see if these drugs together reduced the risk for fatal heart attacks as well as nonfatal heart attacks and stroke; however, they found this combination did not reduce the risk of such events. See CARDIOVASCULAR DISEASE for further information.

Oral Medications for Treatment of Type 2 Diabetes

Oral medications for Type 2 diabetes fall into several primary classes, including the following: alpha-glucosidase inhibitors; BIGUANIDES;

d-phenylalanine derivatives; dipeptidyl pepti-dase-4 (DPP-4) inhibitors; MEGLITINIDES; SULFO-NYLUREAS, and THIAZOLIDINEDIONES.

Alpha-glucosidase inhibitors Medications in the alpha-glucosidase inhibitor class work to slow down the body's digestion of glucose and thus delay the absorption of some carbohy-drates. This in turn acts to flatten the peaks of glucose that can occur within the bloodstream after eating meals. This type of medication par-ticularly slows down the digestion of foods that are high in carbohydrates, such as bread, milk, and fruit.

The two alpha-glucosidase inhibitors that are approved by the Food and Drug Administra-tion (FDA) to treat diabetes in the United States as of this writing are acarbose (Precose) and miglitol (Glyset). These medications are taken with meals. They are often used to treat elderly individuals with diabetes. The primary side effect of alpha-glucosidase inhibitors is that they may sometimes cause gastrointestinal disturbances, such as gas and loose stools. These side effects generally decrease after three or four weeks, when the body has adjusted to the medication.

According to D. M. Nathan et al. in their 2009 article on diabetes medications in *Dia-betologia*, one study has shown that acarbose unexpectedly reduced severe cardiovascular outcomes, although this possible benefit needs to be more thoroughly explored through addi-tional research. (Further research will help to determine if these findings were an anomaly or if the medication truly does improve the cardio-vascular outcome of patients with diabetes.)

Biguanides Medications in the biguanide class work to decrease the glucose production of the liver, thus lowering the blood sugar levels. The biguanide also lessens insulin resis-tance, or the inability of the body to efficiently use all of the insulin that the pancreas makes. The only biguanide in the United States that is approved by the FDA is METFORMIN (Gluco-phage, Glucophage XR, and Riomet). Gluco-phage XR is a long-acting form of metformin, and Riomet is a liquid form.

Metformin does not have a risk for causing HYPOGLYCEMIA, as do some other diabetes medi-cations, particularly sulfonylureas, nor does the medication cause weight gain. Since many peo-ple with Type 2 diabetes have a major problem with OBESITY, this is an important asset.

Metformin may cause nausea, and it can also initially lead to changes in bowel habits, espe-cially loose stools, in about a third of all users. Taking the pill with a meal and slowly titrating the dose up to 2,000 to 2,550 milligrams per day often diminishes these side effects. Metformin should not be used in patients with renal insuf-ficiency or moderate-to-severe liver dysfunction, nor should it be used in patients with congestive heart failure. Individuals with severe infections should not use metformin.

The drug should not be restarted after any procedure that involves the injection of contrast dye such as X-ray or CT scans (they may cause a change in kidney function) or after any major surgery until it has been determined that the patient's kidney function is adequate (usually by rechecking the blood creatinine level).

In a consensus statement from the American Diabetes Association and the European Associa-tion for the Study of Diabetes by D. M. Nathan et al. in *Diabetologia*, metformin is recommended as the initial therapy for Type 2 diabetes. Generic metformin was recommended because of its lower price when compared to branded forms of metformin. If gastrointestinal symptoms appear, physicians can decrease the medication dosage and attempt to increase the dosage at a later time. They recommended the medication be taken either once or twice a day and with meals.

Metformin generally should be avoided in individuals who are alcoholics or who have advanced kidney or liver disease. The drug is not approved for pregnant or breast-feeding women.

According to Edwin Gale, M.D., coauthor of an epidemiologic study presented at the European Association for the Study of Diabetes (EASD) 45th Annual Meeting in October 2009, metformin was found to reduce the risk for pan-creatic and colon cancers in patients with Type 2 diabetes. Their observational study showed the risk of developing colon cancer over five years with insulin and with metformin. They found that patients on insulin were twice as likely to develop colon carcinomas than were those on metformin. In addition, pancreatic cancer patients on insulin alone had 4.5 times the risk. The researchers suggest that metformin could play a significant role in preventing pancreatic cancer, which is a particularly lethal form of cancer.

D-phenylalanine derivatives This class of medication causes the body to create more insulin for a brief period of time, and thus it is taken before each meal. Nateglinide (Starlix) is the one FDA-approved medication in this class. This medication can cause hypoglycemia in some individuals. Nateglinide has a more rapid onset than its meglitinide counterpart, repaglinide. It also lasts for a shorter time in the body, which makes the drug less likely to cause hypoglycemia than repaglinide. However, some patients need a longer duration of action, especially when eating meals with high fat content.

Nateglinide may cause mild weight gain (three to four pounds) and dizziness in some individuals.

Meglitinides Medications in this class are considered short-acting insulin secretagogues because they induce the pancreas to secrete greater amounts of insulin than it would normally produce. (In contrast, sulfonylurea medications are longer-acting secretagogues.) Meglitinides as well as the sulfonylureas and nateglinide mentioned above, are sometimes referred to as insulin secretagogues. The medication in this particular class is repaglinide (Prandin). This drug is taken prior to eating each meal.

The primary side effect of repaglinide is a risk for hypoglycemia, although it may also cause back pain, stomach pain, and minimal weight gain (two to four pounds).

Some individuals should avoid this medication, such as those with liver disease or women who are pregnant, planning to become pregnant, or breast-feeding.

Sulfonylureas Sulfonylureas were the first oral agents used to treat Type 2 diabetes, and the first sulfonylurea, tolbutamide, was introduced in 1955. (Tolbutamide is still available as a generic medication, although few doctors prescribe this medication today.) Medications in the sulfonylurea class are long-acting secretagogues that are usually taken once a day. They often cause mild weight gain (three to five pounds). Sulfonylureas may also cause severe hypoglycemia in some individuals, particularly in the elderly or in those with renal insufficiency.

Individuals who are allergic to sulfa drugs typically are advised to avoid sulfonylurea medications, though the science and validity of the observation is tenuous at best even after many years of study and observation.

Some examples of sulfonylureas are the following FDA-approved medications: glimepiride (Amaryl), glyburide (DiaBeta, Glynase, Micronase), chlorpropamide (Diabinese), and glipizide (Glucotrol, Glucotrol XL). Glimepiride may cause sun sensitivity. Chlorpropamide may cause a flushed face if the individual uses alcohol. It may also cause hyponatremia (low blood sodium levels).

Although not FDA-approved, many practitioners are now using the sulfonylurea glyburide during pregnancy as it has been found to be effective and does not cross the placental-blood barrier.

Thiazolidinediones Medications in the thiazolidinediones (TZD) class make the individual's body more sensitive to the existing insulin that his or her pancreas produces, allowing it to move glucose from the bloodstream into the cells more effectively. The drug takes 12 to 16 weeks to reach its maximal effects. Examples of drugs in this class are Avandia (rosiglitazone) and Actos (pioglitazone). When used alone, TZDs almost never cause hypoglycemia.

When used as monotherapy (the taking of only one drug), TZDs lower hemoglobin HgbA1c levels by about 1 to 2 percent. The amount of lowering is very dependent upon the starting level of HgbA1c (the higher the HgbA1c at the start, the greater the effect; this tends to be true of all the oral anti-diabetic agents). TZDs are often used along with metformin.

TZDs can have some serious side effects; for example, they may lead to weight gain (an average of about four to eight pounds), as well as to anemia, and edema (swelling) in the legs and the ankles. They may also interact with some forms of birth control pills, making them less efficacious, and consequently, they are not recommended for women taking birth control pills unless women check with their doctors to ensure that their contraceptive is unaffected by taking TZDs. In rare cases, individuals have reported vision changes caused by the swelling of the eyes when taking rosiglitazone.

Medications in this class of diabetes drugs should not be used in patients who have been diagnosed with coronary heart disease or those who are at risk for heart failure. The medication may increase the risk for heart attacks, and it can also cause pain from blocked blood vessels. There is considerable controversy regarding this issue but some studies have shown a tendency for more heart attacks in the group treated with rosiglitazone, while in other studies those treated with pioglitazone had fewer deaths, heart attacks, and strokes.

On the plus side, TZDs may have other beneficial effects in addition to their effect on glucose; for example, they may slow the development of ATHEROSCLEROSIS and thus, prevent serious cardiovascular events, such as heart attack and stroke. In addition, some research studies have shown that TZDs are effective anticancer agents, preventing against lung cancer and breast cancer.

As of this writing in late 2010, considerable controversy surrounds the use of TZDs, especially rosiglitazone, although the drug remains on the market at this time. The controversy stems from conflicting research, including some research that indicates that rosiglitazone elevates the risk for myocardial ischemia, which is, simply put, a heart attack. As a result, a black box warning was placed on the label of this drug as illustrated below.

WARNING: CONGESTIVE HEART FAILURE AND MYOCARDIAL ISCHEMIA
See full prescribing information for complete boxed warning.

- Thiazolidinediones, including rosiglitazone, cause or exacerbate congestive heart failure in some patients. After initiation of AVANDIA, and after dose increases, observe patients carefully for signs and symptoms of heart failure (including excessive, rapid weight gain, dyspnea, and/or edema). If these signs and symptoms develop, the heart failure should be managed according to current standards of care. Furthermore, discontinuation or dose reduction of AVANDIA must be considered.

- AVANDIA is not recommended in patients with symptomatic heart failure. Initiation of AVANDIA in patients with established NYHA Class III or IV heart failure is contraindicated.

- A meta-analysis of 42 clinical studies (mean duration 6 months; 14,237 total patients), most of which compared AVANDIA to placebo, showed AVANDIA to be associated with an increased risk of myocardial ischemic events such as angina or myocardial infarction. Three other studies (mean duration 41 months; 14,067 total patients), comparing AVANDIA to some other approved oral antidiabetic agents or placebo, have not confirmed or excluded this risk. In their entirety, the available data on the risk of myocardial ischemia are inconclusive.

In July 2010, the Endocrinologic and Metabolic Drug Advisory Committee (EMDAC) and the Drug Safety and Risk Committee of the Food and Drug Administration (FDA) met again to decide whether rosiglitazone should be removed from the market, and it was voted that the drug would be kept on the market for the time being.

Available research indicates that rosiglitazone is linked to an elevated risk for cardiovascular disease among users, including heart attack. However, other studies show no increased cardiovascular risk from rosiglitazone, and one study showed the drug was actually protective against heart attack. Another study compared rosiglitazone with pioglitazone and found that rosiglitazone was linked to a 25 percent greater risk of a cardiovascular event or death compared with pioglitazone. (A cardiovascular event includes such problems as heart attack, heart failure, and stroke.)

Confusing things further, a study published in August 2010 in *Circulation* indicated that both rosiglitazone and pioglitazone elevated the risk for cardiovascular events and death. Some of the reasons for the differing results appear to be that a large cohort of older individuals were included, and older individuals generally have a higher risk for cardiovascular events and death than younger individuals. However, other studies included individuals of all ages.

According to Clifford J. Rosen, M.D., who has been actively involved in this issue, and a voting member who decided in 2010, with reservations, to keep rosiglitazone on the market, black box warnings are insufficient and, for example, the FDA could create a registry for the compassionate use of the drug. Compassionate use refers to allowing only individuals who particularly need a drug to take it.

In 2010, more restrictions were added to the use of Avandia by the FDA, and experts say that it is clear that this drug will not be a first-line drug of treatment in diabetes. The drug has been banned in some European countries.

In September 2010, GlaxoSmithKline added the following important safety information on Avandia on their Web site at www.avandia.com, as listed below:

AVANDIA can cause or worsen heart failure. If you have severe heart failure (very poor pumping ability of the heart) you cannot be started on AVANDIA. AVANDIA is also not recommended if you have heart failure with symptoms (such as shortness of breath or swelling), even if these symptoms are not severe.

AVANDIA may increase your risk of other heart problems that occur when there is reduced blood flow to the heart, such as chest pain (angina) or heart attack (myocardial infarction).

This risk appeared higher in patients taking medicines called nitrates or insulin.

If you have chest pain or a feeling of chest pressure, you should seek immediate medical attention, regardless of what diabetes medications you are taking. If you take AVANDIA, tell your doctor right away if you have swollen legs or ankles, a rapid increase in weight or difficulty breathing, or unusual tiredness; experience changes in vision; become pregnant.

As a result, it is clear that anyone already taking Avandia or who is considering taking Avandia should have a consultation with their physician with a complete review of their medical history and consideration of any risk factors for heart disease.

DPP-4 inhibitors The DPP-4 inhibitor is a recent entry to the medication arsenal of the person with Type 2 diabetes. The DPP-4 inhibitors affects both the alpha and beta cells that regulate glucose levels from the pancreas. As of this writing, only two DPP-4 inhibitors have been FDA-approved: sitagliptin (Januvia) and saxagliptin (Onglyza). They both work by inhibiting the breakdown of the incretins GLP-1 and GIP, both gastrointestinal hormones. This leads to an increased insulin secretion (lowering glucose levels) and a decreased glucagon secretion (preventing the further synthesis of glucose and the further breakdown of stored glucose in the liver). The HbA1c lowering effects of both drugs are similar.

Sitagliptin and saxagliptin should be avoided by women who are pregnant or who seek to become pregnant and breast-feeding their infants.

Saxagliptin (Onglyza) was approved by the FDA in 2009 and is categorized as a third-line medication for the treatment of Type 2 diabetes by the American Diabetes Association. It is used either as a monotherapy (the only diabetes drug used for treatment) or in combination with other diabetes drugs, such as metformin. According to a 2010 article in the *Journal of Pharmacy Technology*, based on a review of existing studies, saxagliptin has proven effective in lowering the HbA1c levels of patients, with the best results found with patients who took both metformin and saxagliptin, and decreased their average HgbA1c by 2.5 percent or from 9.7 percent to 7.2 percent. The risk for hypoglycemia (low blood sugar) is low, with this risk mainly seen when saxagliptin is combined with a sulfonylurea drug.

According to Jill K. Logan and Alisa K. Escaño in their article for the *Journal of Pharmacy Technology,* saxagliptin inhibits glucagon-like-peptide-1 (GLP-1) in three different ways. First, it stimulates the pancreas to produce insulin when food is eaten. Second, it slows the intestinal absorption of nutrients. Third, it inhibits the pancreas from releasing glucagon, which in turn reduces the fasting glucose levels. This inhibition also enables the liver to produce glucose if needed in the case of hypoglycemia. As a result, the rate of hypoglycemia is very low. (These benefits are also present with sitagliptin.)

Saxagliptin may lead to weight loss, and studies of the drug show weight losses of 1.1 kg in the monotherapy group (about 2.5 pounds) and 1.8 kg in the saxagliptin and metformin group (about 4 pounds).

Some individuals may develop headaches or hypertension with saxagliptin. Patients with moderate kidney disease should take only the lower dose of saxagliptin, and the drug should be used with caution.

Individuals who take sitagliptin or saxagliptin may experience coldlike side effects, such as a runny nose, sore throat, and headache.

Individuals who take sitagliptin or saxagliptin should be monitored for kidney disease before they start taking the drug and periodically during the use of the medication. Kidney function should be measured before initiation of DPP-4, and periodically thereafter.

Combination medications   Because many people with Type 2 diabetes need more than one medication to control their hyperglycemia successfully, and also because many people have trouble remembering to take more than one medication, there are combination medications for diabetics which include two different types of diabetes drugs. See Table 1 for examples of combination medications.

Combination pills have the same effect as each drug would have alone and sometimes their effects are potentiated; for example, the risk for hypoglycemia may be greater with some combination medications.

Injectable Medications

There are also injectable medications that are used by individuals with Type 2 diabetes, which can be divided into subgroups of amylin analogs and incretin mimetics, such as glucagon-like peptide 1 (GLP-1) analogs, which are available in an injected form and a pen injector.

Amylin analogs   In addition to being deficient in insulin, patients with diabetes are also deficient in the amylin that is also made in the pancreas. A newer injectable medication that is used for patients with either Type 1 or Type 2 diabetes, pramlintide helps to control the diabetic individual's blood sugar by slowing down digestion, thus slowing the entry of calories into the bloodstream. This allows the insulin to "catch up," decreasing the amount of glucose that the liver makes (gluconeogenesis) and perhaps by inducing satiety (a feeling of fullness) and causing the patient to eat less.

Symlin (pramlintide) is available in vials for injection and via a pen-injector drug under the name SymlinPen. This medication is used mainly in diabetics who already use insulin, as is true for some individuals with Type 2 diabetes, particularly those with long-term diabetes.

The most common side effect of the pramlintide is nausea, especially during the first weeks of therapy. Severe hypoglycemia is another side effect if this medication is used with insulin, as it commonly is used.

Note that it is very important for diabetic individuals to use a separate syringe for the injection of insulin and for injecting the pramlintide.

Incretin mimetics   Medications that stimulate the incretin system, a newly discovered system that affects glucose metabolism, are known as incretin mimetics, and they include two classes of drugs: glucagon-like peptide-1 (GLP-1) medications.

(text continues on page 266)

TABLE 1: CLASSES OF TYPE 2 MEDICATIONS AND BENEFITS AND SIDE EFFECTS

Category of medication	Generic Names	Brand Names	Major Benefits	Most Common side Effects	Who Should Consider Avoiding This Medication
Alpha-glucosidase inhibitors	acarbose miglitol	Precose Glyset	Flattens glucose peaks that can occur with eating meals.	May cause gas, bloating, and loose stools. Hypoglycemia may occur if the patient also takes insulin or other diabetes medications that cause low blood glucose levels.	Pregnant women should not take these medications.
Amylin mimetic	pramlintide acetate	Symlin (injectable) Symlinpen (pen injector)	Causes food to move more slowly in the stomach, thereby preventing blood glucose from going too high. Also keeps the liver from moving stored glucose into the blood. Note that this is a medication for people who already use insulin.	Can cause nausea and vomiting, headache, decreased appetite, stomach pain, indigestion, dizziness, and tiredness. May cause swelling, redness, or itching at the injection site.	This medication can cause hypoglycemia and should be used only with extreme caution in those who have had hypoglycemic episodes. It should be avoided in those with hypoglycemic unawareness, who cannot recognize the symptoms of hypoglycemia in themselves.
Biguanides	metformin	Glucophage, Glucophage XR, and Riomet	Does not cause obesity. Effective at controlling hyperglycemia in many patients. Metformin is usually the first medication prescribed to treat newly diagnosed patients with Type 2 diabetes	Nausea, loose stools, upset stomach. Can cause a subclinical decrease in vitamin B_{12} levels. May cause ovulation in previously non-ovulating women	Patients with kidney insufficiency should avoid this medication, as should patients with mild to severe liver disease. Individuals with congestive heart disease should also avoid metformin, the only biguanide approved in the United States Alcoholic individuals should avoid this medication. Pregnant women should not use this medication. Note: In very rare cases, this medication can cause lactic acidosis. Symptoms include: weakness, dizziness, feeling cold, difficulty breathing, unusual pain, stomach problems. Call the doctor if these signs occur.
D-phenyl-alanine derivatives	nateglinide	Starlix	This medication causes the body to make more insulin for a brief period of time and prevents glucose levels from rising too fast after eating meals.	Mild hypoglycemia, mild weight gain, dizziness.	Patients with liver disease should not take this medication. Pregnant women should avoid this medication.

(table continues)

TABLE (continued)

Category of medication	Generic Names	Brand Names	Major Benefits	Most Common side Effects	Who Should Consider Avoiding This Medication
Dipeptidyl Peptidase-4 inhibitors (DPP-4 inhibitors)	sitagliptin saxagliptin	Januvia Onglyza	Causes the body to make more insulin, especially after eating meals. Prevents the liver from moving glucose into the blood	Can cause cold symptoms such as a runny nose, sore throat, and a headache. Saxagliptin may cause hypertension.	This medication should be used with caution in individuals with kidney disease. Should be avoided by those with Type 1 diabetes who have had diabetes ketoacidosis (DKA). Pregnant women should avoid this medication.
Incretin mimetic	exenatide	Byetta	Moves food more slowly in the stomach, thus keeping blood glucose from going too high. Also keeps the liver from moving stored glucose into the blood.	May prevent hunger and cause weight loss. May also cause nausea and vomiting, generally at the onset of use. May also cause headache, diarrhea, and dizziness. May cause acid stomach or nervousness. May cause hypoglycemia if used in combination with insulin or with other diabetes medications that cause hypoglycemia.	Not for individuals with severe stomach or digestive problems, as well as those with severe kidney disease or who are on dialysis. Not for those with Type 1 diabetes. Pregnant women should avoid this medication.
	liraglutide	Victoza			Not recommended for patients with significant liver problems.
Meglitinides	repaglinide	Prandin	Helps the body make more insulin for a short period of time after meals.	Can cause hypoglycemia, weight gain, upset stomach, back pain, and headache.	Individuals with liver disease should avoid this medication. Pregnant women should not use this medication.
Sulfonylureas	glimepiride glyburide chlorpropamide glipizide Available in generic form only: tolazamide, tolbutamide	Amaryl DiaBeta, Glynase, Micronase Diabinese Glucotrol, Glucotrol XL	This medication causes the body to make more insulin.	Can cause severe hypoglycemia. Can also cause upset stomach, skin rash, and weight gain.	Should be avoided by individuals who have had episodes of hypoglycemia. Should be avoided by individuals allergic to sulfa drugs. Pregnant women should not use this medication

Category of medication	Generic Names	Brand Names	Major Benefits	Most Common side Effects	Who Should Consider Avoiding This Medication
Thiazolid-inediones	rosiglitazone pioglitazone	Avandia Actos	This medication treats insulin resistance. May prevent the development of cardiovascular disease through delaying atherosclerosis.	Weight gain; anemia; edema; interaction with some contraceptives causing them to fail. Increase risk for bone fractures among women.	Rosiglitazone (Avandia) has special warnings from the FDA. Read more in the text about the black box warning and other concerns for those at risk for heart disease. Should be avoided by those with liver disease. Rarely may cause or worsen macular edema, a serious eye disease. Pregnant women should avoid this medication. Should be avoided by patients with coronary heart disease because it can increase the risk for heart attacks. It may cause congestive failure or worsen it. Warning signs of heart failure include: • swelling in the legs and ankles • a rapid weight gain over a short period of time • trouble breathing • having a cough • being very tired Call the doctor immediately in the event of any signs of liver disease, such as nausea and vomiting, stomach pain, dark-colored urine, appetite loss, and severe fatigue.
Combination pills	pioglitazone + metformin rosiglitazone + metformin rosiglitazone + glimepiride pioglitazone + glimepiride glyburide + metformin sitagliptin + metformin glipizide + metformin	Actoplus Met Avandamet Avandary Duetact Glucovance Janumet Metaglip	See individual medications for what they treat.	Increased risk of bone fractures. Increased risk of bone fractures Increased risk of bone fractures. See individual medications for other side effects.	See individual medications for who should not take components included within the combined medication.

(text continued from page 262)

Exenatide (Byetta) is an FDA-approved GLP-1 incretin mimetics, and it is given by injection. It is often used in combination with either metformin or a sulfonylurea drug.

Exenatide may cause hypoglycemia when it is combined with a sulfonylurea medication. Nausea is a common side effect with the initial use, but this reaction usually subsides over time. Other side effects with exenatide are dizziness, headache, and acidic stomach. The drug may also decrease appetite and cause a decrease in body weight.

In November 2009, the U.S. FDA approved exenatide as a first-line therapy when combined with good nutrition and exercise in the treatment of Type 2 diabetes. Unfortunately, in addition, the FDA also warned that they had received 78 reports of changes in kidney function, some as severe as kidney failure, over a 3.5 year period.

As a result, the FDA recommended that exenatide not be started in any patient with a creatinine clearance < 30 cc/minute or those who already had kidney failure (end-stage renal disease, ESRD). In addition they recommended that doctors use extreme caution in using exenatide in patients with creatinine clearances between 30 and 50 cc/minute. They suggested that doctors carefully monitor blood creatinine levels and asked patients to be sure to report changes in pattern of urination, fluid retention, poor appetite, low backache, or increased blood pressure. Liraglutide (Victoza) is a once-a-day injectable glucagon-like peptide-1 agonist approved by the FDA in 2010 for the treatment of Type 2 diabetes mellitus. Like exenatide (Byetta), it increases insulin secretion, decreases glucagon secretion, and slows stomach emptying, thus improving blood glucose level. It also seems to decrease appetite somewhat and leads to weight loss when compared to the sulfonylurea drug glimepiride. Animal studies have shown that it may help delay the death of beta cells and in fact may stimulate growth of beta cells in the pancreas. It can be injected one time per day subcutaneously, as it has a fatty acid attached to it that allows it to bind to albumin in the blood and circulate for a longer period (half-life of approximately 12 hours). It also has a black box warning from the FDA concerning the growth of C-cell tumors in animals, which states, "Because of the uncertain relevance of the rodent thyroid C-cell tumor findings to humans, prescribe Victoza only to patients for whom the potential benefits are considered to outweigh the potential risk."

Some experts also consider the DPP-4 inhibitor as an incretin mimetic, while others separate it in their descriptions, as was done here.

Tailoring the Medication to the Patient's Primary Symptoms

In his chapter on considering the patient's individual issues when choosing the diabetes medication to prescribe in the *Joslin's Diabetes Deskbook,* author Richard S. Beaser, M.D., says that various factors should be considered by the doctor in determining which medication to prescribe, such as the patient's age, other illnesses that may be present, and the severity of the illness. He also notes some clinical markers that should be considered; for example, a person with a large belly who has been diagnosed with diabetes is likely to be insulin resistant and need a medication that boosts the production of insulin. In addition, the older the person is, the more likely that he or she is insulin resistant, also needing a medication that decreases insulin resistance in the bloodstream.

In contrast, a person with long-term Type 2 diabetes may be deficient in insulin, and medications that boost insulin production will not work because the pancreas cannot produce sufficient insulin. Beaser also notes that individuals with diseases such as hypertension, dyslipidemia, or gout are likely to be insulin resistant.

Some medications, such as biguanides or TZDs, improve insulin action; however, there must be a sufficient level of insulin available for these medications to work effectively.

Another factor in considering which medication the doctor prescribes is the medication itself. In general, physicians do not wish to prescribe a medication that often increases weight in obese patients. In addition, if the patient has preexisting illnesses, such as liver disease, the doctor will want to avoid drugs that can lead to hepatic toxicity.

Medications that reduce insulin resistance include drugs in the categories of biguanides and thiazolidinediones (TZDs). In contrast, alpha-glucosidase inhibitors are medications that slow down the absorption of glucose into the bloodstream. Some medications increase the secretion of insulin, such as drugs that are sulfonylureas, meglitinides, and D-phenylalanines. Other medications increase the incretin effect, which is the stimulation of the body to produce more insulin.

It is important to keep in mind, however, that the prescribing of diabetes medications is a medical skill and also that often trial and error enters the equation; for example, the doctor may believe that he or she has prescribed the ideal medication based on a very thorough analysis, yet the patient develops unanticipated severe side effects and consequently, the medication must be changed.

Questions to Ask Physicians about Diabetes Medications

In their pamphlet on diabetes medications, the National Institute on Diabetes and Digestive and Kidney Diseases (NIDDK), recommends that patients should ask their doctors questions about their medications when they are prescribed and before they begin taking the drug. Some questions that are wise to ask in advance are as follows:

1. What is the brand name and the generic name of the medication?
2. What does my medicine do?
3. When should I start taking this medicine?
4. How long will it take for this medicine to work?
5. What is the strength of the medicine (such as how many milligrams, which is often written as mg)?
6. How many times a day should I take my medicine?
7. At what times should I take my medicine?
8. Should I take the medicine before, with, or after a meal?
9. Should I avoid any foods or other medicines when I take it?
10. Should I avoid alcoholic beverages when I take it?
11. Are there any times when I should change the amount of medicine that I take?
12. What should I do if I forget to take my medicine?
13. If I am sick and cannot keep food down, should I still take my medicine?
14. Can my diabetes medicine cause low blood glucose (hypoglycemia)?
15. What should I do if my blood glucose is too low?
16. What side effects does this medicine cause?
17. What should I do if I have side effects?
18. How should I store this medicine?

Newer Medications versus Older Medications

In an analysis of more than 216 controlled studies, researchers Shari Bolen, M.D., and colleagues reported in *Annals of Internal Medicine* in 2007 that older agents such as metformin and some sulfonylureas to treat Type 2 diabetes had either similar or superior effects on glycemic control compared to newer medications such as TZDs, alpha-glucosidase inhibitors, and meglitinides, although they noted the risk for hypoglycemia with sulfonylurea medications. They also noted that metformin and second-generation sulfonylureas were lower in cost, had been used longer by physicians, and had received more scrutiny in long-term studies.

Medication Compliance Is Often a Problem

Diabetes medications cannot work unless individuals with diabetes actually take them. This sounds self-evident but the reality is that compliance is a problem among many people with diabetes. They may forget to take the medication, choose not to take it, or may fail to take the drug for various reasons; for example, they may mistakenly believe that they do not need to take their medications when they are sick, risking such emergency problems as DIABETIC KETOACIDOSIS.

Peggy Soule Odegard and Kam Capoccia performed an analysis of issues that are related to medication adherence based on numerous studies of medication adherence among patients with diabetes, publishing their results in *Diabetes Educator* in 2007. The researchers found that major specific barriers to medication compliance included such factors as patient fears about gaining weight or of developing hypoglycemia, a lack of patient confidence in the immediate or future benefits of taking the medication, and problems with patients remembering to take their medication.

Some factors about the medication itself were also found to be relevant to adherence, such as the complexity of the regimen, with compliance falling as the medication regimens become more complicated; the frequency of dosing (with two or more dosages a day related to poorer compliance), and the cost or the adverse effects related to a medication. Depression was also found to be related to poor medication compliance.

See also EMERGENCY ISSUES IN DIABETES; HYPERTENSION.

Beaser, Richard S., M.D. "Pharmacotherapy of Type 2 Diabetes: Medications to Match the Pathophysiology." In *Joslin's Diabetes Deskbook: A Guide for Primary Care Providers,* edited by Richard S. Beaser, M.D., and the Staff of Joslin Diabetes Center, 173–247. 2nd ed. Boston: Joslin Diabetes Center, 2007.

Bolen, Shari, M.D., et al. "Systematic Review: Comparative Effectiveness and Safety of Oral Medications for Type 2 Diabetes Mellitus." *Annals of Internal Medicine* 147 (2007): 386–399.

Endocrine Society, American Association of Clinical Endocrinologist, American Diabetes Association. "Joint Statement for Health Care Providers—Re: FDA Advisory Panel Avandia Recommendation." July 15, 2010. Available online. URL: http://professional.diabetes.org/News_Display.aspx?TYP=9&CID=82299. Accessed August 30, 2010.

European Association for the Study of Diabetes (EASD) 45th Annual Meeting. Presented October 1, 2009.

Garber, Alan et al. Liraglutide versus glimepiride monotherapy for type 2 diabetes. Lancet 373: (2009); 473–81.

Logan, Jill K., and Alisa K. Escaño. "Saxagliptin: New Therapy for Type 2 Diabetes." *Journal of Pharmacy Technology* 26 (2010): 123–128.

Nathan, D. M., et al. "Medical Management of Hyperglycemia in Type 2 Diabetes Mellitus: A Consensus Algorithm for the Initiation and Adjustment of Therapy." *Diabetologia* 52, no. 1 (2009): 17–30.

National Institute of Diabetes and Digestive and Kidney Diseases (NIDDK). *What I Need to Know about Diabetes Medicines.* March 2008. Available online. URL: http://diabetes.niddk.nih.gov/dm/pubs/medicines_ez/meds.pdf. Downloaded October 10, 2009.

Soule Odegard, Peggy, and Kam Capoccia. "Medication Taking and Diabetes: A Systematic Review of the Literature." *Diabetes Educator* 33, no. 6 (2007): 1,014–1,029.

meglitinides A class of medication prescribed for people with Type 2 diabetes in order to maintain glycemic control. As of this writing, Prandin (repaglinide) is the only FDA-approved drug in this class. A meglitinide drug is a "secretagogue" medication, which means that it induces a greater secretion of insulin. Sulfonylurea drugs also are secretatogues but they act differently.

Prandin helps restore "first phase insulin" secretion, which is important to control glucose levels after meals. The rates of HYPOGLYCEMIA and weight gain are lower with Prandin than is seen with sulfonylurea medications. Thus, it appears safer although slightly less effective. Prandin is usually prescribed to be taken three to four times a day in dosages ranging from 0.5 mg to 4.0 mg (0.5 mg three to four times a day up to 4.0 mg for three to four times per day.)

The drug is taken with the first bite of a meal. It can be used in patients with renal insufficiency and mild liver disease.

menopause Refers to the process of the cessation of ovulation and the end of menstruation in middle-aged or older women. It begins with a lowering of production of estrogen and progesterone and occurs over five to 16 years. If the woman has not menstruated for over a year and is over age 45, the probability is high that she has experienced menopause, although she should consult with a physician and request confirming laboratory tests to verify if this is true. Women with diabetes may have more difficulty with menopause than nondiabetics.

The average age for menopause is 51 years. In addition, if women have had both their ovaries surgically removed, an artificial menopause will occur at whatever age the surgery is performed.

Menopause may upset glycemic control and a perimenopausal woman (woman in early menopause) may need to consult with her diabetes care team to review her program. As progesterone levels fall, women become less insulin resistant. However, many perimenopausal women exercise less and consequently will gain weight. As a result, this is an important time for women with diabetes to review their exercise program.

Hormone replacement therapy Many physicians prescribe HORMONE REPLACEMENT THERAPY (HRT) to women who are menopausal. There are many pros and cons to this choice and each woman should discuss this decision with her gynecologist. In addition, the woman with diabetes should remind her gynecologist about her diabetes, in the event that a medication might affect her glucose levels.

The number of incidents of urinary tract infections, vaginitis, and yeast infections may also increase during menopause, as the lack of estrogen leads to vaginal lining atrophy. Eating low fat yogurt with active cultures (acidophilus) may help.

menstruation Refers to the monthly flow of menstrual blood that occurs after puberty and continues regularly until interrupted by pregnancy, menopause, or the removal of the uterus in a hysterectomy. Diabetic control may become more difficult for a female during menstruation, because hormonal changes can drastically affect the hormonal balance and make tight control even more difficult than at other times. Typically, glucose levels tend to rise just prior to menstruation and then drop when bleeding starts, although this is not always the case.

Good GLYCEMIC CONTROL is associated with more normal menstrual cycles in adolescent girls, based on a study reported in a 2000 issue of *The Journal of Reproductive Medicine.*

Researchers reported on their retrospective review of the medical records of 46 adolescent females with Type 1 diabetes, including 37 girls (81 percent) with normal cycles and nine girls (19 percent) with menstrual problems. The girls were seen every three to six months, at which time their menstrual function, glycemic level, and any problem areas were evaluated. The girls were similar in BODY MASS INDEX and the age when they began menstruating. The average blood glucose levels were significantly higher for the girls with menstrual difficulties. The researchers also noted that as glucose levels of the girls increased, problems with menstruation also increased. In addition, the girls with menstrual problems had a higher rate of hospital admissions for DIABETIC KETOACIDOSIS (DKA).

The researchers noted that menstrual problems may be greater among females with diabetes than among the general population.

In a study of females with Type 1 diabetes, researchers found that 61 percent had an increase in their blood glucose prior to menstruation, causing 36 percent of them to change their insulin dosing.

Women who do not have diabetes have also been found to have an increase in insulin resistance prior to menstruation. Some clinicians hypothesize that some women may increase their intake of carbohydrates prior to menstruation.

To date, there is no evidence that women with diabetes suffer more from premenstrual syndrome (PMS) or from premenstrual dysphoric disorder (PMDD) than nondiabetic women. When such a problem does occur, antidepressants such as Prozac (fluoxetine) or Zoloft (sertraline) have been found to work effectively to combat these symptoms.

See also WOMEN WITH DIABETES.

Roumain, Janine, M.D., et al., "The Relationship of Menstrual Irregularity to Type 2 Diabetes in Pima Indian Women." *Diabetes Care* 21, no. 3 (1998): 346–349.
Schroeder, Betsy, et al. "Correlation between Glycemic Control and Menstruation in Diabetic Adolescents." *Journal of Reproductive Medicine* 45, no. 1 (January 2000): 1–5.

men with diabetes Adult males with Type 1 or Type 2 diabetes. Both men and women are at risk for diabetes; however, men have a higher risk for DEATH from diabetes. In the United States, about 12 million men ages 20 years and older have diabetes, or 11.2 percent of all men; however, an estimated one-third do not know that they have diabetes. Most adult males with diabetes have Type 2 diabetes.

Attitudes and Emotions toward Their Illness

Some researchers have found that men report feeling more in control of their illness than women, and they are more confident that they can affect the outcome of their diabetes. These beliefs are also carried through in behaviors; for example, men seem to be less likely to delay eating meals or injecting their INSULIN than women, and they are also less likely to engage in binge eating than females or to misuse insulin to lose weight. Men also generally have fewer complications related to diabetes, with the exception of ERECTILE DYSFUNCTION. Erectile dysfunction may be caused by DIABETIC NEUROPATHY or by peripheral vascular disease or both.

Erectile Dysfunction, Retrograde Ejaculation, and Low Levels of Testosterone

Men with diabetes typically develop erectile dysfunction about 10 to 15 years before their nondiabetic peers. According to Konstantinos Hatzimouratidis in his 2007 article on male sexual dysfunction in the *American Journal of Men's Health,* the rate of erectile dysfunction (ED) is higher among men with Type 2 diabetes than it is among men with Type 1 diabetes.

The risk for ED also increases with the risk for the presence of other disorders, such as heart disease, kidney disease, diabetic neuropathy, and DIABETIC RETINOPATHY. In addition, ED in male diabetics is related to BODY MASS INDEX (with a greater body mass index being linked to more problems) and age (older age is correlated with an increased risk for the development of ED). Men who have had Type 2 diabetes for 20 years or more have an increased risk for ED.

According to Brendan Lloyd and colleagues in their 2004 article on ED and diabetes published in the *British Journal of Diabetes and Vascular Dis-*

ease, the presence of diabetes increases the risk for ED by an estimated 1.5 to 2.0 times greater than the rate found among nondiabetic males. However, many diabetic men with this problem fail to seek help for this condition out of embarrassment, and it is also true that doctors may fail to ask men if ED is a problem for them.

Yet according to Lloyd et al., ED is also linked to CARDIOVASCULAR DISEASE, and thus it is an important problem, not only for the man's sexual life but also for his cardiovascular health. ED may be an early clinical marker of cardiovascular disease, which, if known, could be treated.

In their study of 159 males with diabetes, ages 18–75 years and from the United Kingdom, Lloyd and colleagues sought information about their ED treatment (or lack of treatment). Most of the subjects (88.9 percent) were married and most (92.8 percent) had Type 2 diabetes.

The researchers found that the overwhelming majority of the men were aware of sildenafil (Viagra) as a treatment for ED, but only about 10 percent knew of other medications or treatments for ED. Among the subjects who said that they had ED, 53 percent said that they had been offered at least one treatment for the disorder, but the other men said that no treatment had been offered to them.

Of those treated with sildenafil for their ED, they were more likely to receive treatment if they were young; for example, all of the men ages 40–49 years had been prescribed sildenafil, while 64.3 percent ages 50–59 were offered the drug, and 44.8 percent ages 60–69 years were prescribed sildenafil. The rate for men ages 70 and older who were prescribed sildenafil for their ED was 25.0 percent.

The researchers also discussed quality of life (QOL) among the subjects, and said that the QOL was significantly worse for men who said that their relationships had been affected by their ED.

Low testosterone levels A low testosterone level may be the cause of the early development of erectile dysfunction. (However, overall it is an uncommon cause of ED; it is more specifically associated with reduced libido and muscle mass.) In such cases, men with diabetes may have testosterone levels that are one-third to one-half lower than men without diabetes.

In an analysis of 26 studies of males and levels of testosterone, JoAnne B. Farrell and colleagues analyzed the results in a 2008 issue of the *Diabetes Educator*. The analysis found that there was a link between low testosterone levels and both OBESITY and insulin resistance. Thus, there was evidence that low testosterone levels (hypogonadism) correlated with both METABOLIC SYNDROME and Type 2 diabetes.

According to the researchers, up to 50 percent of men with Type 2 diabetes may have hypogonadism, which is about twice the risk that is found among nondiabetic men. Often this condition is not identified by doctors. It is not known whether male diabetics have a greater risk for having hypogonadism than other males primarily due to their age (most men who are diagnosed with Type 2 diabetes are older than 40 years) or if this problem is one that is specific to diabetes itself.

Hypogonadism is diagnosed when the total testosterone level is equal to or less than 300 ng/dL and the patient also has signs and symptoms of hypogonadism, although experts report that symptoms may be vague, such as decreased energy, mood swings, increased body fat, and so forth.

Testosterone levels should be measured in the morning when they are likely to be at their highest levels. Testosterone is an extremely important male hormone; it affects male sexual desire as well as mood, and even bone development in the developing male. Primary hypogonadism refers to testicular failure and is characterized by not only low testosterone levels but also poor sperm production, thus affecting the male's fertility.

Men who are deficient in testosterone may be treated with medications, such as pills, injections, gels, pellets, transdermal patches, and even a buccal tablet that is inserted into the mouth by the gums surrounding the incisor tooth. Note that older men who are testosterone-deficient should be screened for prostate cancer prior to the institution of testosterone therapy, and screening should include at least a digital rectal examination as well as a prostate specific anti-

gen (PSA) blood test, because if prostate cancer is present, testosterone increases its growth rate. Men with other conditions such as benign prostatic hyperplasia (which involves an enlarged prostate gland and frequent urgency and urination) as well as severe urinary tract symptoms should also avoid treatment with testosterone.

According to Farrell and colleagues, if testosterone treatment is given, then "laboratory parameters that should be monitored during treatment include PSA, hemoglobin, hematocrit, lipid profiles, and liver function tests. Patients should also be monitored for signs of edema, gynecomastia [enlarged male breasts], sleep apnea, lower urinary tract symptoms, and low bone mineral density."

Men with diabetes may also suffer from retrograde ejaculation. This means that with intercourse and orgasm, the semen is secreted backwards into the bladder. This can affect fertility. If a man has such a problem, he should be evaluated by a urologist.

Other Risks with Diabetes for Adult Males

Men who develop diabetes before the age of 30 years are more likely than women with diabetes to develop diabetic retinopathy, which can lead to blindness if it is not diagnosed and treated. Men with diabetes also face a risk of AMPUTATION that is at least double the risk suffered by women who have diabetes.

Cardiovascular Disease

The Quebec Cardiovascular Study followed 4,376 men aged 35 to 64 years old from 1974 (none had previously been diagnosed with cardiovascular disease) until 1998. By the end of the study, the risk of death in diabetics was about 3.5 times that of the subjects who had not developed diabetes nor cardiovascular disease.

The authors concluded in their article in the *Canadian Medical Association Journal*, "The implications of these findings underscore the importance of optimal management of this disease and its associated cardiovascular conditions, as well as the importance of pursuing research to prevent type 2 diabetes altogether."

See also DIABETES MELLITUS; WOMEN WITH DIABETES.

Dagenais, Gilles R., Annie St-Pierre, Patrick Gilbert, Benoît Lamarche, Jean-Pierre Després, Paul-Marie Bernard, and Peter Bogaty. "Comparison of Prognosis for Men With Type 2 Diabetes Mellitus and Men With Cardiovascular Disease." *Canadian Medical Association Journal* 180, no. 1 (2009): 40–47.

Farrell, JoAnne B., Anjali Deshmukh, and Ali A. Baghaie. "Low Testosterone and the Association with Type 2 Diabetes." *Diabetes Educator* 34 (2008): 799–806.

Greene, Michael A. "Diabetes Legal Advocacy Comes of Age." *Diabetes Spectrum.* Available online. URL: http://spectrum.diabetesjournals.org/content/19/3/171.full. Accessed August 28, 2010.

Hatzimouratidis, Konstantinos. "Epidemiology of Male Sexual Dysfunction." *American Journal of Men's Health* 1 (2007): 103–125.

Lloyd, Brendan, Rhys Williams, and Jörg Huber. "Erectile Dysfunction and Diabetes: A Study in Primary Care." *British Journal of Diabetes and Vascular Disease* 4 (2004): 387–392.

metabolic syndrome A common cluster of medical symptoms that can result in severe health problems if these symptoms are not identified and treated. These health problems, particularly CARDIOVASCULAR DISEASE and cerebrovascular diseases such as heart attack (myocardial infarction) and stroke, are often associated with Type 2 DIABETES MELLITUS. A person with metabolic syndrome has about twice the risk of developing heart disease as that which is experienced by a person without metabolic syndrome. Individuals with metabolic syndrome also have about five times the risk of developing diabetes as those without metabolic syndrome.

Metabolic syndrome can also lead to the development of ATHEROSCLEROSIS (which is colloquially known as "hardening of the arteries"), kidney disease (such as DIABETIC NEPHROPATHY), and other severe medical problems. In addition, some research has indicated that the risk for the development of breast cancer is increased among women who have metabolic syndrome, according to the American Association for Cancer Research. The

National Heart, Lung, and Blood Institute (NHLBI) reports that an estimated 51 million adults have metabolic syndrome in the United States.

Some individuals with metabolic syndrome already have been diagnosed with Type 2 diabetes, and they are currently taking medications for the disease, according to the Centers for Disease Control and Prevention (CDC), although they may not yet have been diagnosed with metabolic syndrome itself.

Individuals with metabolic syndrome often have *prediabetes,* which is a fasting blood glucose level of 100–125 on a glucose tolerance test (GTT). Those with prediabetes are at high risk for developing Type 2 diabetes unless their glucose levels and the other symptoms of metabolic syndrome (especially OBESITY) are treated and resolved.

Based on a sample of 3,424 adults ages 20 years and older by R. Bethene Ervin and colleagues and reported in 2009 in the *National Health Statistics Reports,* about 34 percent of Americans may have metabolic syndrome. These subjects were drawn from the National Health and Nutrition Examination Survey (NHANES) 2003–06. Not all races and ethnicities were studied, and the research was limited to three racial/ethnic groups, including non-Hispanic whites, non-Hispanic blacks, and Mexican Americans. However, it is also known that AMERICAN INDIANS and Pacific Islanders have a high rate of obesity, hypertension, prediabetes or diabetes, and other conditions that are often associated or occur concurrently with metabolic syndrome.

Symptoms and Diagnostic Path

According to the Centers for Disease Control and Prevention (CDC), metabolic syndrome includes three or more of the following features, and the more features that are present, the more likely it is that the individual will develop cardiovascular disease and/or diabetes. These features include

- abdominal obesity or a waist line circumference of greater than 40 inches in men and 35 inches in women

- insulin resistance, which is defined by a blood glucose metabolism of greater than or equal to 100 mg/dL (or the use of a medication to lower the blood glucose level)

- a high level of blood triglycerides (hypertriglyceridemia) that is greater than or equal to 150 mg/dL

- a low level of high density lipoproteins (HDLs), or the "good" form of CHOLESTEROL; a low level is defined as less than 40 mg/dL for men and less than 50 mg/dL for women

- A blood pressure equal to or greater than 135/85 mm Hg

At the European Society for the Study of Diabetes 2009 annual meeting, the International Diabetes Federation (IDF), the National Heart, Lung, and Blood Institute (NHLBI), the World Heart Federation, the International Atherosclerosis Society, and the American Heart Association (AHA) together attempted to eliminate some of the confusion regarding how to identify patients with the syndrome. The new guidelines attempt to simplify the issues surrounding waist circumference. The criteria are now country- and population-specific. The American Diabetes Association did not completely concur with these changes.

Many of the organizations have been arguing about how to think about and treat metabolic syndrome as well as how to advise patients. Most of the arguments involve semantics; that is, one side wanting to speak of a syndrome or a constellation of signs and symptoms known as metabolic syndrome, while the counter argument is to focus on individual signs and symptoms. Thus the conclusion reached and agreed to by these organizations in addition to the nuancing of the criteria on waist circumference includes the notion that the metabolic syndrome is a clustering of signs and symptoms and not a "disease" and that it should not be used to estimate risks for cardiovascular and/or cerebrovascular disease.

However, in practice clinicians do both, that is, they note that a patient has one or more of the signs and symptoms of metabolic syndrome, and they advise the patient about how best to treat each specific issue. For the most part, good nutrition, weight loss, and consistent physical activity will improve or normalize the signs and symptoms that make up the metabolic syndrome.

Metabolic syndrome may be present for as long as 10 years before the symptoms finally become distinct and apparent enough to the physician for diagnosis and treatment. The diagnosis is made on the basis of the symptoms.

Some conditions that may be associated with metabolic syndrome are polycystic ovarian syndrome (a tendency to develop multiple cysts on the ovaries), fatty liver disease (excessive triglycerides and other fats in the liver), gallstones, and breathing problems during sleep, such as sleep apnea.

Treatment Options and Outlook

Metabolic syndrome is treated by treating an individual's problematic symptoms; for example, if he or she is obese, then the individual is advised to lose weight. (Weight loss alone may resolve most or all of the other signs of metabolic syndrome, such as hypertension, prediabetes, etc.) According to the NHLBI, individuals with metabolic syndrome who are overweight or obese are advised to reduce their weight by 7 to 10 percent in the first year of treatment; thus, someone weighing 300 pounds should lose 21 to 30 pounds.

If the patient is primarily hypertensive, then appropriate medications will be prescribed, as they also are when the individual has hypertriglyceridemia. It is also important for individuals who smoke to stop SMOKING, because smoking increases triglyceride levels, decreases HDL cholesterol levels, and is also an exacerbating factor for atherosclerosis.

Risk Factors and Preventive Measures

Some groups have a greater risk for the development of metabolic syndrome than others, and Native Americans, Mexican Americans, and ASIANS/PACIFIC ISLANDERS are all groups that are at high risk for the development of metabolic syndrome. In general, females have a greater risk for developing metabolic syndrome than males. There are other gender differences, such as the prevalence of specific symptoms. For example, as seen in Table 1, nearly 61 percent of

TABLE 1: PREVALENCE OF INDIVIDUAL RISK FACTORS FOR METABOLIC SYNDROME AMONG ADULTS 20 YEARS AND OLDER BY SELECTED CHARACTERISTIC: UNITED STATES, 2003–2006

Characteristic	Number of subjects	Abdominal obesity	Hypertriglyceridemia	Low HDL cholesterol	High blood pressure or medication use for hypertension	High fasting glucose or medication use for diabetes
Total	3,423	53.2	31.4	24.7	40.0	39.0
Gender						
Male	1,794	44.8	35.6	21.6	43.4	45.8
Female	1,629	60.7	26.5	27.8	35.2	31.3
Male						
Age						
20–39 years	607	32.0	29.6	21.4	24.1	28.8
40–59 years	546	52.1	41.5	23.0	44.5	50.3
60 years and older	641	55.2	36.7	19.5	74.4	67.8
Race and ethnicity						
Non-Hispanic white	967	47.4	36.6	22.6	43.5	44.8
Non-Hispanic black	346	36.0	21.2	11.5	51.3	40.9
Mexican American	364	37.6	43.7	26.0	35.5	49.8
Body Mass Index (BMI)						
Underweight and normal weight	532	Not available	18.0	9.4	32.0	35.0
Overweight	701	35.1	37.7	22.6	40.3	45.0
Obese and extremely obese	557	94.4	48.6	31.3	57.5	55.5
Female						
Age						
20–39 years	488	49.8	17.8	29.4	6.8	13.4
40–59 years	542	64.1	27.3	29.4	43.2	35.5
60 years and older	599	74.0	40.1	22.7	71.0	55.1
Race and ethnicity						
Non-Hispanic white	846	58.0	27.3	27.6	33.0	28.7
Non-Hispanic black	348	76.3	14.4	26.8	53.4	38.7
Mexican American	306	74.9	34.6	39.6	32.1	41.7
Body Mass Index (BMI)						
Underweight and normal weight	519	13.6	12.9	12.9	26.4	15.8
Overweight	474	77.7	32.3	30.5	31.7	31.2
Obese and extremely obese	634	99.6	36.8	43.1	46.8	46.9

Adapted from Ervin, R. Bethene. "Prevalence of Metabolic Syndrome Among Adults 20 Years of Age and Over, by Sex, Age, Race and Ethnicity, and Body Mass Index: United States, 2003–2006." *National Health Statistics Reports* 13 (May 5, 2009), p. 6.

the female subjects had abdominal obesity, compared to about 45 percent of the male subjects. However, when considering those with prediabetes or diagnosed diabetes, nearly 46 percent of the males had this symptom, compared to about 31 percent of the females.

Table 2 shows further data by illustrating the odds ratio for the development of metabolic syndrome based on age, race and ethnicity, and body mass index, for both males and females. For example, for males 60 years and older, 51.5 percent have metabolic syndrome and their risk is more than four times higher than among those ages 20–39 years. In considering body mass index, 65.0 percent of the male NHANES subjects with metabolic syndrome were either obese or extremely obese. Their risk for metabolic syndrome was nearly 32 times the risk for those who were underweight or of normal weight. Among the females, 56.1 percent were obese and extremely obese and their risk for metabolic syndrome was more than 17 times the risk of those females who were underweight or of normal weight. In considering race and ethnicity, both Mexican American males and females had the highest rates of hypertriglyceridemia for their gender, or 43.7 percent for Mexican American males and 34.6 percent for Mexican American females.

The study also showed that females age 60 years and older were more than six times as likely as the youngest adults to have metabolic syndrome and males ages 60 years and older were more than four times as likely to have metabolic syndrome. (See Table 2 for further details.)

Other groups at risk for the development of metabolic syndrome include those with a parent or sibling with this syndrome as well as individuals with diabetes and women with polycystic ovarian syndrome. In addition, some individuals are at risk for the development of metabolic syndrome because of the type of medications that they take, which may cause changes in their blood pressure, cholesterol, or blood sugar levels. These primarily include medications that are taken for inflammation, allergies, the human immunodeficiency virus (HIV), DEPRESSION and some other forms of mental illness, such as

TABLE 2: PREVALENCE OF METABOLIC SYNDROME AND ODDS RATIOS FOR PREVALENCE OF METABOLIC SYNDROME AMONG ADULTS 20 YEARS OF AGE AND OLDER BY SELECTED CHARACTERISTICS: UNITED STATES, 2003–2006

Characteristic	Percent	Odds Ratio
Total	34.4	—
Gender		
Male	35.1	1.00
Female	32.8	0.89
Male		
Age		
20–39 years	20.3	1.00
40–59 years	40.8	2.70
60 years and older	51.5	4.18
Race and ethnicity		
Non-Hispanic white	37.2	1.00
Non-Hispanic black	25.3	0.54
Mexican American	33.2	0.78
Body Mass Index (BMI)		
Underweight and normal weight	6.8	1.00
Overweight	29.8	6.17
Obese and extremely obese	65.0	31.92
Female		
Age		
20–39 years	15.8	1.00
40–59 years	37.2	3.20
60 years and older	54.4	6.44
Race and ethnicity		
Non-Hispanic white	31.5	1.00
Non-Hispanic black	38.8	1.44
Mexican American	40.6	1.55
Body Mass Index		
Underweight and normal weight	9.3	1.00
Overweight	33.1	5.48
Obese and extremely obese	56.1	17.14

Adapted from Ervin, R. Bethene. "Prevalence of Metabolic Syndrome Among Adults 20 Years of Age and Over, by Sex, Age, Race and Ethnicity, and Body Mass Index: United States, 2003–2006." *National Health Statistics Reports* 13 (May 5, 2009), p. 7.

schizophrenia or bipolar disorder, as when these individuals take the so-called atypical antipsychotic medications. Note that it is not the diseases that increase the risk for metabolic syndrome but rather the side effects of the medications taken to treat these diseases that cause problems.

There are no known preventive measures against the development of metabolic syndrome other than avoiding obesity and maintaining a healthy diet and exercise plan, but when metabolic syndrome is present, it should be treated to avoid the greater risk of cardiovascular disease. For example, in a study of 2,559 subjects ages 25–64 who were followed up for more than seven years, reported by Carlos Lorenzo, M.D., and colleagues in *Diabetes Care* in 2007, the researchers found that the presence of metabolic syndrome was significantly linked to a risk for cardiovascular disease, especially among men 45 years and older and women 55 years and older.

Metabolic syndrome was also predictive for the development of diabetes. This was true whether varying definitions of metabolic syndrome were used, such as the definitions used by the National Cholesterol Education Program, the International Diabetes Federation, and the World Health Organization.

Alberti, K. G., et al. "Harmonizing the Metabolic Syndrome. A Joint Interim Statement of the International Diabetes Federation Task Force on Epidemiology and Prevention; National Heart, Lung, and Blood Institute; American Heart Association; World Heart Federation; International Atherosclerosis Society; and International Association for the Study of Obesity." *Circulation* 120, no, 6 (2009): 1,640–1,645.

Ervin, R. Bethene. "Prevalence of Metabolic Syndrome among Adults 20 Years of Age and Over, by Sex, Age, Race and Ethnicity, and Body Mass Index: United States, 2003–2006." *National Health Statistics Reports* 13 (May 5, 2009): 1–8.

Lorenzo, Carlos, M.D., et al. "The National Cholesterol Education Program-Adult Treatment Panel III, International Diabetes Federation, and World Health Organization Definitions of the Metabolic Syndrome as Predictors of Incident Cardiovascular Disease and Diabetes." *Diabetes Care* 30, no. 1 (2007): 8–13.

metabolism The series of chemical and physical processes that all cells use to maintain life. One part of metabolism is catabolism, which refers to the breakdown of chemicals (including foods) to release energy. The other part of metabolism is anabolism, which refers to the process during which the body uses food to either build up or to mend damaged cells. Insulin is an essential part of the anabolic process.

When patients with Type 1 diabetes have inadequate insulin, they are in a catabolic state, i.e., they are unable to store amino acids in protein, fatty acids in triglycerides, or convert glucose into glycogen and thus, their bodies begin breaking down the muscle protein and fat.

Anabolism is the process in which the body integrates simple molecules into larger ones. This is a healthy build-up state. This is also the reason why a person with poorly controlled diabetes and who then becomes well-controlled will gain weight. He or she goes from a catabolic state to an anabolic state and is able to store energy.

metformin One of the medications in the BIGUANIDE class that is used to treat people with Type 2 diabetes. Metformin has been available worldwide for many years but became available as Glucophage (produced by Bristol-Myers Squibb) in the United States in about 1995. The drug is only effective if a person's body still makes some insulin, thus it is not helpful for patients with Type 1 diabetes.

Metformin works by decreasing the amount of glucose that the liver produces and thus, it has a good effect on fasting glucose levels. Sophisticated studies have shown that this effect is most likely due to the suppression of the synthesis of new glucose (gluconeogenesis). By improving glucose levels, the drug will diminish glucose toxicity and indirectly will also decrease resistance to insulin. Because it does not cause an increase in insulin secretion when used alone (as monotherapy), it will not cause HYPOGLYCEMIA (low blood glucose).

If metformin is added to insulin or to an insulin secretagogue (a compound that stimulates the pancreas to make more insulin), this addition can contribute to hypoglycemia. In such a case, the physician will usually decrease the dose of either the insulin or the secretagogue.

Because it does not cause weight gain, metformin is favored as the first line therapy for overweight patients with Type 2 diabetes. (Most Type 2 diabetes patients are either overweight or obese.) Some patients with diabetes who are taking metformin lose a few pounds. In nondiabetic patients, the drug has not been effective in aiding with weight loss.

The primary adverse effect of metformin is gastrointestinal upset and it may cause diarrhea and a change in bowel habits. These effects can be minimized by starting the patient on a low dose and slowly titrating upwards to the maximally tolerated and effective dose.

Formulations of Metformin

Glucophage is available in the United States in dosages of 500-, 850-, and 1,000-mg tablets. The maximum allowed dose is 2,550 mg/day, generally given in two doses, although clinical studies have shown that most people achieve a maximal effect at a dose of 2,000 mg per day. The drug is also available as a sustained release preparation, known as Glucophage XR, which comes in 500-mg tablets that can be taken in one dose. This preparation seems to be as effective as Glucophage and causes fewer side effects.

Metformin is also available in a combination medication called Glucovance, which contains both metformin and the sulfonylurea drug, glyburide. It is formulated in a glyburide/metfor-min combination in tablets of 1.25/250 mg, 2.5/500 mg, and 5/500 mg. Many patients who were on the two medications are pleased to take one pill instead of two and to have one insurance co-payment (if they have copayments). Studies have also revealed that MEDICATION ADHERENCE/COMPLIANCE is also better with this regimen.

In the UNITED KINGDOM PROSPECTIVE DIABETES STUDY (UKPDS), patients treated with metformin had the lowest cardiac mortality of all treatment groups.

Patients Who Should Avoid Metformin

Metformin should not be used in patients with active congestive heart failure, significant liver disease, or in patients with renal insufficiency. It should also be used cautiously in patients over the age of 80 years. If a patient has had surgery or a radiological procedure that used contrast dye, the metformin should be withheld for 48 hours to ensure adequate urine flow. It is customary to recheck the patients' blood creatinine level 48 hours after the procedure.

One rare and very serious adverse effect of metformin is lactic acidosis. This is fatal in up to half of the patients who develop it. It is almost always seen in patients who have liver or kidney disease and in those who should not have been taking metformin.

See also CANCER.

microalbuminuria Minute amounts of albumin found in the urine and which may be early indicators of DIABETIC NEPHROPATHY (kidney disease) or even atherosclerosis. If a standard urine dipstick is negative, the patient with diabetes should be tested for microalbuminuria. This can be done in the office with a color-coded dipstick or it can be sent to a lab for a more precise radioimmunoassay measurement.

Microalbuminuria is defined as 30–300 mg of albumin per g of creatinine, as measured in a spot urine sample. Less than 30 is normal and greater than 300 is overt albuminuria/proteinuria.

Poor glycemic control, fever, and exercise can cause transient increases in albumin excretion. Generally, the level is determined two to three times before committing a patient to therapy. Generally an ACE inhibitor drug is prescribed, even if the patient has normal blood pressure.

In patients with Type 1 diabetes, microalbuminuria is an indication of early kidney damage, even within the first five years of diagnosis. In patients with Type 2 diabetes, microalbuminuria is also predictive of progression to overt proteinuria. In addition, for Type 2 patients, microalbuminuria is also a risk for the development of early cardiovascular disease.

The microalbuminuria syndrome has been associated with hypertension, abnormal lipid profiles, insulin resistance, an increased prevalence of "silent killer" heart disease, diabetic neuropathy, and peripheral vascular disease, as well as a variety of clotting and cellular abnormalities.

Mattock, M. B., et al. "Prospective Study of Microalbuminuria as a Predictor of Mortality in NIDDM." *Diabetes* 41 (1992): 736.

Messent, J., et al. "Prognostic Significance of Microalbuminuria in Insulin-Dependent Diabetes: A Twenty-three Year Followup Study." *Kidney International* 41 (1992): 836.

myocardial infarction   Refers to the death of the myocardial cells (the muscle cells) of the heart and usually associated with ATHEROSCLEROSIS; also known as a heart attack. Myocardial infarction, along with angina (chest pain) is a problem experienced by people with CORONARY HEART DISEASE (CHD). Patients with long-term diabetes are more prone to myocardial infarctions and other manifestations of cardiac diseases. A heart attack is a life and death emergency and an ambulance should be called immediately for a person exhibiting symptoms of a heart attack.

According to the American Heart Association (AHA), the following symptoms are the most common warning signs of a heart attack:

- an uncomfortable pressure, fullness, squeezing, or pain in the center of the chest that lasts longer than a few minutes
- pain that spreads to the shoulders, neck, or arms
- chest discomfort that is accompanied by light-headedness, fainting, sweating, nausea, or shortness of breath

The AHA says that there are also some less common indicators of a heart attack, such as:

- unusual pain in the chest, stomach, or abdomen
- nausea or dizziness
- difficulty with breathing or shortness of breath
- heart palpitations
- a cold sweat or paleness
- unexplained anxiety, fatigue, or weakness

See also CARDIOVASCULAR DISEASE; COMPLICATIONS OF DIABETES AND ASSOCIATED DISORDERS.

nephrologist Medical doctor who specializes in treating diseases of the kidneys, such as DIABETIC NEPHROPATHY and END-STAGE RENAL DISEASE (ESRD). Nephrologists generally train for three years in internal medicine and then an additional two to three years in a nephrology fellowship.

When patients with diabetes have a creatinine level of 1.8 mg/dL or greater, then a nephrology consultation should be considered. Nephrologists also evaluate structural problems of the kidneys and bladder. (Patients with kidney and bladder problems may also see a urologist.)

The nephrologist also treats patients with a PROTEINURIA level that is greater than 1,000 mg or 1 g per day, or one that has changed rapidly. In addition, they treat patients with hard to control blood pressure and other unexplained abnormalities seen on urinalysis (red blood cells, casts, and other findings).

nephropathy See DIABETIC NEPHROPATHY.

nephrotic syndrome A kidney disorder that is often caused by DIABETIC NEPHROPATHY. It is marked by damage to the glomeruli of the kidneys. These are blood vessels that filter waste and extra water from the blood and transport them to the kidney in the form of urine.

Key characteristics of nephrotic syndrome are:

- high levels of protein in the urine (PROTEINURIA) that exceed 3.5 grams
- swelling of the body, especially around the feet, hands, and eyes
- high levels of cholesterol

The treatment for nephrotic syndrome depends on the cause. If the main problem is high blood pressure, then the physician will work with the patient to control HYPERTENSION. If there is a possibility of glomerulonephritis, then a kidney biopsy is usually needed and the patient may also require immunosuppressive therapy. All patients with this syndrome should be referred to a NEPHROLOGIST.

Neurontin (gabapentin) An antiseizure medication that is also used to treat people with DIABETIC NEUROPATHY because it can alleviate neuropathic pain symptoms. The exact mechanism of the medicine is unknown. If the medication is started at lower doses, it is generally well tolerated. The patient may eventually need 3,000 to 7,000 mg a day to relieve pain symptoms. Neurontin can cause some side effects, such as sleepiness, fatigue, dizziness, and irritability. It has been studied for its use in treating seizures.

Backonja, M., et al. "Gabapentin for the Symptomatic Treatment of Painful Diabetic Neuropathy in Patients with Diabetes Mellitus: A Random Controlled Trial." *JAMA* 280 (1998): 1,831–1,836.

neuropathy See DIABETIC NEUROPATHY.

nocturnal hypoglycemia Low blood glucose experienced at night, especially while an individual with diabetes is asleep. Nearly 50 percent of severe hypoglycemia occurs when patients are asleep and thus, their response to it is much slower. Testing blood glucose levels at bedtime is critically important.

People with Type 1 diabetes need to be vigilant about their food intake and blood glucose levels and to be especially watchful that they work to avoid a lapse into hypoglycemia while asleep. To avert such a problem, most people with Type 1 diabetes are advised to eat a small snack before bedtime, especially if the glucose level is less than 140 mg/dL. Milk and crackers is one commonly recommended snack.

Working with their physicians and registered dietitians, people with nocturnal hypoglycemia may adjust the timing and dosage of their insulins to avoid HYPOGLYCEMIA. If the nocturnal hypoglycemia is recurrent, the use of the continuous glucose monitor may be helpful.

non-insulin-dependent diabetes mellitus (NIDDM) The former name for what is now called Type 2 diabetes. This name was changed because it was misleading. Many people with Type 2 diabetes do not require insulin injections and may manage their diabetes with medication, diet, and exercise. However, as most people with Type 2 diabetes age, and their pancreas secretes less insulin, most will eventually require insulin therapy.

noninvasive monitor/testing A device that can measure blood glucose levels without pricking the skin and drawing blood. Because most people don't like to prick their fingers with a sharp instrument (LANCET), they may fail to test their blood glucose level as frequently as their doctor recommends (or they may fail to test their blood at all). For this reason, researchers have been working on noninvasive and nonpainful methods to attain the same information about glucose levels. For example, some devices can extract blood from the forearm or other body parts where nerve endings are less sensitive than the finger. The Glucowatch, developed by Cygnus Therapeutics, can actually test blood through the skin using special sensors. It was on the market in 2002 in the United States. Other researchers are working with infrared technologies to measure glucose levels.

nursing homes See ELDERLY; SKILLED NURSING FACILITIES.

nutrition Intake of food. People with both Type 1 and Type 2 diabetes need to pay attention to eating a healthy and balanced diet, while at the same time maintaining good GLYCEMIC CONTROL through regular blood testing and acting on the results of the test. One problem is that the average American, including people with and without diabetes, does not eat the recommended five or more servings of fruits and vegetables per day. According to the Centers for Disease Control and Prevention (CDC), poor nutrition and also lack of regular exercise is responsible for an estimated 300,000 deaths in the United States per year, second only to smoking as a cause of death.

Rates of good nutrition vary from state to state. Of those adults not eating recommended amounts of fruits and vegetables, Arizona is the worst, at 91 percent of all adults. Although still not eating sufficient levels of fruits and vegetables, Minnesota scores the best, at 68 percent of adults who fail to maintain good nutritional habits.

Portion control is a critical aspect of nutrition for patients with diabetes. Many patients initially need to weigh and measure foods in order to learn how to accurately estimate their portions.

See also CARBOHYDRATES AND MEAL PLANNING; DIETITIAN.

American Diabetes Association. "Position Statement: Nutrition Recommendations and Principles for People with Diabetes Mellitus." *Diabetes Care* 24, Supp. 1 (2001): 544–547.

Karlsen, Marie, et al. "Efficacy of Medical Nutrition Therapy: Are Your Patients Getting What They Need?" *Clinical Diabetes* 14, no. 4 (May–June 1996): 54–61.

obesity Excessive body fat for an individual's height and build. The federal government in the United States uses a term called BODY MASS INDEX (BMI) to denote both overweight and also obesity, which is a more extreme problem than "overweight." BMI is a gender-neutral term, which takes into account both weight and height. Thus, individuals who have a BMI of 25.0 to 29.9 are overweight, and individuals who have a BMI of 30.0 or more are obese. See the entry on DIABETES MELLITUS for information on screening for diabetes that includes specific heights and weights and the corresponding body mass index among individuals who are overweight or obese. Table 1 in this entry shows the BMIs that correspond to individuals who are underweight to those who are morbidly obese.

According to research reported in *Diabetes Health* in 2009, one in five adults with Type 2 diabetes is "morbidly obese," with a body mass index of 40.0 or greater. Among African Americans, the situation is even worse; one in three African Americans with Type 2 diabetes is morbidly obese. Morbidly obese individuals are at least 100 pounds overweight, and they are also at serious risk for developing the complications of

diabetes, such as DIABETIC NEPHROPATHY, DIABETIC NEUROPATHY, and many other complications.

An estimated 25 percent of all adult Americans are obese, according to the Centers for Disease Control and Prevention (CDC). However, about 80 percent of individuals with Type 2 diabetes are obese, and many (an estimated 20 percent) are morbidly obese.

Usually a chronic disease, obesity can become very dangerous because it may lead to the development of Type 2 diabetes as well as to a variety of other medical problems, such as heart disease, gallbladder disease, and even cancer. Obesity causes INSULIN RESISTANCE, or the inability of the body to efficiently and effectively use all the insulin that is produced, a problem which can progress to diabetes. Weight loss can markedly reduce the risk for developing Type 2 diabetes. Sometimes weight loss causes a remission of diabetes in those who have been recently diagnosed with the disease.

Obesity is rarely found among people with Type 1 diabetes, although the use of INSULIN to treat the disease may cause an average weight gain of 5–10 pounds. Some adolescents and even adults may manipulate their insulin use in order to lose weight; such a practice is very dangerous. (See ADOLESCENTS WITH DIABETES.) Some medications prescribed for people with Type 2 diabetes may also cause an increase in weight, especially medications in the THIAZOLIDINEDIONE (TZD) class.

Medical Issues Associated with Obesity and Diabetes

Patients with obesity have increased rates of insulin resistance, HYPERTENSION, hyperlipidemia,

TABLE 1: BMI AND OVERWEIGHT AND OBESITY

BMI	Weight Status
Less than 18.5	Underweight
18.5 to 24.9	Normal weight
25.0 to 29.9	Overweight
30.0 to 39.9	Obese
40.0 and greater	Morbidly obese

and a generalized increased level of inflammation, especially in the blood vessels. They also often have an altered immune function and an increased risk of blood clots (referred to as a *prothrombotic state*). All of these changes likely help to lead to an increased risk for the development of Type 2 diabetes, cardiovascular disease, and also the development of preeclampsia in pregnant women.

Obesity is linked to many other serious illnesses, such as CORONARY HEART DISEASE and STROKE. When an individual loses weight, often these other medical problems will also improve, such as hypertension, dyslipidemia, or diabetes.

According to the National Cancer Institute (NCI), obesity is linked to some forms of cancer, such as colorectal cancer, breast cancer, pancreatic cancer, gallbladder cancer, and ovarian cancer. The combination of obesity and physical inactivity may account for up to 30 percent of such cancers as colon cancer, breast cancer, kidney cancer, and esophageal cancer, reports the NCI.

Obesity is also associated with an increased incidence for gallstones, osteoarthritis, sleep apnea, and irregular menstrual cycles and infertility in women.

People who routinely sleep less than five hours per night have a greater risk for the development of obesity than those who sleep greater than seven hours per night, possibly because they produce more of a hormone called ghrelin (which stimulates the appetite) and less of a hormone called leptin (which helps to suppress the appetite).

Treating Obesity

Obesity is usually treated with a combination of diet and exercise, and some individuals benefit from weight loss medications. However, most people who are obese fail to maintain a weight loss with either or both diet and diet drugs. For this reason, many diabetes experts are increasingly looking at bariatric surgery as an option for the treatment of obesity and the subsequent improvement of or remission from Type 2 diabetes.

Bariatric surgery Some people who are 100 pounds or more overweight have BARIATRIC SURGERY, which is surgery that limits the amount of food that their stomachs can take in and process. Bariatric surgery is often considered for people with a BMI of over 40 (about 100 pounds overweight) or for people with a BMI that is over 35 and who also have concurrent medical problems, such as diabetes and/or hypertension. Of course, such individuals must be healthy enough to withstand major surgery and its risks.

Patients need to receive extensive physical screening before bariatric surgery, as well as a psychiatric consultation. The psychiatric consultation is needed to rule out existing psychiatric problems that could impede success with bariatric surgery, such as depression, anxiety disorders, or adult attention deficit/hyperactivity disorder (ADHD). Some evidence indicates that adults with untreated ADHD do poorly with bariatric surgery, failing to adhere to the required regimens.

The after-surgery regimen is not a simple one, and the individual must take vitamin pills and follow a strict diet that is even more rigid than that which is followed by most people with diabetes. In addition, some people who have bariatric surgery regain the weight at a later date. However, despite these caveats, research has demonstrated that bariatric surgery is effective in the majority of obese individuals with diabetes.

A study by Marney A. White and colleagues that was published in the *Primary Care Companion* in 2009 considered 361 subjects who had had gastric bypass surgeries. These subjects were surveyed both before and after the surgeries with regard to factors that were predictive of weight loss success as well as of psychological problems.

The researchers found that a preoperative loss of control with regard to eating was *not* significantly related to success with weight loss subsequent to the bariatric surgery. However, a postsurgical loss of control with eating *was* predictive for a poorer weight loss in the 12 and 24 months after surgery. The researchers noted, "Since LOC [loss of control] following bariatric surgery significantly attenuated postsurgical improvements, it may signal a need for clinical attention."

Other researchers have found that the majority of individuals who have bariatric surgery lose a significant amount of weight, and most keep the weight off. As a result, in 2009, the American Diabetes Association recommended bariatric surgery as a possible treatment for obesity in individuals who meet specific parameters.

Some physicians remain skeptical about bariatric surgery as the answer for obese individuals with diabetes. In an article in Medscape published in 2009, diabetologist John Buse told experts at the European Association for the Study of Diabetes (EASD) 45th annual meeting, "We do need to remember that surgical approaches to medical problems have been fraught with their fits and starts. Lobotomy was widely viewed as a reasonable therapy for behavioral disorders, and now it's considered an abomination."

Others interviewed for this article disagreed; for example, endocrinologist Nick Finer said, "The take-home message about bariatric surgery is, here we have a treatment that, let's be dramatic, 'cures' many people with diabetes. Why are not the diabetologists hammering at the door to get their patients access to this treatment?"

Weight loss medications Some individuals have had some success with medications for weight loss. The two prescribed medications approved by the Food and Drug Administration (FDA) are Xenical (orlistat) and Meridia (sibutramine). There is also an over-the-counter (OTC) version of orlistat, which is about half the dosage of the prescribed formulation, and which may be purchased by consumers.

In late 2009, the FDA issued an early communication about a possible elevated risk for cardiovascular disease among patients taking sibutramine. A preliminary study of about 10,000 patients with either Type 2 diabetes or stable heart disease found that 11.4 percent of the subjects who took sibutramine experienced cardiovascular events, compared to 10 percent of the subjects who took a placebo. This is a small difference between the study group and the placebo group, but it is also one of concern. The FDA advised that health care professionals should evaluate the risks and benefits of sibutramine by taking into account the health histories of individual patients.

Sibutramine is a norepinephrine and serotonin reuptake inhibitor (SNRI), and in addition to the possible aforementioned cardiovascular risks, it has other side effects; for example, it can raise blood pressure. It can also cause constipation, headache, insomnia, and other side effects.

Orlistat is a gastric, intestinal, and pancreatic lipase inhibitor, which by preventing the breakdown of fats limits their absorption by approximately 30 percent. The primary side effect of orlistat is an oily stool, and it can cause fecal urgency or even fecal incontinence (accidents).

There are also a myriad of over-the-counter drugs and supplements that purportedly enable the individual to lose a great deal of weight. These items rarely work, and if the person does lose any weight, it is usually quickly regained.

Some research reported in *Lancet* in 2009 by Arne Astrup has shown that the diabetes drug liraglutide (Victoza) plus dieting caused more weight loss than diet alone. It also improved obesity-related risk factors and lowered the rate of prediabetes over a 20-week trial. Further research should help to confirm or refute these findings.

Exercise Exercise is another important treatment for weight loss; however, people with diabetes need to test their glucose levels before and after strenuous physical activity in order to avoid a problem with HYPOGLYCEMIA. Experts say that exercise need not be difficult or even especially strenuous; for example, walking for 20 minutes a day can make a significant difference in weight as well as in the health of the individual.

Specific diets Many individuals have tried to succeed with a variety of diets, far too many to describe here. However, research has shown that the majority of people who lose considerable weight with a particular diet will gain the weight back at a later date.

A study of Pima Indians and whites without diabetes demonstrated that those who were night-time eaters had a greater risk of weight gain. Thus it is likely good advice to have those with diabetes avoid night-time eating and snacks unless they are specifically prescribed by the dietitian as part of the patient's overall caloric intake.

An Internet success story   In an interesting study of 4,209 "completers" who participated in an Internet-based weight loss club program, published in the *Scandinavian Journal of Public Health* in 2009, J. Jonasson and colleagues found that 16 percent of the completers changed their weight category from overweight or obese to normal weight. The researchers said that this was equivalent to 29 percent losing 5–9.9 percent of their initial body weight and 20 percent losing 10 percent of more of their body weight. The average weight loss was about 5 percent of the initial body weight. The researchers found that the strongest predictors of weight loss were activity as measured by the number of logins to the Internet and diary entries.

The Web site provided balanced meals and choices for weekly menus, and members were advised to measure all food consumed and enter it into a food diary. Once entered, the program provided immediate feedback.

The researchers said, "The participants in the club could access the Internet at any time to request information, or to introduce their new data on weight and height. The members were recommended to measure their weight and waist once a week. They could also participate in a chat, either with other members of the club or at given times with experts, where questions of varying types were answered by a physician, a dietician, an exercise specialist, and also occasionally by other members of the staff, e.g. doctors. Sometimes, successful members of the weight loss club would report about their experience and the methods that they had applied." According to the researchers, individuals from more than 50 countries had joined the club.

The researchers concluded that the low cost and the 24/7 availability of the Internet program made it an attractive alternate for some consumers who needed to lose weight.

Racial Risk Factors for Obesity

Some racial groups and ethnicities have a worse problem with obesity than others. For example, as can be seen from Table 2, more than a third (35.7 percent) of all non-Hispanic black adults are obese, compared to 28.7 percent of Hispanic adults and 23.7 percent of white adults. Black females have the greatest problem with obesity, and 39.2 percent of this group are obese. Blacks also have a high rate of Type 2 diabetes, which is largely linked to their obesity.

As noted by Gertraud Maskarinec and colleagues in a 2009 issue of *Ethnicity & Disease*, the prevalence of diabetes and body mass index vary considerably in terms of ethnicity. In their study, the researchers analyzed obesity by ethnicity in 187,439 subjects in California and Hawaii, drawn from five ethnic groups. They found that the age-adjusted diabetes prevalence ranged from 6.3 percent for whites/Caucasians to a high of 16.1 percent for Native Hawaiians. Rates for other groups were as follows: 10.2 percent among Japanese subjects; 15.0 percent among African Americans; and 15.8 percent among Latinos.

The researchers reported that the prevalence of diabetes was at least twice as high in non-white groups. The researchers also noted that the Japanese subjects in the United States were twice as likely to have diabetes as were Japanese who lived in Japan, indicating an environmental impact was at work.

In addition, the researchers also noted high rates of diabetes among minorities, despite the body mass index of the subjects. They concluded, "The high diabetes prevalence across minority populations with significantly different BMIs warrants further investigation into etiologic pathways, body fat distribution, and genetics. As the incidence and prevalence of type 2 diabetes continue to rise, current strate-

TABLE 2: PREVALENCE OF OBESITY AMONG ADULTS, BY BLACK/WHITE RACE OR HISPANIC ETHNICITY, CENSUS REGION AND SEX, 2006–2008, BY PERCENTAGE

Census Region	White, non-Hispanic (n = 900,629)	Black, non-Hispanic (n = 84,838)	Hispanic (n = 63,825)
Both sexes	23.7	35.7	28.7
Men	25.4	31.6	27.8
Women	21.8	39.2	29.4
Northeast			
Both sexes	22.6	31.7	26.6
Men	25.0	26.5	26.9
Women	20.0	36.1	26.0
Midwest			
Both sexes	25.4	36.3	29.6
Men	27.0	32.1	29.7
Women	23.8	40.1	29.2
South			
Both sexes	24.4	36.9	29.2
Men	26.3	32.6	28.3
Women	22.5	40.6	29.7
West			
Both sexes	21.0	33.1	29.0
Men	22.1	34.1	27.3
Women	19.8	32.0	30.4

Source: Adapted from Centers for Disease Control and Prevention. "State-Specific Prevalence of Obesity Among Adults—United States, 2007." *Morbidity and Mortality Weekly Report* 57, no. 28 (July 17, 2009): 741.

gies related to diabetes diagnosis and prevention may require modifications in order to consider the importance of sex and ethnicity related to diabetes risk."

States in the United States and obesity In looking at the rates of obesity by race and ethnicity from state to state, there is considerable variation between states. For example, 45.1 percent of blacks in Maine were obese, the highest rate among states. Among whites, the highest rate of obesity was found in West Virginia, or 30.2 percent. Last, among Hispanics, the highest rate of obesity was found in Tennessee, or 36.7 percent. See Table 3 for more information.

Note that Table 4 includes general information on states and obesity; for example, according to the CDC, in 2008, the highest percentage of obese individuals lived in Mississippi (32.8 percent), followed by Alabama (31.4 percent). States that had the lowest percentage of obese people were Colorado (18.5 percent) and Connecticut (21.0 percent).

Causes of Obesity

It would seem obvious that the primary cause of obesity is that an individual takes in more calories than are expended, thereby increasing stored food. However, it is not a simple problem for those people who are obese. Some obese

**TABLE 3: STATE BY STATE PERCENTAGE OF ADULTS CATEGORIZED AS OBESE,
BY BLACK/WHITE RACE OR HISPANIC ETHNICITY, UNITED STATES, 2006–2008, BY PERCENTAGE**

State	White, non-Hispanic	Black, non-Hispanic	Hispanic	State	White, non-Hispanic	Black, non-Hispanic	Hispanic
Alabama	27.3	40.4	29.0	Montana	21.0	unknown	22.9
Alaska	25.0	30.8	30.8	Nebraska	25.7	35.9	29.0
Arizona	21.7	35.9	31.4	Nevada	22.8	28.7	29.1
Arkansas	27.1	37.6	25.5	New Hampshire	22.9	23.0	32.3
California	19.8	34.3	29.2	New Jersey	21.9	33.0	24.1
Colorado	16.2	26.2	25.1	New Mexico	19.5	31.9	27.6
Connecticut	19.9	31.2	24.6	New York	22.8	29.7	27.1
Delaware	24.3	39.2	29.0	North Carolina	24.9	38.8	25.3
District of Columbia	9.0	32.9	22.6	North Dakota	25.1	unknown	31.9
Florida	20.9	35.1	26.0	Ohio	26.6	42.5	25.9
Georgia	23.5	36.0	26.1	Oklahoma	27.3	32.7	30.7
Hawaii	16.4	26.0	26.7	Oregon	24.6	41.6	23.0
Idaho	23.6	unknown	28.7	Pennsylvania	25.0	36.5	31.3
Illinois	23.4	33.3	30.7	Rhode Island	20.1	30.1	26.0
Indiana	26.1	35.7	26.6	South Carolina	25.1	38.8	27.0
Iowa	25.5	35.7	27.5	South Dakota	25.3	unknown	28.6
Kansas	25.7	39.8	31.7	Tennessee	27.0	38.0	36.7
Kentucky	27.4	38.5	27.0	Texas	23.5	37.8	32.3
Louisiana	24.9	35.9	24.4	Utah	22.6	34.9	21.6
Maine	23.6	45.1	27.8	Vermont	21.2	unknown	24.4
Maryland	22.4	34.0	21.0	Virginia	23.6	34.5	24.7
Massachusetts	20.0	30.0	27.1	Washington	24.0	29.7	29.9
Michigan	26.2	37.4	31.2	West Virginia	30.2	36.3	26.1
Minnesota	24.3	32.5	27.9	Wisconsin	24.5	36.4	27.3
Mississippi	27.6	40.4	26.0	Wyoming	22.5	36.9	28.6
Missouri	26.5	36.1	28.8				

Source: Adapted from Centers for Disease Control and Prevention. "State-Specific Prevalence of Obesity Among Adults—United States, 2007."
Morbidity and Mortality Weekly Report 57, no. 28 (July 17, 2009): 742.

people insist that they eat no more than others, and in some cases, this is verifiable. In other cases, some individuals may have a genetic predisposition to overeat, and research in 2009 revealed that some extremely obese children have a genetic risk for excessive eating. This was important because child protective authorities had assumed that the obesity was their par-ents' fault, who presumably had compelled or allowed the children to overeat. The genetic risk data apparently refuted this allegation.

In contrast to a genetic risk for gaining weight, many people apparently may have the "thrifty gene," wherein their body works very effectively to keep them at a stable weight. As they eat less, their bodies then adjust to use

TABLE 4: 2008 STATE OBESITY RATES: PERCENT OF OBESE INDIVIDUALS IN EACH STATE

State	%	State	%	State	%	State	%
Alabama	31.4	Illinois	26.4	Montana	23.9	Rhode Island	21.5
Alaska	26.1	Indiana	26.3	Nebraska	26.6	South Carolina	30.1
Arizona	24.8	Iowa	26.0	Nevada	25.0	South Dakota	27.5
Arkansas	28.7	Kansas	27.4	New Hampshire	24.0	Tennessee	30.6
California	23.7	Kentucky	29.8	New Jersey	22.9	Texas	28.3
Colorado	18.5	Louisiana	28.3	New Mexico	25.2	Utah	22.5
Connecticut	21.0	Maine	25.2	New York	24.4	Vermont	22.7
Delaware	27.0	Maryland	26.0	North Carolina	29.0	Virginia	25.0
Washington, DC	21.8	Massachusetts	20.9	North Dakota	27.1	Washington	25.4
Florida	24.4	Michigan	28.9	Ohio	28.7	West Virginia	31.2
Georgia	27.3	Minnesota	24.3	Oklahoma	30.3	Wisconsin	25.4
Hawaii	22.6	Mississippi	32.8	Oregon	24.2	Wyoming	24.6
Idaho	24.5	Missouri	28.5	Pennsylvania	27.7		

Source: Centers for Disease Control and Prevention. *Obesity and Overweight for Professionals: Data and Statistics: U.S. Obesity.* Available online. URL: http://www.cdc.gov/obesity/data/trends.html. Accessed December 8, 2009.

the food more efficiently and to maintain their weight. Thus, some people need to severely limit their calories in order to lose weight. However, most people will lose weight when they reduce their caloric intake.

Medical problems that may cause obesity In some rare cases, the obese individual may have an underlying medical problem such as a THYROID DISEASE or CUSHING'S SYNDROME that is contributing to their excessive weight. Hypothyroidism (low levels of thyroid hormone) is a common problem, but it rarely causes obesity. Cushing's syndrome is quite rare and is associated with truncal (in the trunk of the body) obesity.

Medications may cause or contribute to obesity Many medications are associated with causing weight gain or even obesity, including some antidiabetic agents (INSULIN, SULFONYLUREAS, and thiazolidinediones); some antihypertensive medications (alpha-1 blockers and beta blockers); some antipsychotics (clozapine, olanzapine, mirtazapine, and risperidone); and some antiseizure drugs (valproate, gabapentin, and carbamazepine). The mood stabilizing drug lithium, which is given to treat bipolar disorder, may

also cause weight gain. (Other mood-stabilizing drugs can be prescribed that do not cause such an extreme weight gain.) Steroids may also cause weight gain, such as hormonal contraceptives and especially corticosteroid medications (such as prednisone and cortisone).

When individuals take medications that are likely to (or do) increase their weight, it is a good idea for doctors to monitor these patients, particularly when they have diabetes or are at risk for developing diabetes, as with prediabetes. This is also important advice in the case of children who take medications that may increase their weight. Some experts recommend that before a child or adolescent is started on such a medication, a family history is taken of diabetes, heart disease, or obesity. The child should also be weighed on each patient encounter.

Children and Obesity

Of concern is that increasing numbers of children and adolescents in the United States are increasingly overweight and obese, which may later lead to the development of Type 2 diabetes. In some cases, children have already been diagnosed with Type 2 diabetes, although most children with diabetes have been diagnosed with Type 1 diabetes. (See CHILDREN WITH DIABETES, SCHOOL-AGE.) Very few adolescents are treated with bariatric surgery (about 300) each year, probably because of the medical risks and the costs associated with the surgery in children.

The body mass index of children is computed differently from those of adults. Children are classified by percentile of BMI for age: <5th percentile is considered underweight, 5–85 percent is normal weight, 85–95 percent is at risk for overweight, and >95 percent is overweight. Also see Appendix X for information on body mass index and the BMIs among children and adolescents.

See also CARBOHYDRATES AND MEAL PLANNING; LIFESTYLE ADAPTATIONS.

Astrup, Arne, M.D., et al. "Effects of Liraglutide in the Treatment of Obesity: A Randomised, Double-Blind, Placebo-Controlled Study." *Lancet* 374, no. 9701 (2009): 1,606–1,616.

Centers for Disease Control and Prevention. "Differences in Prevalence of Obesity among Black, White, and Hispanic Adults—United States, 2006–2008." *Morbidity and Mortality Review* 58, no. 27 (July 17, 2009): 740–744.

Centers for Disease Control and Prevention. "U.S. Obesity Trends." Available online. URL: http://www.cdc.gov/obesity/data/trends.html. Accessed October 21, 2009.

Gluck, M.E., C.A. Venti, A.D. Salbe, et al. "Nighttime Eating: Commonly Observed and Related to Weight Gain in an Inpatient Food Intake Study." *American Journal of Clinical Nutrition* 88 (2008): 900–905.

Idelevich, Evgeny, Wilhelm Kirch, and Christoph Schindler. "Current Pharmacotherapeutic Concepts for the Treatment of Obesity in Adults." *Therapeutic Advances in Cardiovascular Disease* 3 (2009): 75–90.

Jonasson, J., et al. "An Internet-Based Weight Loss Programme: A Feasibility Study with Preliminary Results from 4209 Completers." *Scandinavian Journal of Public Health* 37 (2009): 75–82.

Maskarinec, Gertraud, et al. "Diabetes Prevalence and Body Mass Index Difference by Ethnicity: The Multiethnic Cohort." *Ethnicity & Disease* 19 (2009): 49–55.

Nainggolan, Lisa. "Experts Debate Bariatric Surgery as a Cure for Diabetes." Medscape Conference Coverage, based on selected sessions at the European Association for the Study of Diabetes (EASD) 45th Annual Meeting." December 1, 2009. Available online to subscribers. URL: http://www.medscape.com/viewarticle/71382_print. Accessed December 9, 2009.

Totty, Patrick. "One in Five Type 2s Is 'Morbidly Obese'—100 or More Pounds Overweight." *Diabetes Health.* December 5, 2009. Available online. URL: http://www.diabeteshealth.com/read/2009/12/03/6468/diabetes-surgery-summit-issues-call-to-use-bariatric-surgery-as-a-type-2-treatment-/. Accessed December 9, 2009.

White, Marney A., et al. "Loss of Control Over Eating Predicts Outcomes in Bariatric Surgery Patients: A Prospective, 24-Month Follow-Up Study." *Journal of Clinical Psychiatry* 7, no. 2 (2010): 175–184.

onset of diabetes Some individuals may be diagnosed with diabetes as children (as with Type 1 diabetes, although the illness may not be diagnosed until adolescence or adulthood), while others are not diagnosed until they are adults or even elderly individuals. In general, when the individual has Type 1 diabetes, the onset is usually sudden and severe, and it is clear that the person is very ill. Often there has been considerable weight loss and other apparent symptoms.

In contrast, when adults (and some children and adolescents) are diagnosed with Type 2 diabetes, they may have no symptoms for years until they exhibit such symptoms as extreme thirst, excessive urination, and other classic symptoms of diabetes.

Unfortunately, damage may have already occurred prior to the time of diagnosis.

ophthalmologist A surgical doctor who specializes in diagnosing and treating diseases of the eye both medically and surgically, such as CATARACTS, GLAUCOMA, MACULAR EDEMA, or DIABETIC RETINOPATHY.

Many experts believe that eye exams should begin within five years for patients with Type 1 diabetes. Patients with Type 2 diabetes should be examined shortly after diagnosis. It's best to have a dilated eye examination, in which the doctor inserts special eye drops that enlarge the pupils of the eyes so that the doctor can see the entire retina. Patients often will need to wear sunglasses home after such an exam because their dilated eye will be extremely sensitive to light. They may prefer to have someone drive them home.

Children who have been diagnosed with Type 1 diabetes should receive regular eye exams within five years after diagnosis. Children with Type 2 diabetes may need screening exams sooner because they may have metabolic abnormalities that precede the diagnosis of their diabetes.

Interestingly, it is quite rare for children with Type 1 diabetes to develop any complications prior to puberty even with poor glycemic control (other than a possible delayed growth and/ or feeling ill).

See also BLINDNESS; BLURRED VISION; DIABETIC EYE DISEASES.

oral glucose tolerance test (OGTT)   A test to determine if a person has diabetes. After fasting for eight to 14 hours, plasma glucose levels are measured and levels are taken again about one or two hours later and after the individual ingests 75 g of glucose provided by the person administering the test. An alternative test is the fasting plasma glucose (FPG) test.

Extending the test to three, four, or five hours is not necessary. In fact, a large number of people with normal glucose metabolism will become hypoglycemic between the third and fifth hour. Thus, the OGTT should *never* be used to diagnose hypoglycemia.

Generally, urine measurement of the level of glucose provides no significant extra information.

TABLE 1

	Fasting Glucose	2-Hour Glucose
Normal	Less than 110 mg/dL	Less than 140 mg/dL
Impaired Fasting Glucose	110–125 mg/dL	140–199 mg/dL
Diabetes	≥126 mg/dL	>200 mg/dL

orthostatic hypotension   Refers to a decrease in blood pressure that may occur when the afflicted person changes position, for example from lying down to sitting, from sitting to standing or from lying down to standing. The result may be fainting (syncope).

Individuals with diabetes are at greater risk for orthostatic hypotension than are nondiabetics, primarily because they are more likely to have autonomic DIABETIC NEUROPATHY and are also more susceptible to DEHYDRATION. Other risk factors for experiencing orthostatic hypotension are

- medications
- atherosclerosis
- prolonged bed rest

Symptoms of orthostatic hypotension are dizziness or lightheadedness, as well as blurred vision. The person may also feel off-balance or experience vertigo.

Treatment depends on the cause of the orthostatic hypotension; for example, if the physician believes a medication is the cause, he or she may change the dosage or prescribe another medicine. If the problem is dehydration, the patient receives fluids and salts intravenously and, when discharged from the hospital or emergency room, will be encouraged to consume copious quantities of fluids.

Sometimes medications are used, such as Florinef, a synthetic steroid that helps the body retain both salt and water and also helps to constrict the blood vessels. Alpha agonists such as midodrine (Proamatine) may also be used to constrict the blood vessels. In addition, patients are counseled to move slowly from a lying down position to a sitting position, and then to a standing position.

osteoporosis   A medical condition in which not only is total bone mass decreased but there are also microarchitectural abnormalities in the bones that lead to an increased risk for fractures. People with diabetes have a slightly increased risk for developing osteoporosis compared to nondiabetics.

About 80 percent of those with osteoporosis are female. The hip fractures that osteoporosis can cause are especially dangerous and about 20 percent of these patients die within a year and 50 percent lose their independence.

Anyone can have osteoporosis although people with Type 1 diabetes have a slightly greater risk for developing this problem. Often still thought of as a disease of the elderly, the reality is that osteoporosis can occur in middle-aged or younger people. Some experts have expressed concern, however, that osteoporosis among men has been virtually ignored as an issue.

According to the National Institute of Arthritis and Musculoskeletal and Skin Diseases, 10 million people in the United States have osteoporosis. Eighteen million more experience decreased bone mass and they are at risk for osteoporosis. The disease causes 1.5 million fractures per year in the United States, including about 300,000 hip fractures, 700,000 spinal fractures, 250,000 wrist fractures, and 300,000 fractures found elsewhere in the body.

Symptoms and Diagnostic Path

The doctor may strongly suspect a patient has osteoporosis because of a fracture from a minor fall or because he or she has risk factors for the disease. The only way to know for sure if the patient has osteoporosis is to run tests and most doctors order bone mass density tests. In most cases, the dual-energy X-ray absorptiometry (DXA) is used to measure bone density, although other tests are available.

Treatment Options and Outlook

Medications are usually the treatment for osteoporosis. Many doctors prescribe estrogen for postmenopausal women, although studies indicate estrogen may serve better as a prevention from osteoporosis rather than a treatment for the disease after it is known to occur. All patients should be on adequate calcium and vitamin D, 1000–1500 mg/day and 400–800 IU respectively. Other drugs that are prescribed are:

- Fosamax (alendronate) if the osteoporosis was drug-induced by taking glucocorticoid medications
- Actonel (risedronate)
- Evista (raloxifene)
- Miacalcin (calcitonin)

Other treatments under investigation are vitamin D metabolites, sodium fluoride, and injectable parathyroid hormone, which may become available in 2002.

Causes of Osteoporosis

Aging is clearly one factor in the development of osteoporosis, although middle-aged and younger people can develop osteoporosis. The disease may also be due to a genetic predisposition. For example, according to the National Institutes of Health, one study showed that women age 65 and older who had the apolipoprotein E gene on chromosome 19 had twice the risk of those without the gene to experience fractures of the hip and wrist. The loss of naturally occurring sex steroid hormones, such as estrogen in women and testosterone in men, play a pivotal role in the development of osteoporosis.

Lifestyle factors clearly play a role and less active people are more likely to develop osteoporosis.

Secondary causes of osteoporosis   A study of 56 patients with Type 1 diabetes, 68 patients with Type 2 diabetes and 498 nondiabetic control subjects, reported in a 1999 issue of *Diabetes Care*, revealed that those with Type 1 diabetes faced a significantly greater risk for osteoporosis, unexplained by insulin treatment or other factors. Other secondary causes of osteoporosis include anorexia nervosa, ACROMEGALY, alcoholism, steroid use, malnutrition, primary hyperparathyroidism, and hypogonadism.

Risk Factors and Preventive Measures

According to the National Resource Center for Osteoporosis and Related Bone Diseases, a subsection of the National Institutes of Health, the key risk factors for developing osteoporosis are

- gender (females are at greater risk)
- thin or small-boned stature
- age (risk increases with age)
- a family history of osteoporosis
- postmenopausal status
- eating disorders such as anorexia nervosa or bulimia
- diets low in calcium
- medications such as corticosteroids and anticonvulsants
- inactive life
- smoking cigarettes
- race (greatest risks are for Caucasians or Asians)

See also ELDERLY; HORMONE REPLACEMENT THERAPY; MENOPAUSE.

Lambing, Cheryl L., M.D. "Osteoporosis Prevention, Detection, and Treatment: A Mandate for Primary Care Physicians." *Postgraduate Medicine* 107, no. 7 (June 2000): 37–41, 47–48.

McGarry, Kelly A., M.D., et al. "Postmenopausal Osteoporosis: Strategy for Preventive Bone Loss, Avoiding Fracture." *Postgraduate Medicine* 108, no. 3 (September 2000): 79–82, 85–88, 91.

Tumoninen, Jussi T., et al. "Bone Mineral Density in Patients with Type 1 and Type 2 Diabetes." *Diabetes Care* 22, no. 7 (July 1999): 1,196–1,200.

Pacific Islanders See ASIANS/PACIFIC ISLANDER AMERICANS.

pain Moderate or severe discomfort. When patients have diabetes, their pain from the disease most commonly stems from DIABETIC NEUROPATHY. This pain is usually treated with analgesics such as aspirin or acetaminophen and more serious pain may be treated with prescribed analgesic medications or even narcotics.

Sometimes physicians prescribe tricyclic antidepressants (TCAs) for the pain of neuropathy and other chronic pain. In the book *Pain: What Psychiatrists Need to Know*, physician Augusto Caraceni and colleagues describe studies in which patients who were depressed and in pain were compared to nondepressed patients who had pain. Both groups were given tricyclic antidepressants. The results revealed that TCAs were successful at decreasing pain for both groups, although it is not entirely clear how the medications worked. Imipramine is one form of TCA that has been shown to be successful at reducing the pain of diabetic neuropathy. Currently, Elavil (amitriptyline) and Pamelor (nortriptyline) are most commonly used.

In addition, drugs in the adrenergic agonist class, such as Catapres (clonidine) and tizanidine have also proven effective at decreasing pain from diabetic neuropathy and other forms of chronic pain.

An antiseizure drug, NEURONTIN, is also frequently used for pain. Tegretol (carbamazepine) is another antiseizure medication that is often tried when a person has lightning-like pain.

Sometimes it is the absence of pain rather than its presence that presents a problem to the person with diabetes; for example, if neuropathy is advanced, then when part of the body is injured, there is no pain. The person with diabetes is particularly at risk for harming the foot and should be vigilant about FOOT CARE. If an unnoticed infection continues, the person may suffer from GANGRENE and may require an AMPUTATION of a limb.

Caraceni, Augusto, M.D., et al. "Pain Management: Pharmacological and Nonpharmacological Treatments." In *Pain: What Psychiatrists Need to Know*. Washington, D.C.: American Psychiatric Press, 2000.

pancreas A vital digestive organ that is located in the mid-posterior abdomen, behind the stomach. Malfunction of the beta cells in the pancreas leads to diabetes.

The pancreas is an endocrine (it secretes hormones) gland as well an exocrine (secretes digestive enzymes) organ. It secretes insulin, glucagon, somatostatin, and a variety of other hormones. The enzymes it makes include lipase and amylase.

Individuals cannot survive without a pancreas, although it is possible to have a TRANSPLANT of a donor pancreas. In the case of people with Type 1 diabetes, their pancreas fails to produce insulin. As a result, they must self-inject insulin in order to live. However, people with Type 1 diabetes have some normal endocrine function.

It is the pancreas that contains the BETA CELLS, and those cells produce the much-needed insu-

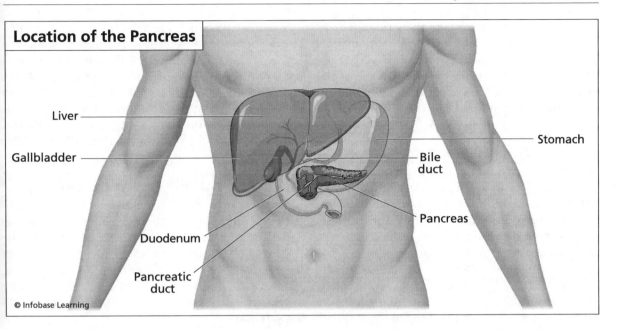

Location of the Pancreas

Liver

Gallbladder

Stomach

Bile
duct

Pancreas

Duodenum

Pancreatic
duct

© Infobase Learning

lin. The alpha cells in the pancreas control the release of GLUCAGON into the blood. The delta cells make a substance called somatostatin. There are also other pancreatic functions about which little is known, although research continues.

As can be seen from the drawing, the pancreas is in close proximity to the liver and the gallbladder. Pancreatitis is an inflammation of the pancreas that can be caused by gallstones, alcohol, or very high triglyceride levels.

pediatric endocrinologist A pediatric medical doctor who specializes in treating endocrine disorders (diabetes, thyroid diseases, growth problems, abnormal puberty, and others) that are suffered by children and adolescents. Pediatric endocrinologists usually train for three years in pediatrics and then an additional two to three years in endocrinology. They will generally treat children until the children are in their late teen years and sometimes into their early 20s, at which time most then switch to an adult endocrinologist who has had training in internal medicine.

There are very few pediatric endocrinologists nationwide and many of them have full-time academic appointments at medical schools. When treating children with diabetes, the pediatric endocrinologist usually works with a diabetes team (registered nurse, registered dietitian, social worker, etc.) to care for children with diabetes.

See also ADOLESCENTS WITH DIABETES; CHILDREN WITH DIABETES, SCHOOL-AGE; ENDOCRINOLOGIST; INFANTS AND PRESCHOOL CHILDREN WITH DIABETES.

periodontal disease Bacterial infections that cause inflammation and, if untreated, result in destruction of the soft tissues and bone that surround the teeth and gums. As a result of this damage, the teeth are not held as firmly and the disease can lead to the loss of teeth. People with diabetes are at greater risk for developing periodontal disease than nondiabetics.

According to the National Institutes of Health, about 22 percent of adults who are ages 35–44 have periodontitis, an advanced gum disease. GINGIVITIS, an inflammation and infection of the gums, is an early stage of periodontal disease that always comes before periodontitis. If treated, gingivitis usually will not get any worse. Some very controversial research indicates that the bacterium that is linked to periodontal disease may be associated with a greater risk for heart disease and STROKE.

Symptoms of Periodontitis

There are often no symptoms at all until the periodontal disease is advanced. (Periodontal disease can be detected in a dental examination, which is a key reason why people with diabetes should have dental checkups twice a year or more frequently, if the dentist recommends it.) At that point, the individual will feel pain and loosening of at least some of the teeth. The patient will need the services of a periodontist and may also need surgery as well. Regular brushing of the teeth and flossing will no longer be sufficient, as it would have been when the disease was gingivitis.

Diabetes and Periodontitis

Periodontal disease is a frequent problem among people with diabetes, many of whom fail to see a dentist even annually, although they are at greater risk for gum and tooth disease than nondiabetics. Unfortunately, research has revealed that many individuals with diabetes are apparently unaware of the importance of regular dental visits. Dentists can detect cavities and gum diseases and are also educated to detect oral cancers.

Diagnosis and Treatment

The severity of destructive periodontal disease is measured by the loss of the surrounding tissue attachment to the teeth and by the depth of gum pockets. Special treatments can minimize tissue damage if they are done in time. For example, in the early stages of periodontitis, the dentist or a technician can perform deep cleaning of the gum surfaces and can also smooth the damaged root surfaces of the teeth.

When the disease is advanced, the person will usually need gum surgery to save the teeth. The surgery will be performed by a periodontist,

a dentist who has special training in this area. An antibiotic may also be ordered to stem any further bacterial growth. Before receiving treatment for periodontitis, the person with diabetes should ask his or her medical doctor to contact the dentist and provide information on the medical status before any complicated procedures are started. Tight glycemic control will aid in the healing of tissue and infection.

Prevention of Periodontal Disease

The best prevention is an annual dental examination, or more frequent examinations, if the dentist recommends them. An annual examination often can enable the dentist to detect and treat problems before they become severe. Yet, only about 58 percent of those over age two who have diabetes have an annual dental examination.

Education clearly plays a role in those who have an annual dental examination. Only 40 percent of those with less than a high school education have their teeth checked once a year. That percentage rises to 52 percent for the high school graduate and still further to 65 percent for the person with diabetes who has at least some college education.

Only 42 percent of persons with diabetes who have disabilities get an annual exam, compared to 66 percent without disabilities. Apparently healthier people with diabetes are more likely to see their dentists; however, it is important for all to have annual checkups. Also, sicker people probably are in even greater need of a checkup.

As for age discrepancies, the probability of having an annual dental examination decreases with age. Sixty percent of people with diabetes who are 18–44 years old see their dentist annually. The percentage falls to only 50 percent for people ages 45 to 64 and continues to fall with age.

peripheral neuropathy   Refers to nerve damage that is directly caused by diabetes and that usually involves sensory nerves or sometimes motor nerves. DIABETIC NEUROPATHY is a form of peripheral neuropathy. Peripheral neuropathy can also be caused by other diseases, such as AIDS, alcoholism, or nutritional deficiencies, such as an insufficiency of vitamin B$_{12}$. People with diabetes are at greater risk of experiencing peripheral neuropathy than nondiabetics.

People experiencing peripheral neuropathy have varied complaints ranging from numbness and tingling to pain and burning, and the loss of sensation. Patients may also have abnormal sensations, such as feeling like they are walking on balls or that there is an extra sock in their shoe, even though the patient knows that nothing is there. The cause is believed to be an excess of glucose in the nerve, which results in changes in the cell that make it unable to nourish itself. In essence, the nerve cell's "battery" runs down.

The most common complaint voiced by those suffering from a peripheral neuropathy is that their bedding bothers their feet at night, and they feel compelled to get up and walk around or at least remove their feet from under the sheets. This type of neuropathy can cause a great deal of suffering. It is treated by pain medications, based on its severity. They range from aspirin and acetaminophen to antidepressant medications, antiseizure drugs, or narcotics.

Peripheral neuropathy may also cause weakness, particularly occurring in the legs and feet, although it may also occur in the hands or arms.

In its most extreme case, peripheral neuropathy may lead to ulceration, which, if due to a lack of feeling, can then lead to GANGRENE. At that point, amputation of the affected limb is the only treatment.

Another form of peripheral neuropathy involves the lateral femoral cutaneous nerves in the upper thigh. It can cause numbness, tingling, or pain in the legs. It generally disappears on its own, but can be very annoying while the person experiences the problem. Often this form of peripheral neuropathy occurs in both legs.

Early symptoms of peripheral sensory neuropathy are aches and pains in the feet and hands that tend to be worse when the patient is inactive, especially when they go to bed. Patients should avoid SMOKING, maintain tight GLYCEMIC CONTROL, and also keep their blood pressure down to as close as normal as possible.

Both the DIABETES CONTROL AND COMPLICATIONS TRIAL (DCCT) and the UNITED KINGDOM PROSPECTIVE DIABETES STUDY (UKPDS) revealed that tight glycemic control can help prevent the development and progression of peripheral sensory neuropathy.

See also PAIN.

Benbow, S. J., et al. "Diabetic Peripheral Neuropathy and Quality of Life." *QJM: Monthly Journal of the Association of Physicians* 91, no. 11 (1998): 733–737.

peripheral vascular disease (PVD) Disease of the large blood vessels found in the arms, legs, and feet. This is also known as a "macrovascular" disease. People with long-term diabetes are most prone to developing PVD. Symptoms include pain and aching in the arms, legs and feet, especially during walking (intermittent claudication) and may also lead to foot ULCERS that are slow to heal.

PVD is best prevented by preventive FOOT CARE as well as by avoiding or quitting SMOKING, keeping HYPERTENSION under control, and maintaining good GLYCEMIC CONTROL.

Physicians evaluate a patient's blood flow by palpating the pulses in the feet, groin and arms. They also inspect for the presence or absence of hair as well as the health of fingernails and the general skin condition. This inspection helps the doctor make a clinical assessment for PVD because people with PVD lose hair and their fingernails are less healthy and grow less well. A noninvasive evaluation can also be done with blood pressure cuffs and Doppler ultrasound to measure pressure and wave forms.

Patients who appear to have PVD are typically referred to a vascular surgeon, who will often request a standard angiography or magnetic resonance imaging (MRI) to delineate the extent of the disease. Some diseases can be improved with balloon angioplasty while others require bypass surgery. Medication therapy includes aspirin and clopidogrel (both antiplatelet agents), pentoxiphyllin, and cilostazol.

Patients are encouraged to walk until pain occurs, then rest and walk again. This process will encourage new arterial blood growth around the blocked area.

Pima Indians A tribe of Native Americans. In Arizona, they have been studied by researchers from the National Institutes of Health since 1965. The Pima Indians suffer from the highest known rate of diabetes in the world. About half of all U.S. Pima Indians develop Type 2 diabetes after the age of 35 years. The children of Pima parents who have DIABETIC NEPHROPATHY appear to inherit their parents' risk for the disease.

Experts believe that the high rate of Type 2 diabetes among the Pima Indians is partly a function of genetics but also stems from such environmental factors as obesity and a sedentary lifestyle. They point to the Pima Indians living in Mexico (who still apparently have an agrarian, active lifestyle, a low fat diet and overall, much lower BMIs) whose prevalence of diabetes is very low.

Pima Indians in the United States are also at much greater risk of suffering from diabetic complications such as END-STAGE RENAL DISEASE, BLINDNESS, AMPUTATIONS, and other complications related to diabetes.

With Pima Indians, an elevation in blood pressure before the onset of diabetes predicts abnormal PROTEINURIA.

See also AMERICAN INDIANS/ALASKA NATIVES; COMPLICATIONS OF DIABETES AND ASSOCIATED DISORDERS.

pneumonia See IMMUNIZATIONS.

podiatrist A specialist in diseases of the foot. Some people with diabetes, particularly those who have had long-term diabetes, experience problems with their feet stemming from DIABETIC NEUROPATHY, such as pain, lack of feeling, or tingling. They may need to see a podiatrist for regular foot examinations. Individuals with diabetes should also regularly check their feet for cuts or infections.

It should be noted that some podiatrists concentrate on routine care while others are more likely to specialize in surgery or other aspects of foot care.

Many insurance plans, including MEDICARE, will cover regular podiatric visits for patients with diabetes who have problems such as ulcer, pre-ulcerative callus, use of anticoagulant medications, or the presence of neuropathy or PERIPHERAL VASCULAR DISEASE.

See also FOOT CARE.

polycystic ovarian syndrome (PCOS) A condition that, if untreated, causes enlarged cystic ovaries. It is frequently accompanied by irregular MENSTRUATION and infertility. Women who have INSULIN RESISTANCE syndrome or Type 2 diabetes are at greater risk for this medical problem. See DIABETES MELLITUS.

Previously known as Stein-Leventhal syndrome, PCOS is more common among women who are obese. Other co-occurring syndromes are ACANTHOSIS NIGRICANS and HYPERTENSION. Many also have HYPERLIPIDEMIA. The women with this condition also have a problem with excessive body hair (hirsutism). Treatment is aimed at lowering insulin resistance with medications such as METFORMIN, rosiglitazone, or pioglitazone, although these drugs are not FDA-approved for this indication. An overweight woman who has not menstruated or who menstruated erratically and who is then placed on one of these drugs is advised to use BIRTH CONTROL unless pregnancy is her intention. The drugs may alleviate years of infertility.

Treatment will decrease the levels of male hormones and thus the hirsutism will decrease.

postprandial blood glucose levels Blood glucose levels that are tested from one to two hours after eating and that may give a better picture of the person's glycemic control than only pre-meal testing could provide. In a person with normal digestive and stomach emptying functions (and who does not have GASTROPARESIS), the peak glucose level generally occurs one hour after the start of a meal.

The advent of bioengineered and very rapidly acting human insulin, such as insulin lispro (HUMALOG) and insulin Aspart (NovoLog) has been a great help to improve GLYCEMIC CONTROL. This is primarily because the level of these insulins peaks one hour after injection and thus, coincide with the peak of the blood glucose rise. As a result, the increased insulin levels can meet the increased levels of glucose after meals.

Postprandial glycemia is better correlated with macrovascular complications (versus microvascular complications), such as heart attack (MYOCARDIAL INFARCTION) and STROKE, as well as death. In 1987, the Honolulu heart study showed that there was a significantly increased risk of fatal coronary heart disease in those patients who had the highest blood glucose levels after having an oral glucose tolerance test.

If premeal glucose levels seem well controlled and the hemoglobin HgbA1c level is elevated (i.e., it is not consistent with the glucose levels), then the physician will request that the patient measure postprandial glucose levels.

prediabetes See DIABETES MELLITUS.

pregnancy Gestation of a fetus. Pregnancy may bring many fears and joys to a woman. When her pregnancy is complicated by the presence of diabetes in the form of either Type 1 or Type 2 diabetes or GESTATIONAL DIABETES (diabetes that is diagnosed during pregnancy and which usually remits after the child is delivered), then the woman's concerns are usually magnified. The realization that the health of her baby is heavily dependent on her ability to maintain good glucose levels can be a frightening burden. The additional medical treatment, more frequent testing, and other requirements of managing diabetes may also seem very daunting to the woman, although all of these actions are extremely important, not only to the health of the developing fetus but to the mother's health as well.

HOME BLOOD GLUCOSE MONITORING is important for all people with diabetes, but it becomes even more important for the pregnant woman. Depending on the individual, the doctor may ask that the woman screen her blood as frequently as eight times per day, as well as adjust her diet and exercise plans based on the results of the blood tests. This frequent screening also has the advantage that it will help the woman to know if she may have a problem with hypoglycemia.

According to Margaret J. Evans in her article on pathology in pregnancy among women diabetics, published in the *British Journal of Diabetes and Vascular Diseases* in 2009, diabetic mothers may be divided into four key groups, including those who are dependent on insulin prior to their pregnancy, and who may benefit from prepregnancy planning; those with Type 2 diabetes prior to pregnancy who develop hyperglycemia in pregnancy that continues after the delivery; those with gestational diabetes in whom diabetes ends after the delivery; and those with prediabetes or a glucose rate that is high but not sufficiently high to diagnose diabetes. Mothers in this last group may have late stillbirths, according to Evans.

She further notes that diabetes is linked to an abnormal coiling of the umbilical cord, which can affect the maturation of the placenta. It is also linked to fetal anomalies that may be avoided by improved preconception glycemic control. Evans notes that delivery at the normal weeks (normal gestation is about 40 weeks) of gestation seems to provide protection against some of the adverse effects of macrosomia (large size of the baby).

To face the special challenges of diabetes and pregnancy, experts emphasize a team management approach to help the pregnant woman with diabetes. It is best if she consults not only with an obstetrician, but also with an endocrinologist, a registered dietitian, and any other experts that her physicians deem necessary, such as a neonatologist, a nephrologist (doctor expert in kidney diseases), and an ophthalmologist (physician expert in eye disease).

Preconception Planning Is Important Whenever Possible

Excellent GLYCEMIC CONTROL, or a blood sugar that is as close to normal as possible, is critical in the first weeks of pregnancy, and most experts prefer that women with diabetes seek medical advice even before conception occurs. Some experts report that poor glycemic control in very early pregnancy is predictive of the baby's longer stay in a neonatal intensive care unit after the birth. Inadequate glycemic control is also predictive of infant malformations and even of infant death.

When women with diabetes receive medical advice about pregnancy even before conception occurs, major advantages accrue; for example, their babies have a rate of congenital malformations that is about equal to women who do not have diabetes, or about 2 percent or less. However, when women with diabetes do not receive preconception care, the rate of small to severe birth defects among their infants can be as high as 11 percent. Also, studies have found lower death rates among the newborns of mothers with diabetes when the mothers had received preconception care. Clearly, preconception care is very important for the children of women with diabetes.

Some researchers have studied the cost effectiveness of preconception care and have found a financial savings of thousands of dollars. Healthier mothers and babies incur fewer medical expenses.

Demographic Data on Pregnant Women with Diabetes

According to the National Center for Health Statistics in their 2009 report, the rate of diabetes during pregnancy (including diabetes diagnosed both before and during the pregnancy) was a rate of 42.3 per 1,000 women, or about 4 percent, of all births (a total of 4,265,555 births) in 2006. This was an increase from a rate of 38.5 per 1,000 in 2005.

Maternal age was a major factor in the risk for diabetes, and the older that the mother was, the greater the risk for diabetes. For example, mothers under age 20 had the lowest rate of diabetes, or 13.3 per 100,000, while women ages 40–54 years had a dramatically higher rate of diabetes, or 94.3 per 100,000 women of all races and ethnicities. However, the rate of diabetes among women of this age was even higher for black women, or 99.7 per 100,000. Rates were highest for Hispanic mothers of this age, or 127.7 per 100,000 women. (See Table 1.)

The rate of diabetes also varied considerably by maternal race and ethnicity, and considering pregnant women of all ages, it was the highest among Asian or Pacific Islander pregnant women (7.1 percent), followed by American Indian/Alaska Native women who were pregnant (6.4 percent). Rates were 4.3 percent for Hispanic pregnant women, 4.0 percent for non-Hispanic whites and 3.7 percent for non-Hispanic blacks. Among subgroups of Hispanics, the lowest rate was 4.0 for Cuban women who were pregnant, and the highest was 4.9 percent for pregnant Puerto Rican women.

Women with Type 1 Diabetes

Researchers have looked at the risk for pregnancy complications among women with Type 1 diabetes, and have found that some women are more at risk for developing preeclampsia, a dangerous condition that is related to the combination of HYPERTENSION, PROTEINURIA, and edema. Women who are the most at risk are those with their first pregnancies (nulliparous), and also women with the following factors:

• preexisting DIABETIC NEPHROPATHY (kidney disease), including a proteinuria rate of 190–499 mg/d before 20 weeks of pregnancy and/or microalbuminuria before pregnancy

TABLE 1: NUMBER AND RATE OF LIVE BIRTHS TO MOTHERS WITH DIABETES DURING PREGNANCY, BY AGE, RACE, AND HISPANIC ORIGIN OF MOTHER, UNITED STATES, 2006

	Number of all births	Number of women with reported diabetes	Rate of diabetes: All ages	Rate: Under 20 years	Rate: 20–24 years	Rate: 25–29 years	Rate: 30–34 years	Rate: 35–39 years	Rate: 40–54 years
All races	4,265,555	179,898	42.3	13.3	24.2	40.0	56.2	74.5	94.3
Non-Hispanic white	2,308,640	92,263	40.1	14.9	25.1	36.8	48.5	63.5	76.8
Non-Hispanic black	617,247	22,839	37.1	11.3	22.0	39.9	61.5	81.0	99.7
Hispanic	1,039,077	44,814	43.0	12.4	22.7	42 .1	65.8	95.1	127.7

Adapted from: Martin, Joyce A., et al. "Births: Final Data for 2006." *National Vital Statistics Reports* 57, no. 7 (January 7, 2009): 63–64.

- elevated HbgA1c level in early pregnancy
- chronic hypertension
- longer duration of maternal diabetes (the longer that the woman has had diabetes, then the greater is the risk)

It is also clear that aggressive control of maternal hypertension and blood sugars before and during the pregnancy is extremely important, although medications must be carefully regulated and often require altering from medications that were used prior to the occurrence of the pregnancy.

Women with Type 2 Diabetes

Although many people consider Type 1 diabetes to be a far more serious condition than Type 2 diabetes, both conditions can be very dangerous to a developing fetus. Some studies indicate a high risk of death among the babies of women with Type 2 diabetes, particularly if the women are obese.

It is important to note that the risks are as high with Type 2 diabetes as they are with Type 1 diabetes, although often glycemic control is not as rigorous among pregnant women with Type 2 diabetes. In an analysis of 33 studies of pregnant women with Type 1 and Type 2 diabetes and their outcomes, researcher Montserrat Balsells and colleagues reported in the *Journal of Clinical Endocrinology and Metabolism* in 2009 that women with Type 2 diabetes had about

the same level of perinatal outcomes (outcomes of their newborn babies) as did women with Type 1 diabetes. Thus, whether the woman has Type 1 or Type 2 diabetes prior to pregnancy, she requires specialized care and needs to carefully comply with the recommendations of physicians.

Poor outcomes with Type 2 diabetes Helen R. Murphy, Rosemary C. Temple, and Jonathan M. Roland in their 2007 article in the *British Journal of Diabetes and Vascular Disease* on pregnancy in women with diabetes, state key reasons why the outcomes of pregnant women with Type 2 diabetes may be poor, particularly in the case of women with poor glycemic control.

The authors say, "Many women with Type 2 diabetes receive routine diabetes care in the community and, unlike women with Type 1 diabetes, may not be aware of the importance of optimal glycaemic control at the time of conception and the 6–7 critical weeks thereafter. The health care provider may also be less aware of the importance of good risk of poor glycaemic control in early pregnancy."

In his 2008 article for *Obstetric Medicine*, E. Keely, M.D., noted that hypertension associated with pregnancy, including preeclampsia, is more common among women with Type 2 diabetes than nondiabetics, and this problem may be linked to obesity, chronic hypertension, and insulin resistance. Keely says, "The profound insulin resistance associated with pregnancy makes it unlikely that women will maintain glycaemic control with diet/exercise or oral hypoglycaemic agents throughout pregnancy. For women who are still on oral agents when they achieve pregnancy, it is important to continue them in the first trimester until insulin can be initiated, otherwise severe hyperglycaemia may occur during organogenesis [the development of fetal organs]."

Keely added, "There is an urgent need to reinforce the seriousness of T2DM [Type 2 diabetes mellitus] in women of childbearing age and to their care-providers. Close collaboration between primary care-providers, obstetricians, obstetric internists, endocrinologists, paediatricians and the patient, will be critical to the success of any interventions. Serious adverse outcomes can be reduced through preconception glycemic control, folate ingestion and optimization of management for chronic complications. Care during pregnancy should be as rigorous as that provided for women with T1DM [Type 1 diabetes mellitus], including multidisciplinary specialized clinics and close surveillance."

Risks to the Child

The children born to women with diabetes have a higher rate of birth defects when maternal blood glucose levels are not optimal. The types of birth defects may vary from cleft palate or cleft lip to heart, lung, or intestinal problems as well as developmental or motor delays. These malformations are found more frequently among the babies of women who have not had good prenatal care and who did not work to attain close to normal glucose levels, although risks can present even among women with good glycemic control.

Fetal deaths and abnormalities Even with good glycemic control of the pregnant woman, the risk for fetal deaths caused by abnormalities is elevated (although it is much worse when glycemic control is poor). Said Oded Langer in the book *The Diabetes in Pregnancy Dilemma*, "Although it was demonstrated that the rate of anomalies [in the fetus] can be decreased in patients who achieved targeted levels of glycemic control, the

majority of studies report an incidence of 8–9 percent. This is [a] three-to-five-fold increase in comparison to non-diabetic pregnancies (2–3 percent). Certain system anomalies occur in a disproportionately higher frequency. Cardiac anomalies and, in particular, ventricular septal defects [heart defects] and complex lesions such as transposition of the great vessels occur about five times more frequently, and central nervous system malformation, in particular, neural tube defect and holoproscencephaly occur about 10 times more frequently. The sacral agenesis/caudal dysplasia complex is reported to occur up to 400 times more commonly among fetuses of mothers with diabetes."

Langer also described the case of a 42-year-old pregnant woman with Type 2 diabetes who came to the obstetrics office for the first time when she was seven weeks pregnant. Although her glycemic levels were kept in good control throughout her pregnancy, the baby ultimately died, and an autopsy report showed that the fetus had oversized organs, with a fetal heart that was 168 percent of normal size, a liver that was 178 percent of normal size and a brain that was 110 percent of the normal size. This case illustrates the major importance of preconception planning, particularly among older pregnant women, who have a high risk of both maternal and fetal issues complicated by diabetes.

Obesity in the mother OBESITY is also associated with risks to the fetus and the newborn child, according to Anjum Doshani and Justin C. Konje in their article in 2009 for the *British Journal of Diabetes and Vascular Disease*. They note that obese women spend nearly five days more in the hospital and have increased risk of complications during pregnancy and needed interventions in labor. In addition, babies who are born to obese mothers have a 3.5 times greater risk of requiring admission to a neonatal intensive care unit. The authors also said, "Pregnant women with pre-gestational type 1 and type 2 diabetes are more likely to have Caesarean deliveries, macrosomic infants, congenital malformations and preterm deliveries. GDM [gestational diabetes mellitus] has also been associated with adverse pregnancy outcomes, including pre-term birth, macrosomia and associated shoulder dystocia, and Caesarean deliveries."

According to the International Diabetes Federation in their 2009 guidelines, "Weight loss diets are in general not recommended during the course of a pregnancy. However, at least for women with GDM who are considerably overweight, reducing energy intake by no more than 30% of habitual intake is not associated with ketosis [diabetic ketoacidosis] and does not cause harm."

Treatment: Medications

All women with Type 1 diabetes as well as many women with Type 2 diabetes will require insulin during their pregnancy. According to the International Diabetes Federation, "Insulin has been used in pregnancy since 1922. It is essential for women with type 1 diabetes and is still widely considered the drug of choice for women with either type 2 diabetes or GDM who are not meeting treatment goals with lifestyle modification and/or oral glucose-lowering agents." (After the pregnancy, many women with Type 2 diabetes may return to taking their oral medications.) Women who need insulin during their pregnancies will also usually require insulin intravenously during labor and delivery, to protect both the mother and her baby. Some women with diabetes may require other medications as well, and doctors will work to balance any possible dangers that medication may present to both mother and child during the pregnancy.

It should be noted that in their 2009 guidelines on pregnancy, the International Diabetes Federation recommended that women taking calcium channel blockers should use these drugs only with caution, if at all, because they can cause fetal hypoxia (insufficient oxygen to the fetus). In addition, congenital malformations in the fetus have been reported with the use of statin medications. The International Diabetes Federation recommends that statin medications [used for the treatment of elevated cholesterol levels (LDL)] should be stopped during prepregnancy planning or as soon as a pregnancy is identified. Blood pressure control can be maintained with other medications, such as labetalol. ACE and ARB drugs should not be used in the treatment of blood pressure in pregnant women as they are associated with urogenital tract abnormalities.

Treatment: Tests

Many doctors rely on ultrasound imaging tests to determine the size and the health of the fetus. The fetal Biophysical Profile (BPP) is one form of ultrasound test that has been used successfully with pregnant women who have diabetes. It can ascertain the volume of the amniotic fluid, and it can also identify malformations that may be present. This test looks at various aspects of the fetus, such as fetal breathing, gross body motions, fetal tone, and amniotic fluid and awards points for normal, below-normal, and so forth.

A normal and healthy fetus scores eight out of 10 possible points on the BPP. A fetus that may be in trouble scores six points or lower. One study of 98 women with Type 1 diabetes revealed that the BPP was predictive of normal Apgar scores (scores that are given to newborns at birth) in 99 percent of the cases. This means that if the BPP said that the baby was normal, in almost every case the infant *is* normal upon delivery. The reverse is also true; if the BPP indicates the baby is abnormal, then the baby usually does have abnormalities.

Another testing option is Doppler velocimetry, which measures uterine waveform data and can also help determine if there is a problem with the pregnancy.

Some physicians rely upon the nonstress (monitoring the baby's heart rate while he/she is resting versus active) test to determine the fetal heart rate and identify possible problems. The test may be given at 32 weeks, or it may be administered earlier if the woman also has hypertension or other medical problems in addition to diabetes. If the woman is using insulin, the test may be performed twice a week after the 32-week point.

Medical Risks to the Mother and Child

The pregnant woman with diabetes incurs risks to her own body as well as to her fetus or newborn child. For example, the risks for developing DIABETIC RETINOPATHY are increased with pregnancy, as is the risk for already existing retinopathy to worsen with pregnancy. Tight glycemic control can prevent such a worsening.

Pregnancy can also exacerbate any preexisting medical problems of the pregnant woman with diabetes. For example, if the pregnant woman has kidney disease stemming from her diabetes, then her pregnancy outcome is affected as well. The experts report that nearly all of the infants of the mother with diabetic nephropathy will survive but they may have problems with developmental delays (such as mental retardation) or with motor delays.

Overly strict glycemic control   Although a consensus of physicians agrees that tight glycemic control during pregnancy is critically important, there are some physicians who worry that the overall definition of good glycemic control is too vague. They are also concerned that pregnant women who rigidly adhere to glucose control guidelines run a greater risk of developing hypoglycemia. In addition, these physicians say that not enough attention is paid to the fact that women with diabetes may have babies who are small for their gestational age (SGA), and such babies are at risk for developing diabetes as adults.

Cesarean deliveries   Some studies have shown that women with diabetes have about a four times greater risk of having a cesarean section (C-section) compared to nondiabetic women. The reason for this may be that the fetus is overly large, and it is determined by her physician that it is safer to perform a C-section. Some doctors are also more likely to perform cesarean sections on women with diabetes because of

health concerns and risks, even when the infant is normal-sized.

Induction of labor   Even if a vaginal delivery is planned, sometimes doctors will induce labor, particularly if they are concerned that the child is large or will become too large by the time of delivery. Prior to induction, an amniocentesis test on the fetus is usually performed to determine the maturity of the lungs.

After Delivery of the Baby

Once the child is safely delivered, it is checked for any signs of diabetes, respiratory difficulty, jaundice, and other possible medical problems. If the child was large, it is also checked for SHOULDER DYSTOCIA and other problems that might occur with a difficult childbirth. The child is also checked for symptoms of hypoglycemia. If the baby weighs over nine pounds, then the calcium and magnesium levels are checked to learn if the infant needs to receive supplemental calcium or magnesium.

The mother is also checked thoroughly and often given insulin intravenously. Her glucose levels are taken and she is evaluated for hypoglycemia and any other medical problems that may have developed during the delivery.

In summary, the two most important things to keep in mind about pregnant women who have diabetes are that (1) preconception planning and consulting with physicians prior to the pregnancy have enormous benefits to both the mother and the child, and (2) careful glycemic control, by working with medical experts and self-monitoring, greatly increase the probability of having a healthy and normal child.

See also CHILDREN OF DIABETIC MOTHERS; DIABETES MELLITUS; FERTILITY; HYPOGLYCEMIA; INSULIN; INSULIN PUMP.

Balsells, Montserrat, et al. "Maternal and Fetal Outcomes in Women with Type 2 versus Type 1 Diabetes Mellitus: A Systematic Review and Meta-analysis." *Journal of Clinical Endocrinology and Metabolism* 94, no. 1 (2009): 4,284–4,291.

Doshani, Anjum, and Justin C. Konje. "Diabetes in Pregnancy: Insulin Resistance, Obesity and Placental Dysfunction." *British Journal of Diabetes and Vascular Disease* 9 (2009): 208–212.

Evans, Margaret J. "Diabetes and Pregnancy: A Review of Pathology." *British Journal of Diabetes and Vascular Disease* 9 (2009): 201–206.

International Diabetes Federation. Global Guideline: Pregnancy and Diabetes. Available online. URL: http://www.idf.org/global-guideline-pregnancy-and-diabetes. Accessed October 27, 2009.

Keely, E., M.D. "Type 2 Diabetes in Pregnancy: Importance of Optimized Care before, during and after Pregnancy." *Obstetric Medicine* 1 (2008): 72–77.

Langer, Oded. "Fetal Testing in Pregnancies Complicated by Diabetes Mellitus: Why, How, and For Whom?" In *The Diabetes in Pregnancy Dilemma: Leading Change with Proven Solutions*, edited by Oded Langer, 304–326. Lanham, Md.: University Press of America. 2006.

Martin, Joyce A., et al. "Births: Final Data for 2006." *National Vital Statistics Reports* 57, no. 7 (January 7, 2009).

Murphy, Helen R., Rosemary C. Temple, and Jonathan M. Roland. "Improving Outcomes of Pregnancy for Women with Type 1 and Type 2 Diabetes." *British Journal of Diabetes and Vascular Disease* 7 (2007): 38–42.

prevention of diabetes   See DIABETES MELLITUS.

prosthesis   A device, such as an artificial leg or arm, that is used to replace a limb that has been amputated. The term may also refer to an implant of a hip, knee, or other body part. A prosthesis may also be a device used to supplement body functioning, such as a hearing aid. People with diabetes have a high rate of AMPUTATIONS, primarily due to foot ULCERs that have progressed to GANGRENE.

After an amputation it is often critical that patients with diabetes work with a rehabilitation team to properly fit the prosthesis and to learn how to use it properly. This usually involves using the assistance of physical therapists and physical medicine medical doctors known as physiatrists, as well as prosthetists, specialists in prosthetic devices.

proteinuria   Protein in the urine, which is usually a sign of kidney disease. (Exercise and fever can sometimes temporarily increase the protein levels in the urine.) When detected early enough, the underlying abnormality may be treated; however, when there are large amounts of proteinuria, this indicates that the person has a kidney or cardiovascular disease and may be in danger of kidney failure, stroke, or heart attack. The individual may also have diabetes, HYPERTENSION, or other illnesses (or the patient may have two or more illnesses, such as having both hypertension and diabetes or another combination of ailments).

Proteins are processed by the body and they are usually too large to pass through the kidney into the urine. As a result, they normally cannot be found in urinalysis. However, in the case of early damage to the kidneys, the two major types of proteins that may be found in the urine are albumin and globulins. Of these, albumin is smaller and more likely to be seen than are globulins.

When a person has either Type 1 or Type 2 diabetes, even a small amount of albumin in the urine (microalbuminuria) is an indication of early kidney malfunction.

Testing for Proteinuria

There are no specific symptoms that are experienced by those with proteinuria, and, consequently, the only way to tell if the problem exists is to test the urine. One such test is done with a urinary dipstick that tests for albumin. If the urine dipstick is negative, then the patient should have a yearly spot urine test for microalbumin by radioimmunoassay. This is a very sensitive test to detect tiny amounts of protein (30–300 mg protein/every 1,000 mg creatinine).

Another test for proteinuria is a 24-hour urine collection, in which urinary protein excretion is measured over a 24-hour period. Kidney function and protein loss can be quantified by a 24-hour collection. In general, the 24-hour test is used on adults and adolescents rather than on children, because it is usually more difficult to collect the child's urine for such a long time-frame and spot tests provide reasonable data.

If protein is found in the urine, then blood tests are usually ordered. The doctor will generally order a test for creatinine and urea nitrogen levels. The reason for this testing is that creatinine and urea nitrogen are normally removed from the blood by the kidneys. However, if there are high levels of creatinine and urea nitrogen in the blood, this is an indication that the kidneys are not functioning normally.

Physicians recommend that testing for proteinuria be done annually on people who have already been diagnosed with hypertension or with Type 1 or Type 2 diabetes. Others who fall into certain risk groups should receive periodic testing as well, according to the determination of the individual's physician.

Some groups of people are more likely than others to have proteinuria, including:

- people with diabetes (both Type 1 and Type 2)
- people with hypertension
- African Americans
- American Indians
- Hispanic Americans
- Pacific Islander Americans
- elderly individuals
- obese individuals
- those with a family history of kidney disease

Treatment of Proteinuria

After diagnosing proteinuria, the medical goal usually is to determine and treat the underlying cause. For example, if the primary problem is hypertension, the goal is to reduce the blood pressure. Some people do not have hypertension but they do have proteinuria. The doctor should work to determine the cause and treat the proteinuria. The person with diabetes should work to normalize blood pressure, improve glucose control, and adjust his or her diet.

The more copious the protein in the urine, the more important it is to bring blood pressure levels under control. For example, if the proteinuria exceeds 1 g per 24 hours, the National Heart, Lung, and Blood Institute recommends that the blood pressure be maintained below 125/75 mm Hg. **Note:** 125/75 is considered a normal and not hypertensive level, however, when the person has proteinuria that is caused by diabetes, then attaining an even lower blood pressure will work to improve the prognosis for the individual.

If diabetes is the main cause of the proteinuria rather than hypertension, then the goal will be to attain glycemic control. Doctors may also recommend dietary changes such as cutting back on salt and protein and may have other recommendations.

If the individual has both diabetes and hypertension, the doctor may prescribe a medication from the angiotensin-converting enzyme (ACE) inhibitor class of drugs, which are more protective of the kidneys than are other medications for blood pressure control.

ACE drugs should be used as soon as tests reveal that a person has microalbuminuria, a condition that precedes proteinuria. Normal levels of albumin in the urine are less than 30 mg/g creatinine. When the levels are 30–300 mg albumin/g creatinine, that is defined as microalbuminuria. An even greater problem is proteinuria, in which levels greater than 300 mg albumin/g creatinine. When the person receives medication when the problem is still at the microalbuminuria level, the protein levels may still be pushed back into the normal range. But if treatment does not occur until proteinuria is present, then medication can only diminish the rate of decline—rather than stopping the decline altogether, as can be done at earlier stages of the problem.

Some people cannot tolerate ACE drugs, and in that case, ANGIOTENSIN RECEPTOR BLOCKER (ARB) medications may be used as a good second choice. It should also be noted that either of these medications may also be used in a person who does not have hypertension, but who does have microalbuminuria or overt proteinuria.

For further information, contact the following organizations:

American Kidney Fund
6110 Executive Boulevard
Suite 1010
Rockville, MD 20852
(800) 638-8299 (toll-free) or (301) 881-3052
www.akfinc.org

National Kidney Foundation
30 East 33rd Street
New York, NY 10016
(800) 622-9010 (toll-free) or (212) 889-2210
www.kidney.org

Hogg, Ronald J., M.D., et al. "Evaluation and Management of Proteinuria and Nephrotic Syndrome in Children: Recommendations from a Pediatric Nephrology Panel Established at the National Kidney Foundation Conference on Proteinuria, Albuminuria, Risk, Assessment, Detection, and Elimination (PARADE)." *Pediatrics* 105, no. 6 (June 2000): 1,242–1,249.
National Kidney and Urologic Diseases Information Clearinghouse. "Proteinuria." NIH Pub. No. 01-4732, May 2000.

pumps   See INSULIN PUMP.

race/ethnicity See AFRICAN AMERICANS WITH DIABETES; AMERICAN INDIANS/ALASKA NATIVES; ASIANS/PACIFIC ISLANDERS; HISPANICS/LATINOS; PIMA INDIANS.

reagent strips Chemically treated strips that change color when exposed to blood, urine, or other substances. People with diabetes use these reagent strips to test their blood glucose levels. The glucose levels in the patient's urine are rarely tested by the patient at home or the doctor in the clinic, because blood testing provides much more accurate information. The most common urine test for a patient with diabetes to check at home is for urinary KETONES. (See also SICK DAY RULES.)

Physicians use reagent strips in the office to test patients' urine for protein, blood, and signs of infection. More sophisticated reagent strips allow physicians and patients to test their own fructosamine levels at home as well as to test for ketones in their blood.

The reagent strips come with a color code to compare the used strip. The color code allows the person to determine their own levels and whether they are within the normal range or not.

One caution: reagent strips may be sensitive to extreme weather conditions. As a result, they should be stored in the airtight container that they come in unless they are individually foil wrapped. The expiration date on the bottle should be noted as well.

A diagnosis of diabetes should not be made *solely* on the results of a reagent strip analysis.

Instead, the individual should also have a fasting blood glucose level or an ORAL GLUCOSE TOLERANCE TEST (OGTT).

See also HOME BLOOD GLUCOSE MONITORING.

religion/spirituality Spiritual belief in a higher power, which may include practices in the rituals that are associated with an organized religious group, such as prayer, singing, or other religious practices. For the majority of Americans, religion plays an important part in their lives, and 62 percent attend religious services at least monthly. For many people in other countries, religion also plays a key role. Religion may enable people to cope more effectively with their illnesses, including diabetes.

Several studies have indicated that individuals who are regular attendees at their place of worship actually live longer. In one such study, 2,025 Marin County, California residents over age 55 were followed for five years. Researchers found that the best predictor for those who were still alive at the end of the study was weekly attendance at religious services.

The researchers attempted to determine the cause for the enhanced longevity of the religious attendees. They factored out chronic diseases such as diabetes, as well as sex, race, and other variables, but they still could not discover the reason for the increased life expectancy of the religious attendees. The authors said, "Even after controlling for six classes of potential confounding and intervening variables, we were unable to explain the protection against mortality offered by religious attendance."

Some experts believe that places of worship may also be an effective place to provide individuals with information on diabetes and even to offer screening to them. In an article published in the *American Journal of Health Studies* in 1998, researcher Michael Kelly reported on a study of individuals screened for diabetes at four Catholic churches on the West Texas/Mexico border. Many of the attendees were Hispanics, a group at high risk for diabetes. Many American Diabetes Association affiliates have formed relationships with African-American churches for the same purpose.

Kelly concluded, "Some churches are becoming more receptive to secondary health intervention, such as diabetes and heart disease screening. . . . Still more progressive churches are exploring the realm of primary health intervention, better known as health education and promotion."

When Faith and Medicine Clash

Sometimes a person's religious beliefs may interfere with what a physician believes to be medically best or even necessary. Confronted with such a conflict, the physician may discuss the situation in the context of the patient's spirituality or enlist the aid of a clergyperson. However, sometimes those options are not available or possible or they do not work.

In some cases, the courts or law enforcement may be drawn in. For example, in 1996, a 16-year-old girl with diabetes died at her home in Altoona, Pennsylvania, because her parents had refused to provide her with medical treatment and relied instead upon prayer. The girl, whose blood sugar level was 18 times the norm, died and her parents were charged with manslaughter. The Pennsylvania Supreme Court upheld their conviction in 2000.

See also ABUSE/NEGLECT.

Associated Press. "Faith-Healing Parents Convicted of Manslaughter." *St. Louis Post-Dispatch*, November 29, 2000.

Kelly, Michael P. "Diabetes Screening and Health Education at Roman Catholic Churches Along the West Texas Mexico Border." *American Journal of Health Studies* 14, no. 1 (January 1998): 48.

Larson, David B., M.D., et al. "Patient Spirituality in Clinical Care: Clinical Assessment and Research Findings: Part One." *Primary Care Reports Archives* (October 2, 2000).

Oman, Douglas, and Dwayne Reed. "Religion and Mortality among the Community-Dwelling Elderly." *American Journal of Public Health* 88, no. 10 (1998): 1,469–1,475.

repaglinide See MEGLITINIDES.

research See CLINICAL STUDIES/RESEARCH.

retinopathy See DIABETIC EYE DISEASES; DIABETIC RETINOPATHY.

S

Scandinavian Simvastatin Survival Study (4-S Study) A study of 4,444 patients ages 35–70 years who had prior CORONARY HEART DISEASE and high CHOLESTEROL levels. The subjects included people with and without diabetes. They were given either drug therapy with Zocor (Simvastatin) to lower their cholesterol levels or they were given a placebo. This study is significant for people with diabetes because of the high rate of heart disease that occurs among people with diabetes. Also, the data on the patients with diabetes were reported on as a subgroup and then compared to the total group.

The subjects were followed for about five years. The medication was extremely effective and reduced the risk of death from coronary heart disease among patients with previous MYOCARDIAL INFARCTION. The drug also reduced the risk of major coronary events (fatal and near fatal myocardial infarctions).

The patients with diabetes showed even more dramatic improvements than nondiabetic coronary heart patients. The patients with diabetes reduced their cholesterol levels and also showed a 54 percent risk reduction in major coronary events. In contrast, patients without diabetes had only a 32 percent risk reduction. This study proved the importance of cholesterol levels to the person with diabetes as well as the effectiveness of medication to counteract high levels of cholesterol.

See also HDL; LDL.

Pedersen, T. R., et al. "Baseline Serum Cholesterol and Treatment Effect in the Scandinavian Simvastatin Survival Study." *The Lancet* 345, no. 8960 (May 20, 1995): 1,274–1,275.

Pedersen, T. R., et al. "Safety and Tolerability of Cholesterol Lowering with Simvastatin During 5 Years in the Scandinavian Simvastatin Survival Study." *Archives of Internal Medicine* 156 (October 14, 1996): 2,085–2,092.

school See CHILDREN WITH DIABETES, SCHOOL-AGE.

screening for diabetes See DIABETES MELLITUS.

self-care/self-monitoring Personal management of a medical problem, such as diabetes. Although physicians, diabetes nurse educators, and other experts can provide a great deal of advice and information, the reality is that people with diabetes must take charge of their own self-care. This includes periodic blood testing, monitoring the diet, often taking prescribed medication and visiting their physician on a regular basis. Both patient and doctor need to perform monitoring for any signs or symptoms that the diabetes has gone beyond the normal range. However, patients must do most monitoring themselves.

Such monitoring is extremely important and often can mean the difference between relative stability as well as the avoidance of serious complications.

The failure to adequately monitor glucose levels can ultimately lead to a variety of very severe conditions such as blindness, amputation of limbs, kidney and heart disease, and even death. It may also lead to DIABETIC KETOACIDOSIS (DKA), a very dangerous condition requiring hospitalization.

Because of the importance of self-care among people with diabetes, experts say that physicians must take on much more of a partnership role, and one that is very different from what they may be used to maintaining with their other patients. According to a manual called "Basic Practice Guidelines for Diabetes Mellitus," jointly prepared by the South Dakota Diabetes Control Program and the South Dakota Diabetes Advisory Council in 1999,

> This represents a major paradigm shift in which new roles are required from both the patient and provider. Patients need to understand and accept that diabetes care is their personal responsibility. In addition, professionals need to assume their 'new' role as consultant and view the patient as the decision maker.

The physician must also help patients develop strategies to work out changes themselves, rather than depending on flat directives issued by their doctors. The South Dakota experts said,

> The tendency to solve problems for the patients rather than helping them work through a problem is another barrier. If the person is in need of technical expertise, for instance, making the glucose meter work, such behavior is warranted. On the contrary, most challenges facing people are more psychosocially based than technical, for example, 'it is very hard for me to cut back on fat in my diet, when my family insists on eating fried foods all of the time.' In this situation, the solution needs to be addressed by the patient, with selected input from the provider. It is the process of helping the patient discover the capacity to creatively think and find solutions to their work problems. This empowerment creates and reinforces their self-efficacy and responsibility for the treatment of their diabetes.
>
> In order for the professionals to use the empowerment approach with success, patients need to believe that they are viewed as the 'driver' in the diabetes care process.

South Dakota Diabetes Control Program and South Dakota Diabetes Advisory Council. "Basic Practice Guidelines for Diabetes Mellitus." February 1999.

sexuality and sexual problems The impact of diabetes on sexual desire or sexual problems experienced by men and women. Adults with diabetes may experience a variety of sexual problems that stem from their illness, although according to the American Diabetes Association, the topic of sexual problems is often avoided by both patients with diabetes and their physicians. The subject may embarrass them or the patient may believe that there is nothing that can be done. However, in many cases, doctors do (or should) know about ways to assist patients struggling with sexual problems related to their diabetes.

The most prominent sexual problem that men with diabetes may suffer from is ERECTILE DYSFUNCTION. Both men and women with diabetes may also experience a lack of sexual desire.

WOMEN WITH DIABETES may have problems with vaginal lubrication or pain that occurs during sex (dyspareunia) because of dryness or another reason. The doctor may recommend a vaginal lubricant and may also advise the woman to try Kegel exercises, which are muscle-tightening exercises in the pelvic area.

Women with diabetes may also suffer from neurogenic bladder, or bladder spasms and leakage of urine. Doctors may advise women with such problems to urinate before and then again after having sex. This practice will also help the woman to prevent vaginal and bladder infections, which is important, since many women with diabetes are prone to such infections.

shoulder dystocia A birthing crisis in which the baby's shoulder and arm are trapped on the pelvic bone of the mother. This can harm the baby's neck and cause paralysis in one or both arms. This injury is referred to as a "brachial plexus injury." The baby may also suffer from ERB'S PALSY.

Mothers with diabetes or GESTATIONAL DIABETES are at risk for having a baby with shoulder dystocia. Other risk factors are:

- having a large baby (nine pounds or more)
- obesity of the mother
- excessive weight gain of the mother during pregnancy (over 35 pounds)
- a baby that is overdue: more than 40 weeks in gestation

To decrease the risk of the baby experiencing shoulder dystocia, pregnant women should work with their obstetricians and their diabetes specialists, such as endocrinologists, registered dietitians, and nurses. The physician may also suggest an implantable pump for better glycemic control.

See also PREGNANCY.

sick day rules Encompasses the general management concepts to use during illness which physicians/nurses/dietitians teach patients who have diabetes. These concepts will help them when they are sick with other illnesses in addition to diabetes, such as a severe cold, the flu, or another ailment that makes it difficult to eat or drink or to take normal care of themselves.

Some people think that when people with diabetes are ill, they need not worry about their diet or fluid intake. This is not true because sickness can cause blood sugar to rise due to a lack of food or fluid intake. It is also very important for the sick person to continue to take diabetes medication as well as to test blood sugars and write down the results, so that the information can be reported to the doctor. Ill people with diabetes are at risk for the extremes of either HYPOGLYCEMIA or DIABETIC KETOACIDOSIS (DKA)/HYPEROSMOLAR COMA, both of which can be life-threatening conditions.

It is almost inevitable that at some point, the person with diabetes will develop an illness. As a result, it is important to develop a plan for what to do *before* the person becomes sick. A written checklist may be helpful, because many people do not think as clearly as normal when they are feeling ill. If they can instead refer to a simple checklist, it is more likely that they will be able to follow it. If the patient wishes to develop such

a list, it should be reviewed with their physician. (A very simplified list of basic "to do" items are included in this essay.)

Principles Underlying Sick Day Rules

Patients with diabetes need a basic understanding of the fact that when people are sick, they are also under stress from their own bodies, in response to the bacteria, virus or other medical problem they are experiencing.

An illness is a form of physiological stress (mental or physical, or both) that will induce the release of stress hormones. Some examples of these stress hormones are adrenaline (epinephrine), noradrenaline (norepinephrine), cortisol, growth hormones, and GLUCAGON. Stress hormones are also released when a person becomes ill and/or feverish.

Avoiding risk of ketone buildup If stress levels continue to increase (i.e. an increase in insulin resistance or decrease in insulin sensitivity), the body becomes less able to utilize glucose and to store fatty acids in fat and instead, begins to break down fat into fuel for the body. The breakdown product of these fats is ketone bodies or ketoacids. As a result, when a person with diabetes is ill, he or she needs to test their urine for KETONES to avoid further complications such as diabetic ketoacidosis or hyperosmolar coma. Over-the-counter REAGENT STRIPS can measure these ketone levels.

If a significant amount of ketones is found in the urine, then the person who takes insulin needs more insulin. If the person is unable to eat or drink because of nausea and vomiting, and glucose levels are falling because the person has injected insulin, then he or she needs to go to a hospital emergency room for an intravenous infusion of both insulin and glucose.

If the Patient Takes Insulin

Unfortunately for the person with diabetes who uses insulin, all of these stress hormones counteract the effects of INSULIN. They either cause insulin to work less well than usual or they cause more glucose to enter the circulation from where it was stored in the liver. Either way, the glucose in the system tends to increase. Even if a person has not eaten anything and may have been vomiting and/or had diarrhea, blood glucose levels tend to increase.

As mentioned, many people think that if they are not eating anything, then they don't have to worry about coping with their diabetes. This is a serious mistake that could lead to acute diabetic complications necessitating emergency room visit or hospitalization. In fact, when a person is sick, he or she may need *more* than their normal dose of insulin, even when not eating.

If the Patient Is on Oral Medications

Even if a person with diabetes does not need insulin, it is still important to establish Sick Day Rules. The effect of the illness can throw the system off and put the patient at risk for a more serious illness than whatever temporary medical problem he or she is experiencing.

Avoiding Dehydration Is Important

Another problem that may occur when a person with diabetes is ill is that as glucose levels rise, the person may develop GLYCOSURIA (glucose in the urine) and experience DEHYDRATION. This dehydration will worsen rising glucose levels. As a result, a second principle for patients with diabetes is that when they are sick, they need to push themselves to drink fluids in order to stay well hydrated. Most patients who are sick are told to drink plenty of fluids, whether they have diabetes or not. But this advice is even more important for people with diabetes. The ill person should drink 6–8 ounces of fluid every waking hour. Recommended fluids include: water, diet ginger ale, broth or decaffeinated tea. If the ill person cannot eat, nondiet liquids should be consumed every other hour, such as 4 ounces of apple juice or Gatorade.

If the Ill Person Cannot Follow Meal Plans or Cannot Eat at All

When people with diabetes cannot follow their normal meal plans, experts say that they may replace the carbohydrate portion of meals by eating items such as orange juice (½ cup), regular yogurt with fruit (⅓ cup), regular ice cream (½ cup) and honey (1 tablespoon). One or two of these items can be eaten every one to two hours.

Contacting the Physician Right Away

People with diabetes who are sick should call their doctor right away if any of the following conditions are present:

- diarrhea for more than 24 hours
- blood sugar levels above 300 in two or more tests
- low blood sugar
- vomiting or inability to keep any fluids down for two to three hours

If a Patient Cannot Comply with Sick Day Rules

If the patient is so sick that he or she cannot comply with these recommendations, then another family member or other person should provide such care. If sick day rules are not followed, the person with diabetes may need hospitalization, depending on how long the sickness lasts, how severe it is and how debilitated the patient was before the illness.

Summarizing the Basics

In summary, the patient with diabetes who is also sick with another illness that makes them unable to perform their normal activities, such as illnesses that cause nausea and vomiting, should:

- Check glucose levels every one to three hours, depending upon the situation and severity of illness.
- Check and recheck urine ketones until they are negative and the person is feeling much better.
- Continue taking insulin, preferably short-acting insulin.

- Push fluids, drinking as much as tolerated to avoid lightheadedness/dizziness. Patients often may need to drink high calorie beverages that they typically avoid in order to take in some nutrition at this time.
- Contact the physician for diagnosis and advice on how to treat the underlying illness as well as advice on any recommended variations of the insulin dosage and or oral medications.

Joslin Diabetes Center affiliate at New Britain General Hospital, New Britain, Connecticut and Joslin Diabetes Clinic, Boston, Massachusetts. "Sick Day Guidelines Nutrition Management." 1995.

skilled nursing facilities (SNFs, nursing homes)
Refers to long-term care facilities for the aged and disabled. Some nursing facilities also offer temporary rehabilitative services to those who are not ill enough to remain in the hospital but who are too sick to return home. Many skilled nursing facilities receive payments for their residents from MEDICARE or MEDICAID. The rules for who may be admitted to a SNF under Medicare or Medicaid rules vary, as well as the rules on how long individuals may stay in a facility.

Because diabetes is a very common ailment among older people, SNF staffs need to be aware of the symptoms of diabetes, glucose testing, and symptoms of an individual who may be in danger. They also should be very knowledgeable about the medications used by people with diabetes as well as side effects and differences in reactions that older individuals may have to medications.

Many older people have problems with slow stomach emptying (GASTROPARESIS) and many also have more than one illness, such as the combination of HYPERTENSION and diabetes. It is important for the staff to be very aware of these illnesses as well as problems with medication interactions.

See also ASSISTED LIVING FACILITIES; ELDERLY.

skin problems Pain or itching of the skin. Some individuals with diabetes have a serious problem with dry and itchy skin and, consequently, need to use skin moisturizers on a regular basis. It is also important for people with diabetes to perform regular checks of their feet because they are more prone to developing problems, which can become very serious, particularly if the person suffers from DIABETIC NEUROPATHY and/or PERIPHERAL VASCULAR DISEASE.

Some examples of skin problems that may occur in people with diabetes are:

- acanthosis nigricans
- acquired perforating dermatosis (a condition of small dome-shaped papules (flat lesions) or nodules (small bumps) with a crust-filled center)
- diabetic bullae (blisters)
- granuloma annulare (fleshy red papules or plaques arranged like pearls on strings in a semicircle. Center is unaffected and borders are raised. Most commonly seen on backs of hands or on feet or legs)
- xerosis (very dry skin)
- fungal infections, such as Tinea pedis (feet), Tinea cruris (groin), and Tinea capitis (scalp)

One uncommon form of skin disorder in some people with diabetes is necrobiosis lipoidica diabeticorum. This disease was first described in 1929 and is strongly associated with Type 1 diabetes. The disease is four times more common in women than men. Sixty percent of those with the disorder have diabetes and most of the remaining patients have impaired glucose tolerance or impaired fasting glucose levels. In 10–20 percent of the cases, the problem resolves on its own. No therapies are effective.

Scleroderma diabeticorum is another skin condition associated with diabetes. It slowly evolves without preceding infection or trauma. It typically starts as a nonpitting thickening in the neck area and can involve the neck, back, trunk, and even legs. It is four times more common in men, usually those with long-term diabetes. It is usually not painful and there is no known treatment. The cause is unknown.

See also FOOT CARE.

smoking The use of tobacco products that are smoked, usually cigarettes but also other tobacco products such as cigars and pipe tobacco. Smoking is especially unhealthy for people with diabetes and typically exacerbates many complications of the disease. Smoking is the one most preventable cause of death among both diabetics and nondiabetics. Some studies have indicated that smoking is linked to the development of diabetes.

Millions of people worldwide smoke, making them at risk for a broad array of severe ailments, including CARDIOVASCULAR DISEASE, cancer, respiratory ailments, DIABETIC RETINOPATHY, DIABETIC NEUROPATHY, and other illnesses, as well as an increased risk for the AMPUTATION of a limb.

In addition to the well-known health risks of smoking for the average person, smoking further increases an already elevated risk for the person with diabetes in the development of heart and/ or kidney disease. It also raises the probability of the individual ultimately suffering from BLINDNESS, cancer, heart attacks, STROKE, amputations of limbs, and a broad array of other ailments.

Sometimes being diagnosed with diabetes as an adult is sufficient to motivate a person to quit smoking. Presumably this is due at least partly to a physician urging a newly diagnosed person to end their smoking habit immediately to avoid the array of future severe health risks.

Smokers tend to be of lower income and are less educated than the general population. Individuals with less than a high school education are more likely to be smokers, and there is an inverse relationship between years of education and smoking. That is, college graduates are less likely to smoke than high school graduates. Individuals with diabetes appear to smoke at about the same level as people who do not have diabetes, although, as mentioned, smoking is

even more of a health hazard for people who are diabetic.

Smoking May Cause Diabetes

In an analysis of 25 studies reported in the *Journal of the American Medical Association* in 2007, analysts Carole Willi, M.D., and colleagues found that smoking was associated with the later development of diabetes. It is unknown if there is a causal mechanism at work, and further research will be required to determine the relationship between smoking and the subsequent escalated risk for diabetes. It is possible that smokers are generally less healthy than nonsmokers, or other factors may be at work.

It is also possible, as the analysts suggest, that smoking could affect the beta cells of the pancreas. It is known that cigarette smoking is associated with both pancreatic cancer and chronic pancreatitis, so the possibility of harm to the pancreas from smoking seems feasible, although as yet unproven.

Diabetic Smokers Compared to Nonsmoking Diabetics

From a study of 188 diabetic smokers compared to 1,264 nonsmoking diabetics, researchers Leif I. Solberg, M.D., and colleagues reported their findings in 2004 in the *Annals of Family Medicine*. The researchers found that the smokers were significantly more likely to report themselves as being in fair or poor health (30.3 percent) than the nonsmokers (26.2 percent). They were also more likely to report feeling frequently depressed (27.7 percent) than the nonsmokers (17.2 percent), and they had a higher percentage of mental health visits (19.2 percent) than the nonsmokers (10.5 percent).

The smokers had gone to fewer eye examinations and dental checkups, and they reported wanting and receiving less support from their family and friends for diabetic self-management. The diabetic smokers were also less willing to give up smoking than other populations.

In addition, the smokers were less likely to have had at least one foot check in the past year

(54.8 percent) than the nonsmokers (65.0 percent), and the smokers were also less likely to have had a dilated eye examination in the past year (51.6 percent) compared to the nonsmokers (63.8 percent). The smokers were also less likely to have had an influenza immunization in the past year (57.4 percent for the smokers versus 65.2 percent for the nonsmokers) or ever to have had a pneumonia immunization (14.9 percent of the smokers versus 22.8 percent of the nonsmokers).

The researchers concluded, "These data suggest that diabetes patients who smoke are more likely to report often feeling sad or depressed; but even after adjusting for this factor, they are less likely to be active in self-management or to comply with diabetes care recommendations. Thus, diabetic patients who smoke are special clinical challenges and are likely to require more creative and consistent interventions and support."

In another study that compared 2,261 diabetic smokers and 2,261 diabetic nonsmokers, reported by Akiho S. Hosler and colleagues in *Diabetes Care* in 2007, the researchers found that the diabetic smokers had significantly lower rates for having a biannual HgbA1c blood test (48.9 percent for the smokers versus 57.4 percent for the nonsmokers) and lower rates for having an annual professional foot examination (39.6 percent for the smokers compared to 47.8 percent for the nonsmokers); they were less likely to have had an annual dilated eye examination (60.9 percent for the smokers vs. 68.1 percent for the nonsmokers) and less likely to receive an annual flu shot (52.2 percent for the smokers vs. 62.8 percent for the nonsmokers).

Other Research

A study reported in 2005 by Sharon L. Eason and colleagues in the *Journal of the American Board of Family Practice* found that smoking diabetics had an increased risk for asymptomatic peripheral arterial disease (PAD). In a study of 403 patients with and without diabetes who were screened for PAD, the researchers found of those who neither had diabetes nor did they smoke, the

risk was 1 percent. Of those without diabetes who smoked, the risk was 8 percent. Of those with diabetes alone, the risk was 12 percent. However, the presence of diabetes and smoking at least a pack of cigarettes per day increased the risk to 15 percent.

Smoking Cessation Medications

There are a variety of medications that smokers may use to withdraw from cigarettes. Smoking cessation medications in the form of nicotine replacement are available in the form of gum, nasal spray, transdermal patch, or inhaler. Good success has also been found with medications such as bupropion (Zyban).

In addition to nicotine replacement therapy and Zyban, some smokers find success with using hypnotherapy or with group or individual psychotherapy.

At the 56th Annual Meeting of the American Academy of Child and Adolescent Psychiatry in 2009, data was presented that analyzed the results from combined therapy with bupropion and contingency management (CM). With CM, money was paid to those who tested negative for nicotine at visits done two times per week. The researchers found that CM was more successful in getting adolescents to quit smoking than was monotherapy or placebo. The study included 143 patients ages 14–21. At one month, those on dual therapy had about 3.6 to 4.1 times the odds of remaining abstinent from nicotine compared to the other groups. The obvious limitation is that it was a short term study.

"There is a real need for evidence-based treatments for nicotine-dependent adolescents, especially since most adult smokers started smoking as adolescents," lead investigator Kevin M. Gray, M.D., child and adolescent psychiatrist and assistant professor at the Medical University of South Carolina in Charleston, told *Medscape Psychiatry*. "What we found in our study was that basically, the combination treatment of bupropion SR and [CM] beat the single treatments, at least in the acute setting, for smoking cessation in adolescents."

American Academy of Child Adolescent Psychiatry 56th Annual Meeting: Abstract 2.26. Presented October 28, 2009.

Eason, Sharon L., et al. "Diabetes Mellitus, Smoking, and the Risk for Asymptomatic Peripheral Arterial Disease: Whom Should We Screen?" *Journal of the American Board of Family Practice* 18 (2005): 355–361.

Hosler, Akiko S., Theresa M. Hinman, and Harlan R. Juster. "Disparities in Diabetes Care Between Smokers and Nonsmokers." *Diabetes Care* 30, no. 7 (2007): 1,883–1,885.

Solberg, Leif I., M.D., et al. "Diabetic Patients Who Smoke: Are They Different?" *Annals of Family Medicine* 2, no. 1 (2004): 26–32.

Willi, Carole, et al. "Active Smoking and the Risk of Type 2 Diabetes: A Systematic Review and Meta-analysis." *Journal of the American Medical Association* 298, no. 22 (2007): 2,654–2,664.

Social Security Disability Disability payment that is usually accompanied by MEDICARE coverage for eligible individuals. For example, if a person has been employed in the past and has now become disabled due to BLINDNESS or another disability, then he or she may be eligible for a Social Security disability payment prior to attaining retirement age. Some adults younger than age 65 are eligible for SSA disability as are some widowed individuals. The person must formally apply for this disability and provide documentation to support the claim.

See also DISABILITY/DISABILITY BENEFITS; MEDICAID.

SSI (Supplemental Security Insurance) A public assistance program for indigent and disabled individuals. Launched in 1974, SSI is funded by federal and state funds and provides the individual with a monthly check and MEDICAID benefits as well. The amount of payments is based on the individual's income in a formula that is used by the Social Security Administration. As of December 2000, there were 39,996 people with diabetes receiving SSI benefits, according to statistics provided by the Social Security Administration.

Most SSI recipients are disabled (79 percent). Twenty percent are aged and 1 percent are blind. Most recipients (56 percent) are between the ages of 18 and 64, followed by 31 percent who are ages 65 or older and 13 percent who are under age 18. Most SSI recipients (59 percent) are females. Disabled individuals receiving SSI benefits are re-evaluated at least every three years to verify that they are still disabled and poor.

See also DISABILITY/DISABILITY BENEFITS.

stress tests/exercise tolerance tests Tests that are administered on a treadmill and other devices and which help determine a person's overall physical stamina and the heart's response to exercise. Before people with diabetes undergo an EXERCISE regimen, their physicians may recommend a stress test to ensure they are healthy enough to undergo the type of exercise they have chosen. This is particularly true if they have or are at risk for CARDIOVASCULAR DISEASE.

People who are able to walk may have a simple treadmill test, with monitoring of the heart, blood pressure, and pulse. For those unable to walk well or for as long as six to 12 minutes, the cardiologist may administer a nuclear stress test with thallium or sestamibi to take pictures of the heart. In addition, medications such as dipyridamole and dobutamine may be given to artificially "stress" the heart.

stroke A sudden and life-threatening loss of blood flow to a part of the brain that results in damage or death of brain cells and may be fatal. Also known as a "brain attack." People with diabetes have a greater risk for stroke, particularly those with DIABETIC NEPHROPATHY (kidney disease that is associated with diabetes) and HYPERTENSION. They also have at least twice the risk of death from stroke compared to nondiabetics.

Very prompt medical attention often means the difference between life and death for the person who has had a stroke. If patients receive medical attention within one to three hours of a stroke, then their chances of survival are much greater because the patient may be given a medication that dissolves the blood clots that obstruct arteries, a common cause of a stroke. Immediate medical attention may also improve the prognosis for later health and decrease the severity of problems with long-term disability that many stroke patients suffer.

A stroke may cause the following medical consequences:

- temporary or permanent paralysis
- cognitive (thinking) problems
- language deficits
- pain
- emotional problems
- death: about 15 percent of stroke victims die soon after the stroke and stroke is a leading cause of death in the United States

Symptoms and Diagnostic Path

A person who has one or more of any of the following symptoms should seek immediate emergency attention. In the United States, the individual or others should call 911 for emergency assistance. The patient should not drive, nor should others take the person to the hospital. Instead, in most cases, an ambulance is best because it will provide the fastest medical attention.

The danger symptoms of stroke are:

- sudden confusion in understanding speech or in speaking
- sudden numbness in the face, leg, or arm, especially if it is on one side of the body only
- sudden blindness or difficulty seeing in one or both eyes
- sudden inability to walk or severe difficulty in walking

When an individual has possible stroke symptoms, doctors generally use radiologic imaging methods to verify whether the person has actu-

ally had a stroke and, if a stroke has occurred, to determine the degree of the severity, type, and location of the stroke. Physicians may use computed tomography (CT) scans of the brain to determine if an acute stroke has occurred. Another diagnostic device is the magnetic resonance imaging (MRI) scan, which can detect the tiny after-effects of a stroke, such as an increase in the water content of the brain tissue, also called *cytotoxic edema.*

Physicians may use ultrasound to image the carotid arteries. These images will assist the doctor in identifying blockages or clots. *Magnetic resonance angiography* (MRA) is rapidly replacing conventional angiography as a technique to look for blockages in the blood vessels in the brain, including blockages of both the carotid arteries (anterior) and the vertebral arteries (posterior). The MRA is a way of using MRI (magnetic resonance imaging) to look at a blood vessel but without the traditional intravenous "dye" contrast that can potentially damage the kidneys in a patient with diabetes.

Treatment Options and Outlook

The stroke victim requires hospitalization and stabilization of vital signs, especially of the blood pressure. Medications such as antiplatelet agents and anticoagulants are often prescribed. Two common anticoagulants, as of this writing, are warfarin (Coumadin) and heparin. Neuroprotectant medications may also be prescribed, such as calcium channel blocker medications, as well as newer medications.

If the patient is over age 50, after stabilization, his or her physician may choose to place the patient on long-term baby aspirin therapy to reduce the risk of further strokes. If the patient was already on aspirin prior to the stroke, he or she may be changed to another drug plus the aspirin.

In rare cases, the stroke patient may require surgery to treat an acute stroke or to repair damage that has already occurred. This is generally required only with intracranial bleeds and is performed to relieve the pressure on the brain.

Many patients will require at least some degree of rehabilitation, including physical therapy, occupational therapy, and speech therapy. Psychological help may also be needed to help the patient cope with anxiety and depression.

Physical therapists can assist the patient in regaining lost abilities in such basic skills as walking, sitting, moving from one position to another, and similar important activities of daily living (also known as ADLs).

Occupational therapists may be needed to help the stroke victim relearn a variety of tasks, ranging from reading and writing to bathing, dressing, and other activities of daily living that must be mastered again.

Speech therapists can often help the patient who can think rationally but who has difficulty in physically getting the words to come out right or enunciating them (dysarthria). Some patients also have mental rather than physical trouble understanding verbal language (aphasia). These therapists can also help patients relearn swallowing and how to avoid aspiration.

Psychological counseling may help a patient deal with anxiety, anger, frustration, and the other emotions that accompany the trauma of recovering from a stroke. Many patients require antidepressants.

Risk Factors and Preventive Measures

People with diabetes are at a greater risk for experiencing a stroke than the general population. Other risk factors for stroke include:

- hypertension (high blood pressure)
- a history of heart disease, particularly atrial fibrillation (a very irregular heartbeat which can lead to clots in the left upper chamber of the heart that can break free and travel to the brain)
- history of transient ischemic attacks (TIAs), or mini-strokes
- cigarette smoking: heavy smokers are at greatest risk
- race: African Americans have a risk of stroke that is nearly twice that of Caucasians. In addition, African Americans who are between the ages of 45 and 55 years and who have a stroke face a five to six times greater risk of dying from a stroke than a white American of the same age who has had a stroke.
- age greater than 65 years old
- a high count of low-density lipoprotein (LDL) cholesterol count (in patients with diabetes the goal is less than 100 mg/dL)
- alcoholism or ALCOHOL ABUSE
- the use of illegal drugs, especially ones that can elevate blood pressure, cause irregular heart rhythms, or cause blood vessels to constrict such as cocaine and amphetamines

If the stroke victim was a smoker, physicians will urge him or her to stop smoking immediately and permanently, in order to reduce the risk of any further strokes. A broad array of other lifestyle recommendations may be made, depending on the individual needs of the patient.

In addition, good blood pressure control is critically important. Generally, blood pressure can be lowered to normal with medication and lifestyle changes; however, a major acute drop in blood pressure may potentially worsen the decreased blood flow to the damaged area.

Important Precautions for People with Diabetes

Because of the risks that are related to stroke, it is very important for everyone who has diabetes to maintain excellent control of their blood sugar, working to attain as near to normal a blood sugar as is possible without causing other issues, especially hypoglycemia. The Diabetes Control and Complications Trial (DCCT), which included 1,441 patients with Type 1 diabetes, showed that intensive treatment reduced the risk of any CARDIOVASCULAR DISEASE event by 42 percent and the risk of nonfatal myocardial infarction, stroke, or death from cardiovascular disease by 57 percent.

Tobacco products should be avoided altogether because tobacco increases the risk of stroke. It is also important to keep lipids at goal levels set by the physician, in order to avoid a first stroke as well as to decrease the probability of another stroke.

See also ELDERLY.

Diabetes Control and Complications Trial/Epidemiology of Diabetes Interventions and Complications (DCCT/EDIC) Study Research Group. *New England Journal of Medicine* 353, no. 25 (2005): 2,643–2,653.

sulfonylureas   A class of oral medications used to treat some individuals with Type 2 diabetes. The drugs in this class promote the pancreatic secretion of insulin and thus lower blood glucose levels. They are also known as "secretagogues" along with medications in the meglitinide and phenylalanine classes. All three classes of drugs directly stimulate the pancreatic beta cell to secrete insulin. About 5 percent of patients treated with sulfonylureas each year fail to respond to the medication (secondary failure).

Sulfonylureas do NOT cause the pancreas to lose its ability to secrete insulin any sooner nor do they protect the beta cell. Patients in the UNITED KINGDOM PROSPECTIVE DIABETES STUDY (UKPDS) who were treated with sulfonylureas gained an average of six pounds. Although there is a theoretical concern that sulfonylureas can increase the risk of heart attack, no increased risk was seen in the UKPDS study subjects.

These medications are broken down into first generation agents and second generation agent sulfonylureas. The first four drugs in this class were Diabinese (chlorpropamide), Tolinase (tolazamide), Orinase (tolbutamide), and Dymelor (acetohexamide). These drugs are rarely used today. The first-generation agents are generally less potent, have a wider side-effect profile, and have a slightly greater risk of interactions with other medications that the patient may be taking.

Second-generation agents, which are used more frequently today, include glyburide (with brand names of DiaBeta, Glynase PresTab, and Micronase), glipizide (Glucotrol), glipizide-GITS (Glucotrol XL), and glimepiride (Amaryl).

All sulfonylurea drugs have the common side effect of potentially causing HYPOGLYCEMIA. They may also cause weight gain, stomach upset, and skin rash or itching. Hypoglycemia is most common with glyburide and chlorpropamide, due to their long half-lives (which means, they remain in the body for a long time) and active metabolites. The ingestion of alcohol with sulfonylureas can lead to a flushing Antabuse-like reaction. (Antabuse is a drug given to alcoholics, which induces vomiting if the alcoholic person consumes any alcohol.)

Sulfonylureas can cause weight gain and the average weight gain over the course of a year is 4 to 6 pounds. These drugs provide 80 to 90 percent of their maximal effect at 50 percent of their maximal dose.

These drugs should absolutely not be used by patients who have Type 1 diabetes, because, by definition, they have no beta cell function, and thus cannot cause increased secretion of insulin from the pancreas.

The United Kingdom Prospective Diabetes Study showed that the use of sulfonylureas did not increase cardiovascular morbidity (illness) and mortality (death).

These drugs should not be used in women who are pregnant or in people who have Type 1

TABLE 1: MOST COMMONLY USED SULFONYLUREA MEDICATIONS				
Name	How Supplied	Starting Dose	Max	Dosing
Glyburide	1.25, 1.5, 2.5, 3.0, 5.0, 6.0, 10 mg	Usu 2.5–5.0	20 mg	Gen daily
Glipizde	2.5, 5.0, 10.0	Usu 2.5–5.0	40 mg/day	Usu 2x/day
Glimepiride	1.0, 2, 4	0.5–2.0	8 mg/day	Daily

diabetes. They should also be avoided by patients who are allergic to sulfa drugs. Patients with some liver failure or with kidney disease should also avoid them.

Sulfonylureas lower glucose levels within two to three days and lower HgbA1c by 1 to 2 percent. The most common side effect is hypoglycemia, found more frequently with chlorpropamide and glyburide. These are older "first generation" drugs that are not commonly used. Second-generation drugs are less likely to cause hypoglycemia, although it can occur. Another effect that can occur if the patient also consumes alcohol is a flushing syndrome. Alcohol consumption is not recommended with this class of drugs.

symptoms of diabetes Physical indicators of either Type 1 or Type 2 diabetes. There are specific symptoms that are commonly found in many people who have diabetes. If a person has such symptoms, he or she should check with a medical doctor to find out if diabetes is present. A person may have some but not all of these symptoms. It is also possible to have Type 2 diabetes and experience few or no symptoms. In addition, it is also possible to have some or all of the following symptoms and yet the person does not have diabetes.

Common symptoms of diabetes include:

- blurred vision
- constant thirst
- frequent skin or other infections
- frequent urination
- increased hunger
- excessive fatigue for no apparent reason
- unexplained weight loss is a symptom of Type 1 diabetes

When some or all of the above symptoms are seen in a person along with other characteristics that are found among many people with diabetes, the physician is even more suspicious of

diabetes. For example, OBESITY is a very common factor found among people with Type 2 diabetes. In addition, people who are of African-American or Native American descent are more likely to have Type 2 diabetes than are people of other races. Age is another factor: individuals who are over age 65 have a much greater risk of developing diabetes than do people of younger ages.

Syndrome X See METABOLIC SYNDROME.

syringe Device used to inject liquid medications into the body. The syringe is a hollow device with a plunger inside and it may include an attached needle. The medicine is placed into the syringe. When the syringe includes a needle and the plunger is depressed, the needle forces the insulin into the body. All people with Type 1 diabetes and some people with Type 2 diabetes need to inject insulin to control their blood glucose levels.

Nearly all syringes are made from plastic and are disposable. They are manufactured in three typical sizes, 0.3 cc, 0.5 cc, and 1.0 cc, and hold a maximum of 30, 50, and 100 units of insulin respectively. All insulin on the market is U-100, which means there are 100 units per one cc. If a patient needs U-500 insulin, it must be specially ordered.

The needles attached to the syringes have become ever sharper and smaller and most now are 29-, 30-, and 31-gauge (the larger the number, the smaller the needle). Needles are also silicon-coated to allow them to pass through the skin almost painlessly. Experts advise patients against wiping the needle with alcohol because this may remove the silicon coating.

Reuse of Needles

Many patients reuse their syringes and needles in order to save money. Although it is not recommended, this practice can work for some patients when they are very cautious and are sure to keep their skin very clean, and recap the needle after each usage.

Disposal of Syringes and Needles

There is no standard approach to the disposal of needles and syringes. The traditional teaching has been to have patients fill an old plastic bleach bottle with syringes and needles, and when it was full, to recap the bottle, tape it up, and place it in a standard trash container. It should be labeled "non-recyclable." There are also devices available on the market that can safely remove the needle from the syringe and prevent any inadvertent needle sticks as well as prevent someone else from reusing the needle.

Many patients prefer prefilled insulin pen devices, because dosing is easier and more accurate. The needles on the pen devices tend to cause far less discomfort, because the insulin is already inside the syringe. As a result, the patient does not need to push the needle through a rubber stopper on an insulin bottle to draw up insulin; this very act decreases the sharpness of the needle. A duller needle causes more pain upon injection.

systolic blood pressure Refers to the peak pressure generated by the left ventricle as the heart contracts. Systolic pressure is the numerator (top number) that is reported when blood pressure results are given. For example, if the blood pressure were 120/80, the 120 would be the systolic pressure. The lower number is the diastolic pressure. The heart spends about ⅔ of its time in diastole (at rest, i.e., between beats) and ⅓ in systole.

Individuals with both Type 1 and especially Type 2 diabetes are at high risk for developing high levels of both diastolic and systolic blood pressure, or HYPERTENSION. People with diabetes are more likely to suffer from hypertension. The combination of diabetes and hypertension can directly lead to or exacerbate both microvascular and macrovascular complications.

The microvascular complications that clearly are affected by hypertension include DIABETIC RETINOPATHY and DIABETIC NEPHROPATHY, while the macrovascular complications include myocardial infarction (heart attack), STROKE, ERECTILE DYSFUNCTION, and peripheral vascular disease (clinical syndrome of intermittent claudication, i.e., pain in the legs or buttocks with walking).

In the recent past, it was felt that the systolic blood pressure was *less* important than the diastolic blood pressure. This assumption is now known to be incorrect. Increased systolic blood pressure correlates better with a risk of stroke. Increased diastolic blood pressure actually correlates better with a risk for heart attack. Both measures are important.

Isolated systolic hypertension (ISH) in the elderly is common and should be treated. Studies such as the SHEP (Systolic Hypertension in the Elderly Program) trial have demonstrated that the treatment of ISH in patients who are over age 65 dramatically lowers complications these individuals experience.

See also DIASTOLIC BLOOD PRESSURE.

team management of diabetes The concept of using a group of medical experts that assists an individual with diabetes in managing diabetes. This concept was developed by Dr. Joslin in the early 20th century and is still considered very important today by leading diabetes experts. Unfortunately, due to managed care and cost constraints, it may be difficult for patients to receive treatment from an entire team. Yet good team treatment is essentially cost-effective because it can prevent severe and costly consequences such as AMPUTATIONS, STROKES, and other complications of diabetes.

As a result, most medical experts believe that, whenever possible, individuals with diabetes should be treated by a team of medical experts, including a physician, registered dietitian, certified diabetes educator, and other diabetes practitioners. Other possible members of the health care team may be neurologists, NEPHROLOGISTS, podiatrists, social workers, psychologists, exercise physiologists, and OPHTHALMOLOGISTS. Also, if a woman with diabetes becomes pregnant, she needs to coordinate the care provided by her obstetrician with the expertise that her other "team members" provide.

Some research has indicated that team management provided to people with diabetes results in lower costs due to less frequent hospitalizations.

thiazolidinediones (TZDs) The newest class of oral medications used to treat people with Type 2 diabetes. These drugs only work in patients who still make some insulin. TZDs make the body more sensitive to existing insulin, allowing it to move glucose from the bloodstream into the cells more effectively and giving the body more energy. The drug takes 12 to 16 weeks to reach its maximal effects. When used as monotherapy (one drug), TZDs can lower glucose levels by about 1 to 2 percent.

Examples of drugs in this class are Avandia (rosiglitazone) and Actos (pioglitazone). Rezulin (troglitazone) was a drug in this class but the Food and Drug Administration (FDA) removed it from the market in 2000 after reports of liver toxicity in some patients. TZDs work to directly improve the problem of INSULIN RESISTANCE. Thus, TZDs do not cause a greater output of insulin but instead enable the body to more efficiently use the insulin that is produced.

TZDs can cause weight gain (four to eight pounds), anemia (mild and dilutional, due to fluid retention) and edema (swelling) in the legs and the ankles. They can also interact with BIRTH CONTROL pills, making them less efficacious and are not often used with women taking birth control pills.

Sometimes thiazolidinedione drugs are taken in combination with other medications for diabetes, such as METFORMIN or insulin.

Although the FDA and the manufacturers recommend testing the liver prior to the use of TZDs, and every two months for the first year of use, there has been *no* significant evidence of liver toxicity with the remaining two drugs in this class that are still on the market.

These drugs should not be used in patients with coronary heart disease but can be used in patients with kidney failure.

TZD drugs have also been used to treat women with POLYCYSTIC OVARIAN SYNDROME, in order to treat excessive hairiness (hirsutism) and to improve fertility. These are not FDA-approved indications.

As of this writing in late 2010, considerable controversy surrounds the use of rosiglitazone. Some studies, such as by Nissen, have shown that the drug is linked to heart attacks while other studies have shown that this medication does not statistically increase the risk for heart attack. The Food and Drug Administration (FDA) evaluated the existing studies in July 2010 and decided to keep rosiglitazone on the market. Based on the joint advice of the Endocrine Society, the American Diabetes Association, and the American Association, of Clinical Endocrinologists, individuals should not stop taking rosiglitazone unless their physicians tell them to do so. However, if they need to change medications, there are other good choices to maintain good glucose control. There are black box warnings associated with rosiglitazone, and this drug should be used only with caution among those at risk for heart disease.

See also MEDICATIONS FOR TREATMENT OF TYPE 2 DIABETES.

Nissen, S. E., and K. Wolski. "Rosiglitazone Revisited." *Archives of Internal Medicine* 170, no. 14 (2010): 1,191–1,201.

thyroid disease An abnormality of the thyroid, which is a butterfly-shaped gland that is located in the neck. The key thyroid disorders are hyperthyroidism, which is an excess of thyroid hormone and hypothyroidism, which is due to insufficient thyroid hormone. Hypothyroidism is more common among people with diabetes. Graves' disease, an autoimmune disorder, is the most common cause of hyperthyroidism.

About 6 percent of the nondiabetic population has a thyroid disorder and the risk further increases to 10 percent for people with diabetes. According to Patricia Wu, M.D., in her 2001 article for *Diabetes Self-Management,* the risk further increases to 30 percent for WOMEN WITH DIABETES.

Others who are at risk to develop thyroid disorders include:

- women (who develop hypothyroidism about five times as often as men)
- those with other family members with thyroid disease
- people over age 50 (aging brings an increased risk of hypothyroidism)
- those who take medications that can decrease thyroid levels, such as lithium
- existence of another autoimmune disorder such as Type 1 diabetes, pernicious anemia, vitiligo, Addison's disease

Causes of Thyroid Disease

Many thyroid diseases are autoimmune disorders, which means that the body mistakenly attacks the thyroid as it would a foreign invader. In fewer cases, the body may react to medications such as lithium (for manic depression), or amiodarone (for some heart conditions), which may trigger hypothyroidism. Much more rarely, a disorder of the hypothalamus or the pituitary gland may cause hypothyroidism.

Symptoms of Hyperthyroidism

Hyperthyroidism may be detected by a physician when a patient has some or all of the following symptoms below. **Note:** these symptoms may also indicate many other diseases and thus, only an experienced physician can perform the diagnosis.

- elevated heart rate (pulse) of over 100 beats per minute
- enlarged thyroid
- increased requirement for insulin and worsening of blood glucose levels, if the person has diabetes
- insomnia/nightmares
- weight loss despite a greater appetite

- heavy sweating
- extreme nervousness and irritability/anxiety
- heat intolerance
- shaking hands
- decreased menstruation or no menstruation, prior to menopause or surgical removal of the uterus

Symptoms of Hypothyroidism

There are basic symptoms common to many people whose thyroid levels are low. However, these symptoms may also indicate other diseases. Common symptoms of hypothyroidism are:

- chronic constipation
- puffy face, especially under the eyes
- dry and itchy skin, doughy skin
- depression/lack of energy/apathy
- sensitivity to cold temperatures
- decreased need for insulin in those who have diabetes
- heavier menstruation
- muscle cramps and aches
- more frequent bowel movements (although not diarrhea)

The most common form of hypothyroidism is Hashimoto's thyroiditis. This is an autoimmune condition in which the body mistakenly makes antibodies (proteins) against the enzyme in the thyroid. Initially, it can cause hyperthyroidism because excess thyroid hormone is released from the damaged thyroid cells (Hashitoxicosis). More frequently, however, it will cause hypothyroidism. This is due to ongoing damage to the thyroid gland.

Diagnosis of Thyroid Disease

If the doctor believes a person has thyroid disease based on the symptoms displayed, then he or she will usually order a blood test known as a thyroid stimulating hormone (TSH) assay. This will determine if levels are high, low or in the normal range. The lower the TSH outside the normal range, the more hyperthyroid a person is. The higher the TSH outside the normal range, the more hypothyroid the person is.

Treating Thyroid Disease

The treatment depends on the cause. Treatment may be very simple, such as prescribing supplemental thyroid hormone to the hypothyroid patient and following up with periodic blood tests to ensure the blood levels of thyroid are in the normal range. Conversely, if the person has excessive levels of thyroid, the physician may attempt to suppress thyroid function through various means, such as with prescribing antithyroid pills or radioactive iodine. In some cases, surgery will become necessary. The primary test used to diagnose thyroid disease, the TSH (thyroid-stimulating hormone) has numerical levels that are inversely related to thyroid function. This means that numbers that are high indicate hypothyroidism and numbers that are very low indicate hyperthyroidism.

When the person with thyroid disease also has diabetes, then blood glucose levels must be monitored even more carefully than usual until the doctor believes the patient has achieved a stable level of thyroid function. After that point, regular glucose monitoring should continue. Glucose levels are more unstable with hyperthyroidism than with hypothyroidism.

If people with diabetes are hypothyroid, however, this increases the risk for lipid abnormalities, such as an increase in low-density lipoproteins, otherwise known as "bad cholesterol." Therefore, patients with elevated levels of cholesterol should be screened for hypothyroidism.

Wu, Patricia, M.D. "Thyroid Disease and Diabetes." *Diabetes Self-Management* 18, no. 3 (Winter 2000): 6–12.

travel Leaving home to go to another site, usually for a day or more and for business or pleasure. Many people with diabetes enjoy traveling.

The importance of GLYCEMIC CONTROL, however, does not take a holiday and is still an issue for people with both Type 1 and Type 2 diabetes.

According to Davida F. Kruger, author of *The Diabetes Travel Guide: How to Travel with Diabetes—Anywhere in the World,* it's important for people with diabetes to see their physicians at least four to six weeks before a trip. This will enable the person with diabetes to have a physical examination and receive advice from the physician. It is also a good idea to obtain a letter from the doctor that states the person has diabetes and what medications the person takes.

Medication Preparation

The person with diabetes should bring sufficient medication for the duration of the trip. Kruger says it is also a good idea to ask the doctor to write a prescription for generic medication, in case the patient needs but is unable to obtain the specific usual form of medication at the travel site. It is unlikely that it will be possible to fill a prescription in a foreign country; however, the prescription will enable a physician in that country to write a prescription, if necessary.

It is not advisable to check luggage that has medication packed inside it because luggage may be misplaced or lost. Instead, if traveling by plane, it is best to bring medication in a carry-on bag or in another container that will fit under the seat.

It is also a good idea to buy and wear a medical identification necklace, bracelet, or anklet that includes key information about the person with diabetes, such as that he or she has diabetes and what medication is taken. ID cards inserted into wallets are not useful in emergencies because they are often not searched immediately when a person becomes seriously ill. A medical ID, in contrast, will reveal important information immediately to emergency medical experts and others.

People with diabetes who need injected insulin should consider a plan to dispose of their syringes and medications, such as a personal size disposal box. It can be dangerous and even illegal to dispose of syringes and lancets by throwing them in a public trash can.

Food Snacks

Regardless of how well an individual with diabetes manages the illness, it is still a good idea to bring some basic snacks along on a trip, to avoid any possibility of HYPOGLYCEMIA. These items should be placed in sealable plastic bags to decrease the probability of spoilage. People with diabetes should not assume that airlines will have nutritious snacks. (Individuals with diabetes may request a diabetic meal two to three days before the flight.)

Emergency Medical Assistance

If the person with diabetes becomes ill when faraway from home or in another country, he or she should ask the hotel concierge for assistance, being sure to explain that he or she has diabetes. If in a foreign country, the ill individual may also need to contact the consul office for their country. U.S. citizens can obtain a list of consulates by calling the U.S. State Department ahead of time or visiting their Web site: http://travel.state.gov.

Whether in the country or out of the country, it is important for all people with diabetes to wear EMERGENCY MEDICAL IDENTIFICATION, so that treatment can occur quickly if it is needed.

Dendinger, M. J. "Traveling with Diabetes: Business as Usual." *Diabetes Self-Management* 15, no. 3 (1998): 7–8, 11–13.

Kruger, Davida F. *The Diabetes Travel Guide: How to Travel with Diabetes—Anywhere in the World.* Alexandria, Va: American Diabetes Association, 2000.

Peragallo-Dittko, V. "Planes, Trains, and Diabetes: A Guide to Safe Travel." *Diabetes Self-Management* 14, no. 3 (1997): 32–33, 35, 38–40.

"Traveling with Diabetes." *Postgraduate Medicine* 105, no. 2 (1999): 233–234.

triglyceride A form of fat that is found in the blood. Insulin helps store fat and when diabetes is well-controlled, triglycerides are efficiently removed. When diabetes is not controlled, triglyceride levels increase and the individual has an increased risk for developing vascular diseases and pancreatitis. (Pancreatitis is a significant risk if triglycerides exceed 1,000 mg/dL.) Additionally, when a person's triglyceride level increases, low density lipoprotein (LDL, or "bad cholesterol") levels tend to become more atherogenic (more likely to cause clots or breakages).

Other forms of fats are high density lipoproteins (HDLs).

See also HDL; LDL.

Type 1 diabetes One of the two prevailing forms of diabetes and far less common than Type 2 diabetes. Formerly known as "insulin-dependent diabetes mellitus" or "juvenile-onset diabetes." This type was renamed Type 1 diabetes because the disease may be diagnosed in adults as well as in children. In addition, children diagnosed with Type 1 diabetes continue to have the illness into adulthood and throughout their lives.

Individuals with Type 1 diabetes constitute an estimated 5–10 percent of all cases of diabetes found in North America. In the United States, there are about 900,000 children and adults who have Type 1 diabetes and an estimated 13,000 new cases are diagnosed each year.

Type 1 diabetes is generally considered an autoimmune disease in which the afflicted individual's own immune system destroys the beta cells in the pancreas. These are the cells that make insulin. As a result, people with Type 1 diabetes must take INSULIN in order to survive.

The delivery of insulin may be by injection via standard syringes, a "pen" device, or an insulin pump. It is also critically important that people with Type 1 diabetes carefully monitor their blood glucose levels at least several times daily, depending on the advice provided by their physicians. They also need to monitor their diets and may need to do carbohydrate counting.

Many studies, most prominently the DIABETES CONTROL AND COMPLICATIONS TRIAL (DCCT), have proven that glucose levels that are as close to normal as possible will greatly reduce the risk for an individual with Type 1 diabetes to develop one or more of the serious COMPLICATIONS OF DIABETES. Some examples of such complications are:

- amputations
- blindness
- cardiovascular disease
- death
- diabetic nephropathy
- diabetic neuropathy
- diabetic retinopathy
- stroke

Women with Type 1 diabetes who experience PREGNANCY should consult with their physicians for the best ways to keep themselves and their unborn babies healthy. Studies also indicate that preconception planning is a critical course of action for women with diabetes and will greatly reduce the risk of miscarriage and fetal abnormalities.

See also DIABETES MELLITUS.

Type 2 diabetes The more common form of diabetes, accounting for at least 90 percent of all cases of diabetes in the United States. Formerly called non-insulin-dependent (NIDDM) diabetes, or adult onset diabetes mellitus (AODM) the illness was renamed "Type 2 diabetes" in the latter part of the 20th century because researchers felt that the name of the illness should not depend on the treatment or age at diagnosis, as it is now being diagnosed in children and adolescents. In addition, some individuals who have Type 2 diabetes may need to use insulin. In the United States about 7.4 percent of adults had Type 2 diabetes in 1995, and the prevalence was expected to increase to about 9 percent by 2025.

Type 2 diabetes is most common among certain racial groups, such as AFRICAN AMERICANS and Native Americans. The risk for developing Type 2 diabetes also rises with advancing age.

Certain conditions, such as OBESITY and lack of physical activity, are associated with the development of Type 2 diabetes. In addition, diet and nutrition play a role as well; for example, the PIMA INDIANS in Arizona have very high rates of Type 2 diabetes; however, Pima Indians in Mexico have very low rates. The Mexican Pima Indians are generally slender and very active in contrast to the obese and sedentary Pima of Arizona.

Some women are at risk for developing Type 2 diabetes, including women who have had GESTATIONAL DIABETES MELLITUS (GDM) or women who have had polycystic ovary syndrome. Men and women with HYPERTENSION, DYSLIPIDEMIA, or IMPAIRED GLUCOSE TOLERANCE (IGT) have an increased risk of developing Type 2 diabetes.

Genetics is another factor in the development of Type 2 diabetes and the disease clearly "runs in" families. If a parent or sibling has the disease, the risk is heightened for other family members. However, environmental constraints also play a role. For example, the parent or sibling with Type 2 diabetes may eat a very high carbohydrate and high calorie diet, which diet is shared by other family members.

Type 2 diabetes is on the rise among affluent populations and is also increasingly found among adolescents and even children in developed and affluent societies where inactivity is the rule and food is plentiful. As of this writing, the only approved treatment for diabetes in children is the use of INSULIN or METFORMIN (Glucophage).

GLYCEMIC CONTROL is important for any person with diabetes and affected individuals should test their blood at least once daily and make adjustments based on the results. Study after study has demonstrated that glycemic control can reduce the risk for serious complications of diabetes such as DIABETIC RETINOPATHY, DIABETIC NEPHROPATHY, or DIABETIC NEUROPATHY. The most prominent and largest study of this nature was the UNITED KINGDOM PROSPECTIVE DIABETES STUDY (UKPDS).

Many people with diabetes suffer from hypertension, and the combination of hypertension and diabetes causes a greatly increased risk for CARDIOVASCULAR DISEASE.

People with diabetes should see a physician on a regular basis. They should also check their feet on a daily basis for any damage. In addition, an annual dilated-eye examination will help detect any serious eye diseases before it is too late and avoid BLINDNESS.

See also DIABETES MELLITUS.

ulcer A break or sore in the skin, which may become infected if untreated. People with diabetes are at greater risk for developing ulcers of the foot or legs that result from skin that is accidentally abraded in minor scrapes. The most common risk factor is neuropathy leading to loss of sensation. In the worst cases, an untreated ulcer may lead to GANGRENE and the subsequent need for AMPUTATION of the affected limb.

Regular FOOT CARE can prevent the many cases of ulcers that lead to infection and HOSPITALIZATION each year. For example, patients with diabetes should remove their shoes and socks every time they see their doctor before he arrives in the room. This will help the doctor to remember to check the feet.

People with diabetes should never go barefoot, even in the house, lest they step on an object that harms their feet. They should also examine their own feet carefully every day.

Ultralente insulin Long-acting form of insulin. There are also short and medium-acting forms of insulin. Ultralente insulin action does not work until about four to six hours after injection. It continues to work for about 24 to 28 hours. It has lower peak activity than NPH insulin or Lente insulin, and thus, may bring less of a risk for hypoglycemia. However, Ultralente insulin may also be a bit more variable in its absorption rates.

When it was available in the past as animal insulin, Ultralente insulin was often used once per day as a "basal" insulin and then regular insulin was used to cover meals. Now Ultralente insulin is available only as recombinant human insulin. It may still be used once per day but it is also often used two to three times per day and combined with rapid or short-acting insulin.

See also INSULIN.

United Kingdom Prospective Diabetes Study (UKPDS) A massive study performed in the United Kingdom of over 5,000 patients recently diagnosed with Type 2 diabetes in 23 centers within the United Kingdom. The average patient was followed for 10 years. This study definitively proved that control of hyperglycemia and hypertension among people with diabetes dramatically reduced the subjects' risk for a variety of common complications faced by people with diabetes, such as DIABETIC RETINOPATHY, DIABETIC NEPHROPATHY, heart attack, STROKE, and death.

The study concentrated on the impact of tight glucose control on individuals with Type 2 diabetes and whether intensive medication therapy using insulin, metformin, glibenclamide (such as glyburide) and chlorpropamide would provide clinical benefits. In a substudy, patients with high blood pressure also received either an ACE inhibitor drug or a beta-blocker medication.

The study definitively proved that tight control greatly decreased the likelihood of later complications from diabetes, such as diabetic retinopathy and diabetic nephropathy. The study also showed that for every percentage point decrease in HgbA1c, there was a corresponding decrease in deaths and fatal or nonfatal MYOCARDIAL INFARCTIONS. In addition, the study proved that decreased hypertension was significantly correlated with a corresponding decreased risk for stroke, death related to diabetes, heart failure, BLINDNESS, and other COMPLICATIONS OF DIABETES.

Hypertension risks Follow-up studies of smaller subsets of the UKPDS group also revealed significant findings. For example, in a study of 1,148 male newly diagnosed hypertensive patients drawn from the UKPDS group, reported in a 1998 issue of the *British Medical Journal,* one group was assigned to the "tight" blood pressure control group and achieved an average pressure of 144/82 mmHg. The standard treatment group achieved an average pressure of 154/87 mmHg. Subjects were treated with beta blockers and ACE drugs as well as others as clinically needed.

Compared to the standard group, the tight control group had marked reduction in deaths from diabetes (down 32 percent), strokes (down 44 percent), and diabetic retinopathy (34 percent). The tight control group had a risk of 3.6 risk events per 1,000 patient years for heart failure, compared to 8.1 for the less tight control group. The risk of death from kidney failure was lower for the tight control group, whose members had a risk of 0.3 of death from kidney failure, compared to 1.0 for the nontight group. The tight control group had a lower risk of fatal stroke (1.5) versus 3.6 for the nontight group. The tight group had a lower risk of fatal myocardial infarction (heart attack), at 9.8 versus 13.8 for the less controlled group.

Clearly, control of HYPERTENSION among patients with diabetes is crucial to their continued lives and health.

American Diabetes Association. "Implications of the United Kingdom Prospective Diabetes Study." *Diabetes Care* 21 (1998): 2,180–2,184.

Turner, R. C., et al. "Risk Factors for Coronary Artery Disease in Non-Insulin Dependent Diabetes Mellitus: United Kingdom Prospective Diabetes Study (UKPDS): 23." *British Medical Journal* 316 (March 14, 1998): 823–828.

UK Prospective Diabetes Study Group. "Tight Blood Pressure Control and Risk of Macrovascular and Microvascular Complications in Type 2 Diabetes: UKPDS 38." *British Medical Journal* 317 (September 12, 1998): 703–713.

urinary tract infection (UTI) A commonly used generic term which may indicate several different urological problems, including pyelonephritis (inflammation of the kidney), CYSTITIS (inflammation of the bladder) or urethritis (inflammation of the urethra, the tube leading from the bladder and through which urine travels to be voided). However, the most common use of the phrase "urinary tract infection" is to indicate bladder INFECTIONS. These infections are often caused by *E. coli* bacteria or other organisms that are known to be associated with infections of the bladder.

According to research by Kees J. Gorter and colleagues and published in 2010 in *Family Practice Advance Access,* women with diabetes have an elevated risk for both urinary tract infections and recurrent urinary tract infections. This study included 340 women with diabetes and compared them with 6,618 nondiabetic women. For example, about 16 percent of the women with diabetes had recurring infections compared to only 4 percent of the women without diabetes. Women who had diabetes for five years or longer had an elevated risk of recurrent urinary infections.

Urinary tract infections are common problems experienced by people with diabetes, especially women. (Women in general are more prone to UTIs than men, primarily because of the shortness of the urethra, which is the tube that leads to the bladder.)

Symptoms and Diagnostic Path
Common symptoms and signs of a urinary tract infection include the following:

- pain and burning with urination
- a feeling of urgency even after urination
- back pain
- microscopic or visible blood in the urine

Cultures of the urine can determine what type of bacteria are present and can also indicate what antibiotics would be most effective to eliminate the infection. However, often doctors prescribe medications the first time for infrequent UTIs, without ordering cultures or seeing results based on a urinalysis alone. The reason for this action is that doctors know there are specific bacteria that are commonly found in the urinary tract and the physician may assume that the bacteria causing the current infection is one of these. However, in people who have recurrent UTIs, a urine culture should be done.

Risk Factors and Preventive Measures

In a study reported in a 2000 issue of *Diabetes Care,* researchers studied women with both Type 1 and Type 2 diabetes. Among the women with Type 1 diabetes, 115 women or 20 percent of the total population, developed a urinary tract infection and many patients developed repeated infections.

For the women with Type 1 diabetes, 34 of the 241 women (14 percent) developed UTIs. Researchers found that the most common risk factor for the development of urinary tract infections was having had sexual intercourse the week before the study. A lesser risk factor was the use of oral contraceptives.

Of the women with Type 2 diabetes, 81 of the 348 women, or 23 percent, developed a urinary tract infection. For these women, the only significant risk was the existence of asymptomatic bacteria that was present in their urine when they joined the study. The authors concluded, "The risk factors for UTI development in diabetic women are the same as those reported for women without diabetes."

Urologists advise people with recurrent UTIs to drink plenty of fluid, especially water, every day. Some urologists also advise women who are prone to UTIs to urinate before and again after having sexual intercourse. Women may also be given medications that are bladder anesthetics in addition to antibiotics. The reasons for this is it may take several days before the antibiotic alleviates the symptoms. It is important for the entire course of medication to be taken to avoid recurrences.

Geerlings, Suzanne E., M.D., et al. "Risk Factors for Symptomatic Urinary Tract Infection in Women with Diabetes." *Diabetes Care* 23, no. 12 (December 2000): 1,737–1,741.

Gorter, Kees J., et al. "Risk of Recurrent Acute Lower Urinary Tract Infections and Prescription Pattern of Antibiotics in Women with and without Diabetes in Primary Care." *Family Practice Advance Access* 27, no. 4 (2010): 379–385.

urine testing   Laboratory testing of urine for diabetes, infection or other purposes. In the past, physicians tested individuals for diabetes by urinalysis, using REAGENT STRIPS. The problem with relying upon urinalysis for diagnosis is that an individual with diabetes may have fairly severe hyperglycemia well before any evidence actually appears in the person's urine. As a result, blood testing is far more reliable and is considered the "gold standard" for those with diabetes. However, urine testing is still an essential part of SICK DAY RULE management and is also essential if the physician suspects DIABETIC KETOACIDOSIS (DKA), a potentially fatal condition. KETONES are easily tested for in the urine.

Urine testing can be done for other purposes as well. For example, a urinalysis or urine culture is commonly performed to determine if a person has a URINARY TRACT INFECTION (the physician will test for red blood cells, white blood cells, and the presence of nitrates, an enzyme that will indicate the presence of bacteria). Sometimes, because of problems with DIABETIC NEUROPATHY, a person with diabetes who has a UTI may not have the common problems of pain and urgency that would be felt by a person without diabetes.

Urine testing is frequently done on patients with diabetes at office visits to test for protein in the urine (PROTEINURIA or MICROALBUMINURIA). If a routine urine reagent strip is used and it does not reveal the presence of proteins, then the physician may do a second test in the urine to screen for very tiny amounts of protein in the urine (microalbuminuria). Many times, a sample of urine will then be sent to the laboratory to quantitatively measure the very small amounts of protein, using a method called radioimmunoassay. This test can be followed serially by the physician to determine whether or not the patient's renal function is improving, stabilizing, or worsening.

vaginitis Infection in the vaginal area, often a fungal infection. Over 10 million office visits each year are attributed to vaginal discharge complaints. There are three very common causes: bacterial vaginosis (BV), vulvovaginal candidiasis (VC), and trichomoniasis.

Candidiasis causes about 50 percent of all vaginal infections. In about 85–90 percent of the cases of infections caused by yeast, the infection is caused by *Candida albicans* (this yeast is also normally found in the genital tracts of women of reproductive years). In recurrent or complicated cases of fungal vaginitis, the problem may be caused by *C. glabrata* or *C. tropicalis,* both of which are more difficult to treat. Diabetes by itself is a risk factor for colonization (presence of the organism without signs or symptoms of infection) of the vulvovaginal tract with candida. WOMEN WITH DIABETES are more likely to develop vaginal infections than are nondiabetics because of their elevated glucose levels. It is not uncommon for a gynecologist to diagnose women who have recurrent vaginal infections with diabetes.

Should the woman become pregnant, the physician needs to be informed, because it will affect the decision on what to prescribe; for example, oral antifungal medications could be dangerous during pregnancy.

Symptoms and Diagnostic Path
Some common symptoms of vaginal infection are

- unusual discharge (which, if yeast, often is characterized by a white or cottage cheese appearance to the discharge)
- pain with urination (this may also be a symptom of a URINARY TRACT INFECTION)
- pain with sexual intercourse (dyspareunia)
- itching/irritation/discomfort in the vaginal and/or vulvar area
- unusual odor in the vaginal area

It is also possible that a vaginal discharge or other symptom associated with a common form of vaginitis could instead be a sign of a sexually transmitted disease. For this reason, it is very important for the woman with diabetes who has symptoms of vaginitis to be examined by a medical doctor rather than attempting to self-medicate with over-the-counter drugs. The gynecologist can readily identify the source of the problem and determine the correct treatment. Typically the patient with true VC has redness, normal pH in the vagina, and a microscopic exam of the discharge that is consistent with Candida infection.

Cultures are rarely done as 15 percent or more of women may be colonized with yeast. In one study only 34 percent of women with vaginitis symptoms who thought they had VC actually had a confirmed diagnosis (cultures and microscopic examinations) after examination.

Treatment Options and Outlook
Treatment depends on the cause. If the physician believes the cause of the vaginitis is fungal, then he or she will prescribe an antifungal medication. The medication may come in the form of a cream or suppository to be inserted into the vaginal area or it may be an oral medication that is prescribed to eradicate a systemic fungal infection. One oral dose may be sufficient or a longer course may be needed. Some antifungal medications may be purchased over the counter. The medication

331

TABLE 1: TREATMENT REGIMENS FOR VULVOVAGINAL CANDIDIASIS APPROVED BY THE CDC

	Brand Name	Dosage (qhs)	Duration
Intravaginal agents (one of the following)			
Butoconazole 2% cream	Mycelex 3	5 g intravaginally	3 days*
Butoconazole 2% sustained release tablet	Gynazole-1	5 g intravaginally	Single dose
Clotrimazole 1% cream	Gyne-Lotrimin-7; Mycelex-7	5 g intravaginally	7–14 days*†
Clotrimazole 100 mg tablet	Gyne-Lotrimin-7	1 tablet intravaginally	7 days
Clotrimazole 100 mg tablet	Gyne-Lotrimin-7	Place 2 tablets intravaginally	3 days
Miconazole 2% cream	Monistat-7	5 g intravaginally	7 days*†
Miconazole 100 mg suppository	Monistat-7	1 suppository intravaginally	7 days*
Miconazole 200 mg suppository	Monistat-3	1 suppository intravaginally	3 days
Miconazole 1200 mg suppository	Monistat-1	1 suppository intravaginally	Single dose*
Nystatin 100,000 unit vaginal tablet	Mycostatin	1 tablet intravaginally	14 days
Tioconazole 6.5% ointment	Vagistat 1	5 g intravaginally	Single dose*
Terconazole 0.4% cream (45 gms)	Terazol-7	5 g intravaginally	7 days†
Terconazole 0.8% cream (25 gms)	Terazol-3	5 g intravaginally	3 days
Terconazole 80 mg suppository	Terazol-3	1 suppository intravaginally	3 days
Oral agents			
Fluconazole	Diflucan	150 mg oral tablet	Single dose

Source: Centers for Disease Control and Prevention. "Sexually Transmitted Diseases Treatment Guidelines." *Morbidity and Mortality Weekly Report Recomm Rep* 55 (2006).
*Available over-the-counter. †Recommended during pregnancy.

should provide relief fairly quickly in 80–90 percent of confirmed cases but the entire course of medication should be taken. If the woman has recurrent fungal infections, physicians may opt to instruct a patient to use an OTC medication if the exact same signs and symptoms recur, and after treating the most recent infection, the physician may prescribe low-dose preventive oral antifungal medications for as long as six months. See Tables 1 and 2 for more information on specific treatments.

TABLE 2: TREATMENT REGIMENS FOR BACTERIAL VAGINOSIS APPROVED BY THE CDC

Medication	Dose	Duration
Metronidazole	500 mg orally twice daily	7 days
Metronidazole gel 0.75%	One intravaginal application daily	5 days
Clindamycin cream 2%	One intravaginal application daily	7 days
Alternate Regimens*		
Clindamycin	300 mg orally bid	7 days
Clindamycin ovules	100 g once daily	3 days

*A 2 g oral dose of metronidazole is no longer recommended as an alternative for treating BV.

Centers for Disease Control and Prevention. "Sexually Transmitted Diseases Treatment Guidelines." *Morbidity and Mortality Weekly Report Recomm Rep* 55 (2006).

Many of the antifungal therapies used vaginally contain oils that may weaken condoms and/or diaphragms, and thus patients need to abstain from intercourse during therapy or use an alternative contraceptive method. Treatment of partners in uncomplicated cases is not recommended and is controversial even in complicated or recurrent VC.

Risk Factors and Preventive Measures

Tight glycemic control is critical for the woman with diabetes who has frequent bouts of vaginitis. Without it, infections are likely to recur.

See also TYPE 1 DIABETES; TYPE 2 DIABETES.

Mashburn, J. "Etiology, Diagnosis, and Management of Vaginitis." *Journal of Midwifery and Women's Health* 51, no. 6 (2006): 423–430.

Owen, M. K., and T. L. Clenney. "Management of Vaginitis." *American Family Physician* 70 (2004): 2,125–2,132.

veterans (military)   According to the Department of Veterans Affairs within the U.S. Veterans Administration, diabetes is more prevalent among military veterans than in the general population. This may be because many military veterans are older/retired men. An estimated 16 percent of military veterans, or about 500,000, have diabetes, versus about 6 percent of the general public. In addition, of the 5,900 AMPUTATIONS performed by the VA in 1999, 75 percent were performed on patients with diabetes. About 98 percent of these veterans were male and most were over age 65. (Most older military veterans are male.)

Veterans who developed or were diagnosed with diabetes during their military service or within one year after leaving the military may be eligible for additional compensation. Also, special rules apply to Vietnam veterans who have developed Type 2 diabetes since their discharge from military service.

Vietnam Veterans

Some evidence from the Institute of Medicine (IOM) has indicated a possible linkage between an exposure to Agent Orange and other herbicides that were used during the Vietnam War, and the subsequent development of Type 2 diabetes in veterans who served in Vietnam. The IOM report also noted that traditional risk factors for diabetes, such as OBESITY, sedentary lifestyle, and other factors common to the veterans, outweighed the Agent Orange–induced risk for diabetes.

However, as a result of the report, in November of 2000, the U.S. Department of Veterans Affairs (VA) ruled that military veterans who had served in Vietnam and were since diagnosed with Type 2 diabetes may be eligible to apply for disability compensation. According to VA estimates, an estimated 178,000 veterans may be eligible for this compensation.

In addition to Type 2 diabetes, the VA considers other conditions as service-connected for veterans who served in Vietnam, including prostate and respiratory cancers, acute or subacute PERIPHERAL NEUROPATHY (associated with diabetes), and other illnesses.

For further information, contact the local office of the Veterans Administration or the national office at its toll-free number, (800) 827-1000, or visit the Web site at www.va.gov.

vitamins   Fat or water soluble organic compounds that are required in very small amounts for normal cellular function and growth. Some vitamins, such as vitamin E, may cause an improvement in diabetic symptoms or in symptoms related to problems that stem from diabetes. However, clinical studies are ongoing and definitive health benefits are yet to be proven.

Vitamin B_1 and B_6 have been occasionally helpful in treating DIABETIC NEUROPATHY. Epidemiological data suggest that an increased intake of antioxidants can decrease cardiovascular disease risk. Patients with diabetes seem to have more oxidative damage. Thus, many patients and medical doctors use antioxidant vitamins such as vitamin C and vitamin E for patients with diabetes, although there is no long-term care data showing that these antioxidants clearly decrease hard endpoints such as heart attack or stroke.

waist to hip ratio (WHR) A comparison of waist size to hip size and a measure of obesity. The waist equals midway between the iliac crest, which is the top part of the pelvic bone, and the lowest rib. The hips are measured at the widest point.

Many studies have measured abdominal fat by comparing the waist size to the hip measurements. However, waist circumference alone appears to be a better measure of both abdominal fat and the risk of developing Type 2 diabetes than the WHR. People who have an "apple" shape (with enlarged abdomens) are at greater risk for health problems than overweight or obese people with "pear" shapes (who carry their fat in the hip area rather than the abdomen). Acceptable values are 0.8 to 1.0 for men and 0.7 to .85 for women.

Studies have found that when obese people with diabetes lose weight and consequently have a decrease in their abdominal fat, such people also show a related improvement in both glucose tolerance and insulin action.

See also BODY MASS INDEX; EATING DISORDERS; OBESITY.

whites/Caucasians Light-skinned individuals who are not of Hispanic, African-American, or Asian origin. Whites have an elevated risk for Type 1 diabetes; for example, data from the SEARCH for Diabetes in Youth Study revealed that the prevalence of Type 1 diabetes among whites ages 0–19 years was 2.0 per 100,000 subjects. (Prevalence is a statistical concept that refers to everyone who has a disease, no matter when they were diagnosed.) According to

researchers Ronny A. Bell and colleagues in their 2009 article in *Diabetes Care,* the prevalence of Type 2 diabetes was 0.18 per 1,000 white individuals ages 10–19 years. The incidence (the number of new cases in a year) of Type 1 diabetes for white subjects ages 0–19 years was 23.6 per 100,000 subjects, and the incidence of Type 2 diabetes among this group was 3.7 per 100,000 subjects in this age group. Note also that increasing numbers of researchers are concerned about OBESITY in American youths, which is likely to further escalate the rate of Type 2 diabetes among some children and adolescents.

In considering only adults with diabetes, according to the Centers for Disease Control and Prevention (CDC), 6.6 percent of non-Hispanic white adults age 20 and older have been diagnosed with diabetes. This is the lowest rate of diagnosed diabetes among the various rates and ethnicities; for example, the rate was 7.5 percent for Asian Americans, 10.4 percent for Hispanics, and 11.8 percent for African Americans.

Youths with Diabetes

In considering youths ages 0–19 years old, data from the SEARCH for Diabetes in Youth Study revealed that the incidence of Type 1 diabetes among non-Hispanic whites is one of the highest rates in the world. According to Bell and colleagues Type 1 diabetes occurs most frequently among individuals who are of northern European descent; for example, the rates of Type 1 diabetes among youths in a World Health Organization study showed that the worldwide rates of Type 1 diabetes ranges from about 40.9 per 100,000 youths in Finland, 30.6 per 100,000 youths in Italy, and 29.4 per 100,000 youths in Sweden among youths ages 14 and younger. In contrast, the rates of Type 1 diabetes are only 0.1 per 100,000 youths in both China and Venezuela. Thus, youths in Finland, Italy, and Sweden have about a 350 times greater rate of Type 1 diabetes than youths in Venezuela and China, say the researchers.

Adults with Diabetes

Among adults, non-Hispanic whites continue to have the highest rate of Type 1 diabetes. However, with regard to Type 2 diabetes, African American, American Indian, and Hispanic adults all have higher rates. Individuals of other races and ethnicities also have a higher rate of suffering from serious complications of diabetes; for example, according to the National Kidney Disease Education Program (NKDEP), among new patients with kidney failure that was caused by diabetes, nearly a third (31.3 percent) are African American. African Americans are also much more likely than non-Hispanic whites to have high blood pressure (hypertension), and African American males ages 30–39 years have 14 times greater risk of kidney failure caused by hypertension than Caucasian men in the same age group.

Many adults have both diabetes and hypertension, further escalating the risk for kidney disease and kidney failure. According to the NKDEP, diabetes and high blood pressure together account for 70 percent of new cases of kidney failure. (See DIABETIC NEPHROPATHY.)

See also AFRICAN AMERICANS WITH DIABETES; AMERICAN INDIANS/ALASKA NATIVES; ASIANS/PACIFIC ISLANDER AMERICANS; DIABETES MELLITUS; HISPANICS/LATINOS.

Bell, Ronny A., et al. "Diabetes in Non-Hispanic White Youth." *Diabetes Care* 32, Supplement 2 (2009): S102–S111.

Mayer-Davis, Elizabeth, et al. "The Many Faces of Diabetes in American Youth: Type 1 and Type 2 Diabetes in Five Race and Ethnic Populations: The SEARCH for Diabetes in Youth Study." *Diabetes Care* 32, Supplement 2 (2009): S99–S101.

National Diabetes Information Clearinghouse. National Diabetes Statistics, 2007. Available online. URL: http://diabetes.niddk.nih.gov/DM/PUBS/statistics/DM_Statistics.pdf. Downloaded October 23, 2009.

whole grain foods Foods that contain items such as oats and whole wheat. Some research has indicated that eating whole grain foods such as oatmeal and whole grain breads can significantly reduce the risk for developing Type 2 diabetes. In a 2000 study in the *American Journal of Public Health,* conducted by researchers at Harvard University on the diets of more than 75,000 women over 10 years, researchers found that one serving of cooked oatmeal eaten two to four times per week was linked to a 16 percent reduction in the risk for developing Type 2 diabetes. In addition, the study also revealed that consuming one serving of oatmeal five or six times per week was linked to a 39 percent reduction in risk.

The researchers said, "The overall protective effect of whole grains (on risk for Type 2 Diabetes) was observed for individual whole-grain foods, including dark bread, whole grain breakfast cereal, popcorn, oatmeal, brown rice, wheat germ, bran and other grains."

Whole grain contains FIBER, which may be another reason why it has healthful preventive effects against Type 2 diabetes.

See also CARBOHYDRATES AND MEAL PLANNING; DIET.

Liu et al. "A Prospective Study of Whole-Grain Intake and Risk of Type 2 Diabetes Mellitus in U.S. Women." *American Journal of Public Health* 90, no. 9 (2000): 409–415.

Wisconsin Diabetic Retinopathy Study (WESDR)

A study that occurred between July 1979 and June 1980 on patients with diabetes in Wisconsin, with the purpose of identifying risk factors for the development of DIABETIC RETINOPATHY. The researchers also looked at the number of patients who required CATARACT surgery at a later date.

The WESDR study divided patients into two groups. One group of 1,210 patients, the "younger-onset" group, were diagnosed with diabetes before the age of 30 and were also using insulin. The other group was comprised of 1,770 patients who were diagnosed after age 30, the "older-onset" group. In the older group, 824 patients were using insulin and 956 patients were not. The subjects were followed four years later and then again, ten years later. (Not all subjects participated in follow-ups. Some had died or relocated or were not interested in participating.)

Cataract Surgery

Over a 10-year period, the researchers found that 27 percent of the people with diabetes in the "younger-onset" group (who were 45 years or older at follow-up) needed cataract surgery. They also found that 44 percent of the "older-onset" group who were age 75 or older had already had cataract surgery.

Factors associated with needing cataract surgery were as follows among the younger-onset group:

- severity of diabetic retinopathy
- high systolic blood pressure
- proteinuria (equal to or less than 0.30 g)
- use of thiazide diuretics
- use of central antiadrenergic agents

Among the older-onset patients with diabetes, the primary associated factor for requiring cataract surgery was the use of thiazide diuretics.

Study Findings

The WESDR demonstrated that increased levels of cholesterol were associated with an increased severity of retinal hard exudates (a leakage of fat and protein into the retina). Epidemiological follow-up data revealed that 90 percent of the patients with Type 1 diabetes who were diagnosed at over 30 years old had retinopathy after 10–15 years of diabetes. Proliferative retinopa-thy was seen in 25 percent of Type 1 patients after 10–15 years.

For patients over 30 years old who were diagnosed with Type 2 diabetes, they had been diagnosed less than five years ago. Forty percent of the patients who were taking insulin and 24 percent who were taking oral medication had retinopathy.

Aspirin use in patients with proliferative retinopathy did not increase the risk of vitreous hemorrhage and was associated with a 17 percent decrease in cardiovascular disease and death. Therefore, the existence of proliferative retinopathy is not a contraindication for aspirin.

The study also showed that high cholesterol levels were associated with an increased risk of retinopathy. In addition, it showed that early laser therapy in older patients with severe nonproliferative and early proliferative retinopathy was effective at reducing vision loss.

In addition, the study demonstrated that laser therapy was beneficial for patients who had macular edema involving or threatening to involve the center of the macula.

See also DIABETIC EYE DISEASES; DIURETICS.

The Diabetes Control and Complications Trial Research Group. "A Comparison of the Study Populations in the Diabetes Control and Complications Trial and the Wisconsin Epidemiologic Study of Diabetic Retinopathy." *Archives of Internal Medicine* 155 (April 10, 1995): 745–754.

Klein, Barbara E. K. "Incidence of Cataract Surgery in the Wisconsin Epidemiologic Study of Diabetic Retinopathy." *American Journal of Ophthalmology* 119, no. 3 (March 1995): 295–301.

women with diabetes Females with Type 1 or Type 2 diabetes. About 11.5 million women in the United States have diabetes according to the American Diabetes Association, or 10.2 percent of all adult women age 20 years and older. However, nearly 25 percent of them have not yet been diagnosed with the disease. Most women with diabetes, about 90–95 percent, have Type 2 diabetes.

Generally, females with Type 1 diabetes have an onset of the disease during their childhood or adolescence, while the onset of Type 2 diabetes often occurs during adulthood. However, it is possible for Type 1 diabetes to appear in adulthood. GESTATIONAL DIABETES MELLITUS (GDM) is diabetes that occurs during pregnancy. However, most women with gestational diabetes have risk factors for Type 2 diabetes.

Female Diabetics Compared to Male Diabetics and Nondiabetic Women

Diabetes affects both genders, but women are affected in several unique ways. For example, women with diabetes are at much greater risk of death from coronary heart disease than nondiabetic men or women; middle-aged women with diabetes ages 45–64 years are three to seven times more likely to have coronary heart disease. The risk for coronary heart disease among diabetic women is even greater than for diabetic men, the reverse of the situation for nondiabetics, where men have the higher risk.

Women with diabetes also have a greater risk for developing HYPERTENSION than nondiabetic people as well as than men with diabetes. In addition, women with diabetes are also at a higher risk of dying from CARDIOVASCULAR DISEASE than are nondiabetics or men with diabetes.

As might be expected, women with diabetes have a shorter life expectancy than nondiabetic women. In addition, women with diabetes have a greater risk for suffering from BLINDNESS than nondiabetics, and they also have a greater risk for blindness than men with diabetes. At least part of the reason for this is that women live longer than men, but diabetes is also a pacing factor.

If they become pregnant, women with diabetes require careful monitoring during PREGNANCY to avoid harm to the fetus and also to themselves. In addition, some women who have not previously been diagnosed with diabetes may have gestational diabetes mellitus (GDM) during the pregnancy only. This illness should be carefully monitored by the patient and her physician because of serious potential harm that may come to both mother and child if glucose levels are not kept under good control.

Women with diabetes are prone to developing a variety of medical problems that nondiabetic women face at a much lower rate, such as vaginitis or infections. Women with diabetes also have a risk of developing DIABETIC KETOACIDOSIS (DKA) that is an estimated 50 percent greater than the risk faced by men. In addition, women with diabetes are also nearly eight times more likely to suffer from peripheral vascular disease (a diminished blood and oxygen flow to the feet and lungs, causing pain) than are men.

The risk of STROKE that women with diabetes face is four times greater than the risk found among men with diabetes.

Most older women with Type 2 diabetes are obese, and 70 percent of them are 20 percent or more over their desired weight. Physical inactivity is another risk factor for Type 2 diabetes, and many older people have significantly decreased levels of physical activity.

In a study of thousands of patients in a diabetes registry versus control group subjects, reported by Gregory A. Nichols and colleagues in 2009 in *Diabetes Care*, the researchers found that diabetes was a predictive factor for atrial fibrillation (irregular heartbeat) in women only. The researchers said, "Diabetes was not a significant predictor of atrial fibrillation among men after controlling for other risk factors but was highly significant among women." They said their findings were new and needed further exploration.

The sexual dysfunction that occurs in women with diabetes is felt to be a neurological complication. It can lead to diminished desire, decreased arousal, an inability to climax, and a failure to lubricate adequately, leading to painful intercourse (dyspareunia). There are no easily done or established tests to confirm the diagnosis. The diagnosis is primarily made via the medical history, and many women are not comfortable discussing this subject with a male primary care physician or endocrinologist, although many will discuss it with their gynecologists.

Problematic Behaviors

SMOKING is a risk behavior that increases the risk of cardiovascular disease among the already high-risk females with diabetes. Yet many young adults smoke, and some research indicates that people with diabetes are more likely to smoke than nondiabetics. According to the Centers for Disease Control and Prevention (CDC), almost half (47 percent) of women with diabetes have a BODY MASS INDEX (BMI) that is greater than 30, indicating obesity, compared to 25 percent of all women with the same BMI.

Racial and Ethnic Differences among Women with Diabetes

Women of some races and ethnicities have a greater risk for the development of diabetes; for example, American Indian women pass everyone when it comes to risk for developing diabetes. The Pima Indians are at very high risk for diabetes and the majority (70 percent) of middle-aged Pima women have diabetes. About 41 percent of middle-aged Navajo women have diabetes.

Psychological Impact of Diabetes

Some research indicates that women are troubled by their diabetes, and particularly by weight gain that may be associated with medications for diabetes. Some young women with Type 1 diabetes reportedly purposely allow their blood sugar levels to go high by not taking their insulin so that they can lose weight. This is very dangerous and can result in the need for a hospitalization.

In a 2007 study of 100 diabetic women from India ranging in age from 30–65 years, Purnima Awasthi and R. C. Mishra analyzed the women's responses to psychological measures. They found that women who used "approach" (proactive) methods of coping with their diabetes scored lower on feelings of interpersonal, psychological, and physiological consequences of their illness, and they also scored high in their belief in themselves and also in their physician with regard to their diabetes. (In other words, they apparently felt more in control.)

In contrast, women who used avoidance methods of coping with their diabetes scored high on measures that indicated a belief of problems with interpersonal, psychological, and physiological consequences of their diabetes. In addition, this group scored lower in their belief in themselves and their doctors.

In another study which concentrated on young women with Type 1 diabetes, reported by Catharine Kay and colleagues in 2009 in the *Journal of Health Psychology,* the researchers performed semi-structured interviews with nine women ages 19–25 years in the United Kingdom, then analyzed the results. One of the themes which emerged was the women's concern about their weight, and all of the women said that they wanted to lose weight. One of the women compared purposely having high blood sugar levels to extreme dieting. Another theme centered on the personal challenges of having diabetes, and the researchers said, "There was a strong sense that the women felt restricted or disadvantaged at times compared with other people who don't have diabetes."

A third theme was how their diabetes affected their relationships with others, and the participants were concerned with how they were viewed by other people. Some of the women felt that their identity was affected by the diabetes, and they said they did not want to be seen primarily as a person with diabetes. In addition, the participants said they did not feel understood by nondiabetics. However, when they were able to speak to another person with diabetes, this was important and helpful. The researchers said, "There was much evidence of change and adjustment to life with diabetes in the women's accounts, which ranged from young women trying to live their lives as if they did not have diabetes (as much as possible) to feeling beaten by diabetes and feeling it had a very damaging effect socially."

See also MEN WITH DIABETES.

Awasthi, Purnima, and R. C. Mishra. "Role of Coping Strategies and Social Support in Perceived Illness Consequences and Controllability Among Diabetic Women." *Psychology and Developing Societies* 19, no. 2 (2007): 179–197.

Kay, Catharine, et al. "An Exploration of the Experiences of Young Women Living with Type 1 Diabetes." *Journal of Health Psychology* 14 (2009): 242–250.

Nichols, Gregory A., Kyndaron Reinier, and Sumeet S. Chugh, M.D. "Independent Contribution of Diabetes to Increased Prevalence and Incidence of Atrial Fibrillation." *Diabetes Care* 32 (2009): 1,851–1,856.

yeast infections Fungal infections, usually of the genitals or the mouth, but which can also be found in other parts of the body. People with diabetes are more susceptible to yeast infections than are nondiabetics. WOMEN WITH DIABETES are more likely than nondiabetics to develop vaginal yeast infections. Individuals who have been on antibiotic regimens are also susceptible to developing a yeast infection, particularly when they have been on more than one course of antibiotics.

These infections are treated with prescribed or over-the-counter antifungal creams, suppositories, or oral medications. Sometimes infections are also treated with ALTERNATIVE MEDICINE such as acidophilus tablets, which may also be used as a preventive remedy in some cases.

The most common forms of yeast infections are thrush, esophageal yeast infection, Candida balanitis and Candida VAGINITIS. Thrush is an oral infection, characterized by a white or black tongue and throat. The key symptom of an esophageal yeast infection is painful swallowing. Candida balanitis is an infection of the foreskin of the penis. Candida vaginitis is a yeast infection of the vaginal area.

youths See ADOLESCENTS WITH DIABETES.

zinc A trace element needed by humans and usually obtained through food. Individuals with diabetes, particularly those who are elderly, may experience a deficiency of zinc. Zinc aids in the healing of wounds and a deficiency could lead to an increased probability of pressure ulcers, particularly in homebound individuals or those confined to their beds. Experts recommend that individuals with diabetes who are experiencing pressure ulcers should be supplied with supplemental zinc.

When people with diabetes develop low zinc levels, it has often been felt to be secondary to either poor intake or increased excretion associated with poor glycemic control. Improvement in glycemic control can help improve zinc levels.

APPENDIXES

APPENDIX I
IMPORTANT ORGANIZATIONS

AARP
601 E Street NW
Washington, DC 20049
(888) 687-2277
http://www.aarp.org

Administration on Aging
Department of Health and Human Services
330 Independence Avenue SW
Washington, DC 20201
(202) 619-0724
http://www.aoa.gov

Alzheimer's Association
225 North Michigan Avenue
Floor 17
Chicago, IL 60611
(312) 335-8700
(800) 272-3900 (toll-free)
http://www.alz.org

American Academy of Ophthalmology
P.O. Box 7424
San Francisco, CA 94120-7424
(415) 561-8500
http://www.aao.org

American Academy of Optometry
6110 Executive Boulevard
Suite 506
Rockville, MD 20852
(301) 984-1441
http://www.aaopt.org

American Academy of Pediatrics
141 Northwest Point Boulevard
Elk Grove Village, IL 60007
(847) 434-4000
http://www.aap.org

American Association for Marriage and Family Therapy
112 South Alfred Street
Alexandria, VA 22314
(703) 838-9808
http://www.aamft.org

American Association of Clinical Endocrinologists (AACE)
245 Riverside Avenue
Suite 200
Jacksonville, FL 32202
(904) 353-7878
http://www.aace.com

American Association of Diabetes Educators (AADE)
200 West Madison Street
Suite 800
Chicago, IL 60606
(800) 338-3633
http://www.diabeteseducator.org

American Association of Sex Educators, Counselors and Therapists
P.O. Box 1960
Ashland, VA 23005-1960
(804) 752-0026
http://www.aasect.org

American Bar Association Commission on Mental and Physical Disability Law
740 15th Street NW
Washington, DC 20005-1009
(202) 666-1000
http://www.abanet.org/disability

American Board of Medical Specialties
1007 Church Street
Suite 404
Evanston, IL 60201
(847) 491-9091
http://www.abms.org

American Chronic Pain Association
P.O. Box 850
Rocklin, CA 95677-0850
(800) 533-3231
http://www.theacpa.org

The American College of Foot and Ankle Surgeons (ACFAS)
8725 West Higgins Road
Suite 555
Chicago, IL 60631
(773) 693-9300
http://www.acfas.org

American Council of the Blind
2200 Wilson Boulevard
Arlington, VA 22201
(202) 467-5081
(800) 424-8666 (toll-free)
http://www.acb.org

American Diabetes Association (ADA)
National Call Center
1701 North Beauregard Street
Alexandria, VA 22311
(800) 342-2383
http://www.diabetes.org

American Dietetic Association
120 South Riverside Plaza
Suite 2000
Chicago, IL 60606
(800) 877-1600
http://www.eatright.org

American Foundation for the Blind
11 Penn Plaza
Suite 300
New York, NY 10001
(212) 502-7634
http://www.afb.org

American Heart Association/American Stroke Association
7272 Greenville Avenue
Dallas, TX 75231-4596
(800) AHA-USA1 (242-8721)
http://www.americanheart.org

American Medical Association
515 North State Street
Chicago, IL 60654
(800) 621-8335
http://www.ama-assn.org

American Optometric Association
1505 Prince Street
Suite 300
Alexandria, VA 22314
(800) 365-2219
http://www.aoanet.org

American Pharmacists Association
1100 15th Street NW
Suite 400
Washington, DC 20005-1707
(800) 237-APhA (2742)
(202) 628-4410
http://www.pharmacyandyou.org/

American Podiatric Medical Association (APMA)
9312 Old Georgetown Road
Bethesda, MD 20814-1621
(301) 571-9200
http://www.apma.org

American Printing House for the Blind
1839 Frankfurt Avenue
P.O. Box 6085
Louisville, KY 40206
(502) 895-2405
(800) 223-1839 (toll-free)
http://www.aph.org/

American Psychiatric Association
1000 Wilson Boulevard
Suite 1825
Arlington, VA 22209
(888) 35-PSYCH (77924) (toll-free)
http://www.psych.org

American Psychological Association
750 First Street NE
Washington, DC 20002-4242
(202) 336-5500
http://www.apa.org

American Society of Human Genetics
9650 Rockville Pike
Bethesda, MD 20814
(301) 634-7300
http://www.ashg.org

American Society of Nephrology (ASN)
1725 I Street NW
Suite 510
Washington, DC 20006
(202) 659-0599
http://www.asn-online.com

American Urological Association (AUA)
1000 Corporate Boulevard
Linthicum, MD 21090
(410) 687-3700
http://www.auanet.org

Association for Glycogen Storage Disease
P.O. Box 896
Durant, IA 52747
(563) 785-6038
http://www.agsdus.org

Association of American Indian Physicians
1235 Sovereign Row
Suite 103
Oklahoma City, OK 73108
(405) 946-7072
http://www.aaip.org

Association of Asian Pacific Community Health Organizations
300 Frank H. Ogawa Plaza
Suite 620
Oakland, CA 94612
(510) 272-9536
http://www.aapcho.org

Centers for Disease Control and Prevention (CDC)
1600 Clifford Road
Atlanta, GA 30333
(877) 232-4636
http://www.cdc.gov

Centers for Medicare and Medicaid Services (formerly the Health Care Financing Administration)
7500 Security Boulevard
Baltimore, MD 21244
(800) 633-4227
http://www.cms.hhs.gov

Diabetes Action Research and Education Foundation
426 C Street NE
Washington, DC 20002
(202) 333-4520
http://www.diabetesaction.org

Diabetes Exercise and Sports Association (DESA)
P.O. Box 1935
Litchfield Park, AZ 85340
(623) 535-4593
(800) 898-4322 (toll-free)
http://www.diabetes-exercise.org

Disability Rights Education and Defense Fund, Inc.
2212 6th Street
Berkeley, CA 94710
(510) 644-2555 (voice and TDD)
(800) 348-4232 (toll-free)
http://www.dredf.org

Easter Seals Disability Services
233 South Wacker Drive
Suite 2400
Chicago, IL 60606
312-726-6200
http://www.easterseals.com

Eldercare Locator
National Association of Area Agencies on Aging
1730 Rhode Island Avenue NW
Suite 1200
Washington, DC 20036
(202) 872-0888
http://www.n4a.org/

Endocrine Society
8401 Connecticut Avenue
Suite 900
Chevy Chase, MD 20815
(301) 941-0200
http://www.endo-society.org

Family Caregiver Alliance
1 Montgomery Street
Suite 1100
San Francisco, CA 94104
(415) 434-3388
http://www.caregiver.org/caregiver/jsp/home.jsp

Food and Nutrition Information Center
National Agricultural Library/USDA
10301 Baltimore Avenue
Room 105
Beltsville, MD 20705
(301) 504-5719
http://fnic.nal.usda.gov/nal_display/index.
    php?info_center=4&tax_level=1

The Genetic Alliance
4301 Connecticut Avenue NW
Suite 404
Washington, DC 20008-2304
(202) 966-5557
http://www.geneticalliance.org

The Glaucoma Foundation
80 Maiden Lane
Suite 700
New York, NY 10038
(212) 285-0080
http://www.glaucomafoundation.org/

Indian Health Service Headquarters
Diabetes Program
5300 Homestead Road NE
Albuquerque, NM 87110
(505) 248-4182
http://www.his.gov/MedicalPrograms/Diabetes

**Juvenile Diabetes Research Foundation
    (JDF) International**
120 Wall Street
19th Floor
New York, NY 10005

(800) 533-CURE (2873) (toll-free)
http://www.jdf.org

National Alliance for Hispanic Health
1501 16th Street NW
Washington, DC 20036
(202) 387-5000
http://www.hispanichealth.org

National Amputation Foundation
38–40 Church Street
Malverne, NY 11565
(516) 887-3600
http://www.nationalamputation.org/

**National Association for Visually
    Handicapped (East Coast)**
22 West 21st Street
New York, NY 10010
(212) 889-3141
http://www.navh.org

**National Certification Board for Diabetes
    Educators**
330 East Algonquin Road
Suite 4
Arlington Heights, IL 60005
(847) 228-9795
http://www.ncbde.org

National Council on Aging
1901 L Street NW
4th Floor
Washington, DC 20036
(202) 479-1200
http://www.ncoa.org

National Diabetes Education Program
1 Diabetes Way
Bethesda, MD 20892
(800) 438-5383 (toll-free)
http://www.ndep.nih.gov

**National Diabetes Information
    Clearinghouse (NDIC)**
1 Information Way
Bethesda, MD 20892-3560
(800) 860-8747 (toll-free)
http://www.niddk.nih.gov/health/ diabetes.
    ndic.htm

National Digestive Diseases Information Clearinghouse
1 Information Way
Bethesda, MD 20892
(800) 891-5389 (toll-free)
http://www.digestive.niddk.nih.gov

National Eye Institute
Information Office
31 Center Drive, MSC 2510
Bethesda, MD 20892-2510
(301) 496-5248
http://www.nei.nih.gov

National Family Caregivers Association
10400 Connecticut Avenue
Suite 500
Kensington, MD 20895-3944
(301) 942-6430
(800) 896-3650 (toll-free)
http://www.nfcacares.org

National Federation of the Blind
1800 Johnson Street
Baltimore, MD 21230
(410) 659-9314
http://www.nfb.org

National Glycohemoglobin Standardization Program
Department of Child Health
University of Missouri Hospital & Clinics
1 Hospital Drive N712
Columbia, MO 65212
(573) 882-6882
http://www.ngsp.org

National Heart, Lung and Blood Institute
Information Center
P.O. Box 30105
Bethesda, MD 20824-0105
(301) 592-8573
http://www.nhlbi.nih.gov

National Information Center for Children and Youth with Disabilities (NICHCY)
P.O. Box 1492
Washington, DC 20013

(800) 695-0285
http://www.nichcy.org

National Institute of Diabetes and Digestive and Kidney Diseases (NIDDK)
National Institutes of Health
Building 31, Room 9A06
31 Center Drive, MSC 2560
Bethesda, MD 20892-2560
(301) 496-3583
http://www.niddk.nih.gov

National Institute on Aging
Building 31, Room 5C27
31 Center Drive, MSC 2292
Bethesda, MD 20892
(301) 496-1752
http://www.hih.gov/nia

National Kidney and Urologic
Diseases Information Clearinghouse (NKUDIC)
3 Information Way
Bethesda, MD 20892-3580
(800) 891-5390 or (301) 654-4415
http://www.niddk.nih.gov/health/ kidney/ kidney.htm

National Kidney Disease Education Program
3 Kidney Information Way
Bethesda, MD 20892
(866) 454-3639
http://www.nkdep.nih.gov

National Kidney Foundation, Inc.
30 East 33rd Street
New York, NY 10016
(800) 622-9010
http://www.kidney.org

National Library Service for the Blind and Physically Handicapped
Library of Congress
1291 Taylor Street NW
Washington, DC 20011
(202) 707-5100
(202) 707-0744 (TDD)
http://www.loc.gov/nls/

National Organization for Rare Disorders
55 Kenosia Avenue
P.O. Box 1968
Danbury, CT 06813-1968
(203) 744-0100
http://www.rarediseases.org

National Osteoporosis Foundation
1232 22nd Street NW
Washington, DC 20037
(202) 223-2226
http://www.nof.org

National Rehabilitation Information Center
8201 Corporate Drive
Suite 600
Landover, MD 20785
(800) 346-2742 (toll-free)
http://www.naric.com

National Stroke Association
9707 East Easter Lane
Englewood, CO 80112-3747
(303) 649-9299
(800) STROKES (toll-free)
http://www.stroke.org

Office of Minority Health Resource Center
P.O. Box 37337
Washington, DC 20013
(800) 444-6472 (toll-free)
http://www.omhrc.gov

Pedorthic Footwear Association (PFA)
2025 M Street NW
Suite 800
Washington, DC 20036
(202) 367-1145
(800) 673-8447 (toll-free)
http://www.pedorthics.org

President's Council on Physical Fitness and Sports
200 Independence Avenue SW
Room 7384
Washington, DC 20201

(202) 272-3421
http://www.fitness.gov

Prevent Blindness America
211 West Wacker Drive
Suite 1700
Chicago, IL 60606
(800) 331-2020
http://www.preventblindness.org

Recording for the Blind and Dyslexic
20 Riszel Road
Princeton, NJ 08540
(866) 732-3585
http://www.rfhd.org

The Seeing Eye Inc.
P.O. Box 375
Morristown, NJ 07943-0375
(973) 539-4425
http://www.seeingeye.org

Transplant Recipient International Organization
2100 M Street NW, #170-353
Washington, DC 20037-1233
(202) 293-0980
(800) TRIO-386 (toll-free)
http://www.trioweb.org/

United Network for Organ Sharing
P.O. Box 2484
Richmond, VA 23218
(804) 782-4800
http://www.unos.org

Veterans Health Administration
Program Chief, Diabetes
810 Vermont Avenue NW
Washington, DC 20420
(202) 273-5400
http://www1.va.gov/diabetes/#veterans

Weight-control Information Network
1 WIN Way
Bethesda, MD 20892-3665
(877) 946-4627
http://www.win.niddk.nih.gov/

APPENDIX II
DIABETES PERIODICALS

Clinical Diabetes
American Diabetes Association
1701 N. Beauregard Street
Alexandria, VA 22311
(800) 806-7801 (toll-free)

Diabetes
American Diabetes Association
1701 N. Beauregard Street
Alexandria, VA 22311
(800) 806-7801 (toll-free)

Diabetes Care
American Diabetes Association
1701 N. Beauregard Street
Alexandria, VA 22311
(800) 806-7801 (toll-free)

Diabetes Forecast
American Diabetes Association
1701 N. Beauregard Street
Alexandria, VA 22311
(800) 806-7801

Diabetes Self-Management
R.A. Rapaport Publishing, Inc.
150 West 22nd Street
New York, NY 10011
(800) 234-0923 (toll-free)

Diabetes Spectrum
American Diabetes Association
1701 N. Beauregard Street
Alexandria, VA 22311
(800) 806-7801 (toll-free)

Diabetic Cooking
Publications International, Ltd.
7373 North Cicero Avenue
Lincolnwood, IL 60712

APPENDIX III
DIABETES RESEARCH AND TRAINING CENTERS (DRTCs)

The National Institute of Diabetes and Digestive and Kidney Diseases (NIDDK) supports the research, seminars, and training materials of six diabetes research and training centers nationwide.

Albert Einstein College of Medicine DRTC
Department of Medicine (Endocrinology)
Department of Epidemiology and Population
   Health
701 Belfer Building, Room 705
1300 Morris Park Avenue
Bronx, NY 10461
(718) 430-3242
(718) 430-8557 (fax)

Indiana University DRTC
Indiana University School of Medicine
National Institute for Fitness and Sport
Room 122
250 North University Boulevard
Indianapolis, IN 46202
(317) 278-0905
(317) 278-0911 (fax)

University of Chicago DRTC
Howard Hughes Medical Institute
University of Chicago
Bell Laboratory
5812 South Ellis Street
Chicago, IL 60637
(773) 702-1334
(773) 702-4292 (fax)

University of Michigan DRTC
Michigan Diabetes Research and Training
   Center
University of Michigan Medical School
300 NIB, 3DO6, Box 0489
Ann Arbor, MI 48109
(734) 936-9237
(734) 936-8967 (fax)

Vanderbilt University DRTC
Director, Division of Diabetes, Endocrinology,
   and Metabolism
Division of Diabetes, Endocrinology and
   Metabolism
2220 Pierce Avenue, 715 PRB
Nashville, TN 37232
(615) 936-1649
(615) 936-1667 (fax)

Washington University DRTC
Psychology, Medicine, and Pediatrics
Division of Health Behavior Research
Washington University
4444 Forest Park Avenue
St. Louis, MO 63108
(314) 286-1900
(314) 286-1919 (fax)

APPENDIX IV
DIABETES ENDOCRINOLOGY RESEARCH CENTERS (DERCs)

Joslin Diabetes Center DERD
One Joslin Place
Boston, MA 02215
(617) 732-2635
(617) 732-2487 (fax)
http://www.joslin.harvard.edu

Massachusetts General Hospital DERC
Diabetes Unit Medical Service
Wellman 8
55 Fruit Street
Boston, MA 02114
(617) 726-6909
(617) 726-6909 (fax)

University of Colorado DERC
Barbara Davis Center for Childhood Diabetes
1775 North Ursula Street
P.O. Box 6511
Mail Stop Box B-140
Aurora, CO 80045
(303) 724-6837
http://www.uchsc.edu/misc/diabetes/DERC/
index.htm

University of Iowa DERC
Iowa Diabetes-Endocrinology Research Center
VA/JDF Diabetes Research Center
3E19 VA Medical Center
Iowa City, IA 52246
(319) 338-0581, extension 7625
(319) 339-7025 (fax)
http://www.int-med.uiowa.edu/faculty.htm

University of Massachusetts Medical School DERC
373 Plantation Street
Suite 218
Worcester, MA 01605
(508) 856-3800
(508) 856-4093 (fax)
http://www.umassedu.diabetes

University of Pennsylvania DERC
Division of Endocrinology, Diabetes and
Metabolism
611 Clinical Research Building
415 Curie Boulevard
Philadelphia, PA 19104
(215) 898-0198
(215) 898-5408 (fax)
http://www.uphs.upenn.edu/endocrin/faculty/
lazar.htm.

University of Washington DERC
DVA Puget Sound Health Care System
1660 South Columbian Way
Seattle, WA 98109
(206) 764-2688
(206) 764-2693 (fax)

Yale University School of Medicine DERC
Department of Internal Medicine
P.O. Box 208020
333 Cedar Street
New Haven, CT 06520
(203) 785-4183
(203) 737-5558 (fax)

APPENDIX V
DIABETES CONTROL PROGRAMS IN U.S. STATES AND TERRITORIES

ALABAMA

Alabama Diabetes Prevention and Control Program
Bureau of Health Promotion & Chronic Disease
State of Alabama Department of Public Health
201 Monroe Street
Suite 976
Montgomery, AL 35104
(334) 206-5300
(334) 206-5609 (fax)
http://www.adph.org/diabetes

ALASKA

Alaska Diabetes Prevention and Control Program
P.O. Box 240249
3601 C Street
Suite 722
Anchorage, AK 99524-0249
(907) 269-8035
(907) 269-5446 (fax)
http://www.hss.state.ak.us/dph/chronic/diabetes/default.htm

ARIZONA

Arizona Diabetes Control & Prevention Coordinator
Arizona Department of Health Services
150 North 18th Avenue
Suite 310
Phoenix, AZ 85007
(602) 542-1214
(602) 542-6512 (fax)
http://www.azdiabetes.gov

ARKANSAS

Arkansas Department of Health
4815 W. Markham, Slot #3
Little Rock, AR 72205
(501) 661-2093
(501) 661-2009 (fax)
http://www.healthyarkansas.com/services/services_diabetes.html

CALIFORNIA

California Department of Public Health
Diabetes Prevention and Control Program, MS 7211
P.O. Box 997377
Sacramento, CA 95899-7377
(916) 552-9942
(916) 552-9988 (fax)
http://www.caldiabetes.org/

COLORADO

Colorado Diabetes Prevention and Control Program
Colorado Department of Public Health and Environment
4300 Cherry Creek Drive South, #A-5
Denver, CO 80246
(303) 692-2577
(303) 691-7900 (fax)
http://www.cdphe.state.co.us/pp/diabetes/index.html

CONNECTICUT

Connecticut Department of Public Health
Health Information Systems and Reporting
    Section
410 Capitol Avenue
Hartford, CT 06134-0308
(860) 509-7711
(860) 509-8403 (fax)
http://www.ct.gov/dph

DELAWARE

**Delaware Diabetes Prevention and
    Control Program**
Thomas Collins Building
Suite 10
540 South DuPont Highway
Dover, DE 19901
(302) 744-1020
(302) 739-2544 (fax)
http://www.dhss.delaware.gov/dph/

DISTRICT OF COLUMBIA

**District of Columbia Diabetes Prevention
    and Control Program**
825 North Capitol Street NE
Third Floor
Washington, DC 20002
(202) 671-5000
(202) 442-4825 (fax)
http://doh.dc.gov/doh/cwp/
    view,a,1373,q,582788,dohNav_
    GID,1801,dohNav,l33183l33187l.asp

FLORIDA

**Florida Diabetes Prevention and Control
    Program**
Bureau of Chronic Disease Prevention and
    Health Promotion
Department of Health
4052 Bald Cypress Way
Bin # A-18
Tallahassee, FL 32399-1744
(850) 245-4330
(850) 245-4391 (fax)
diabetes@doh.state.fl.us
http://www.floridadiabetes.org

GEORGIA

**Georgia Diabetes Prevention and Control
    Drive for Sight Programs**
DHR-Chronic Disease Prevention and Health
    Promotion Branch
2 Peachtree Street
Suite 16-293
Atlanta, GA 30303
(404) 657-6313
(404) 657-631 (fax)
http://health.state.ga.us/programs/cardio/
    diabetes.asp

HAWAII

Diabetes Prevention and Control Program
Hawaii State Department of Health
601 Kamokila Boulevard
Room 344
Kapolei, Hawaii 96707
(808) 692-7462
(808) 692-7461 (fax)
diabetes@doh.hawaii.gov
http://www.hawaii.gov/health/diabetes

IDAHO

**Idaho Diabetes Control and Prevention
    Program Coordinator**
Bureau of Health Promotion, Division of
    Health
Department of Health and Welfare
450 West State Street
P.O. Box 83720
Boise, ID 83720-0036
(208) 334-4928
(208) 334-6573 (fax)
http://www.diabetesprogram.idaho.gov

ILLINOIS

Illinois Department of Human Services
Bureau of Family Nutrition
Diabetes Prevention and Control Program
535 West Jefferson Street
Springfield, IL 62702-5058
(217) 782-2166
(217) 785-5247 (fax)
http://www.dhs.state.il.us/page.aspx?item=33873

INDIANA

Diabetes Control Program Coordinator
Indiana Diabetes Prevention and Control
    Program
Indiana State Department of Health
2 North Meridian Street, 6B
Indianapolis, IN 46204
(317) 233-7634
(317) 233-7127 (fax)
http://www.in.gov/isdh/19701.htm

IOWA

**Iowa Diabetes Prevention and Control
    Program**
Iowa Department of Public Health
Lucas Building
321 East 12th Street
Des Moines, IA 50319-0075
(515) 242-6204
(515) 281-6475 (fax)
http://www.idph.state.ia.us/hpcdp/diabetes.asp

KANSAS

**Kansas Diabetes Prevention and Control
    Program**
Office of Health Promotion
Kansas Department of Health and Environment
1000 SW Jackson
Suite 230
Topeka, KS 66612
(785) 291-3739
(785) 296-8059 (fax)
http://www.kdheks.gov/diabetes/index.htm

KENTUCKY

**Kentucky Diabetes Prevention and
    Control Program**
Chronic Disease Prevention and Control
    Branch
275 East Main Street, HS2W-E
Frankfort, KY 40621-0001
(502) 564-7996
(502) 564-4667 (fax)
http://chfs.ky.gov/dph/ach/cd/diabetes.htm

LOUISIANA

Louisiana Diabetes Program
628 North 4th Street
P.O. Box 3118
Baton Rouge, LA 79821-3118
(225) 342-2663
(225) 342-2652 (fax)
http://www.dhh.louisiana.gov

MAINE

**Maine Diabetes Prevention and Control
    Program**
Division of Chronic Disease
286 Water Street
5th Floor
11 State House Station
Augusta, ME 04333-0011
(207) 287-5380
(207) 287-7213 (fax)
http://www.maine.gov/dhhs/bohdcfh/dcp

MARYLAND

Maryland Diabetes Prevention and Control
201 West Preston Street
Third Floor
Baltimore, MD 21201
(410) 767-3608
(410) 333-5030 (fax)
http://www.fha.state.md.us/cphs/diabetes.cfm

MASSACHUSETTS

**Massachusetts Diabetes Prevention and
    Control Program**
Massachusetts Department of Public Health
250 Washington Street
Fourth Floor
Boston, MA 02108
(617) 624-5429
(617) 624-5075 (fax)
http://www.mass.gov/dph/ (Search *diabetes*)

MICHIGAN

**Michigan Department of Community
    Health Diabetes and Other Chronic
    Diseases Section**
109 West Michigan Avenue

Lansing, MI 48913
(517) 335-8789
(517) 335-9461 (fax)
http://www.michigan.gov/diabetes

MINNESOTA

Minnesota Diabetes Program
Minnesota Department of Health
P.O. Box 64882
St. Paul, MN 55164-0882
(651) 201-5423
(651) 201-5800 (fax)
http://www.health.state.mn.us/diabetes

MISSISSIPPI

**Mississippi Diabetes Prevention and
Control Program**
570 East Woodrow Wilson Drive
Osborne Building
Suite 200
Jackson, MS 39215-1700
(601) 576-7781
(601) 576-7444 (fax)
http://www.msdh.state.ms.us/msdhsite/_
static/43,0,296.html

MISSOURI

**Missouri Diabetes Prevention and Control
Program**
Bureau of Cancer and Chronic Disease Control
Section for Chronic Disease Prevention and
Nutrition Services
Missouri Department of Health and Senior
Services
930 Wildwood
P.O. Box 570
Jefferson City, MI 65102
(573) 522-2861
(573) 522-2898 (fax)
DiabetesMO@dhss.mo.gov
http://www.dhss.mo.gov/diabetes/

MONTANA

Montana Diabetes Project
1400 Broadway
Room C314B

P.O. Box 202951
Helena, MT 59620-2951
(406) 444-6677
(406) 444-7465 (fax)
http://www.diabetes.mt.gov

NEBRASKA

**Nebraska Diabetes Prevention and
Control Program**
Nebraska Department of Heath and Human
Services
301 Centennial Mall South
P.O. Box 95026
Lincoln, NE 68509-5026
(800) 745-9311 (toll-free)
(402) 471-6446 (fax)
http://www.dhhs.ne.gov/dpc/ndcp.htm

NEVADA

**Nevada Diabetes Prevention and Control
Program**
Nevada State Health Division
4150 Technology Way
Suite 101
Carson City, NV 89706
(775) 684-5996
(775) 684-5998 (fax)
http://health.nv.gov/

NEW HAMPSHIRE

**New Hampshire Diabetes Education
Program**
Division of Public Health Services
NH Department of Health and Human Services
29 Hazen Drive
Concord, NH 03301
(603) 271-5173
(603) 271-5199 (fax)
http://www.dhhs.state.nh.us/DHHS/CDPC/dep.
htm

NEW JERSEY

**New Jersey Department of Health &
Senior Services**
Wellness and Chronic Disease Prevention
Program

50 East State Street
P.O. Box 364
Trenton, NJ 08625
(609) 984-6137
(609) 292-9288 (fax)
http://www.state.nj.us/health/fhs/diabetes/
    index.shtml

NEW MEXICO

**New Mexico Diabetes Prevention and
    Control Program**
New Mexico Department of Health
810 West San Mateo Road
Suite 200E
Santa Fe, NM 87505
(505) 476-7615
(888) 523-2966 (toll-free)
(505) 476-7622 (fax)
http://www.diabetesnm.org/

NEW YORK

New York State Department of Health
Bureau of Chronic Disease Services
Diabetes Prevention and Control Program
150 Broadway
Room 350
Albany, NY 12204-0678
(518) 474-1222
(518) 473-0642 (fax)
http://www.nyhealth.gov/diseases/conditions/
    diabetes

NORTH CAROLINA

**North Carolina Diabetes Prevention and
    Control Program**
5505 Six Forks Road
Third Floor
Raleigh, NC 27609
(919) 707-5340
(919) 870-4801 (fax)
http://www.ncdiabetes.org

NORTH DAKOTA

**North Dakota Diabetes and Prevention
    Program**
North Dakota Department of Health

600 East Boulevard Avenue
Department 301
Bismarck, ND 58505-0200
(701) 328-2367
(701) 328-2036 (fax)
http://www.diabetesnd.org

OHIO

**Ohio Diabetes Prevention and Education
    Program**
Ohio Department of Health
Diabetes Unit
246 North High Street
Eighth Floor
Columbus, OH 43266-0588
(614) 466-2144
(614) 644-7740 (fax)
http://www.odh.ohio.gov/odhPrograms/hprr/
    diabete/diab1.aspx

OKLAHOMA

Oklahoma State Department of Health
Diabetes Prevention and Control Program
1000 Northeast 10th Street
Oklahoma City, OK 73117-1299
(405) 271-4072
(405) 271-6315 (fax)
http://www.ok.gov/health/Disease,_
    Prevention,_Preparedness/Chronic_Disease_
    Service/Diabetes_Prevention_and_Control_
    Program/index.html

OREGON

**Oregon Diabetes Prevention and Control
    Program**
Health Promotion and Chronic Disease Preven-
    tion Program
Oregon Department of Human Services, Public
    Health Division
800 N.E. Oregon Street
Suite 730
Portland, OR 97232-2162
(971) 673-0984
(971) 673-0994 (fax)
http://oregon.gov/DHS/ph/diabetes

PENNSYLVANIA

Pennsylvania Diabetes Prevention and Control Program Administrators
Pennsylvania Department of Health
Division of Nutrition and Physical Activity
Health & Welfare Building
Room 1000
7th and Forster Streets
Harrisburg, PA 17120
(717) 787-5876
(717) 783-5498 (fax)
http://www.health.state.pa.us/diabetes

RHODE ISLAND

Rhode Island Diabetes Prevention and Control Program
Rhode Island Department of Health
3 Capitol Hill
Room 409
Providence, RI 02908
(401) 222-6957
(401) 222-4415 (fax)
http://www.health.ri.gov/disease/diabetes/
index.php

SOUTH CAROLINA

South Carolina Diabetes Prevention & Control Program
Bureau of Chronic Disease Prevention and
Home Health Services
SC Department of Health and Environmental
Control
1800 St. Julian Place
Columbia, SC 29204
(803) 545-4471
Program fax number: (803) 545-4921 (fax)
http://www.scdhec.gov/health/chcdp/diabetes/

SOUTH DAKOTA

South Dakota Diabetes Prevention & Control Program
South Dakota Department of Health
615 East 4th Street
Pierre, SD 57501
(605) 773-7046

(800) 738-2301 (toll-free)
(605) 773-5509 (fax)
http://diabetes.sd.gov

TENNESSEE

Diabetes Prevention and Control Program
Tennessee Department of Health, Nutrition and
Wellness
425 5th Avenue North
Cordell Hull Building
Fifth Floor
Nashville, TN 37247
(615) 532-8192
(615) 532-7189 (fax)
http://health.state.tn.us

TEXAS

Texas Diabetes Prevention and Control Program
Texas Department of State Health Services
MC 1965
P.O. Box 149347
Austin, TX 78714-9347
(512) 458-7490
(512) 458-7408 (fax)
http://www.dshs.state.tx.us/diabetes/

UTAH

Utah Diabetes Prevention and Control Program
Utah Department of Health
P.O. Box 142107
Salt Lake City, UT 84114-2107
(801) 538-6141
(888) 222-2542 (toll-free)
(801) 538-9495 (fax)
http://www.health.utah.gov/diabetes

VERMONT

Vermont Diabetes Prevention and Control Program
Vermont Department of Health
108 Cherry Street
P.O. Box 70
Burlington, VT 05402-0070

(802) 865-7708
(802) 651-1634 (fax)
http://healthvermont.gov/prevent/diabetes/
  diabetes.aspx

VIRGINIA
Virginia Department of Health
Division of Chronic Disease Control and
  Prevention
Diabetes Prevention and Control Project
109 Governor Street
10th Floor
Richmond, VA 23219
(804) 864-7877
(804) 864-7880 (fax)
http://www.vahealth.org/cdpc/diabetes

WASHINGTON
**Washington State Diabetes Prevention
  and Control Program**
Washington State Department of Health
P.O. Box 47855
Olympia, WA 98504-7855
(360) 236-3708 (fax)
http://www.doh.wa.gov/cfh/diabetes

WEST VIRGINIA
**West Virginia Diabetes Prevention and
  Control Program**
350 Capitol Street
Room 206
Charleston, WV 25301
(304) 558-0644
(304) 558-1553 (fax)
http://www.wvdiabetes.org

WISCONSIN
**Wisconsin Diabetes Prevention and
  Control Program**
1 West Wilson
P.O. Box 2659
Madison, WI 53701-2659
(608) 261-9422
(608) 266-8925 (fax)
http://dhfs.wisconsin.gov/health/diabetes/

WYOMING
Wyoming Department of Health
Diabetes Prevention & Control Program
6101 Yellowstone Road
Suite 259A
Cheyenne, WY 82002
(307) 777-3579
(307) 777-8604 (fax)
http://wdh.state.wy.us/PHSD/DIABETES/index.
  html

AMERICAN SAMOA
**American Samoa Diabetes Prevention &
  Control Program**
American Samoa Government
Department of Health Services
P.O. Box 5061
Pago Pago, American Samoa 96799
(684) 633-2186
(684) 633-5379 (fax)
esptlevi4@yahoo.com

FEDERATED STATE OF MICRONESIA
**Department of Health, Education and
  Social Affairs**
FSM Diabetes Prevention & Control Program
P.O. Box 70, PS
FMS National Government
Palikir, Pohnpei, FM 96941
(0-11-691) (320) 2619/2643
(0-11-691) 320-5263 (fax)
fsmhealth@mail.fm or mhsamo@mail.fm

GUAM
**Guam Diabetes Control and Prevention
  Program**
Department of Public Health and Social
  Services
P.O. Box 2816
Agana, Guam 96910
(0-11-671) 475-0282
(0-11-671) 477-7945 (fax)
Patrick.luces@dphss.guam.gov

REPUBLIC OF THE MARSHALL ISLANDS

Republic of the Marshall Islands Diabetes Control and Prevention Program
Ministry of Health Services
P.O. Box 16
Republic of the Marshall Islands
Majuro, Marshall Islands 96960
(011-692) 625-3355
(011-692) 625-3432 (fax)
i_debrum@yahoo.com

NORTHERN MARIANA ISLANDS

Commonwealth of the Northern Mariana Islands Diabetes Control and Prevention Program
Department of Public Health
Government of Northern Mariana Islands
P.O. Box 409 CK
Saipan, Commonwealth Northern Mariana Islands 96950
(0-11-670) 234-8950, extension 2005
(0-11-670) 234-8930 (fax)
Taynabc@gmail.com

REPUBLIC OF PALAU

Palau Diabetes Prevention and Control Program Coordinator
Director of Public Health
P.O. Box 6027
Ministry of Health
Koror, Palau PW 96940

(0-11-680) 488-6262
(0-11-680) 488-8667 (fax)
dcp@palaunet.com

PUERTO RICO

Puerto Rico Diabetes Control and Prevention Program
Puerto Rico Department of Health
Secretaría Auxiliar de Promoción y Proteción de la Salud
División de Prevención y Control de Enfermedades Transmisibles
P.O. Box 70184
San Juan, Puerto Rico 00936
(787) 274-5634
(787) 274-5523 (fax)
leperez@salud.gov.pr
http://www.salud.gov.pr

VIRGIN ISLANDS

Virgin Islands Department of Health
Bureau of Health Education & Promotion
Diabetes Prevention & Control Program
3500 Estate Richmond
Charles Harwood Complex
Christiansted, St. Croix USVI 00820-4370
(340) 773-1311 ext. 3144
(340) 773-8354 (fax)
Sandra.charles@USVI-doh.org
http://www.usvidiabetes.org/

APPENDIX VI
WORLD HEALTH ORGANIZATION WORLDWIDE COLLABORATING CENTERS FOR DIABETES

ARGENTINA

WHO Collaborating Centre for Diabetes Research, Education and Care

Dr. Juan Jose Gagliardino
Centro de Endocrinologia Experimental y
 Aplicada (CENEXA)
Facultad de Ceincias Medicas
Universidad Nacional de la Plata
Calle 60 y 120, -1900
La Plata, Argentina
(54-221) 423-6712
(54-221) 422-2081 (fax)
http://www.cenexa.org

AUSTRALIA

WHO Collaborating Centre for the Epidemiology of Diabetes Mellitus and Health Promotion for NCD Control

Paul Zimmet
International Diabetes Institute
260 Kooyong Road
P.O. Box 185
VIC 3162
Victoria
Caulfield, South Australia
(61-3) 9258 5050
(61-3) 9258 5090 (fax)
http://www.diabetes.com.au

BANGLADESH

WHO Collaborating Centre for Research and Rehabilitation in Diabetes, Endocrine and Metabolic Disorders

Hajera, Professor Mahtab

Bangladesh Institute of Research &
 Rehabilitation in Diabetes, Endocrine &
 Metabolic Disorder (BIRDEM)
122, Kazi Nazrul Islam Avenue, 1000
Dhaka Bangladesh
(880-2) 861-7130
(880-2) 861-1138 (fax)
http://www.dab-bd.org

CHILE

WHO Collaborating Centre for Primary Health Care

Dr. Ilta Lange, Dr. Paz Soto
Escuela de Enfermeria Pontificia Universidad
 Catolica de Chile
Pontificia Universidad Catolica de Chile
Vicuna Mackenna 4860- 6904411 Macul
Santiago, Chile
(56-2) 354-5831
(56-2) 354-7025 (fax)

CROATIA

WHO Collaborating Centre for Appropriate Technology in the Control of Diabetes Mellitus

Zeljko Metelko
Vuk Vrhovac University Clinic for Diabetes,
 Endocrinology & Metabolic Diseases
Faculty of Medicine
University of Zagreb
Du I dol 4a, 1000-10,000
Zagreb, Croatia
(385-1) 233-1480
(385-1) 233-1515 (fax)
http://www.idb.hr

CUBA

WHO Collaborating Centre for Integrated Medical Care Services in Diabetes
Dr. Oscar Diaz
Centro de Atencion al Diabetico
Instituto Nacional de Endocrinologia
Zapata y D. Vedado-10400
La Habana Cuba
(53-7) 329 707
(53-7) 333 417 (fax)

GERMANY

WHO Collaborating Centre for Diabetes Treatment and Prevention
Professor Wener A. Scherbaum
Department of Endocrinology and Metabolism
Heinrich Heine University
Aufm Hennekamp 65, D-40225
Dusseldorf, Germany
(49-211) 33 82-0
(49-211) 34 20 80 (fax)

WHO Collaborating Centre for Quality Assurance and Standardization in Laboratory Medicine
Hans Reinauer
Instand e.v. Society for Promotion Quality Assurance in Medical Laboratories
Uberstrasse 20, D-40223
Dusseldorf, Germany
(49-211) 15 92 13-0
(49-211) 15-92-13-32 (fax)
http://www.instand-ev.do

INDIA

WHO Collaborating Centre for Research, Education and Training in Diabetes
Dr. Vijay Viswanathan
Diabetes Research Centre and M.V. Hospital for Diabetes
No. 4, Main Road
Royapuram, Chennai 600 013
India
(91-44) 2595-4913
(91-44) 2595-4919 (fax)
www.http://www.mydiabetes.com

ISLAMIC REPUBLIC OF IRAN

WHO Collaborating Centre for Research and Education on Management of Osteoporosis and Diabetes
Professor Bagher Larijani
Endocrinology and Metabolism Research Center (EMRC)
Tehran University of Medical Sciences
North Kargar Avenue, 14114
Tehran, Iran
(98-21) 8026902-3
(98-21) 802-9399 (fax)
http://www.endocrineweb.org

ISRAEL

WHO Collaborating Centre for the Study of Diabetes in Youth
Professor Zvi Laron
Endocrinology & Diabetes Research Unit
Institute of Paediatric & Adolescent Endocrinology
Schneider Children's Medical Center of Israel
14 Kaplan Street-49202
Petah Tiqva, Israel
(972-3) 939-3610
(972-3) 922-2996 (fax)

ITALY

WHO Collaborating Centre for Community Control of Hereditary Diseases
Professor Renzo Galanello
Struttura Complessa Microcitemie ed altre Malattie Ematologiche ASLB Dipartimento di Scienze Biomediche e Biotechnologie
Universita degli Studi di Cagliari
Via Jennver s/s, I-09121
Cagliari, Italy
(39-70) 609-5508
(39-70) 609-5509 (fax)
http://mcweb.unica.it

JAPAN

WHO Collaborating Centre for Diabetes Treatment and Education
Shigeo Kono
Diabetes Center

Kyoto Medical Center
National Hospital Organization
1-1 Fukakusa Mukaihata-cho, Fushimu-ku
612-8555
Kyoto, Japan
(81-75) 641 9161, extension 6115
(81-75) 645-4339 (fax)
http://www.hosp.go.jp/~kyotolan/

JORDAN

WHO Collaborating Centre for Research, Education and Primary Health Care
Kamol Ajlovni
National Centre for Diabetes, Endocrinology
    and Inherited Diseases
Queen Ranis Astreet
11942 Amman
Amman, Jordan
(962-6) 535-3374
(962-6) 535-3326 (fax)
http://www.ncd.org.jo

LEBANON

WHO Collaborating Centre for Research, Training and Outreach in Food and Nutrition
Dr. Nahla Hwalla
Department of Nutrition and Food Science
American University of Beirut
Riad El South 1107 2020
Beirut, Lebanon
+ 961 1 350000, extension 4540
+ 961 1 744460 (fax)
http://www.aub.edu.lb

NETHERLANDS

WHO Collaborating Centre for Nutrition
Dr. Wanda Bemelmans and Joopran Raaij
Centre for Prevention and Health Services
    Research
National Institute for Public Health and the
    Environment RIVM
P.O. Box 1
3720 BA
Bilthoven, Netherlands
31 302744297

31 302744407 (fax)
http://www.rivm.nl/en/

NEW ZEALAND

WHO Collaborating Centre for Human Nutrition
Jim Mann
Department of Human Nutrition
University of Otago
P.O. Box 56
Dunedin, New Zealand
(64-3) 479-7959
(64-3) 479-7958 (fax)
http://www.otago.ac.nz

OMAN

WHO Collaborating Centre for Research and Training in Diabetes Programme Development
Dr. Mohammed Bin Abdullah
Department of Internal Medicine and
    Endocrinology
National Diabetes Centre
The Royal Hospital
111 Muscat
Seeb, Oman
(968) 592-888, extension 2250
(968) 592-984 (fax)

PAKISTAN

WHO Collaborating Centre for Treatment, Education and Research in Diabetes and Diabetic Pregnancies
Dr. A. Samad Shera
Diabetic Association of Pakistan
5-E/3
Nazimabad, 74600
Karachi, Pakistan
(92-21) 661-6890
(92-21) 668-0959 (fax)
http://www.dap.org.pk/index.htm

POLAND

WHO Collaborating Centre for Nutrition
Zbigniew Szybinski
Department of Endocrinology

Collegium Medicum
Jagiellonian University
Kopernika str 17
31-501
Krakow, Poland
48124247520
48124247399 (fax)

ROMANIA

**WHO Collaborating Centre for Oral Health
  Systems in Transition**
Vasile Burlui and Marcea Rusu
Faculty of Dental Medicine
University of Medicine and Pharmacy
16 Universitatil Street, R-700115
Iasi, Romania
(40-0232) 211 820
(40-0232) 211-820 (fax)
http://www.unfiasi.ro

SUDAN

**WHO Collaborating Centre for Research
  and Training in Educational
  Development**
Diaa Elgaili
Educational Development and Research Centre
  (EDC)
Gezira Medical School
University of Gezira
Faculty of Medicine
P.O. Box 20
Wad Medani, Sudan
(249-511) 53649
(249-511) 43415 (fax)
http://www.edc-gezira.net

SWITZERLAND

**WHO Collaborating Centre for Reference
  and Research in the Field of Education
  and Long-Term Follow-up Strategies
  for Chronic Diseases**
Professor Alain Golay
Division of Therapeutic Education for Chronic
  Disease
University Hospital
24, rue Micheli-du-Crest, 1211

Geneva, Switzerland
(41-22) 372-9726
(41-22) 372-9715 (fax)
http://www.hug-ge.ch/setmc

UNITED KINGDOM

**WHO Collaborating Centre for Training,
  Evaluation & Research in Diabetes**
Nigel Unwin
The Diabetes Research Group
School of Clinical Medical Sciences
University of Newcastle-upon-Tyne Medical
  School
Faculty of Medical Sciences
Medical School
Framlington Place-NE2 4HH
Newcastle upon Tyne, United Kingdom
(44-191) 222-7372
(44-191) 222-8211 (fax)
http://www.nci.ac.uk/biomedicine

UNITED STATES

**WHO Collaborating Centre for
  Community Genetics**
Dr. Victor Penchaszadeh
Department of Epidemiology
Center for Genetics and Global Health
Mailman School of Public Health
Columbia University
722 West 168th Street
16th Floor
New York, NY 10032
(212) 305-7992
(212) 342-5168 (fax)
http://www.mailman.hs.columbia.edu/epi/
  index.html

**WHO Collaborating Centre for Continuing
  Health Professional Education in
  Diabetes**
Charles Clark
Division of Continuing Medical Education
Indianapolis University School of Medicine
714 North Senate Avenue
Suite 200
Indianapolis, IN 46202
(317) 274-0104

(317) 274-5187 (fax)
http://cme.medicine.iu.edu

WHO Collaborating Centre for Diabetes Education, Translation and Computer Technology
Dr. Roger S. Mazze
International Diabetes Center
3800 Park Nicollet Boulevard
Minneapolis, MN 55416
(952) 993-1927
(952) 993-1302 (fax)
http://www.idc.com

WHO Collaborating Center for Disease Monitoring, Telecommunications and the Molecular Epidemiology of Diabetes Mellitus
Roland LaPorte and Janice Dorman
Department of Epidemiology
Graduate School of Public Health
University of Pittsburgh
3512 Fifth Avenue
Pittsburgh, PA 15213-3310
(412) 383-7244
(412) 383-1026 (fax)

APPENDIX VII
WEB SITES THAT INCLUDE DIABETES INFORMATION

American Academy of Neurology
http://www.aan.com/

American Academy of Ophthalmology
http://www.aao.org

American Academy of Pediatrics
http://www.aap.org/

**American Association of Clinical
Endocrinologists**
http://www.aace.com/

**American Association of Diabetes
Educators**
http://www.diabeteseducator.org/

**American College of Foot and Ankle
Surgeons**
http://www.acfas.org/

American Diabetes Association
http://www.diabetes.org

American Dietetic Association
http://www.eatright.org/cps/rde/xchg/ada/
hs.xsl/index.html

**Children with Diabetes On-Line
Community**
http://www.childrenwithdiabetes.com/

**Diabetes Action Research and Education
Foundation**
http://www.diabetesaction.org/site/
PageServer?pagename=index

Diabetes Exercise and Sports Association
http://www.diabetes-exercise.org/index.asp

Endocrine Society
http://www.endo-society.org/

FDA Diabetes Information
http://www.fda.gov/diabetes/

Jewish Diabetes
http://www.jewishdiabetes.org/

**Juvenile Diabetes Research Foundation
International**
http://www.jdrf.org/

**National Diabetes Information
Clearinghouse**
http://diabetes.niddk.nih.gov/

**National Institute of Diabetes and
Digestive and Kidney Diseases (NIDDK)**
http://www2.niddk.nih.gov/

World Health Organization
http://www.who.int/topics/diabetes_mellitus/en/

APPENDIX VIII

WORLDWIDE PERCENTAGE OF INCIDENT PATIENTS WITH ESRD DUE TO DIABETES, 2003–2007

Table 1 provides worldwide data for the years 2003–07 on the incidence of kidney failure (end-stage renal disease) caused by diabetes among individuals in selected countries world-wide, including the United States. As can be seen from the table, in 2007 the United States is fifth after Malaysia, Mexico (listed as "Jalisco"), Hong Kong, and the Republic of Korea in the

TABLE 1. PERCENTAGE OF END-STAGE RENAL DISEASES CASES CAUSED BY DIABETES, BY COUNTRY, 2003-2007

Country	2003	2004	2005	2006	2007
Argentina	—	31.4	34.7	33.8	31.2
Australia	26.0	30.3	31.5	32.6	30.9
Austria	33.5	32.3	33.5	33.0	31.5
Belgium, Dutch speaking	24.0	24.4	23.9	22.2	23.4
Belgium, French speaking	25.0	21.2	23.7	22.6	22.9
Bosnia & Herzegovina	22.9	20.1	20.6	21.5	19.7
Canada	34.2	34.3	34.9	34.4	—
Croatia	26.9	29.0	30.0	—	—
Denmark	22.6	21.5	24.2	24.0	22.6
Finland	34.9	33.2	34.6	35.7	35.3
France	—	—	23.3	34.7	22.2
Germany	36.3	34.2	34.9	34.4	—
Greece	28.0	28.3	29.4	29.4	27.8
Hong Kong	39.9	40.5	41.1	40.2	45.1
Hungary	25.5	29.5	26.2	27.5	29.2
Iceland	0.0	4.3	15.0	28.6	12.0
Israel	39.0	42.2	40.7	41.9	41.8
Italy	16.2	16.2	18.0	—	—
Jalisco (Mexico)	51.0	56.0	60.0	49.9	55.0

(table continues)

TABLE (continued)

Country	2003	2004	2005	2006	2007
Japan	40.6	40.9	41.6	42.5	43.2
Luxembourg	—	—	—	28.2	—
Malaysia	53.9	55.1	55.9	59.2	58.5
Netherlands	16.6	17.4	15.6	16.0	17.9
New Zealand	41.3	40.7	42.0	42.2	41.0
Norway	15.8	17.3	12.8	16.5	13.6
Pakistan	40.0	—	36.3	37.7	—
Philippines	32.8	33.5	36.9	38.5	24.1
Poland	22.6	26.9	27.2	29.6	24.1
Republic of Korea	42.5	43.4	38.5	42.3	44.9
Romania	—	—	10.7	12.3	11.7
Russia	10.7	—	11.0	13.9	—
Scotland	18.9	17.9	21.7	21.6	17.6
Spain	—	17.5	23.2	23.3	21.5
Sweden	24.0	25.1	25.8	26.1	27.1
Taiwan	36.8	40.1	41.8	43.0	43.1
Turkey	23.1	21.3	30.2	23.1	22.8
United Kingdom (England, Wales, and Northern Ireland)	—	19.1	19.0	20.6	19.6
United States	44.9	45.0	44.4	44.4	43.9
Uruguay	29.6	21.8	29.6	22.1	22.1

Adapted from United States Renal Data System. *USRDS 2009 Annual Data Report: Atlas of Chronic Kidney Disease and End-Stage Renal Disease in the United States.* Bethesda, Md.: National Institutes of Health, National Institute of Diabetes and Digestive and Kidney Diseases, 2009, p. 349.

The data reported here have been supplied by the United States Renal Data System (USRDS). The interpretation and reporting of these data are the responsibility of the authors and in no way should be seen as an official policy or interpretation of the U.S. government.

high percentage of the incidence (newly diagnosed cases in a year) of end-stage renal disease (ESRD) caused by diabetes mellitus.

In the United States, nearly 44 percent of all new cases of ESRD in 2007 were caused by diabetes. The rate for Malaysia was 58.5 percent, followed by Mexico (55.0 percent), Hong Kong (45.1 percent), and Korea (44.9 percent).

Some countries had rates of less than 20 percent of ESRD that was caused by diabetes, such as Romania, Iceland, Norway, Scotland, the Netherlands, the United Kingdom, and Bosnia and Herzegovina. (Data is missing for some countries in some years because it was not provided in the original table.)

APPENDIX IX
IMPORTANT BUT OFTEN OVERLOOKED KEY ISSUES IN DIABETES

This appendix lists frequently overlooked points and advice that should be considered by people with diabetes and their families.

1. Not only should people with diabetes receive immunizations against flu or pneumonia, but experts also recommend that family members of individuals with diabetes be immunized as well. This will help protect both the family member and the person with diabetes.
2. Medicare and many other health plans provide once a year coverage for therapeutic shoes for patients with diabetes. Patients need to obtain a prescription for the shoes from their physician.
3. People with diabetes should not get new glasses or contact lenses until their glucose levels have been stable for four to six weeks.
4. A medical identification bracelet is very important for everyone who has diabetes. Symptoms of diabetes are often confused with other illnesses.
5. Everyone with diabetes should have an emergency plan for what to do if blood glucose levels swing out of control.
6. Some people with diabetes should have an exercise stress test before undergoing any moderate or intensive exercise program in order to rule out cardiovascular disease. These include people who fit any one or more of the following groups: over age 35; had Type 2 diabetes for more than 10 years; had Type 1 diabetes for more than 15 years; have kidney disease; have proliferative retinopathy; have peripheral vascular disease; have autonomic neuropathy; or have any other risk factors for coronary artery disease.
7. People with diabetes should check their feet daily, making a foot inspection as much a part of the daily routine as teeth brushing. They should also wear comfortable shoes that were bought at the end of the day when the feet are usually the most swollen.
8. Excellent glycemic control levels are as follows:
   Pre-meal: 80–120
   Pre-bedtime: 100–140
9. Adolescents are most at risk to develop Type 2 diabetes if there is a family history of diabetes and if the adolescents are overweight and inactive.
10. Among people with Type 2 diabetes, the key factor that predicted hospitalization was elevated blood glucose levels in the 2–3 weeks prior to admission.

APPENDIX X

BODY MASS INDEX CHARTS AND CURVES FOR CHILDREN AND YOUNG ADULTS UNDER AGE 20

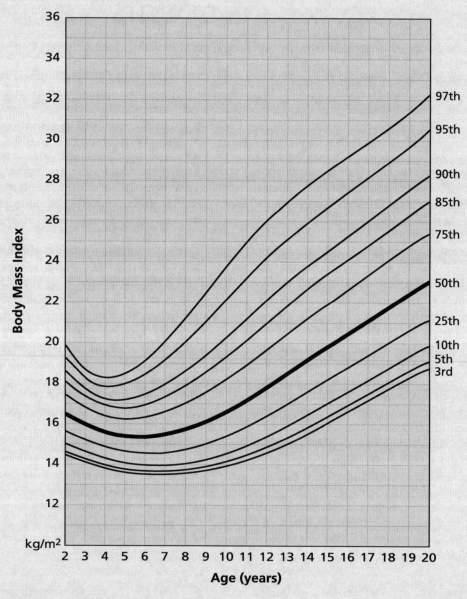

Body Mass Index-for-Age Percentiles: Boys, 2 to 20 Years

Source: Developed by the National Center for Health Statistics in collaboration with the National Center for Chronic Disease Prevention and Health Promotion (2000).

© Infobase Learning

Body Mass Index-for-Age Percentiles: Girls, 2 to 20 Years

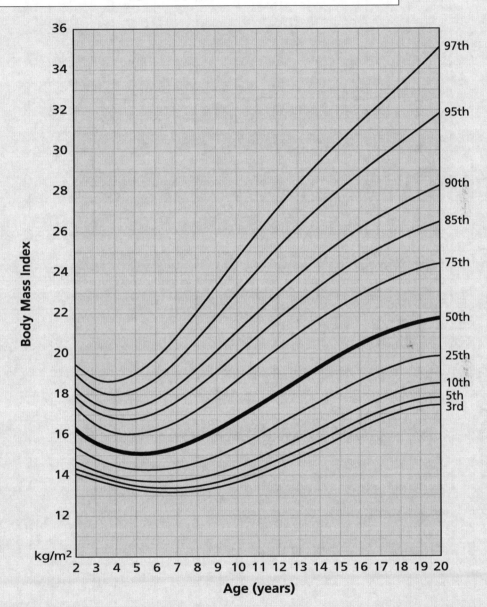

Source: Developed by the National Center for Health Statistics in collaboration with the National Center for Chronic Disease Prevention and Health Promotion (2000).

© Infobase Learning

CALCULATED BODY MASS INDEX   29″–37″ AND 18 LBS.–26 LBS.

Height Cm	Height In	Kg 8.2 / Lb 18	8.4 / 18.5	8.6 / 19	8.8 / 19.5	9.1 / 20	9.3 / 20.5	9.5 / 21	9.8 / 21.5	10.0 / 22	10.2 / 22.5	10.4 / 23	10.7 / 23.5	10.9 / 24	11.1 / 24.5	11.3 / 25	11.6 / 25.5	11.8 / 26
73.7	29	15.0	15.5	15.9	16.3	16.7	17.1	17.6	18.0	18.4	18.8	19.2	19.6	20.1	20.5	20.9	21.3	21.7
74.9	29.5	14.5	14.9	15.3	15.8	16.2	16.6	17.0	17.4	17.8	18.2	18.6	19.0	19.4	19.8	20.2	20.6	21.0
76.2	30	14.1	14.5	14.8	15.2	15.6	16.0	16.4	16.8	17.2	17.6	18.0	18.4	18.7	19.1	19.5	19.9	20.3
77.5	30.5	13.6	14.0	14.4	14.7	15.1	15.5	15.9	16.2	16.6	17.0	17.4	17.8	18.1	18.5	18.9	19.3	19.7
78.7	31	13.2	13.5	13.9	14.3	14.6	15.0	15.4	15.7	16.1	16.5	16.8	17.2	17.6	17.9	18.3	18.7	19.0
80.0	31.5		13.1	13.5	13.8	14.2	14.5	14.9	15.2	15.6	15.9	16.3	16.7	17.0	17.4	17.7	18.1	18.4
81.3	32			13.0	13.4	13.7	14.1	14.4	14.8	15.1	15.4	15.8	16.1	16.5	16.8	17.2	17.5	17.9
82.6	32.5					13.3	13.6	14.0	14.3	14.6	15.0	15.3	15.6	16.0	16.3	16.6	17.0	17.3
83.8	33						13.2	13.6	13.9	14.2	14.5	14.8	15.2	15.5	15.8	16.1	16.5	16.8
85.1	33.5							13.2	13.5	13.8	14.1	14.4	14.7	15.0	15.3	15.7	16.0	16.3
86.4	34								13.1	13.4	13.7	14.0	14.3	14.6	14.9	15.2	15.5	15.8
87.6	34.5										13.3	13.6	13.9	14.2	14.5	14.8	15.1	15.4
88.9	35											13.2	13.5	13.8	14.1	14.3	14.6	14.9
90.2	35.5												13.1	13.4	13.7	13.9	14.2	14.5
91.4	36													13.0	13.3	13.6	13.8	14.1
92.7	36.5															13.2	13.5	13.7
94.0	37																13.1	13.4

Whenever a child's specific height or weight measurement is not listed, round to the closest number in the table.

CALCULATED BODY MASS INDEX 29″–43″ AND 26.5 LBS.–34.5 LBS.

Height Cm	In	Weight Kg 12.0	12.2	12.5	12.7	12.9	13.2	13.4	13.6	13.8	14.1	14.3	14.5	14.7	15.0	15.2	15.4	15.6
		Lb 26.5	27	27.5	28	28.5	29	29.5	30	30.5	31	31.5	32	32.5	33	33.5	34	34.5
73.7	29	22.2	22.6	23.0	23.4	23.8	24.2	24.7	25.1	25.5	25.9	26.3	26.8	27.2	27.6	28.0	28.4	28.8
74.9	29.5	21.4	21.8	22.2	22.6	23.0	23.4	23.8	24.2	24.6	25.0	25.4	25.9	26.3	26.7	27.1	27.5	27.9
76.2	30	20.7	21.1	21.5	21.9	22.3	22.7	23.0	23.4	23.8	24.2	24.6	25.0	25.4	25.8	26.2	26.6	27.0
77.5	30.5	20.0	20.4	20.8	21.2	21.5	21.9	22.3	22.7	23.1	23.4	23.8	24.2	24.6	24.9	25.3	25.7	26.1
78.7	31	19.4	19.8	20.1	20.5	20.9	21.2	21.6	21.9	22.3	22.7	23.0	23.4	23.8	24.1	24.5	24.9	25.2
80.0	31.5	18.8	19.1	19.5	19.8	20.2	20.5	20.9	21.3	21.6	22.0	22.3	22.7	23.0	23.4	23.7	24.1	24.4
81.3	32	18.2	18.5	18.9	19.2	19.6	19.9	20.3	20.6	20.9	21.3	21.6	22.0	22.3	22.7	23.0	23.3	23.7
82.6	32.5	17.6	18.0	18.3	18.6	19.0	19.3	19.6	20.0	20.3	20.6	21.0	21.3	21.6	22.0	22.3	22.6	23.0
83.8	33	17.1	17.4	17.8	18.1	18.4	18.7	19.0	19.4	19.7	20.0	20.3	20.7	21.0	21.3	21.6	22.0	22.3
85.1	33.5	16.6	16.9	17.2	17.5	17.9	18.2	18.5	18.8	19.1	19.4	19.7	20.0	20.4	20.7	21.0	21.3	21.6
86.4	34	16.1	16.4	16.7	17.0	17.3	17.6	17.9	18.2	18.5	18.9	19.2	19.5	19.8	20.1	20.4	20.7	21.0
87.6	34.5	15.7	15.9	16.2	16.5	16.8	17.1	17.4	17.7	18.0	18.3	18.6	18.9	19.2	19.5	19.8	20.1	20.4
88.9	35	15.2	15.5	15.8	16.1	16.4	16.6	16.9	17.2	17.5	17.8	18.1	18.4	18.7	18.9	19.2	19.5	19.8
90.2	35.5	14.8	15.1	15.3	15.6	15.9	16.2	16.5	16.7	17.0	17.3	17.6	17.9	18.1	18.4	18.7	19.0	19.2
91.4	36	14.4	14.6	14.9	15.2	15.5	15.7	16.0	16.3	16.5	16.8	17.1	17.4	17.6	17.9	18.2	18.4	18.7
92.7	36.5	14.0	14.2	14.5	14.8	15.0	15.3	15.6	15.8	16.1	16.4	16.6	16.9	17.2	17.4	17.7	17.9	18.2
94.0	37	13.6	13.9	14.1	14.4	14.6	14.9	15.2	15.4	15.7	15.9	16.2	16.4	16.7	16.9	17.2	17.5	17.7
95.3	37.5	13.2	13.5	13.7	14.0	14.2	14.5	14.7	15.0	15.2	15.5	15.7	16.0	16.2	16.5	16.7	17.0	17.2
96.5	38		13.1	13.4	13.6	13.9	14.1	14.4	14.6	14.9	15.1	15.3	15.6	15.8	16.1	16.3	16.6	16.8
97.8	38.5			13.0	13.3	13.5	13.8	14.0	14.2	14.5	14.7	14.9	15.2	15.4	15.7	15.9	16.1	16.4
99.1	39					13.2	13.4	13.6	13.9	14.1	14.3	14.6	14.8	15.0	15.3	15.5	15.7	15.9
100.3	39.5						13.1	13.3	13.5	13.7	14.0	14.2	14.4	14.6	14.9	15.1	15.3	15.5
101.6	40								13.2	13.4	13.6	13.8	14.1	14.3	14.5	14.7	14.9	15.2
102.9	40.5									13.1	13.3	13.5	13.7	13.9	14.1	14.4	14.6	14.8
104.1	41											13.2	13.4	13.6	13.8	14.0	14.2	14.4
105.4	41.5												13.1	13.3	13.5	13.7	13.9	14.1
106.7	42														13.2	13.4	13.6	13.8
108.0	42.5															13.0	13.2	13.4
109.2	43																	13.1

Whenever a child's specific height or weight measurement is not listed, round to the closest number in the table.

CALCULATED BODY MASS INDEX 29"–43" AND 35 LBS.–43LBS

Height Cm	In	Weight Kg 15.9	16.1	16.3	16.6	16.8	17.0	17.2	17.5	17.7	17.9	18.1	18.4	18.6	18.8	19.1	19.3	19.5
	Lb	35	35.5	36	36.5	37	37.5	38	38.5	39	39.5	40	40.5	41	41.5	42	42.5	43
73.7	29	29.3	29.7	30.1	30.5	30.9	31.3	31.8	32.2	32.6	33.0	33.4	33.9	34.3	34.7			
74.9	29.5	28.3	28.7	29.1	29.5	29.9	30.3	30.7	31.1	31.5	31.9	32.3	32.7	33.1	33.5	33.9	34.3	34.7
76.2	30	27.3	27.7	28.1	28.5	28.9	29.3	29.7	30.1	30.5	30.9	31.2	31.6	32.0	32.4	32.8	33.2	33.6
77.5	30.5	26.5	26.8	27.2	27.6	28.0	28.3	28.7	29.1	29.5	29.9	30.2	30.6	31.0	31.4	31.7	32.1	32.5
78.7	31	25.6	26.0	26.3	26.7	27.1	27.4	27.8	28.2	28.5	28.9	29.3	29.6	30.0	30.4	30.7	31.1	31.5
80.0	31.5	24.8	25.2	25.5	25.9	26.2	26.6	26.9	27.3	27.6	28.0	28.3	28.7	29.1	29.4	29.8	30.1	30.5
81.3	32	24.0	24.4	24.7	25.1	25.4	25.7	26.1	26.4	26.8	27.1	27.5	27.8	28.2	28.5	28.8	29.2	29.5
82.6	32.5	23.3	23.6	24.0	24.3	24.6	25.0	25.3	25.6	26.0	26.3	26.6	27.0	27.3	27.6	28.0	28.3	28.6
83.8	33	22.6	22.9	23.2	23.6	23.9	24.2	24.5	24.9	25.2	25.5	25.8	26.1	26.5	26.8	27.1	27.4	27.8
85.1	33.5	21.9	22.2	22.6	22.9	23.2	23.5	23.8	24.1	24.4	24.7	25.1	25.4	25.7	26.0	26.3	26.6	26.9
86.4	34	21.3	21.6	21.9	22.2	22.5	22.8	23.1	23.4	23.7	24.0	24.3	24.6	24.9	25.2	25.5	25.8	26.2
87.6	34.5	20.7	21.0	21.3	21.6	21.9	22.2	22.4	22.7	23.0	23.3	23.6	23.9	24.2	24.5	24.8	25.1	25.4
88.9	35	20.1	20.4	20.7	20.9	21.2	21.5	21.8	22.1	22.4	22.7	23.0	23.2	23.5	23.8	24.1	24.4	24.7
90.2	35.5	19.5	19.8	20.1	20.4	20.6	20.9	21.2	21.5	21.8	22.0	22.3	22.6	22.9	23.2	23.4	23.7	24.0
91.4	36	19.0	19.3	19.5	19.8	20.1	20.3	20.6	20.9	21.2	21.4	21.7	22.0	22.2	22.5	22.8	23.1	23.3
92.7	36.5	18.5	18.7	19.0	19.3	19.5	19.8	20.1	20.3	20.6	20.8	21.1	21.4	21.6	21.9	22.2	22.4	22.7
94.0	37	18.0	18.2	18.5	18.7	19.0	19.3	19.5	19.8	20.0	20.3	20.5	20.8	21.1	21.3	21.6	21.8	22.1
95.3	37.5	17.5	17.7	18.0	18.2	18.5	18.7	19.0	19.2	19.5	19.7	20.0	20.2	20.5	20.7	21.0	21.2	21.5
96.5	38	17.0	17.3	17.5	17.8	18.0	18.3	18.5	18.7	19.0	19.2	19.5	19.7	20.0	20.2	20.4	20.7	20.9
97.8	38.5	16.6	16.8	17.1	17.3	17.6	17.8	18.0	18.3	18.5	18.7	19.0	19.2	19.4	19.7	19.9	20.2	20.4
99.1	39	16.2	16.4	16.6	16.9	17.1	17.3	17.6	17.8	18.0	18.3	18.5	18.7	19.0	19.2	19.4	19.6	19.9
100.3	39.5	15.8	16.0	16.2	16.4	16.7	16.9	17.1	17.3	17.6	17.8	18.0	18.2	18.5	18.7	18.9	19.2	19.4
101.6	40	15.4	15.6	15.8	16.0	16.3	16.5	16.7	16.9	17.1	17.4	17.6	17.8	18.0	18.2	18.5	18.7	18.9
102.9	40.5	15.0	15.2	15.4	15.6	15.9	16.1	16.3	16.5	16.7	16.9	17.1	17.4	17.6	17.8	18.0	18.2	18.4
104.1	41	14.6	14.8	15.1	15.3	15.5	15.7	15.9	16.1	16.3	16.5	16.7	16.9	17.1	17.4	17.6	17.8	18.0
105.4	41.5	14.3	14.5	14.7	14.9	15.1	15.3	15.5	15.7	15.9	16.1	16.3	16.5	16.7	16.9	17.1	17.3	17.6
106.7	42	13.9	14.1	14.3	14.5	14.7	14.9	15.1	15.3	15.5	15.7	15.9	16.1	16.3	16.5	16.7	16.9	17.1
108.0	42.5	13.6	13.8	14.0	14.2	14.4	14.6	14.8	15.0	15.2	15.4	15.6	15.8	16.0	16.2	16.3	16.5	16.7
109.2	43	13.3	13.5	13.7	13.9	14.1	14.3	14.4	14.6	14.8	15.0	15.2	15.4	15.6	15.8	16.0	16.2	16.4

CALCULATED BODY MASS INDEX 43.5"–48" AND 35 LBS.–43 LBS.

Height Cm	Height In	Kg 15.9 / Lb 35	16.1 / 35.5	16.3 / 36	16.6 / 36.5	16.8 / 37	17.0 / 37.5	17.2 / 38	17.5 / 38.5	17.7 / 39	17.9 / 39.5	18.1 / 40	18.4 / 40.5	18.6 / 41	18.8 / 41.5	19.1 / 42	19.3 / 42.5	19.5 / 43
110.5	43.5	13.0	13.2	13.4	13.6	13.7	13.9	14.1	14.3	14.5	14.7	14.9	15.0	15.2	15.4	15.6	15.8	16.0
111.8	44			13.1	13.3	13.4	13.6	13.8	14.0	14.2	14.3	14.5	14.7	14.9	15.1	15.3	15.4	15.6
113.0	44.5				13.1		13.3	13.5	13.7	13.8	14.0	14.2	14.4	14.6	14.7	14.9	15.1	15.3
114.3	45						13.0	13.2	13.4	13.5	13.7	13.9	14.1	14.2	14.4	14.6	14.8	14.9
115.6	45.5								13.1	13.2	13.4	13.6	13.8	13.9	14.1	14.3	14.4	14.6
116.8	46										13.1	13.3	13.5	13.6	13.8	14.0	14.1	14.3
118.1	46.5											13.0	13.2	13.3	13.5	13.7	13.8	14.0
119.4	47													13.0	13.2	13.4	13.5	13.7
120.7	47.5															13.1	13.2	13.4
121.9	48																	13.1

Whenever a child's specific height or weight measurement is not listed, round to the closest number in the table.

CALCULATED BODY MASS INDEX   30"–44" AND 43.5 LBS.–51.5 LBS.

Height Cm	In	\	Weight															
		Kg	19.7	20.0	20.2	20.4	20.6	20.9	21.1	21.3	21.5	21.8	22.0	22.2	22.5	22.7	22.9	23.1	23.4
		Lb	43.5	44	44.5	45	45.5	46	46.5	47	47.5	48	48.5	49	49.5	50	50.5	51	51.5
76.2	30		34.0	34.4	34.8														
77.5	30.5		32.9	33.3	33.6	34.0	34.4	34.8											
78.7	31		31.8	32.2	32.6	32.9	33.3	33.7	34.0	34.4	34.8								
80.0	31.5		30.8	31.2	31.5	31.9	32.2	32.6	32.9	33.3	33.7	34.0	34.4	34.7					
81.3	32		29.9	30.2	30.6	30.9	31.2	31.6	31.9	32.3	32.6	33.0	33.3	33.6	34.0	34.3	34.7		
82.6	32.5		29.0	29.3	29.6	30.0	30.3	30.6	31.0	31.3	31.6	32.0	32.3	32.6	32.9	33.3	33.6	33.9	34.3
83.8	33		28.1	28.4	28.7	29.1	29.4	29.7	30.0	30.3	30.7	31.0	31.3	31.6	32.0	32.3	32.6	32.9	33.2
85.1	33.5		27.3	27.6	27.9	28.2	28.5	28.8	29.1	29.4	29.8	30.1	30.4	30.7	31.0	31.3	31.6	32.0	32.3
86.4	34		26.5	26.8	27.1	27.4	27.7	28.0	28.3	28.6	28.9	29.2	29.5	29.8	30.1	30.4	30.7	31.0	31.3
87.6	34.5		25.7	26.0	26.3	26.6	26.9	27.2	27.5	27.8	28.1	28.4	28.6	28.9	29.2	29.5	29.8	30.1	30.4
88.9	35		25.0	25.3	25.5	25.8	26.1	26.4	26.7	27.0	27.3	27.5	27.8	28.1	28.4	28.7	29.0	29.3	29.6
90.2	35.5		24.3	24.5	24.8	25.1	25.4	25.7	25.9	26.2	26.5	26.8	27.1	27.3	27.6	27.9	28.2	28.5	28.7
91.4	36		23.6	23.9	24.1	24.4	24.7	25.0	25.2	25.5	25.8	26.0	26.3	26.6	26.9	27.1	27.4	27.7	27.9
92.7	36.5		23.0	23.2	23.5	23.7	24.0	24.3	24.5	24.8	25.1	25.3	25.6	25.9	26.1	26.4	26.7	26.9	27.2
94.0	37		22.3	22.6	22.9	23.1	23.4	23.6	23.9	24.1	24.4	24.7	24.9	25.2	25.4	25.7	25.9	26.2	26.4
95.3	37.5		21.7	22.0	22.2	22.5	22.7	23.0	23.2	23.5	23.7	24.0	24.2	24.5	24.7	25.0	25.2	25.5	25.7
96.5	38		21.2	21.4	21.7	21.9	22.2	22.4	22.6	22.9	23.1	23.4	23.6	23.9	24.1	24.3	24.6	24.8	25.1
97.8	38.5		20.6	20.9	21.1	21.3	21.6	21.8	22.1	22.3	22.5	22.8	23.0	23.2	23.5	23.7	24.0	24.2	24.4
99.1	39		20.1	20.3	20.6	20.8	21.0	21.3	21.5	21.7	22.0	22.2	22.4	22.6	22.9	23.1	23.3	23.6	23.8
100.3	39.5		19.6	19.8	20.1	20.3	20.5	20.7	21.0	21.2	21.4	21.6	21.9	22.1	22.3	22.5	22.8	23.0	23.2
101.6	40		19.1	19.3	19.6	19.8	20.0	20.2	20.4	20.7	20.9	21.1	21.3	21.5	21.8	22.0	22.2	22.4	22.6
102.9	40.5		18.6	18.9	19.1	19.3	19.5	19.7	19.9	20.1	20.4	20.6	20.8	21.0	21.2	21.4	21.6	21.9	22.1
104.1	41		18.2	18.4	18.6	18.8	19.0	19.2	19.4	19.7	19.9	20.1	20.3	20.5	20.7	20.9	21.1	21.3	21.5
105.4	41.5		17.8	18.0	18.2	18.4	18.6	18.8	19.0	19.2	19.4	19.6	19.8	20.0	20.2	20.4	20.6	20.8	21.0
106.7	42		17.3	17.5	17.7	17.9	18.1	18.3	18.5	18.7	18.9	19.1	19.3	19.5	19.7	19.9	20.1	20.3	20.5
108.0	42.5		16.9	17.1	17.3	17.5	17.7	17.9	18.1	18.3	18.5	18.7	18.9	19.1	19.3	19.5	19.7	19.9	20.0
109.2	43		16.5	16.7	16.9	17.1	17.3	17.5	17.7	17.9	18.1	18.3	18.4	18.6	18.8	19.0	19.2	19.4	19.6
110.5	43.5		16.2	16.3	16.5	16.7	16.9	17.1	17.3	17.5	17.6	17.8	18.0	18.2	18.4	18.6	18.8	18.9	19.1
111.8	44		15.8	16.0	16.2	16.3	16.5	16.7	16.9	17.1	17.2	17.4	17.6	17.8	18.0	18.2	18.3	18.5	18.7

Whenever a child's specific height or weight measurement is not listed, round to the closest number in the table.

CALCULATED BODY MASS INDEX   44.5"–51" AND 43.5 LBS.–51.5 LBS.

Height Cm	In	Kg 19.7 / Lb 43.5	20.0 / 44	20.2 / 44.5	20.4 / 45	20.6 / 45.5	20.9 / 46	21.1 / 46.5	21.3 / 47	21.5 / 47.5	21.8 / 48	22.0 / 48.5	22.2 / 49	22.5 / 49.5	22.7 / 50	22.9 / 50.5	23.1 / 51	23.4 / 51.5
110.5	43.5	13.0	13.2	13.4	13.6	13.7	13.9	14.1	14.3	14.5	14.7	14.9	15.0	15.2	15.4	15.6	15.8	16.0
113.0	44.5	15.4	15.6	15.8	16.0	16.2	16.3	16.5	16.7	16.9	17.0	17.2	17.4	17.6	17.8	17.9	18.1	18.3
114.3	45	15.1	15.3	15.5	15.6	15.8	16.0	16.1	16.3	16.5	16.7	16.8	17.0	17.2	17.4	17.5	17.7	17.9
115.6	45.5	14.8	14.9	15.1	15.3	15.5	15.6	15.8	16.0	16.1	16.3	16.5	16.6	16.8	17.0	17.2	17.3	17.5
116.8	46	14.5	14.6	14.8	15.0	15.1	15.3	15.5	15.6	15.8	15.9	16.1	16.3	16.4	16.6	16.8	16.9	17.1
118.1	46.5	14.1	14.3	14.5	14.6	14.8	15.0	15.1	15.3	15.4	15.6	15.8	15.9	16.1	16.3	16.4	16.6	16.7
119.4	47	13.8	14.0	14.2	14.3	14.5	14.6	14.8	15.0	15.1	15.3	15.4	15.6	15.8	15.9	16.1	16.2	16.4
120.7	47.5	13.6	13.7	13.9	14.0	14.2	14.3	14.5	14.6	14.8	15.0	15.1	15.3	15.4	15.6	15.7	15.9	16.0
121.9	48	13.3	13.4	13.6	13.7	13.9	14.0	14.2	14.3	14.5	14.6	14.8	15.0	15.1	15.3	15.4	15.6	15.7
124.5	49			13.0	13.2	13.3	13.5	13.6	13.8	13.9	14.1	14.2	14.3	14.5	14.6	14.8	14.9	15.1
127.0	50							13.1	13.2	13.4	13.5	13.6	13.8	13.9	14.1	14.2	14.3	14.5
129.5	51											13.1	13.2	13.4	13.5	13.7	13.8	13.9
132.1	52														13.0	13.1	13.3	13.4

Whenever a child's specific height or weight measurement is not listed, round to the closest number in the table.

CALCULATED BODY MASS INDEX   47"–56" AND 52 LBS.–60 LBS.

Height Cm	In	| Weight Kg 23.6 / Lb 52	23.8 / 52.5	24.0 / 53	24.3 / 53.5	24.5 / 54	24.7 / 54.5	24.9 / 55	25.2 / 55.5	25.4 / 56	25.6 / 56.5	25.9 / 57	26.1 / 57.5	26.3 / 58	26.5 / 58.5	26.8 / 59	27.0 / 59.5	27.2 / 60
119.4	47	16.6	16.7	16.9	17.0	17.2	17.3	17.5	17.7	17.8	18.0	18.1	18.3	18.5	18.6	18.8	18.9	19.1
120.7	47.5	16.2	16.4	16.5	16.7	16.8	17.0	17.1	17.3	17.5	17.6	17.8	17.9	18.1	18.2	18.4	18.5	18.7
121.9	48	15.9	16.0	16.2	16.3	16.5	16.6	16.8	16.9	17.1	17.2	17.4	17.5	17.7	17.9	18.0	18.2	18.3
124.5	49	15.2	15.4	15.5	15.7	15.8	16.0	16.1	16.3	16.4	16.5	16.7	16.8	17.0	17.1	17.3	17.4	17.6
127.0	50	14.6	14.8	14.9	15.0	15.2	15.3	15.5	15.6	15.7	15.9	16.0	16.2	16.3	16.5	16.6	16.7	16.9
129.5	51	14.1	14.2	14.3	14.5	14.6	14.7	14.9	15.0	15.1	15.3	15.4	15.5	15.7	15.8	15.9	16.1	16.2
132.1	52	13.5	13.7	13.8	13.9	14.0	14.2	14.3	14.4	14.6	14.7	14.8	15.0	15.1	15.2	15.3	15.5	15.6
134.6	53	13.0	13.1	13.3	13.4	13.5	13.6	13.8	13.9	14.0	14.1	14.3	14.4	14.5	14.6	14.8	14.9	15.0
137.2	54					13.0	13.1	13.3	13.4	13.5	13.6	13.7	13.9	14.0	14.1	14.2	14.3	14.5
139.7	55									13.0	13.1	13.2	13.4	13.5	13.6	13.7	13.8	13.9
142.2	56													13.0	13.1	13.2	13.3	13.5

Whenever a child's specific height or weight measurement is not listed, round to the closest number in the table.

CALCULATED BODY MASS INDEX   35.5"–51" AND 61 LBS.–77 LBS.

		Weight																
Height		Kg	27.7	28.1	28.6	29.0	29.5	29.9	30.4	30.8	31.3	31.8	32.2	32.7	33.1	33.6	34.0	34.5	34.9
Cm	In	Lb	61	62	63	64	65	66	67	68	69	70	71	72	73	74	75	76	77
90.2	35.5		34.0	34.6															
91.4	36		33.1	33.6	34.2	34.7													
92.7	36.5		32.2	32.7	33.2	33.8	34.3	34.8											
94.0	37		31.3	31.8	32.4	32.9	33.4	33.9	34.4	34.9									
95.3	37.5		30.5	31.0	31.5	32.0	32.5	33.0	33.5	34.0	34.5	35.0							
96.5	38		29.7	30.2	30.7	31.2	31.6	32.1	32.6	33.1	33.6	34.1							
97.8	38.5		28.9	29.4	29.9	30.4	30.8	31.3	31.8	32.3	32.7	33.2	33.7	34.2	34.6				
99.1	39		28.2	28.7	29.1	29.6	30.0	30.5	31.0	31.4	31.9	32.4	32.8	33.3	33.7	34.2	34.7		
100.3	39.5		27.5	27.9	28.4	28.8	29.3	29.7	30.2	30.6	31.1	31.5	32.0	32.4	32.9	33.3	33.8	34.2	34.7
101.6	40		26.8	27.2	27.7	28.1	28.6	29.0	29.4	29.9	30.3	30.8	31.2	31.6	32.1	32.5	33.0	33.4	33.8
102.9	40.5		26.1	26.6	27.0	27.4	27.9	28.3	28.7	29.1	29.6	30.0	30.4	30.9	31.3	31.7	32.1	32.6	33.0
104.1	41		25.5	25.9	26.3	26.8	27.2	27.6	28.0	28.4	28.9	29.3	29.7	30.1	30.5	31.0	31.4	31.8	32.2
105.4	41.5		24.9	25.3	25.7	26.1	26.5	26.9	27.4	27.8	28.2	28.6	29.0	29.4	29.8	30.2	30.6	31.0	31.4
106.7	42		24.3	24.7	25.1	25.5	25.9	26.3	26.7	27.1	27.5	27.9	28.3	28.7	29.1	29.5	29.9	30.3	30.7
108.0	42.5		23.7	24.1	24.5	24.9	25.3	25.7	26.1	26.5	26.9	27.2	27.6	28.0	28.4	28.8	29.2	29.6	30.0
109.2	43		23.2	23.6	24.0	24.3	24.7	25.1	25.5	25.9	26.2	26.6	27.0	27.4	27.8	28.1	28.5	28.9	29.3
110.5	43.5		22.7	23.0	23.4	23.8	24.2	24.5	24.9	25.3	25.6	26.0	26.4	26.8	27.1	27.5	27.9	28.2	28.6
111.8	44		22.2	22.5	22.9	23.2	23.6	24.0	24.3	24.7	25.1	25.4	25.8	26.1	26.5	26.9	27.2	27.6	28.0
113.0	44.5		21.7	22.0	22.4	22.7	23.1	23.4	23.8	24.1	24.5	24.9	25.2	25.6	25.9	26.3	26.6	27.0	27.3
114.3	45		21.2	21.5	21.9	22.2	22.6	22.9	23.3	23.6	24.0	24.3	24.7	25.0	25.3	25.7	26.0	26.4	26.7
115.6	45.5		20.7	21.1	21.4	21.7	22.1	22.4	22.8	23.1	23.4	23.8	24.1	24.5	24.8	25.1	25.5	25.8	26.1
116.8	46		20.3	20.6	20.9	21.3	21.6	21.9	22.3	22.6	22.9	23.3	23.6	23.9	24.3	24.6	24.9	25.3	25.6
118.1	46.5		19.8	20.2	20.5	20.8	21.1	21.5	21.8	22.1	22.4	22.8	23.1	23.4	23.7	24.1	24.4	24.7	25.0
119.4	47		19.4	19.7	20.1	20.4	20.7	21.0	21.3	21.6	22.0	22.3	22.6	22.9	23.2	23.6	23.9	24.2	24.5
120.7	47.5		19.0	19.3	19.6	19.9	20.3	20.6	20.9	21.2	21.5	21.8	22.1	22.4	22.7	23.1	23.4	23.7	24.0
121.9	48		18.6	18.9	19.2	19.5	19.8	20.1	20.4	20.8	21.1	21.4	21.7	22.0	22.3	22.6	22.9	23.2	23.5
124.5	49		17.9	18.2	18.4	18.7	19.0	19.3	19.6	19.9	20.2	20.5	20.8	21.1	21.4	21.7	22.0	22.3	22.5
127.0	50		17.2	17.4	17.7	18.0	18.3	18.6	18.8	19.1	19.4	19.7	20.0	20.2	20.5	20.8	21.1	21.4	21.7
129.5	51		16.5	16.8	17.0	17.3	17.6	17.8	18.1	18.4	18.7	18.9	19.2	19.5	19.7	20.0	20.3	20.5	20.8

Whenever a child's specific height or weight measurement is not listed, round to the closest number in the table.

CALCULATED BODY MASS INDEX   52"–64" AND 61 LBS.–77 LBS.

Height Cm	Height In	Weight Kg 27.7 / Lb 61	28.1 / 62	28.6 / 63	29.0 / 64	29.5 / 65	29.9 / 66	30.4 / 67	30.8 / 68	31.3 / 69	31.8 / 70	32.2 / 71	32.7 / 72	33.1 / 73	33.6 / 74	34.0 / 75	34.5 / 76	34.9 / 77
132.1	52	15.9	16.1	16.4	16.6	16.9	17.2	17.4	17.7	17.9	18.2	18.5	18.7	19.0	19.2	19.5	19.8	20.0
134.6	53	15.3	15.5	15.8	16.0	16.3	16.5	16.8	17.0	17.3	17.5	17.8	18.0	18.3	18.5	18.8	19.0	19.3
137.2	54	14.7	14.9	15.2	15.4	15.7	15.9	16.2	16.4	16.6	16.9	17.1	17.4	17.6	17.8	18.1	18.3	18.6
139.7	55	14.2	14.4	14.6	14.9	15.1	15.3	15.6	15.8	16.0	16.3	16.5	16.7	17.0	17.2	17.4	17.7	17.9
142.2	56	13.7	13.9	14.1	14.3	14.6	14.8	15.0	15.2	15.5	15.7	15.9	16.1	16.4	16.6	16.8	17.0	17.3
144.8	57	13.2	13.4	13.6	13.8	14.1	14.3	14.5	14.7	14.9	15.1	15.4	15.6	15.8	16.0	16.2	16.4	16.7
147.3	58			13.2	13.4	13.6	13.8	14.0	14.2	14.4	14.6	14.8	15.0	15.3	15.5	15.7	15.9	16.1
149.9	59					13.1	13.3	13.5	13.7	13.9	14.1	14.3	14.5	14.7	14.9	15.1	15.3	15.6
152.4	60							13.1	13.3	13.5	13.7	13.9	14.1	14.3	14.5	14.6	14.8	15.0
154.9	61									13.0	13.2	13.4	13.6	13.8	14.0	14.2	14.4	14.5
157.5	62												13.2	13.4	13.6	13.7	13.9	14.1
160.0	63														13.1	13.3	13.5	13.6
162.6	64																13.0	13.2

Whenever a child's specific height or weight measurement is not listed, round to the closest number in the table.

CALCULATED BODY MASS INDEX   40.5"–60" AND 78 LBS.–94 LBS.

Height		Weight																
Cm	In	Kg 35.4	35.8	36.3	36.7	37.2	37.6	38.1	38.6	39.0	39.5	39.9	40.4	40.8	41.3	41.7	42.2	42.6
		Lb 78	79	80	81	82	83	84	85	86	87	88	89	90	91	92	93	94
101.6	40	34.3	34.7															
102.9	40.5	33.4	33.9	34.3	34.7													
104.1	41	32.6	33.0	33.5	33.9	34.3	34.7											
105.4	41.5	31.8	32.2	32.7	33.1	33.5	33.9	34.3	34.7									
106.7	42	31.1	31.5	31.9	32.3	32.7	33.1	33.5	33.9	34.3	34.7							
108.0	42.5	30.4	30.8	31.1	31.5	31.9	32.3	32.7	33.1	33.5	33.9	34.3	34.6					
109.2	43	29.7	30.0	30.4	30.8	31.2	31.6	31.9	32.3	32.7	33.1	33.5	33.8	34.2	34.6	35.0		
110.5	43.5	29.0	29.4	29.7	30.1	30.5	30.8	31.2	31.6	32.0	32.3	32.7	33.1	33.4	33.8	34.2	34.6	34.9
111.8	44	28.3	28.7	29.1	29.4	29.8	30.1	30.5	30.9	31.2	31.6	32.0	32.3	32.7	33.0	33.4	33.8	34.1
113.0	44.5	27.7	28.0	28.4	28.8	29.1	29.5	29.8	30.2	30.5	30.9	31.2	31.6	32.0	32.3	32.7	33.0	33.4
114.3	45	27.1	27.4	27.8	28.1	28.5	28.8	29.2	29.5	29.9	30.2	30.6	30.9	31.2	31.6	31.9	32.3	32.6
115.6	45.5	26.5	26.8	27.2	27.5	27.8	28.2	28.5	28.9	29.2	29.5	29.9	30.2	30.6	30.9	31.2	31.6	31.9
116.8	46	25.9	26.2	26.6	26.9	27.2	27.6	27.9	28.2	28.6	28.9	29.2	29.6	29.9	30.2	30.6	30.9	31.2
118.1	46.5	25.4	25.7	26.0	26.3	26.7	27.0	27.3	27.6	28.0	28.3	28.6	28.9	29.3	29.6	29.9	30.2	30.6
119.4	47	24.8	25.1	25.5	25.8	26.1	26.4	26.7	27.1	27.4	27.7	28.0	28.3	28.6	29.0	29.3	29.6	29.9
120.7	47.5	24.3	24.6	24.9	25.2	25.6	25.9	26.2	26.5	26.8	27.1	27.4	27.7	28.0	28.4	28.7	29.0	29.3
121.9	48	23.8	24.1	24.4	24.7	25.0	25.3	25.6	25.9	26.2	26.5	26.9	27.2	27.5	27.8	28.1	28.4	28.7
124.5	49	22.8	23.1	23.4	23.7	24.0	24.3	24.6	24.9	25.2	25.5	25.8	26.1	26.4	26.6	26.9	27.2	27.5
127.0	50	21.9	22.2	22.5	22.8	23.1	23.3	23.6	23.9	24.2	24.5	24.7	25.0	25.3	25.6	25.9	26.2	26.4
129.5	51	21.1	21.4	21.6	21.9	22.2	22.4	22.7	23.0	23.2	23.5	23.8	24.1	24.3	24.6	24.9	25.1	25.4
132.1	52	20.3	20.5	20.8	21.1	21.3	21.6	21.8	22.1	22.4	22.6	22.9	23.1	23.4	23.7	23.9	24.2	24.4
134.6	53	19.5	19.8	20.0	20.3	20.5	20.8	21.0	21.3	21.5	21.8	22.0	22.3	22.5	22.8	23.0	23.3	23.5
137.2	54	18.8	19.0	19.3	19.5	19.8	20.0	20.3	20.5	20.7	21.0	21.2	21.5	21.7	21.9	22.2	22.4	22.7
139.7	55	18.1	18.4	18.6	18.8	19.1	19.3	19.5	19.8	20.0	20.2	20.5	20.7	20.9	21.2	21.4	21.6	21.8
142.2	56	17.5	17.7	17.9	18.2	18.4	18.6	18.8	19.1	19.3	19.5	19.7	20.0	20.2	20.4	20.6	20.8	21.1
144.8	57	16.9	17.1	17.3	17.5	17.7	18.0	18.2	18.4	18.6	18.8	19.0	19.3	19.5	19.7	19.9	20.1	20.3
147.3	58	16.3	16.5	16.7	16.9	17.1	17.3	17.6	17.8	18.0	18.2	18.4	18.6	18.8	19.0	19.2	19.4	19.6
149.9	59	15.8	16.0	16.2	16.4	16.6	16.8	17.0	17.2	17.4	17.6	17.8	18.0	18.2	18.4	18.6	18.8	19.0
152.4	60	15.2	15.4	15.6	15.8	16.0	16.2	16.4	16.6	16.8	17.0	17.2	17.4	17.6	17.8	18.0	18.2	18.4

Whenever a child's specific height or weight measurement is not listed, round to the closest number in the table.

CALCULATED BODY MASS INDEX   61"–71" AND 78 LBS.–94 LBS.

Height Cm	Height In	Weight Kg 35.4 / Lb 78	35.8 / 79	36.3 / 80	36.7 / 81	37.2 / 82	37.6 / 83	38.1 / 84	38.6 / 85	39.0 / 86	39.5 / 87	39.9 / 88	40.4 / 89	40.8 / 90	41.3 / 91	41.7 / 92	42.2 / 93	42.6 / 94
154.9	61	14.7	14.9	15.1	15.3	15.5	15.7	15.9	16.1	16.2	16.4	16.6	16.8	17.0	17.2	17.4	17.6	17.8
157.5	62	14.3	14.4	14.6	14.8	15.0	15.2	15.4	15.5	15.7	15.9	16.1	16.3	16.5	16.6	16.8	17.0	17.2
160.0	63	13.8	14.0	14.2	14.3	14.5	14.7	14.9	15.1	15.2	15.4	15.6	15.8	15.9	16.1	16.3	16.5	16.7
162.6	64	13.4	13.6	13.7	13.9	14.1	14.2	14.4	14.6	14.8	14.9	15.1	15.3	15.4	15.6	15.8	16.0	16.1
165.1	65		13.1	13.3	13.5	13.6	13.8	14.0	14.1	14.3	14.5	14.6	14.8	15.0	15.1	15.3	15.5	15.6
167.6	66				13.1	13.2	13.4	13.6	13.7	13.9	14.0	14.2	14.4	14.5	14.7	14.8	15.0	15.2
170.2	67							13.2	13.3	13.5	13.6	13.8	13.9	14.1	14.3	14.4	14.6	14.7
172.7	68									13.1	13.2	13.4	13.5	13.7	13.8	14.0	14.1	14.3
175.3	69												13.1	13.3	13.4	13.6	13.7	13.9
177.8	70														13.1	13.2	13.3	13.5
180.3	71																	13.1

Whenever a child's specific height or weight measurement is not listed, round to the closest number in the table.

CALCULATED BODY MASS INDEX 44"–68" AND 95 LBS.–112 LBS.

Height Cm	Height In	Kg 43.1 / Lb 95	43.5 / 96	44.0 / 97	44.5 / 98	44.9 / 99	45.4 / 100	45.8 / 101	46.3 / 102	46.7 / 103	47.2 / 104	47.6 / 105	48.1 / 106	48.5 / 107	49.0 / 108	49.4 / 109	49.9 / 110	50.8 / 112
111.8	44	34.5	34.9															
113.0	44.5	33.7	34.1	34.4	34.8													
114.3	45	33.0	33.3	33.7	34.0	34.4	34.7											
115.6	45.5	32.3	32.6	32.9	33.3	33.6	34.0	34.3										
116.8	46	31.6	31.9	32.2	32.6	32.9	33.2	33.6	33.9									
118.1	46.5	30.9	31.2	31.5	31.9	32.2	32.5	32.8	33.2	33.5								
119.4	47	30.2	30.6	30.9	31.2	31.5	31.8	32.1	32.5	32.8	33.1	33.4	33.7	34.1	34.4	34.7		
120.7	47.5	29.6	29.9	30.2	30.5	30.8	31.2	31.5	31.8	32.1	32.4	32.7	33.0	33.3	33.7	34.0	34.3	34.9
121.9	48	29.0	29.3	29.6	29.9	30.2	30.5	30.8	31.1	31.4	31.7	32.0	32.3	32.7	33.0	33.3	33.6	34.2
124.5	49	27.8	28.1	28.4	28.7	29.0	29.3	29.6	29.9	30.2	30.5	30.7	31.0	31.3	31.6	31.9	32.2	32.8
127.0	50	26.7	27.0	27.3	27.6	27.8	28.1	28.4	28.7	29.0	29.2	29.5	29.8	30.1	30.4	30.7	30.9	31.5
129.5	51	25.7	25.9	26.2	26.5	26.8	27.0	27.3	27.6	27.8	28.1	28.4	28.7	28.9	29.2	29.5	29.7	30.3
132.1	52	24.7	25.0	25.2	25.5	25.7	26.0	26.3	26.5	26.8	27.0	27.3	27.6	27.8	28.1	28.3	28.6	29.1
134.6	53	23.8	24.0	24.3	24.5	24.8	25.0	25.3	25.5	25.8	26.0	26.3	26.5	26.8	27.0	27.3	27.5	28.0
137.2	54	22.9	23.1	23.4	23.6	23.9	24.1	24.4	24.6	24.8	25.1	25.3	25.6	25.8	26.0	26.3	26.5	27.0
139.7	55	22.1	22.3	22.5	22.8	23.0	23.2	23.5	23.7	23.9	24.2	24.4	24.6	24.9	25.1	25.3	25.6	26.0
142.2	56	21.3	21.5	21.7	22.0	22.2	22.4	22.6	22.9	23.1	23.3	23.5	23.8	24.0	24.2	24.4	24.7	25.1
144.8	57	20.6	20.8	21.0	21.2	21.4	21.6	21.9	22.1	22.3	22.5	22.7	22.9	23.2	23.4	23.6	23.8	24.2
147.3	58	19.9	20.1	20.3	20.5	20.7	20.9	21.1	21.3	21.5	21.7	21.9	22.2	22.4	22.6	22.8	23.0	23.4
149.9	59	19.2	19.4	19.6	19.8	20.0	20.2	20.4	20.6	20.8	21.0	21.2	21.4	21.6	21.8	22.0	22.2	22.6
152.4	60	18.6	18.7	18.9	19.1	19.3	19.5	19.7	19.9	20.1	20.3	20.5	20.7	20.9	21.1	21.3	21.5	21.9
154.9	61	17.9	18.1	18.3	18.5	18.7	18.9	19.1	19.3	19.5	19.7	19.8	20.0	20.2	20.4	20.6	20.8	21.2
157.5	62	17.4	17.6	17.7	17.9	18.1	18.3	18.5	18.7	18.8	19.0	19.2	19.4	19.6	19.8	19.9	20.1	20.5
160.0	63	16.8	17.0	17.2	17.4	17.5	17.7	17.9	18.1	18.2	18.4	18.6	18.8	19.0	19.1	19.3	19.5	19.8
162.6	64	16.3	16.5	16.6	16.8	17.0	17.2	17.3	17.5	17.7	17.9	18.0	18.2	18.4	18.5	18.7	18.9	19.2
165.1	65	15.8	16.0	16.1	16.3	16.5	16.6	16.8	17.0	17.1	17.3	17.5	17.6	17.8	18.0	18.1	18.3	18.6
167.6	66	15.3	15.5	15.7	15.8	16.0	16.1	16.3	16.5	16.6	16.8	16.9	17.1	17.3	17.4	17.6	17.8	18.1
170.2	67	14.9	15.0	15.2	15.3	15.5	15.7	15.8	16.0	16.1	16.3	16.4	16.6	16.8	16.9	17.1	17.2	17.5
172.7	68	14.4	14.6	14.7	14.9	15.1	15.2	15.4	15.5	15.7	15.8	16.0	16.1	16.3	16.4	16.6	16.7	17.0

Whenever a child's specific height or weight measurement is not listed, round to the closest number in the table.

CALCULATED BODY MASS INDEX   69"–77" AND 95 LBS.–112 LBS.

Height			Weight																
Cm	In	Kg	43.1	43.5	44.0	44.5	44.9	45.4	45.8	46.3	46.7	47.2	47.6	48.1	48.5	49.0	49.4	49.9	50.8
		Lb	95	96	97	98	99	100	101	102	103	104	105	106	107	108	109	110	112
175.3	69		14.0	14.2	14.3	14.5	14.6	14.8	14.9	15.1	15.2	15.4	15.5	15.7	15.8	15.9	16.1	16.2	16.5
177.8	70		13.6	13.8	13.9	14.1	14.2	14.3	14.5	14.6	14.8	14.9	15.1	15.2	15.4	15.5	15.6	15.8	16.1
180.3	71		13.2	13.4	13.5	13.7	13.8	13.9	14.1	14.2	14.4	14.5	14.6	14.8	14.9	15.1	15.2	15.3	15.6
182.9	72			13.0	13.2	13.3	13.4	13.6	13.7	13.8	14.0	14.1	14.2	14.4	14.5	14.6	14.8	14.9	15.2
185.4	73						13.1	13.2	13.3	13.5	13.6	13.7	13.9	14.0	14.1	14.2	14.4	14.5	14.8
188.0	74									13.1	13.2	13.4	13.5	13.6	13.7	13.9	14.0	14.1	14.4
190.5	75												13.1	13.2	13.4	13.5	13.6	13.7	14.0
193.0	76														13.0	13.1	13.3	13.4	13.6
195.6	77																	13.0	13.3

Whenever a child's specific height or weight measurement is not listed, round to the closest number in the table.

CALCULATED BODY MASS INDEX   48"–76" AND 114 LBS.–146 LBS.

Height Cm	Height In	Kg 51.7 / Lb 114	52.6 / 116	53.5 / 118	54.4 / 120	55.3 / 122	56.2 / 124	57.2 / 126	58.1 / 128	59.0 / 130	59.9 / 132	60.8 / 134	61.7 / 136	62.6 / 138	63.5 / 140	64.4 / 142	65.3 / 144	66.2 / 146
121.9	48	34.8																
124.5	49	33.4	34.0															
127.0	50	32.1	32.6	33.2	33.7	34.3	34.9											
129.5	51	30.8	31.4	31.9	32.4	33.0	33.5	34.1	34.6									
132.1	52	29.6	30.2	30.7	31.2	31.7	32.2	32.8	33.3	33.8	34.3	34.8						
134.6	53	28.5	29.0	29.5	30.0	30.5	31.0	31.5	32.0	32.5	33.0	33.5	34.0	34.5				
137.2	54	27.5	28.0	28.5	28.9	29.4	29.9	30.4	30.9	31.3	31.8	32.3	32.8	33.3	33.8	34.2	34.7	
139.7	55	26.5	27.0	27.4	27.9	28.4	28.8	29.3	29.7	30.2	30.7	31.1	31.6	32.1	32.5	33.0	33.5	33.9
142.2	56	25.6	26.0	26.5	26.9	27.4	27.8	28.2	28.7	29.1	29.6	30.0	30.5	30.9	31.4	31.8	32.3	32.7
144.8	57	24.7	25.1	25.5	26.0	26.4	26.8	27.3	27.7	28.1	28.6	29.0	29.4	29.9	30.3	30.7	31.2	31.6
147.3	58	23.8	24.2	24.7	25.1	25.5	25.9	26.3	26.8	27.2	27.6	28.0	28.4	28.8	29.3	29.7	30.1	30.5
149.9	59	23.0	23.4	23.8	24.2	24.6	25.0	25.4	25.9	26.3	26.7	27.1	27.5	27.9	28.3	28.7	29.1	29.5
152.4	60	22.3	22.7	23.0	23.4	23.8	24.2	24.6	25.0	25.4	25.8	26.2	26.6	27.0	27.3	27.7	28.1	28.5
154.9	61	21.5	21.9	22.3	22.7	23.1	23.4	23.8	24.2	24.6	24.9	25.3	25.7	26.1	26.5	26.8	27.2	27.6
157.5	62	20.9	21.2	21.6	21.9	22.3	22.7	23.0	23.4	23.8	24.1	24.5	24.9	25.2	25.6	26.0	26.3	26.7
160.0	63	20.2	20.5	20.9	21.3	21.6	22.0	22.3	22.7	23.0	23.4	23.7	24.1	24.4	24.8	25.2	25.5	25.9
162.6	64	19.6	19.9	20.3	20.6	20.9	21.3	21.6	22.0	22.3	22.7	23.0	23.3	23.7	24.0	24.4	24.7	25.1
165.1	65	19.0	19.3	19.6	20.0	20.3	20.6	21.0	21.3	21.6	22.0	22.3	22.6	23.0	23.3	23.6	24.0	24.3
167.6	66	18.4	18.7	19.0	19.4	19.7	20.0	20.3	20.7	21.0	21.3	21.6	22.0	22.3	22.6	22.9	23.2	23.6
170.2	67	17.9	18.2	18.5	18.8	19.1	19.4	19.7	20.0	20.4	20.7	21.0	21.3	21.6	21.9	22.2	22.6	22.9
172.7	68	17.3	17.6	17.9	18.2	18.5	18.9	19.2	19.5	19.8	20.1	20.4	20.7	21.0	21.3	21.6	21.9	22.2
175.3	69	16.8	17.1	17.4	17.7	18.0	18.3	18.6	18.9	19.2	19.5	19.8	20.1	20.4	20.7	21.0	21.3	21.6
177.8	70	16.4	16.6	16.9	17.2	17.5	17.8	18.1	18.4	18.7	18.9	19.2	19.5	19.8	20.1	20.4	20.7	20.9
180.3	71	15.9	16.2	16.5	16.7	17.0	17.3	17.6	17.9	18.1	18.4	18.7	19.0	19.2	19.5	19.8	20.1	20.4
182.9	72	15.5	15.7	16.0	16.3	16.5	16.8	17.1	17.4	17.6	17.9	18.2	18.4	18.7	19.0	19.3	19.5	19.8
185.4	73	15.0	15.3	15.6	15.8	16.1	16.4	16.6	16.9	17.2	17.4	17.7	17.9	18.2	18.5	18.7	19.0	19.3
188.0	74	14.6	14.9	15.2	15.4	15.7	15.9	16.2	16.4	16.7	16.9	17.2	17.5	17.7	18.0	18.2	18.5	18.7
190.5	75	14.2	14.5	14.7	15.0	15.2	15.5	15.7	16.0	16.2	16.5	16.7	17.0	17.2	17.5	17.7	18.0	18.2
193.0	76	13.9	14.1	14.4	14.6	14.9	15.1	15.3	15.6	15.8	16.1	16.3	16.6	16.8	17.0	17.3	17.5	17.8
195.6	77	13.5	13.8	14.0	14.2	14.5	14.7	14.9	15.2	15.4	15.7	15.9	16.1	16.4	16.6	16.8	17.1	17.3
198.1	78	13.2	13.4	13.6	13.9	14.1	14.3	14.6	14.8	15.0	15.3	15.5	15.7	15.9	16.2	16.4	16.6	16.9

Whenever a child's specific height or weight measurement is not listed, round to the closest number in the table.

CALCULATED BODY MASS INDEX 55"–78" AND 148 LBS.–180 LBS.

Height Cm	In	Kg 67.1	68.0	68.9	69.9	70.8	71.7	72.6	73.5	74.4	75.3	76.2	77.1	78.0	78.9	79.8	80.7	81.6
		Lb 148	150	152	154	156	158	160	162	164	166	168	170	172	174	176	178	180
139.7	55	34.4	34.9															
142.2	56	33.2	33.6	34.1	34.5	35.0												
144.8	57	32.0	32.5	32.9	33.3	33.8	34.2	34.6										
147.3	58	30.9	31.3	31.8	32.2	32.6	33.0	33.4	33.9	34.3	34.7							
149.9	59	29.9	30.3	30.7	31.1	31.5	31.9	32.3	32.7	33.1	33.5	33.9	34.3	34.7				
152.4	60	28.9	29.3	29.7	30.1	30.5	30.9	31.2	31.6	32.0	32.4	32.8	33.2	33.6	34.0	34.4	34.8	
154.9	61	28.0	28.3	28.7	29.1	29.5	29.9	30.2	30.6	31.0	31.4	31.7	32.1	32.5	32.9	33.3	33.6	34.0
157.5	62	27.1	27.4	27.8	28.2	28.5	28.9	29.3	29.6	30.0	30.4	30.7	31.1	31.5	31.8	32.2	32.6	32.9
160.0	63	26.2	26.6	26.9	27.3	27.6	28.0	28.3	28.7	29.1	29.4	29.8	30.1	30.5	30.8	31.2	31.5	31.9
162.6	64	25.4	25.7	26.1	26.4	26.8	27.1	27.5	27.8	28.2	28.5	28.8	29.2	29.5	29.9	30.2	30.6	30.9
165.1	65	24.6	25.0	25.3	25.6	26.0	26.3	26.6	27.0	27.3	27.6	28.0	28.3	28.6	29.0	29.3	29.6	30.0
167.6	66	23.9	24.2	24.5	24.9	25.2	25.5	25.8	26.1	26.5	26.8	27.1	27.4	27.8	28.1	28.4	28.7	29.1
170.2	67	23.2	23.5	23.8	24.1	24.4	24.7	25.1	25.4	25.7	26.0	26.3	26.6	26.9	27.3	27.6	27.9	28.2
172.7	68	22.5	22.8	23.1	23.4	23.7	24.0	24.3	24.6	24.9	25.2	25.5	25.8	26.2	26.5	26.8	27.1	27.4
175.3	69	21.9	22.2	22.4	22.7	23.0	23.3	23.6	23.9	24.2	24.5	24.8	25.1	25.4	25.7	26.0	26.3	26.6
177.8	70	21.2	21.5	21.8	22.1	22.4	22.7	23.0	23.2	23.5	23.8	24.1	24.4	24.7	25.0	25.3	25.5	25.8
180.3	71	20.6	20.9	21.2	21.5	21.8	22.0	22.3	22.6	22.9	23.2	23.4	23.7	24.0	24.3	24.5	24.8	25.1
182.9	72	20.1	20.3	20.6	20.9	21.2	21.4	21.7	22.0	22.2	22.5	22.8	23.1	23.3	23.6	23.9	24.1	24.4
185.4	73	19.5	19.8	20.1	20.3	20.6	20.8	21.1	21.4	21.6	21.9	22.2	22.4	22.7	23.0	23.2	23.5	23.7
188.0	74	19.0	19.3	19.5	19.8	20.0	20.3	20.5	20.8	21.1	21.3	21.6	21.8	22.1	22.3	22.6	22.9	23.1
190.5	75	18.5	18.7	19.0	19.2	19.5	19.7	20.0	20.2	20.5	20.7	21.0	21.2	21.5	21.7	22.0	22.2	22.5
193.0	76	18.0	18.3	18.5	18.7	19.0	19.2	19.5	19.7	20.0	20.2	20.4	20.7	20.9	21.2	21.4	21.7	21.9
195.6	77	17.6	17.8	18.0	18.3	18.5	18.7	19.0	19.2	19.4	19.7	19.9	20.2	20.4	20.6	20.9	21.1	21.3
198.1	78	17.1	17.3	17.6	17.8	18.0	18.3	18.5	18.7	19.0	19.2	19.4	19.6	19.9	20.1	20.3	20.6	20.8

Whenever a child's specific height or weight measurement is not listed, round to the closest number in the table.

CALCULATED BODY MASS INDEX   61"–78" AND 182 LBS.–214 LBS.

Height Cm	In	Kg 82.6 / Lb 182	83.5 / 184	84.4 / 186	85.3 / 188	86.2 / 190	87.1 / 192	88.0 / 194	88.9 / 196	89.8 / 198	90.7 / 200	91.6 / 202	92.5 / 204	93.4 / 206	94.3 / 208	95.3 / 210	96.2 / 212	97.1 / 214
154.9	61	34.4	34.8															
157.5	62	33.3	33.7	34.0	34.4	34.8												
160.0	63	32.2	32.6	32.9	33.3	33.7	34.0	34.4	34.7									
162.6	64	31.2	31.6	31.9	32.3	32.6	33.0	33.3	33.6	34.0	34.3	34.7						
165.1	65	30.3	30.6	31.0	31.3	31.6	32.0	32.3	32.6	32.9	33.3	33.6	33.9	34.3	34.6	34.9		
167.6	66	29.4	29.7	30.0	30.3	30.7	31.0	31.3	31.6	32.0	32.3	32.6	32.9	33.2	33.6	33.9	34.2	34.5
170.2	67	28.5	28.8	29.1	29.4	29.8	30.1	30.4	30.7	31.0	31.3	31.6	32.0	32.3	32.6	32.9	33.2	33.5
172.7	68	27.7	28.0	28.3	28.6	28.9	29.2	29.5	29.8	30.1	30.4	30.7	31.0	31.3	31.6	31.9	32.2	32.5
175.3	69	26.9	27.2	27.5	27.8	28.1	28.4	28.6	28.9	29.2	29.5	29.8	30.1	30.4	30.7	31.0	31.3	31.6
177.8	70	26.1	26.4	26.7	27.0	27.3	27.5	27.8	28.1	28.4	28.7	29.0	29.3	29.6	29.8	30.1	30.4	30.7
180.3	71	25.4	25.7	25.9	26.2	26.5	26.8	27.1	27.3	27.6	27.9	28.2	28.5	28.7	29.0	29.3	29.6	29.8
182.9	72	24.7	25.0	25.2	25.5	25.8	26.0	26.3	26.6	26.9	27.1	27.4	27.7	27.9	28.2	28.5	28.8	29.0
185.4	73	24.0	24.3	24.5	24.8	25.1	25.3	25.6	25.9	26.1	26.4	26.7	26.9	27.2	27.4	27.7	28.0	28.2
188.0	74	23.4	23.6	23.9	24.1	24.4	24.7	24.9	25.2	25.4	25.7	25.9	26.2	26.4	26.7	27.0	27.2	27.5
190.5	75	22.7	23.0	23.2	23.5	23.7	24.0	24.2	24.5	24.7	25.0	25.2	25.5	25.7	26.0	26.2	26.5	26.7
193.0	76	22.2	22.4	22.6	22.9	23.1	23.4	23.6	23.9	24.1	24.3	24.6	24.8	25.1	25.3	25.6	25.8	26.0
195.6	77	21.6	21.8	22.1	22.3	22.5	22.8	23.0	23.2	23.5	23.7	24.0	24.2	24.4	24.7	24.9	25.1	25.4
198.1	78	21.0	21.3	21.5	21.7	22.0	22.2	22.4	22.6	22.9	23.1	23.3	23.6	23.8	24.0	24.3	24.5	24.7

Whenever a child's specific height or weight measurement is not listed, round to the closest number in the table.

CALCULATED BODY MASS INDEX   66″–78″ AND 216 LBS.–250 LBS.

Height		Weight																	
Cm	In	Kg 98.0	98.9	99.8	100.7	101.6	102.5	103.4	104.3	105.2	106.1	107.0	108.0	108.9	109.8	110.7	111.6	112.5	113.4
		Lb 216	218	220	222	224	226	228	230	232	234	236	238	240	242	244	246	248	250
167.6	66	34.9																	
170.2	67	33.8	34.1	34.5	34.8														
172.7	68	32.8	33.1	33.5	33.8	34.1	34.4	34.7	35.0										
175.3	69	31.9	32.2	32.5	32.8	33.1	33.4	33.7	34.0	34.3	34.6	34.9							
177.8	70	31.0	31.3	31.6	31.9	32.1	32.4	32.7	33.0	33.3	33.6	33.9	34.1	34.4	34.7				
180.3	71	30.1	30.4	30.7	31.0	31.2	31.5	31.8	32.1	32.4	32.6	32.9	33.2	33.5	33.8	34.0	34.3	34.6	34.9
182.9	72	29.3	29.6	29.8	30.1	30.4	30.7	30.9	31.2	31.5	31.7	32.0	32.3	32.5	32.8	33.1	33.4	33.6	33.9
185.4	73	28.5	28.8	29.0	29.3	29.6	29.8	30.1	30.3	30.6	30.9	31.1	31.4	31.7	31.9	32.2	32.5	32.7	33.0
188.0	74	27.7	28.0	28.2	28.5	28.8	29.0	29.3	29.5	29.8	30.0	30.3	30.6	30.8	31.1	31.3	31.6	31.8	32.1
190.5	75	27.0	27.2	27.5	27.7	28.0	28.2	28.5	28.7	29.0	29.2	29.5	29.7	30.0	30.2	30.5	30.7	31.0	31.2
193.0	76	26.3	26.5	26.8	27.0	27.3	27.5	27.8	28.0	28.2	28.5	28.7	29.0	29.2	29.5	29.7	29.9	30.2	30.4
195.6	77	25.6	25.9	26.1	26.3	26.6	26.8	27.0	27.3	27.5	27.7	28.0	28.2	28.5	28.7	28.9	29.2	29.4	29.6
198.1	78	25.0	25.2	25.4	25.7	25.9	26.1	26.3	26.6	26.8	27.0	27.3	27.5	27.7	28.0	28.2	28.4	28.7	28.9

Whenever a child's specific height or weight measurement is not listed, round to the closest number in the table.

APPENDIX XI
JOSLIN DIABETES CENTER CLINICS AND AFFILIATES

The Joslin Diabetes Center in Boston has provided care to diabetes patients for over a century and its affiliates nationwide also offer care targeted to patients with diabetes.

CALIFORNIA

Joslin Diabetes Center
Affiliate at University of California, Irvine
Gottschalk Medical Plaza
University of California, Irvine
Irvine, CA 92697
(949) 824-8656

CONNECTICUT

Joslin Diabetes Center
Affiliate at the Hospital of Central Connecticut
100 Grand Street
New Britain, CT 06050
(860) 224-5672
(888) 4-JOSLIN (toll-free)

Joslin Diabetes Center
Affiliate at Lawrence and Memorial Hospital
14 Clara Drive
Suite 4
Mystic, CT 06355
(860) 245-0565
9877-JOSLIN-1
Joslin Diabetes Center
Affiliate at Lawrence and Memorial Hospital
50 Faire Harbour Place
Suite 2E
New London, CT 06320
(860) 444-4737
(877) JOSLIN-1

Joslin Diabetes Center
Affiliate at Lawrence and Memorial Medical
    Office Building in Old Saybrook
633 Middlesex Turnpike
Old Saybrook, CT 06475
(860) 444-4737

ILLINOIS

Joslin Diabetes Center
Affiliate at OSF Healthcare System
8600 North Route 91
Suite 110
Peoria, IL 61615
(309) 683-5051

INDIANA

Joslin Diabetes Center
Affiliate at St. Mary's
3700 Washington Avenue
Evansville, IN 47750
(812) 485-1814

Joslin Diabetes Center
Affiliate at Floyd Memorial Hospital & Health
    Services
1850 State Street
New Albany, IN 47150
(812) 949-5700
(888) 77-FMHHS (toll-free)

IOWA

Joslin Diabetes Center
Education Affiliate at Mercy Medical Center
5264 Council Street NE
Cedar Rapids, IA 52403
(319) 398-6711

MARYLAND

Joslin Diabetes Center
Affiliate at Baltimore Washington Medical
    Center
301 Hospital Drive
Glen Burnie, MD 21042
(410) 787-4940

Joslin Diabetes Center
Affiliate at Doctors Community Hospital
8118 Good Luck Road, MOB
Fifth Floor
Lanham, MD 20706
(301) 552-8661

Joslin Diabetes Center
Affiliate at Maryland General Hospital
821 North Eutaw Street
Baltimore, MD 21201
(443) 552-2960

Joslin Diabetes Center
Affiliate at Shore Health System
119 South Washington Street
Easton, MD 21601
(410) 822-1000, extension 5757

Joslin Diabetes Center
Affiliate at University of Maryland Medical
    System
22 South Greene Street
Suite N5W100
Baltimore, MD 21201
(410) 328-6584

MASSACHUSETTS

Joslin Diabetes Center and Joslin Clinic
One Joslin Place
Boston, MA 02215
(800) 567-5461

**Joslin Diabetes Center at Beth Israel
    Deaconess Hospital—Needham Campus**
148 Chestnut Street
Needham, MA 02192
(781) 453-5231

MICHIGAN

Joslin Diabetes Center
Affiliate at Providence Hospital
47601 Grand River Avenue
Suite A218
Novi, MI 48374
(888) 331-3330 (toll-free)

Joslin Diabetes Center
Affiliate at Providence Hospital
Outpatient Education Services
Providence Pavilion
22255 Greenfield
Suite 130
Southfield, MI 48075
(248) 849-3903

NEW HAMPSHIRE

Joslin Diabetes Center
Affiliate at Southern New Hampshire Medical
    Center
29 Northwest Boulevard
Nashua, NH 03064
(603) 577-5760

Joslin Diabetes Center
Affiliate at Southern New Hampshire Medical
    Center
280 Main Street
Suite 431
Nashua, NH 03060
(603) 577-3290

Joslin Diabetes Center
Affiliate at Frisbie Memorial Hospital
245 Rochester Hill Road
Rochester, NH 03867
(603) 994-0120

NEW YORK

Joslin Diabetes Center
Affiliate at SUNY Update Medical University
3229 East Genessee Street
Suite 1
Syracuse, NY 13214
(315) 464-5726

OHIO

Joslin Diabetes Center
Affiliate at St. Vincent Charity Hospital
2322 East 22nd Street
Suite 310
Cleveland, OH 44115
(216) 363-2732
(800) 834-4917 (toll-free)

Joslin Diabetes Center
Affiliate at Southview Hospital
1989 Miamisburg Centerville Road
Suite 304
Dayton, OH 45459
(937) 224-HOPE

PENNSYLVANIA

Joslin Diabetes Center
Affiliate at Alle-Kiski Medical Center
651 Fourth Avenue
New Kensington, PA 15068
(724) 367-2400

Joslin Diabetes Center
Western Pennsylvania Hospital—Forbes
   Regional Campus

2580 Haymaker Road
P.O. Box 2
Suite 403
Monroeville, PA 15146
(412) 858-4474

Joslin Diabetes Center
Affiliate at Western Pennsylvania Hospital
5140 Liberty Avenue
Pittsburgh, PA 15224
(412) 578-1724

WASHINGTON

Joslin Diabetes Center
Education Affiliate at Swedish Medical Center
910 Boylston Avenue
Seattle, WA 98104
(206) 215-2440
(888)-JOSLIN-1 (toll-free)

WEST VIRGINIA

Joslin Diabetes Center
Education Affiliate at St. Mary's Medical Center
2900 First Avenue
Huntington, WV 25702
(304) 526-8363

BIBLIOGRAPHY

Abbott, Kevin, Emad Basta, and George L. Bakris. "Blood Pressure Control and Nephroprotection in Diabetes." *Journal of Clinical Pharmacology* 44 (2004): 431–438.

Abrams, Paris J. "Pharmacologic Treatments for Pain Associated with Diabetic Peripheral Neuropathies." *Journal of Pharmacy Practice* 20 (2007): 103–109.

Acury, Thomas A., et al. "Complementary and Alternative Medicine Use as Health Self-Management: Rural Older Adults with Diabetes." *Journal of Gerontology: Social Sciences* 61B, no. 2 (2006): S62–S70.

Agency for Healthcare Research and Quality. *Complications and Costs for Obesity Surgery.* Press Release. April 29, 2009. Rockville, Md.: Agency for Healthcare Research and Quality. April 29, 2009. Available online. URL: http://www.ahrq.gov/news/press/pr2009/barsurgpr.htm. Accessed December 9, 2009.

———. *Premixed Insulin for Type 2 Diabetes: A Guide for Adults.* Washington, D.C.: Agency for Healthcare Research and Quality. March 2009. Available online. URL: http://effectivehealthcare.ahrq.gov/repFiles/Insulin_Consumer_Web.pdf. Downloaded October 16, 2009.

Ahmed, A. T., A. J. Karter, and J. Liu. "Alcohol Consumption Is Inversely Associated with Adherence to Diabetes Self-Care Behaviours." *Diabetic Medicine* 23 (2006): 795–802.

Aikens, J. E., et al. "Association between Depression and Concurrent Type 2 Diabetes Outcomes Varies by Diabetes Regimen." *Diabetic Medicine* 25, no. 11 (2008): 1,324–1,329.

"ALF Overview Preview." *Contemporary Longterm Care* 23, no. 6 (June 2000): 9.

"Alzheimer's Disease: Seeking New Ways to Preserve Brain Function: An Interview with Kenneth L. Davis." *Geriatrics* 54, no. 2 (February 1, 1999): 42–47.

American Academy of Family Physicians. "The Benefits and Risks of Controlling Blood Glucose Levels in Patients with Type 2 Diabetes Mellitus: A Review of the Evidence and Recommendations." American Diabetes Association, released August 1999.

American Diabetes Association. "Executive Summary: Standards of Medical Care in Diabetes—2009." *Diabetes Care* 32, Supp. 1 (2009): S6–S12.

Anselm, J. M., et al. "Explanation for the High Risk of Diabetes Related to Amputation in a Caribbean Population of Black African Descent and Potential for Prevention." *Diabetes Care* 27, no. 11 (2004): 2,636–2,641.

Apgar, Barbara. "Spontaneous Vaginal Delivery and Risk of Erb's Palsy." *American Family Physician* 58, no. 4 (1998): 973–976.

Aragon-Sanchez, Javier, et al. "Necrotizing Soft-Tissue Infections in the Feet of Patients with Diabetes: Outcome of Surgical Treatment and Factors Associated with Limb Loss and Mortality." *International Journal of Lower Extremity Wounds* 8, no. 3 (2009): 141–146.

Astrup, Arne, M.D., et al. "Effects of Liraglutide in the Treatment of Obesity: A Randomised, Double-Blind, Placebo-Controlled Study." *Lancet* 374, no. 9701 (2009): 1,606–1,616.

Awasthi, Purnima, and R. C. Mishra. "Role of Coping Strategies and Social Support in Perceived Illness Consequences and Controllability among Diabetic Women." *Psychology and Developing Societies* 19, no. 2 (2007): 179–197.

Baker, R. A., et al. "Atypical Antipsychotic Drugs and Diabetes Mellitus in the U.S. Food and Drug Administration Adverse Event Database: A Systematic Bayesian Signal Detection Analysis." *Psychopharmacology Bulletin* 42, no. 1 (2009): 11–31.

Bakris, George L., M.D., et al. "Preserving Renal Function in Adults with Hypertension and Diabetes: A Consensus Approach." *American Journal of Kidney Diseases* 36, no. 3 (September 2000): 646–661.

Baliga, V., and R. Sapsford. "Diabetes Mellitus and Heart Failure: An Overview of Epidemiology and

Management." *Diabetes and Vascular Disease Research* 6 (2009): 164–171.

Balsells, Montserrat, et al. "Maternal and Fetal Outcomes in Women with Type 2 Versus Type 1 Diabetes Mellitus: A Systematic Review and Meta-analysis." *Journal of Clinical Endocrinology* 94, no. 11 (2009): 4,284–4,291.

Barbour, Marilyn M. "Hormone Replacement Therapy Should Not Be Used as Secondary Prevention of Coronary Heart Disease." *Pharmacotherapy* 20, no. 9 (2000): 1,021–1,027.

Barnes, Patricia M., and Barbara Bloom. "Complementary and Alternative Medicine Use Among Adults and Children: United States, 2007." *National Health Statistics Reports* 18 (December 10, 2008): 1–24.

Barnett, Jeffrey L. "Gut Reactions. (How Diabetes Can Affect the Gastrointestinal Tract.)" *Diabetes Forecast* 50, no. 8 (August 1997): 26–30.

Barr, Elizabeth L. M., et al. "Risk of Cardiovascular and All-Cause Mortality in Individuals with Diabetes Mellitus, Impaired Fasting Glucose, and Impaired Glucose Tolerance: The Australian Diabetes, Obesity, and Lifestyle Study (AusDiab)." *Circulation* 116 (2007): 151–157.

Bash, Lori D., et al. "Poor Glycemic Control in Diabetes and the Risk of Incident Chronic Kidney Disease Even in the Absence of Albuminuria and Retinopathy: Atherosclerosis Risk in Communities (ARIC) Study." *Archives of Internal Medicine* 168, no. 22 (December 8/22, 2008): 2,440–2,447.

Bell, David S., et al. "Diabetes as a Risk Factor for Ischemic Heart Disease." *Clinical Reviews* (Spring 2000): 88–92.

Betschart Roemer, Jean. "Emotional and Psychological Considerations of Children with Diabetes: Tips for School Nurses." *NASN School Nurse* 24 (2009): 60–61.

Brenes, Gretchen A. "Anxiety, Depression, and Quality of Life in Primary Care Patients." *Primary Care Companion to Journal of Clinical Psychiatry* 9, no. 6 (2007): 437–433.

Brethauer, Stacy A., M.D., et al. "Bariatric Surgery as a Treatment for Type 2 Diabetes Mellitus in Obese Patients." *Obesity Management* (2009): 112–118.

Brown, Anne W. "Clinicians' Guide to Diabetes Gadgets and Gizmos." *Clinical Diabetes* 26, no. 2 (2008): 66–71.

Buchwald, Henry, M.D., et al. "Weight and Type 2 Diabetes after Bariatric Surgery: Systematic Review and Meta-analysis." *American Journal of Medicine* 122, no. 3 (2009): 248–256.

Burke, James P., et al. "A Quantitative Scale of Acanthosis Nigricans." *Diabetes Care* 22, no. 10 (October 1999): 1,655–1,659.

Calhoun, Darren, et al. "Relationship between Glycemic Control and Depression among American Indians in the Strong Heart Study." *Journal of Diabetes and Its Complications* 24, no. 4 (2009): 217–222.

Campos, G. M., et al. "Factors Associated With Weight Loss After Gastric Bypass." *Archives of Surgery* 143 (2008): 877–884.

Carnethon, Mercedes R., et al. "Longitudinal Association between Depressive Symptoms and Incident Type 2 Diabetes Mellitus in Older Adults: The Cardiovascular Health Study." *Archives of Internal Medicine* 167 (April 23, 2007): 802–807.

Centers for Disease Control and Prevention. "Differences in Prevalence of Obesity among Black, White, and Hispanic Adults—United States, 2006–2008." *Morbidity and Mortality Review* 58, no. 27 (July 17, 2009): 740–744.

———. "U.S. Obesity Trends." Available online. URL: http://www.cdc.gov/obesity/data/trends.html. Accessed October 21, 2009.

Cheng, Yiling J., M.D., et al. "Association of A1C and Fasting Plasma Glucose Levels with Diabetic Retinopathy Prevalence in the U.S. Population." *Diabetes Care* 32, no. 11 (2009): 2,027–2,032.

Cheung, Ning, et al. "Diabetic Retinopathy and the Risk of Coronary Heart Disease: The Atherosclerosis Risk in Communities Study." *Diabetes Care* 30, no. 7 (2007): 1,742–1,746.

Clay, Daniel, et al. "Family Perceptions of Medication Administration at School: Errors, Risk Factors, and Consequences." *Journal of School Nursing* 24 (2008): 95–102.

Colhoun, H. M., on behalf of the SDRN Epidemiology Group. "Use of Insulin Glargine and Cancer Incidence in Scotland: A Study from the Scottish Diabetes Research Network Epidemiology Group." *Diabetologia* 52 (2009): 1,755–1,765.

Currie, C. J., C. D. Poole, and E. A. M. Gale. "The Influence of Glucose-lowering Therapies on Cancer Risk in Type 2 diabetes." *Diabetologia* 52 (2009): 1,766–1,777.

Dabelea, Dana, M.D., et al. "Diabetes in Navajo Youth: Prevalence, Incidence, and Clinical Characteristics: The SEARCH for Diabetes in Youth Study." *Diabetes Care* 32, Supplement 2 (2009): S141–S147.

Dagenais, Gilles R., Annie St-Pierre, Patrick Gilbert, Benoît Lamarche, Ph.D., Jean-Pierre Després, Paul-Marie Bernard, Peter Bogaty. "Comparison of Prognosis for Men With Type 2 Diabetes Mellitus and Men With Cardiovascular Disease." *Canadian Medical Association Journal* 180, no. 1 (01/01/2009) 40–47.

The Diabetes Control and Complications Trial Research Group. "A Comparison of the Study Populations in the Diabetes Control and Complications Trial and the Wisconsin Epidemiologic Study of Diabetic Retinopathy." *Archives of Internal Medicine* 155 (April 10, 1995): 745–754.

———. "Adverse Events and Their Association with Treatment Regimens in the Diabetes Control and Complications Trial." *Diabetes Care* 18, no. 11 (November 1995): 1,415–1,427.

———. "Baseline Analysis of Renal Function in the Diabetes Control and Complications Research Trial." *Kidney International* 43 (1993): 668–674.

———. "Clustering of Long-Term Complications in Families with Diabetes in the Diabetes Control and Complications Trial." *Diabetes* 46 (November 1997): 1,829–1,839.

———. "Effect of Intensive Diabetes Management on Macrovascular Events and Risk Factors in the Diabetes Control and Complications Trial." *The American Journal of Cardiology* 75 (May 1, 1995): 894–903.

———. "Effect of Intensive Diabetes Treatment on the Development and Progression of Long-Term Complications in Adolescents with Insulin-Dependent Diabetes Mellitus: Diabetes Control and Complications Trial." *The Journal of Pediatrics* 125, no. 2 (August 1994): 177–188.

———. "The Effect of Intensive Treatment of Diabetes on the Development and Progression of Long-Term Complications in Insulin-Dependent Diabetes Mellitus." *The New England Journal of Medicine* 329 (September 30, 1993): 977–986.

———. "Effect of Intensive Therapy on the Development and Progression of Diabetic Nephropathy in the Diabetes Control and Complications Trial." *Kidney International* 47 (1995): 1,703–1,720.

———. "The Effect of Intensive Diabetes Therapy on the Development and Progression of Neuropathy." *Annals of Internal Medicine* 122, no. 8 (April 15, 1995): 561–568.

———. "Epidemiology of Severe Hypoglycemia in the Diabetes Control and Complications Research Trial." *The American Journal of Medicine* 90 (April 1991): 450–459.

———. "Factors in Development of Diabetic Neuropathy: Baseline Analysis of Neuropathy in Feasibility Phase of Diabetes Control and Complications Trial (DCCT)." *Diabetes* 37 (April 1998): 476–481.

———. "Diabetes Control and Complications Trial Research Group (DCCT): Update." *Diabetes Care* 13, no. 4 (April 1990): 427–433.

———. "Early Worsening of Diabetic Retinopathy in the Diabetes Control and Complications Trial." *The Archives of Ophthalmology* 116 (1998): 874–886.

———. "The Effect of Intensive Diabetes Therapy on Measures of Autonomic Nervous System Function in the Diabetes Control and Complications Trial (DCCT)." *Diabetologia* 41 (1998): 416–423.

———. "Effect of Intensive Diabetes Treatment on Nerve Conduction in the Diabetes Control and Complications Trial." *Annals of Neurology* 38, no. 6 (December 1995): 869–880.

———. "Effects of Intensive Diabetes Therapy on Neuropsychological Function in Adults in the Diabetes Control and Complications Trial." *Annals of Internal Medicine* 124 (1996): 379–388.

———. "Effects of Intensive Diabetes Therapy on Neuropsychological Function in Adults in the Diabetes Control and Complications Trial." *Annals of Internal Medicine* 124, no. 4 (February 15, 1996): 379–388.

———. "Expanded Role of the Dietitian in the Diabetes Control and Complications Trial: Implications for Clinical Practice." *Journal of the American Dietetic Association* 93, no. 7 (July 1993): 758–764, 767.

———. "Epidemiology of Diabetes Interventions and Complications (EDIC)." *Diabetes Care* 22, no. 1 (January 1999): 99–111.

———. "Hypoglycemia in the Diabetes Control and Complications Trial." *Diabetes* 46 (February 1997): 271–286.

———. "Influence of Intensive Diabetes Treatment on Quality-of-Life Outcomes in the Diabetes Control and Complications Trial." *Diabetes Care* 19, no. 3 (March 1996): 195–203.

———. "Lifetime Benefits and Costs of Intensive Therapy as Practiced in the Diabetes Control and Complications Trial." *Journal of the American Medical Association* 276, no. 17 (November 6, 1996): 1,409–1,415.

———. "Nutrition Interventions for Intensive Therapy in the Diabetes Control and Complications

Trial." *Journal of the American Dietetic Association* 93, no. 7 (July 1993): 768–772.

———. "Pregnancy Outcomes in the Diabetes Control and Complications Trial." *American Journal of Obstetrics & Gynecology* 174 (1996): 1,343–1,353.

———. "Progression of Retinopathy with Intensive versus Conventional Treatment in the Diabetes Control and Complications Trial." *Ophthalmology* 102, no. 4 (April 1995): 647–661.

———. "The Relationship of Glycemic Exposure (HbA1C) to the Risk of Development and Progression of Retinopathy in the Diabetes Control and Complications Trial." *Diabetes* 44 (August 1995): 968–983.

Dodson, Paul M. "Diabetic Retinopathy: Treatment and Prevention." *Diabetes and Vascular Disease Research* 4 (2007): S9–S11.

Dorsey, Rashida R., et al. "Control of Risk Factors among People with Diagnosed Diabetes, by Lower Extremity Disease Status." *Preventing Chronic Disease* 6, no. 4 (2009): 1–10.

Doshani, Anjum, and Justin C. Konje. "Diabetes in Pregnancy: Insulin Resistance, Obesity and Placental Dysfunction." *British Journal of Diabetes and Vascular Disease* 9 (2009): 208–212.

Evans, Margaret J. "Diabetes and Pregnancy: A Review of Pathology." *British Journal of Diabetes and Vascular Disease* 9 (2009): 201–206.

Evert, Allison, et al. "Continuous Glucose Monitoring Technology for Personal Use: An Educational Program that Educates and Supports the Patient." *Diabetes Educator* 35 (2009): 565–580.

Farrell, JoAnne B., Anjali Deshmukh, and Ali A. Baghaie. "Low Testosterone and the Association with Type 2 Diabetes." *Diabetes Educator* 34 (2008): 799–806.

Fink, Ezekiel, M.D., and Anne Louise Oaklander, M.D. "Diabetic Neuropathy." *Pain Management Rounds* 2, no. 3 (2005): 1–6.

Flatt, Peter R., Caroline Day, and Clifford J. Bailey. "Bariatric Surgery: To Treat Diabesity." *British Journal of Diabetes and Vascular Disease* 9 (2009): 103–107.

Fong, D. S., and R. Contreras. "Glitazone Use Associated with Diabetic Macular Edema." *American Journal of Ophthalmology* 147, no. 4 (2009): 583–586.

Garg, Seema, M.D., and Richard M. Davis, M.D. "Diabetic Retinopathy Screening Update." *Clinical Diabetes* 27, no. 4 (2009): 140–145.

Garrow, Donald, M.D., and Leonard E. Edege, M.D. "Association between Complementary and Alternative Medicine Use, Preventive Care Practices, and Use of Conventional Medical Services among Adults with Diabetes." *Diabetes Care* 29, no. 1 (2006): 15–19.

Gary, Tiffany L., et al. "The Effects of a Nurse Care Manager and a Community Health Worker Team on Diabetic Control, Emergency Department Visits, and Hospitalizations Among Urban African Americans with Type 2 Diabetes Mellitus: A Randomized Controlled Trial." *Archives of Internal Medicine* 169, no. 19 (2009): 1,788–1,794.

Gluck, M. E., C. A. Venti, A. D. Salbe, et al. "Nighttime Eating: Commonly Observed and Related to Weight Gain in an Inpatient Food Intake Study." *American Journal of Clinical Nutrition* 88 (2008): 900–905.

Gobert, Colleen P., and Alison M. Duncan. "Use of Natural Health Products by Adults with Type 2 Diabetes." *Canadian Journal of Diabetes* 32, no. 4 (2008): 260–272.

Gold, Michael S., M.D., and Christine Adamec. *The Encyclopedia of Alcoholism and Alcohol Abuse.* New York: Facts On File, Inc., 2010.

Groop, Per-Henrik, et al. "The Presence and Severity of Chronic Kidney Disease Predicts All-Cause Mortality in Type 1 Diabetes." *Diabetes* 58, no.7 (2009): 1,651–1,658.

Hammond, Peter. "Review: Use of Continuous Subcutaneous Insulin Infusion in Special Populations and Circumstances in Patients with Type 1 Diabetes." *British Journal of Diabetes and Vascular Disease* 8 (2008): S11–S14.

Hatzimouratidis, Konstantinos. "Epidemiology of Male Sexual Dysfunction." *American Journal of Men's Health* 1 (2007): 103–125.

Hemkins, L. G., U. Grouven, R. Bender, et al. "Risk of Malignancies in Patients with Diabetes Treated with Human Insulin or Insulin Analogues: A Cohort Study." *Diabetologia* 52 (2009): 1,732–1,744.

Heron, Melonie, et al. "Deaths: Final Data for 2006." *National Vital Statistics Reports* 57, no. 14 (April 17, 2009): 1–136.

Hite, Pamela F., and Heather F. DeBellis. "Diabetic Kidney Disease: A Renin-Angiotensin-Aldosterone System Focused Review." *Journal of Pharmacy Practice* 22, no. 6 (2009): 560–570.

Home, P. D., and P. Lagarenne. "Combined Randomised Controlled Trial Experience of Malignancies in

Studies Using Insulin Glargine." *Diabetologia* (2009): 1,530–1,535.

Hovind, Peter, et al. "Serum Uric Acid as a Predictor for Development of Diabetic Nephropathy in Type 1 Diabetes: An Inception Cohort Study." *Diabetes* 58, no. 7 (2009):1,668–1,671.

Howe, Carol J., et al. "Weight-Related Concerns and Behaviors in Children and Adolescents with Type 1 Diabetes." *The Journal of the American Psychiatric Nurses Association* 13, no. 6 (2008): 376–385.

Idelevich, Evgeny, Wilhelm Kirch, and Christoph Schindler. "Current Pharmacotherapeutic Concepts for the Treatment of Obesity in Adults." *Therapeutic Advances in Cardiovascular Disease* 3 (2009): 75–90.

International Diabetes Federation. "Global Guideline: Pregnancy and Diabetes." Available online. URL: http://www.idf.org/webdata/docs/Pregnancy_EN_RTP.pdf. Accessed October 27, 2009.

Jacquez, Farrah, et al. "Parent Perspectives of Diabetes Management in Schools." *Diabetes Educator* 34 (2008): 996–1,003.

Jeitler, K., et al. "Continuous Subcutaneous Insulin Infusion versus Multiple Daily Insulin Injections in Patients with Diabetes Mellitus: Systematic Review and Meta-Analysis." *Diabetologia* 51 (2008): 941–951.

Johns, Carla, Melissa Spezia Faulkner, and Lauretta Quinn. "Characteristics of Adolescents with Type 1 Diabetes Who Exhibit Adverse Outcomes." *Diabetes Educator* 34 (2008): 874–885.

Jonasson, J., et al. "An Internet-Based Weight Loss Programme: A Feasibility Study with Preliminary Results from 4209 Completers." *Scandinavian Journal of Public Health* 37 (2009): 75–82.

Jonasson, J. M., R. Ljung, M. Tälback, et al. "Insulin Glargine Use and Short-term Incidence of Malignancies—a Population-based Follow-up Study in Sweden." *Diabetologia* 52 (2009): 1,745–1,754.

Joslin, Elliott P., M.D. *The Treatment of Diabetes Mellitus with Observations Upon the Disease Based Upon Thirteen Hundred Cases.* Philadelphia, Pa.: Lea & Febiger, 1917.

Karvonen, Marjatta, et al. "Incidence of Childhood Type 1 Diabetes Worldwide." *Diabetes Care* 23, no. 10 (October 2000): 1,516.

Katon, Wayne J., M.D. "The Comorbidity of Diabetes Mellitus and Depression." *American Journal of Medicine* 121 (2008): S8–S15.

Kay, Catharine, et al. "An Exploration of the Experiences of Young Women Living with Type 1 Diabetes." *Journal of Health Psychology* 14 (2009): 242–250.

Keely, E., M.D. "Type 2 Diabetes in Pregnancy: Importance of Optimized Care Before, During and After Pregnancy." *Obstetric Medicine* 1 (2008): 72–77.

Kelly, Sarah, et al. "Disordered Eating Behaviors in Youth with Type 1 Diabetes." *Diabetes Educator* 34, no. 4 (2005): 572–583.

Kendall, Claire. "Rosiglitazone (Avandia) and Macular Edema." *Canadian Medical Association Journal* 174, no. 5 (2006): 623.

Kerssen, A., et al. "Effect of Breast Milk of Diabetic Mothers on Bodyweight of the Offspring in the First Year of Life." *European Journal of Clinical Nutrition* 58 (2008): 1,429–1,431.

Khan, Laura Kettel, et al. "Recommended Community Strategies and Measurements to Prevent Obesity in the United States." *Morbidity and Mortality Weekly Report* 58, no. RR-7 (July 24, 2009): 1–30.

Kumar, D., S. Bajaj, and R. Mehrotra. "Knowledge, Attitude and Practice of Complementary and Alternative Medicines for Diabetes." *Public Health* 120 (2006): 705–711.

Kyngäs, Helvi A. "Predictors of Good Adherence of Adolescents with Diabetes (Insulin-Dependent Diabetes Mellitus." *Chronic Illness* 3 (2007): 20–28.

Kyrios, Michael, et al. "The Influence of Depression and Anxiety on Outcomes after an Intervention for Prediabetes." *Medical Journal of Australia* 190 (2009): S81–S85.

Lacey, Brian E., M.D., et al. "The Treatment of Diabetic Gastroparesis with Botulinum Toxin Injections of the Pylorus." *Diabetes Care* 27, no. 10 (2004): 2,341–2,347.

Langer, Oded. "Fetal Testing in Pregnancies Complicated by Diabetes Mellitus: Why, How, and For Whom?" In *The Diabetes in Pregnancy Dilemma: Leading Change with Proven Solutions,* edited by Oded Langer, 304–326. Lanham, Md.: University Press of America, 2006.

Lanting, Loes C., et al. "Ethnic Differences in Mortality, End-Stage Complications, and Quality of Care Among Diabetic Patients." *Diabetes Care* 28, no. 9 (2005): 2,280–2,288.

LaVeist, Thomas A., et al. "Environmental and Socio-Economic Factors as Contributors to Racial Disparities in Diabetes Prevalence." *Journal of General Internal Medicine* 24, no. 10 (2009): 1,144–1,148.

Libby, Gillian, et al. "New Users of Metformin Are at Low Risk of Incident Cancer." *Diabetes Care* 32 (2009): 1,620–1,625.

Liu, Lenna L., M.D., et al. "Type 1 and Type 2 Diabetes in Asian and Pacific Islander U.S. Youth: The SEARCH for Diabetes in Youth Study." *Diabetes Care* 32, Supplement 2 (2009): S133–S140.

Lloyd, Brendan, Rhys Williams, and Jörg Huber. "Erectile Dysfunction and Diabetes: A Study in Primary Care." *British Journal of Diabetes and Vascular Disease* 4 (2004): 387–392.

Longitudinal Assessment of Bariatric Surgery (LABS) Consortium. "Perioperative Safety in the Longitudinal Assessment of Bariatric Surgery." *New England Journal of Medicine* 361, no. 5 (2009): 445–454.

Malagelada, Juan-R., M.D. "Gastrointestinal Syndromes due to Diabetes Mellitus." In *Contemporary Diabetes: Diabetic Neuropathy: Clinical Management*, edited by A. Veves and R. Malik, 433–451. 2d ed. Totowa, N.J.: Human Press, Inc., 2007.

Marschilok, Catherine. "Insulin Pump Therapy." *NASN School Nurse* 24 (2009): 25–26.

Martin, Joyce A., et al. "Births: Final Data for 2006." *National Vital Statistics Reports* 57, no. 7 (January 7, 2009).

Maskarinec, Gertraud, et al. "Diabetes Prevalence and Body Mass Index Difference by Ethnicity: The Multiethnic Cohort." *Ethnicity & Disease* 19 (2009): 49–55.

Mayer-Davis, Elizabeth, J., et al. "Breast-Feeding and Type 2 Diabetes in the Youths of Three Ethnic Groups." *Diabetes Care* 31, no. 3 (2008): 470–475.

Mayer-Davis, Elizabeth J., et al. "Diabetes in African American Youth: Prevalence, Incidence, and Clinical Characteristics: The SEARCH for Diabetes in Youth Study." *Diabetes Care* 32, Supplement 2 (2009): S112–S122.

McVeigh, K. H., F. Mostashari, M.D., and L. E. Thorpe. "Serious Psychological Distress among Persons with Diabetes—New York City, 2003." *Morbidity and Mortality Weekly* 53, no. 46 (2004): 1,089–1,091.

Messer, Laurel, et al. "Educating Families on Real Time Continuous Glucose Monitoring: The DireNet Navigator Pilot Study Experience." *Diabetes Educator* 35 (2009): 124–135.

Minocha, Anil, M.D., and Christine Adamec. *The Encyclopedia of the Digestive System and Digestive Disorders*. New York: Facts On File, 2011.

Moussavi, Saba, et al. "Depression, Chronic Diseases, and Decrements in Health: Results from the World Health Surveys." *Lancet* 370 (2007): 851–858.

Mulvaney, Shelagh A., et al. "Self-Management in Type 2 Diabetes: The Adolescent Perspective." *Diabetes Educator* 34 (2008): 674–682.

Murphy, Helen R., Rosemary C. Temple, and Jonathan M. Roland. "Improving Outcomes of Pregnancy for Women with Type 1 and Type 2 Diabetes." *British Journal of Diabetes and Vascular Disease* 7 (2007): 38–42.

Naimi, Timothy S., M.D., et al. "Binge Drinking among U.S. Adults." *Journal of the American Medical Association* 289, no. 13 (2003): 70–75.

Nainggolan, Lisa. "Experts Debate Bariatric Surgery as a Cure for Diabetes." Medscape Conference Coverage, based on selected sessions at the European Association for the Study of Diabetes (EASD) 45th Annual Meeting. December 1, 2009. Available online to subscribers. URL: http://www.medscape.com/viewarticle/71382_print. Accessed December 9, 2009.

National Institute of Diabetes and Digestive and Kidney Diseases. *Bariatric Surgery for Severe Obesity*. Bethesda, Md.: National Institutes of Health, 2009.

——— (NIDDK). What I Need to Know about Diabetes Medicines. March 2008. Available online. URL: http://diabetes.niddk.nih.gov/dm/pubs/medicines_ez/meds.pdf. Downloaded October 10, 2009.

Nicholas, Amy S., et al. "Treatment Considerations for Diabetes: A Pharmacist's Guide to Improving Care in the Elderly." *Journal of Pharmacy Practice* 22, no. 6 (2009): 575–587.

Nichols, Gregory A., Kyndaron Reinier, and Sumeet S. Chugh, M.D. "Independent Contribution of Diabetes to Increased Prevalence and Incidence of Atrial Fibrillation." *Diabetes Care* 32 (2009): 1,851–1,856.

Noel, Rebecca A., et al. "Increased Risk of Acute Pancreatitis and Biliary Disease Observed in Patients with Type 2 Diabetes." *Diabetes Care* 32, no. 4 (2009): 834–838.

Owen, C. G., et al. "Does Breastfeeding Influence a Risk of Type 2 Diabetes in Later Life? A Quantitative Analysis of Published Evidence." *American Journal of Clinical Nutrition* 84, no. 5 (2006): 1,043–1,054.

Pagan, Jose A., and Jesus Tanguma. "Health Care Affordability and Complementary and Alternative Medicine Utilization by Adults with Diabetes." *Diabetes Care* 30, no. 8 (2007): 2,030–2,031.

Parrish, Carol Lee, and Joyce Green Pastors. "Nutritional Management of Gastroparesis in People with Diabetes." *Diabetes Spectrum* 20, no. 4 (2007): 231–234.

Peters, Christine D., et al. "Victimization of Youth with Type-1 Diabetes by Teachers: Relations with Adherence and Metabolic Control." *Journal of Child Health Care* 12 (2008): 209–220.

Petit, William, Jr., M.D. "Management of Diabetes Mellitus during Pregnancy." In *Self-Assessment Profile in Endocrinology and Metabolism,* edited by Pasquale J. Palumbo, M.D., 102–107. Washington, D.C.: The American Association of Clinical Endocrinologists and the American College of Endocrinology, 2001.

Pineda Olvera, Anna E., et al. "Diabetes, Depression, and Metabolic Control in Latinas." *Cultural Diversity and Ethnic Minority Psychology* 13, no. 3 (2007): 223–231.

Ramsey, Susan E., and Patricia A. Engler. "At-Risk Drinking among Diabetic Patients." *Substance Abuse: Research and Treatment* 3 (2009): 15–23.

Resnick, Helaine, et al. "Diabetes in Nursing Homes, 2004." *Diabetes Care* 31, no. 3 (2008): 287–288.

Rolim, Luiz Clemente de Souza Pereira, et al. "Diabetic Cardiovascular Autonomic Neuropathy: Risk Factors, Clinical Impact and Early Diagnosis." *Arquivos Brasileiras Cardiologia* 90, no. 4 (2008): 323–331.

Rosenstock, J., V. Fonseca, and J. B. McGill, et al. "Similar Risk of Malignancy with Insulin Glargine and Neutral Protamine Hagedorn (NPH) Insulin in Patients with Type 2 Diabetes: Findings from a 5 Year Randomized, Open-Label Study." *Diabetologia* 52 (2009): 1,778–1,788.

Saaddine, Jinan B., M.D., et al. "Projection of Diabetic Retinopathy and Other Major Eye Diseases among People with Diabetes Mellitus: United States, 2005–2050." *Archives of Ophthalmology* 126, no. 12 (2008): 1,740–1,747.

Scheiner, Gary, et al. "Insulin Pump Therapy: Guidelines for Successful Outcomes." *Diabetes Educator* 34 (2009): 29S–41S.

Schönauer, Martin, et al. "Cardiac Autonomic Diabetic Neuropathy." *Diabetes and Vascular Disease Research* 5 (2008): 336–344.

Schram, Miranda, Caroline A. Baan, and François Pouwer. "Depression and Quality of Life in Patients with Diabetes: A Systematic Review from the European Depression in Diabetes (EDID) Research Consortium." *Current Diabetes Reviews* 5, no. 2 (2009): 112–119.

Shah, Bijal M., et al. "Depressive Symptoms in Patients with Type 2 Diabetes in the Ambulatory Care Setting: Opportunities to Improve Outcomes in the Course of Routine Care." *Journal of the American Pharmacists Association* 48, no. 6 (2008): 737–743.

Simon, G. E., et al. "Cost-effectiveness of Systematic Depression Treatment among People with Diabetes Mellitus." *Archives of General Psychiatry* 64 (2007): 65–72.

Singh, Rajiv, et al. "Depression and Anxiety Symptoms after Lower Limb Amputation: The Rise and Fall." *Clinical Rehabilitation* 23 (2009): 282–286.

Sloan, Frank A., et al. "The Growing Burden of Diabetes Mellitus in the US Elderly Population." *Archives of Internal Medicine* 168, no. 2 (2008): 192–199.

Soomro, Hibba, Lesley Burnett, and Nigel Davies. "Quantifying Changes in Retinal Anatomy after Interventions for Diabetic Maculopathy." *British Journal of Diabetes and Vascular Disease* 7 (2007): 181–185.

St. Amand, Scott. "Protecting Neglect: The Constitutionality of Spiritual Healing Exemptions to Child Protection Statutes." *Richmond Journal of the Law and the Public Interest* 12, no. 129 (2009): 139–161.

Stuebe, Alison M., et al. "Duration of Lactation and Incidence of Type 2 Diabetes." *Journal of the American Medical Association* 294, no. 20 (2005): 2,601–2,610.

Tice, Jeffrey A., M.D., et al. "Gastric Banding or Bypass? A Systematic Review Comparing the Two Most Popular Bariatric Procedures." *American Journal of Medicine* 121 (2008): 885–893.

Totty, Patrick. "One in Five Type 2s Is 'Morbidly Obese'—100 or More Pounds Overweight." *Diabetes Health.* December 5, 2009. Available online. URL: http://www.diabeteshealth.com/read/2009/12/03/6468/diabetes-surgery-summit-issues-call-to-use-bariatric-surgery-as-a-type-2-treatment-/. Accessed December 9, 2009.

Tseng, Chin-Lin, et al. "Survival Benefit of Nephrologic Care in Patients with Diabetes Mellitus and Chronic Kidney Disease." *Archives of Internal Medicine* 168, no. 1 (January 14, 2008): 55–62.

United Kingdom Prospective Diabetes Study (UKPDS) Group. "Intensive Blood-Glucose Control with Sulphonylureas or Insulin Compared with Conventional Treatment and Risk of Complications in Patients with Type 2 Diabetes (UKPDS 33)." *Lancet* 352 (1998): 837–853.

Wagner, Heidi, et al. "Eye on Diabetes: A Multidisciplinary Patient Education Intervention." *Diabetes Educator* 34, no. 1 (2008): 84–89.

Whaley-Connell, Adam, et al. "Diabetes Mellitus and CKD Awareness: The Kidney Early Evaluation Program (KEEP) and National Health and Nutrition Examination Survey (NHANES)." *American Journal of Kidney Diseases* 53, no. 4, Supp. 4 (2009): S11–S21.

White, Marney A., et al. "Loss of Control over Eating Predicts Outcomes in Bariatric Surgery Patients: A Prospective, 24-Month Follow-Up Study." *Journal of Clinical Psychiatry* 71, no. 2 (2009):175–184.

Wu, Patricia, M.D. "Thyroid Disease and Diabetes." *Diabetes Self-Management* 18, no. 3 (Winter 2000): 6–12.

Yeh, Gloria Y., M.D., et al. "Systematic Review of Herbs and Dietary Supplements for Glycemic Control in Diabetes." *Diabetes Care* 26, no. 4 (2003): 1,277–1,294.

Ziegler, Dan, M.D. "Painful Diabetic Neuropathy: Advantage of Novel Drugs over Old Drugs?" *Diabetes Care* 32, Supplement 2 (2009): S414–S419.

INDEX

Page numbers in **boldface** indicate a major treatment of a topic. Page numbers followed by *t* denote tables.

computed tomography
  in acromegaly 5
  in Cushing's disease and
    syndrome 96
  in stroke 316
congenital anomalies 190, 194,
  298, 300
"Conquering Diabetes: A Strategic
  Plan for the 21st Century" 93
constipation 147, 148
Contemporary Diabetes 147
Contemporary Longterm Care 41
contingency management in
  smoking cessation 314
contraception **49,** 212–213
  drug interactions in 260, 321
  in polycystic ovarian syndrome
    296
Contreras, R. 127
coping behavior
  of adolescents 9, 10–11
  in depression 106
  of women 338
corns 180, 183
coronary artery disease (CAD)
  93, 251. *See also* coronary heart
  disease
coronary heart disease (CHD) 63,
  88–89, **93,** 251
  ACE inhibitors in 2–3
  CARE Trial on 66
  cholesterol levels in 81, 89–90
  death from 63
  and diabetic retinopathy 128
  diuretics in 151
  glucose levels in 116
  metformin in xxiii
  myocardial infarction in 93,
    278
  in obesity 282
  Scandinavian Simvastatin
    Survival Study on 308
  in women 337
cortisol 94, 95, 96, 123, 310
costs of care 110
  DCCT study on 109
  by endocrinologist 167–168
  in gingivitis 198
  in immunizations 224
  in insulin pump 237
  preconception 298
  in team approach 321

cough
  from ACE inhibitors 3, 37, 135
  drug-alcohol interactions in 24*t*
  in flu and pneumonia 225
  in gastroesophageal reflux 186
Coumadin. *See* warfarin
counseling
  in adolescence 10
  in alcohol abuse 18
  in amputation 36
  behavioral modification in 48
  in denial of diabetes 99
  in depression 102–103, 106
  in stroke 317
  in summer camps 56
counterregulatory hormones **94,**
  97, 200
Coustan, D. R. 190
COX-2 inhibitors 185
Cozaar. *See* losartan
C-peptide **94,** 229
cranial mononeuropathy 140
creatinine levels 86, **94–95,** 131,
  135, 168, 169
  in ACE inhibitor therapy 3
  and albumin levels 304
  and amputation risk 35
  in elderly 159
  for nephrologist referral 279
critically ill nondiabetic patients,
  hyperglycemia in **95**
Cuellar, Norma G. 92
Cullen, William xiii
*Cultural Diversity and Ethnic Minority
  Psychology* 105
Current Diabetes Reviews 104
Cushing's disease and syndrome 3,
  95–96, 287
Cutfield, Wayne S. 205
Cygnus Therapeutics 280
Cymbalta. *See* duloxetine
cystitis **96,** 122, 227, 328, 329

D

Dabelea, Dana 33
dairy products 59, 60, 61, 62
Daneman, Denis 227
Davies, Nigel 127
Davis, Catherine 193
Davis, Richard M. 142–143
dawn phenomenon 55, **97**
Day, Caroline 47

daycare centers xxii, 34, 244
death **97–98,** 98*t*
  in abuse/neglect 1–2, 307
  of adolescents 10, 98, 236
  of African Americans 13, 97,
    98*t*
  in Alzheimer's disease 31
  in bariatric surgery 44
  in cardiovascular disease 31, 63,
    64–65, 93, 97, 211
  of children 1, 98, 307
  in coma 84, 164
  in complications of diabetes 31
  in coronary heart disease 93
  in depression 100
  in diabetic ketoacidosis 1, 10,
    13, 98, 130
  in diabetic nephropathy 133,
    134
  fetal 192, 194, 300
  in foot ulcers 182
  in hyperglycemic critically ill
    nondiabetic patients 95
  in hypoglycemia 98, 130, 222
  in leprechaunism 244–245
  and life insurance 241
  in macrovascular disease 251
  of men 97, 98*t*, 270
  in myocardial infarction 146
  in smoking 313
  in stroke 316
debridement of foot ulcers 182
DECODE trial 115–116
dehydration **98**
  in adolescents 10
  in diabetes insipidus 110
  and diabetic ketoacidosis 98,
    130, 162
  electrolytes in 161
  and hyperosmolar coma 98, 215
  orthostatic hypotension in 139,
    289
  in sick days 311
delivery. *See* labor and delivery
delta cells 48, 242, 293
dementia **98–99**
  in Alzheimer's disease **30–32,**
    99
demographics of diabetes 111–112
denial of diabetes **99,** 155, 195, 202
denial of medical care, faith-based
  1–2